HEALING
EAST AND WEST

HEALING
EAST AND WEST

Ancient Wisdom and Modern Psychology

Edited by
ANEES A. SHEIKH
KATHARINA S. SHEIKH

JOHN WILEY & SONS, INC.

New York • Chichester • Brisbane • Toronto • Singapore • Weinheim

Library of Congress Cataloging-in-Publication Data:

Healing east and west : ancient wisdom and modern psychology / edited
by Anees A. Sheikh, Katharina S. Sheikh.
        p.   cm.
    Originally published: Eastern and western approaches to healing.
New York : Wiley, c1989.
    Includes bibliographical references and indexes.
    ISBN 0-471-15560-8 (pbk. : alk. paper)
    1. Medicine and psychology—Cross-cultural studies.   2. Medicine,
Oriental.   3. Mind and body.   4. Psychiatry, Transcultural.
I. Sheikh, Anees A.   II. Sheikh, Katharina S.   III. Title: Eastern
and western approaches to healing
R726.5.H42   1996
615.5′3—dc20   96-21085

Printed in the United States of America

10   9   8   7   6   5   4   3   2   1

Foreword to the Paperback Edition

As this century draws to a close, our nation faces the most pressing concerns in modern memory regarding health and healing. Foremost in public consciousness, of course, is the crucial question: How can health care be effectively designed and delivered in a time of conflicting financial demands? Related to this concern are questions vital to the human condition: What is the nature of the elusive healing response? Why has the development of advanced technology and improved understanding of disease only marginally improved general health over the last century? Why has the United States lost its edge in health and longevity compared with other industrialized countries? How is it that anything can cure somebody and nothing cures everybody? What part do mind and spirit play in causing, exacerbating, and curing disease? And finally, are there other systems of healing beyond the standard allopathic approaches and traditional psychotherapeutic interventions that might improve the health of the nation?

More and more health consumers from every level of society are resonating with these questions. We are frustrated by the way health care is sold. With increasing fervor, we ask to be viewed in a more holistic and humane fashion. No longer impressed by credentials, training, and technology, we demand to be active participants in the health-care system.

When this book was first published in 1989 as *Eastern and Western Approaches to Healing*, it was far ahead of its time, and certainly on the frontier of new ideas. Since the book's initial publication, the Public Health

Service released a 700-page report called *Healthy People 2000,* which challenged the nation to move beyond just saving lives. "Good health comes from reducing unnecessary suffering, illness, and disability," the report noted. "It comes from an improved quality of life. Health is thus measured by citizens' sense of well-being." The report charged the country to address these concerns as an economic imperative.

In 1992, in response to consumer and Congressional demands for more information about both ancient and innovative approaches to healing, Congress established the Office of Alternative Medicine within the National Institutes of Health. The office's immediate goal was to facilitate fair, scientific evaluation of alternative therapies and to reduce barriers that might keep promising clinical strategies from coming to light. The goal was to expand the limited view of what is considered effective and legal practice. The title "Alternative" has been challenged and decried. However, I must say that after serving on government committees where practices that were not part of the mainstream were called "unorthodox," "unproven," "unconventional," or, worse yet, "sheer quackery," "alternative" seems like progress. I predict that relatively soon these "alternative" therapies will be referred to as "integral" or "integrated."

In 1992 it was my privilege to co-chair (with Drs. Larry Dossey and Jim Gordon) the NIH's mind/body study panel, and to be responsible for writing a major section in what has come to be known informally as the *Chantilly Report,* its proper title being *Alternative Medicine: Expanding Medical Horizons. A Report to the National Institutes of Health on Alternative Medical Systems and Practices in the United States.* During the first meeting of the mind/body interest section, I was stunned by the unusual and refreshing cooperation and respect demonstrated by the group. Ideas and therapeutics far beyond the usual behavioral mind/body interventions were woven into the discussion and report with grace and ease. These included the power of prayer, the essential spiritual foundations of healing systems, so-called "energy healing," and the transpersonal nature of medicine.

A vast number of the ideas and therapeutics covered briefly in the *Chantilly Report* are described with fine scholarship in *Healing East and West.* Most gratifying to me was the evidence summarized in the *Chantilly Report* suggesting a solid research basis for imagery, biofeedback, hypnosis, and several of the other therapies reported in this book. In fact, the methodology and epistemology in the mind/body field may set a standard for the research in alternative and complementary therapies.

Two other events have occurred since the publication of the original edition of this book which testify to its innovative and important content. In 1993, David Eisenberg and his colleagues published the results of their survey of American health consumers in the *New England Journal of Medicine;* they showed that an estimated 61 million Americans used an alternative therapy, and 22 million saw a provider of alternative therapies for a principal medical condition. The article also showed that Americans appear to make more total visits to practitioners of alternative medicine than to conventional primary-care physicians, and that they spent an estimated $13.7 billion, of which $10.3 billion was out of pocket. This is telling evidence that customers have chosen alternative medical treatments despite stringent government regulations, limited reimbursement, and in many cases, without evidence that the methods were supported in clinical trials. Many of the therapies listed in the Eisenberg survey, including relaxation, meditation, imagery, hypnosis, and Chinese medicine, are covered in depth in *Healing East and West*, and their theoretical underpinnings and efficacious use are clearly demonstrated.

The second development that testifies to the value of the Sheikhs' book is the launching in 1994 and 1995 of five new professional journals on alternative or complementary therapies in the United States, and at least that many abroad. *Alternative Therapies in Health and Medicine,* a peer-reviewed journal that quickly gained a wide audience, has a theme and vision consistent with that of *Healing East and West*. Both espouse the conviction that we must actively redeem the good, the beautiful, and the true from science and the professions to which we owe allegiance. And the two share the hope that creative collaboration, integration, and bridging of language, wisdom, and technologies will bring healing professionals into their next and finest dimensions.

Jeanne Achterberg
Senior Editor
Alternative Therapies in Health and Medicine
Professor of Psychology, Saybrook Institute
Author of *Imagery in Healing, Woman as Healer,*
and co-author of *Rituals of Healing*

Foreword to the Hardcover Edition

The predominant feature in the intellectual scene as we approach the end of the 20th century is the rapid decline—even collapse—of the dualistic-materialistic paradigm that has dominated world thought for several centuries. What may be called the Cartesian-Newtonian-Marxist paradigm, based on an incurable dichotomy between matter and mind, has been shown by the astounding scientific developments that have taken place over the last four decades to be inadequate. With post-Einsteinian physics, quantum mechanics, Heisenberg's uncertainty principle, C. G. Jung's inner cartography of the psyche and numerous other major developments, the whole picture of reality is changing. Matter dissolves into waves of energy, consciousness emerges not as an epiphenomenon of matter but perhaps as the primary principle behind manifestation. The new science seems to be approaching the ancient insights of seers and mystics from all the great traditions of humanity.

This conceptual revolution is having its impact in all spheres of human activity, and the quest for a holistic vision of life is beginning to assume importance in many fields. This is particularly noticeable in the areas of health and healing, because here the old dichotomy between body and mind was most strongly manifested—and most clearly proved obsolete. Western medicine has tended to look upon the body as a sort of machine that can be treated in total isolation from the mind, but even before the major paradigm shifts, it was becoming clear that this mechanical approach was simply not working. This was especially apparent in areas where psychosomatic linkages were showing that the mind does have a major impact upon bodily functions. C. G. Jung was perhaps the first major figure in the West to grasp the deeper implications of Eastern thought for the study and practice of psychology. Subsequently, a whole host of thinkers has pursued this quest for a synthesis between Eastern and Western approaches, as has been ably summed up by Roger Walsh in the last chapter of this book.

That the mental state of the patient can vastly affect the behavior of the body, that the mind exercises a subtle sovereignty over hormonal and other bodily functions, that the power of thought can often achieve what can only be described as miraculous results, that the mind and the body form one indivisible unit, all are insights shared by all the great spiritual teachings of the past, whether Hindu or Greek, Buddhist or Arab. The ancient Indian medical system of Āyurveda clearly reiterates the integral link between the mind and the body, and indeed goes beyond them to try and unravel the transcendent mysteries of the undying spirit within both.

This is an endlessly fascinating field, and the editors of this book— Anees and Katharina Sheikh—are to be congratulated for bringing together a number of fascinating chapters dealing with the various approaches to healing. The range of topics included is impressive, covering Hindu, Buddhist, Islamic, Jewish, and Christian approaches, as well as those of psychology and neurosciences. Reading these chapters is an intellectual treat because they illuminate the eternal mystery of human consciousness from many varied points of view.

To my knowledge, this book is the most comprehensive effort at bringing together the achievements of both Eastern and Western healing traditions, and thus is a very significant step toward a far-reaching integration of the best of both worlds. I feel that the book is too important to remain accessible only to readers of English, and it is my hope that it will be translated into many languages.

As we draw to the end of this terrible and unique century, which has seen more blood shed and suffering than any other in the long and tortuous history of the human race, we seem at last to glimpse a light at the end of the tunnel. The threat of a global nuclear holocaust is gradually decreasing and, although the situation remains volatile and dangerous, there is reason to believe that the human race may, after all, succeed in surviving its own technological ingenuity. At a time like this, a new synthesis between Eastern and Western approaches to healing would be of considerable value, not only in terms of the medical aspect itself, but in the broader context of the growth of a holistic global consciousness. I believe that this book will make a significant contribution to that end.

New Delhi, India   Karan Singh
September, 1989   Indian Ambassador to the U.S.,
                                          Former Minister of Health, India,
                                          and author of *The Religions of India*

The history of science is rich in the examples of the fruitfulness of bringing two sets of techniques, two sets of ideas, developed in separate contexts for the pursuit of truth, in contact with each other.

from J. R. Oppenheimer, *Science and Common Understanding* (New York: Dutton, 1954.)

Acknowledgments

The work on this book began while the first editor was on an Alumni-in-Residence Fellowship at the East-West Center for Cultural and Technical Interchange in Honolulu, Hawaii. When this Center was proposed in 1959 by Lyndon Johnson, he envisioned it as an international university, a meeting place for scholars and students from the East and the West. In September 1960, the East-West Center opened its doors and since then more than 25,000 scholars and students have participated in the Center's programs.

The first editor was a grantee from Pakistan at the Center in 1961 and was delighted to return many years later as an Alumnus-in-Residence. We gratefully acknowledge the Center's support of this project, and we are thrilled at the prospect that this volume may contribute, in a small way, to the Center's mission of encouraging a dialogue between East and West. It is clear that in a world where countless problems await a solution, we cannot afford to continue to wear the blinders of pride in our own accomplishments and ignore the accumulated wisdom of the other half of the world.

We cordially thank the contributors to this book. Each one provided a unique and important segment to the project. The absence of any one of these chapters would have left a noticeable lacuna.

Our gratitude also goes out to the staff of John Wiley & Sons Publishers, and particularly to Herb Reich, who guided this project with sound advice and much patience from idea to reality.

We are deeply grateful to Marion Jablonski for her cheerful and very conscientious typing of many drafts of our chapters. We consider ourselves very fortunate to have had her help. We are also indebted to Marion Palmer and Beth Limberg for their valuable help in preparing the index.

Finally, we wish to thank our wonderful children, Nadeem, Sonia, and Imran, for bearing with us during these hectic months. Their understanding and patience made us very proud of them.

A. A. S.
K. S. S.

Contents

Introduction

ANEES A. SHEIKH AND KATHARINA S. SHEIKH

A Zen master asks his student, "Which would you rather be, a lowly stonecutter chipping away at the base of a mountain, or the mountain itself?" As he asks the question, he taps his foot on the stone floor, representing the clanging sound of the stonecutter chipping at the mountain.

"I would rather be the stonecutter for he is stronger and chips away at the mountain."

"Very good. And now there is a nobleman for whom the stonecutter works. Which would you rather be, the stonecutter or the nobleman?"

"I would rather be the nobleman for he is the boss and master of the stonecutter."

"Very good," the master replied. "Now the nobleman has many fields which are being scorched by the hot, blazing sun. Which would you rather be, the sun, or the nobleman?"

"I would rather be the sun which is more powerful than the nobleman."

"Again, very good. And now a cloud comes and blocks the rays of the sun. Which would you rather be, the cloud, or the sun?"

"I would rather be the cloud, for it is stronger than the rays of the sun."

"Now the cloud moves across the sky and runs into a large mountain which divides the cloud and makes it scatter into

many pieces. Now which would you rather be, the cloud, or the mountain?"

"The mountain, of course, because it is stronger than the cloud."

And with that, the master smiles, again taps his foot on the stone floor, and bows.

A Japanese Folktale in
Shapiro, 1983, pp. 433–434

Attempts to prove the supremacy of Western science over Eastern knowledge or vice versa, though not uncommon, are generally unproductive. It seems preferable to begin this book by simply acknowledging that Eastern and Western philosophies display some very fundamental differences. The dominant Western view was shaped by the Newtonian-Cartesian paradigm, which represents the universe as a mechanical system that is infinitely intricate. Matter is considered to be inert and unconscious, and consciousness and creative intelligence are regarded as unimportant by-products of material development. Eastern systems, on the other hand, portray consciousness and intelligence as fundamental qualities of existence. In the Western view, only objectively observable and measurable phenomena are considered real. In contrast, Eastern disciplines generally acknowledge a complete hierarchy of realities, ranging from those which are manifest to those which ordinarily are hidden. The West's preoccupation with the concrete has fostered a world view in which man is merely a highly developed animal, and the spiritual side of human nature expressed in religion, spirituality, and mysticism is either ignored or termed pathological. Consequently, the major thrust of materialistic and mechanistic Western science has been to alleviate bodily suffering. In contrast, Eastern philosophies are essentially spiritual and portray human beings as reflections of the universe and ultimately divine; hence, their major focus has been the attainment of inner freedom: that is, passing beyond suffering to the experience of one's divinity. Toward this end, Eastern thinkers have developed a rich and challenging collection of spiritual techniques (Grof, 1984).

These philosophical differences between East and West are reflected also in the approaches to health care. Since the time of Descartes, the vast majority of Western health professionals have subscribed to dualism, and, in essence, they have regarded mind and body as separate entities. But Eastern healers have remained faithful to a tradition which has endured for thousands of years; they believe that body, mind, and spirit form an integral whole, and that any treatment of the body cannot be separated from psychological and spiritual dimensions.

Both systems possess unique strengths, but each would benefit from fertilization by the other. The Western scientific approach has largely not accounted for man's need for inner blossoming while the Eastern quest for Nirvana has led to the neglect of pressing practical problems. As Oppenheimer (1954) pointed out: The history of science contains many examples of the fruitfulness of bringing together ideas and techniques, developed in separate contexts. The time now seems ripe for a genuine synthesis of the great achievements of the Eastern and Western healing traditions.

Perhaps due to the political and economic dominance of the West, many Eastern professionals have lost faith in their culture's approaches and have been given to wholesale and uncritical subscription to Western ideas. On the other hand, Western health scientists generally have rejected Eastern approaches without a fair trial and have regarded them "as little more than muddled and fuzzy religious systems, totally devoid of matters that a hard-nosed psychologist ought to consider" (Goleman, 1988, p. 146). Western investigators did come across some startling Eastern conclusions concerning mental processes, consciousness, and ways of promoting psychological well-being. But they tended to dismiss them as mere superstitions. They did so for several reasons. Since Western psychologists ascribed their success largely to an empirical scientific method, they doubted that their Eastern colleagues, who relied primarily on subjective and experiential means, could have much to offer. The major Eastern psychologies were rooted in spiritual systems, such as Hinduism, Buddhism, Taosim, and Sufism, and hence were viewed with suspicion by Western scientists. Also, many of the assumptions, aims, and practices appeared alien and even nonsensical to Western psychologists. They were bemused and bewildered by the Eastern assessment that our customary state of consciousness is permeated by distortion and illusion, that our minds have escaped our control and have reduced us to automata. Of course, the prescribed remedy for this condition, vigorous exercises in self-awareness, such as prolonged periods of concentration upon our breathing, seemed equally farfetched. Hence, it is not surprising that most Western investigators dismissed these traditions after a cursory examination and did not bother undertaking the rigorous practices which Eastern thinkers claim are a prerequisite to appreciating their discipline (Walsh, 1983). Furthermore, the two dominant models of Western psychology of the 20th century—psychoanalysis and behaviorism—were too narrow in scope to permit appreciation of the depth and breadth of the Eastern claims.

Recently, however, interest in Eastern thought has blossomed. This does not represent an entirely new phenomenon, but rather a flowering of seeds sown long ago and nurtured through the ages by those who recognized the awesome potential of the human spirit. Western thinkers were touched by Eastern philosophies since the time of the Greeks. After all, Alexander (356–323 B.C.) and his solders penetrated deep into India and were not impervious to the riches of this ancient culture. One of the early philosophers profoundly influenced by the East was Plotius (205–270 A.D.), and his ideas were echoed for centuries by the Christian mystics, among them St. Anthony, St. John of the Cross, and Meister Eckhardt.

More recently, a number of prominent thinkers and artists have contributed to nurturing Eastern thought in the West. William James, America's most prominent 19th-century psychologist was fascinated by Oriental religions. Carl Jung was an eminent spokesperson for Eastern thought among psychologists. The movement received significant support from the views of such theorists as Gordon Allport, Gordon Murphy, Abraham Maslow, Martin Buber, Eric Fromm, Medard Boss, and Alberto Assogioli. Also, Alan Watts and Joseph Campbell, although not psychologists or psychiatrists, were very effective in bringing Eastern thought to the attention of Western health professionals.

Eastern thought also found expression in Western literature. For example, the works of American writers Emerson, Thoreau, and Whitman are steeped in the concepts of the East. In Europe, prominent spokesmen for Eastern thought include Romain Rolland and Hermann Hesse, a Nobel prize-winning novelist (see *Siddhartha* and *Journey to the East*).

However, the decisive factor in the growing respectability of Eastern concepts ironically has come from psychological science itself. With the loosening of the stranglehold of psychoanalysis and behaviorism in the mid-60s, research efforts extended into areas that had been taboo for a long time. For instance, investigators of altered states of consciousness have uncovered a much wider array of states than had been recognized hitherto; studies of meditation have disclosed a wide spectrum of physiological, biochemical, and psychological shifts; and due to biofeedback, voluntary control of internal states is no longer a wild hypothesis but common practice. Other challenges to the Newtonian-Cartesian model have come from investigation in the areas of mental imagery, psychedelics, thanatology, field anthropology, parapsychology, and experiential and transpersonal psychotherapies.

Furthermore, recent developments in the "hard" sciences have called into question the belief in mechanistic science. As Fritjof Capra outlines in the *Tao of Physics* (1975) and *The Turning Point* (1982), 20th-century physicists have transcended the Newtonian-Cartesian model: they no longer speak of a world of substance, but rather of process, event, and relation; they now regard the objective world as inseparable from the observer. Scientists no longer view the universe as the intricate mechanical clockwork of Newton but as a network of events and relations, and they consider mind, intelligence, and perhaps consciousness, to be integral constituents of existence rather than mere derivatives of matter (Grof, 1984).

The Newtonian-Cartesian model has been challenged not only by modern physics, but also by other sciences. Among the most important challenges are: Ilya Prigogine's (1986) discovery of the principle of "order through fluctuation," Rupert Sheldrake's theory of morphic resonance (1981), David Bohm's holonomic theory of the universe (1980), Karl Pribram's (1971, 1984) holographic principle, and several developments in cybernetics, systems theory, and information theory.

A most remarkable aspect of the recent developments in Western science is the fact that the newly emerging picture of the universe and of human nature appears similar to the one portrayed by ancient traditions. Finally, we may be nearing a profound synthesis of ancient and modern, Eastern and Western, which may have significant implications for life on earth (Grof, 1984).

Perhaps the most meaningful integration of the two traditions will emerge from the efforts of those scholars who openmindedly immerse themselves in both disciplines. Some noteworthy efforts along these lines already have taken place (see Dossey, 1984; Grof, 1984; Walsh & Shapiro, 1983; and Wilber, Engler, & Brown, 1986). We hope that this book, by juxtaposing some of the most significant developments in the two areas, will provide encouragement in this endeavor.

A sincere attempt at synthesis is likely to have a number of crucial consequences: It will sift the chaff from the wheat in the Eastern claims; and it probably will prompt an acknowledgment of our spiritual nature. We will be led to admit that our essence is not expressed in our struggle for physical survival, or in our efforts to make a place for ourselves within our society, but in nurturing the divine spark within us. This vision of man may inspire individuals, societies, and cultures to reach for new levels of understanding and to develop goals worthy of our spiritual nature. As Oliver Wendell Holmes remarked (see Walsh & Shapiro, 1983, p. 273):

> I think it not improbable that man, like the grub that prepares a chamber for the winged thing it neverhas seen but is to be—that man may have cosmic destinies that he does not understand.

References

Capra, F. (1975). *The Tao of physics.* Berkeley, CA: Shambhala.

Capra, F. (1982). *The turning point.* New York: Simon & Schuster.

Dossey, L. (1984). *Beyond illness.* Boston: Shambhala.

Goleman, D. (1988). *The meditative mind.* Los Angeles: Tarcher.

Grof, S. (Ed.). (1984). *Ancient wisdom and modern science.* Albany, NY: State University of New York Press.

Oppenheimer, J. R. (1954). *Science and common understanding.* New York: Dutton.

Pribram, K. (1971). *Languages of the brain.* Englewood Cliffs, NJ: Prentice-Hall.

Prigogine, I. (1980). *From being to becoming: Time and complexity in the physical sciences.* San Francisco: W. H. Freeman.

Shapiro, D. H. (1983). A content analysis of eastern and western, traditional and new age, approaches to therapy, health, and healing. In R. Walsh & D. H. Shapiro (Eds.), *Beyond health and normality.* New York: Van Nostrand Rheinhold.

Sheldrake, R. (1981). *A new science of life: The hypothesis of formative causation.* Los Angeles: Tarcher.

Walsh, R. (1983). *The psychologies of East and West: Contrasting views of the human condition and potential.* In R. Walsh & D. H. Shapiro (Eds.), *Beyond health and normality.* New York: Van Nostrand Rheinhold.

Walsh, R., & Shapiro, D. H. (1983). *Beyond health and normality.* New York: Van Nostrand Rheinhold.

Wilber, K., Engler, J., & Brown, D. (1986). *Transformations of unconsciousness.* Boston: Shambhala.

HEALING
EAST AND WEST

EASTERN PERSPECTIVES

1

Āyurveda: The Science of Long Life in Contemporary Perspective

CROMWELL CRAWFORD

Thou, Agni,
Art the Protector of the body, protect my body.
Thou, Agni,
Art the Bestower of long life, bestow on me long life.
Thou, Agni,
Art the Bestower of intellectual brilliance;
Bestow on me intellectual brilliance.
Whatever, Agni,
Is deficient in my body, make that complete for me.

Yajurveda Vs. 3.17

INTRODUCTION

The classical system of Hindu medicine is known as Āyurveda. The etymology of the word *Āyurveda* summarizes its purpose. It is made up of two parts, *āyus* meaning "life, vitality, health, longevity," and *veda* meaning "science or knowledge" (Stutley & Stutley, 1977, p. 34). Thus, the prime concern of Hindu medicine is not with "healing" in the narrow sense of curing illness, but in the broader sense of promoting health and prolonging life. The goal of this enhanced vitality is the achievement of all the values that life has to offer, both secular and religious.

The contemporary significance of this study is the fact that traditional Indian medicine is alive and well today, unlike other ancient systems of medicine such as those of Babylon, Egypt, Persia, Greece, and Rome (with the exception of China). By some estimates, approximately 80% of India's population, especially those residing in rural areas, "still rely on Āyurvedic remedies . . . supplemented to a certain extent by modern medicines" (Sanyal, 1964, p. 47). To be sure, the mere fact of survival is no guarantee of authenticity, but it is a positive sign when the government of India and members of the scientific community find certain elements in the traditional medicine that they consider worth preserving and promoting. In his preface to *Indian Medicine* by Julius Jolly, C. G. Kashikar reports on the "new impetus" accorded to Āyurveda, since 1947:

> Qualified Āyurvedic Physicians have been and are being registered as medical practitioners. Āyurvedic Colleges have been founded where theoretical and practical training is being imparted to students. A number of medical hospitals have been established where patients are being treated according to the Āyurvedic Science and practical lessons are being given to students. Āyurvedic manuscripts are being published, and books on Āyurvedic subjects and Āyurvedic textbooks have also been published in different languages. Research work in theory and practice of Āyurveda is being conducted to some extent. Thus Āyurvedic studies have received a new impetus. (Kashikar, 1977 p. xv)

In addition to the revival of Āyurveda, attempts are being made to develop "a national medicine of India." This means that greater scientific scrutiny will be accorded to the theory and practice of Āyruveda, which should only serve to update this ancient craft.

The second component in the term *Āyurveda* identifies its origins in the Vedas. *Veda* is knowledge, but with religious underpinnings drawn from the most sacred core of Hindu scriptures. Our purpose is not historically to investigate these origins, but merely to show the evolution of Āyurveda from religio-magical beginnings to a more rational and scientific orientation, embodied in the classical doctrines of the schools of Caraka and Suśruta that flourished in the first few centuries of the common era. The literary character of these scriptures suggests that we take a step back into time because clearly they are compilations with no pretensions to novelty. They revise and reconstruct an ongoing tradition in which Āyurveda is considered an *upāṅga* ("secondary part") of the Atharvaveda and an *upa-veda* ("secondary Veda") of the Ṛg Veda.

The stereotype generally conveyed by philosophers is that the Vedas are preoccupied with questions of spirituality and moral values. Therefore, it is surprising to find that the Vedas are also concerned with the physical and material well-being of individuals and communities, particularly in the area of health care. What follows is a brief résumé of the medical data to be found in the Vedic Saṃhitās. This should serve as the backdrop for our study of classical Hindu medicine.

EARLY INDIAN MEDICINE

The Ṛg Veda is the oldest Indo-European monument of literature containing medical data. Its 1,017 hymns hark back to the middle of the second millennium B.C.E. The Yajur Veda deals with sacrificial formulae, and the Sama Veda deals with melodies. The Atharva Veda, composed toward 1400 B.C.E., though replete with magic formulas, supplies the foundations for later medical science. The Atharva Veda should be studied in conjunction with the *bhaiṣajya* chapters (xxv–xxxii) of the Kauśika Sūtra, which contain the accompanying rituals and practices. "Taken together, the two sources furnish a better picture of primitive medicine than has been preserved in any literature of so early a period" (Bolling, n.d., p. 762). Later, between 1000 and 500 B.C.E., the Brāhmaṇas and Upaniṣads were composed; these were important to us for their cosmo-physiological speculations.

The world of the Ṛg Veda is one of natural immensity, mystery, beauty, order, and inexhaustible riches. The Vedic poet sees himself as part of nature and invokes the deities to grant health and strength. No artificial lines are drawn between spiritual and physical well-being. Life expectancy is set at 100 years. But along with longevity, "the best of treasures" are also desired. The poet sings:

> Bestow on us, Indra, the best of treasures:
> the efficient mind and great brilliance,
> the increase of wealth, the health of bodies,
> the sweetness of speech and the fairness of days.

> (Ṛg Veda, in Bose, 1966, p. 16)

Since the Āryans were a conquering race, the physical and material conditions necessary for that style of life were particularly prized, as expressed in the prayer:

Thou art energy, give me energy;
thou art manliness, give me manliness;
thou art strength, give me strength;
thou art vigour, give me vigour;
thou art wrath, give me wrath;
thou art conquering power, give me conquering power.

(Yajur Veda, in Bose, 1966, p. 16)

Thus, the Āryan's quest for total well-being gives prominence to the role of medicine in the Ṛg Vedic age; and even though it is in its most primitive form, it is precious for its antiquity. Radhakrishnan states: "A study of the hymns of the Ṛg Veda is indispensable for any adequate account of Indian thought. Whatever we may think of them, half-formed myths or crude allegories, obscure gropings or immature compositions, still they are the source of the later practices and philosophies of the Indo-Āryans, and a study of them is necessary for a proper understanding of subsequent thought" (Radhakrishnan & Moore, 1967, p. 3). This is particularly true for a proper understanding of medical studies.

The 1,017 hymns of the Ṛg Veda record the evolution of the religious consciousness of the ancient Āryans from naturalistic polytheism, to monotheism, and to monism. In its polytheistic stage, the gods are central and, in the context of the present study, have medical roles to perform. G. N. Mukhopadhyaya's *History of Indian Medicine* carefully documents the healing prowess of the gods. Most beneficent of all are the Aśvins ("horsemen"), possibly related to the Dioscuri of classical Europe. They are invoked for their powers of rejuvenation and are known to heal blindness, mend fractures, and protect the aged and infirm. Indra is equally beneficent, but the same is not unequivocally true of Rudra and the Maruts. Rudra is hailed "the most eminent of physicians" because while he is feared for his capacity to send punishing disease, he is, by virtue of those same powers, capable of curing disease. Of his many remedies, the *jalasa* is most distinctive, employing cow urine, which is also cited in the Avesta for its medical properties. This is one instance of the linkage of Vedic medicine with a tradition that goes back to Indo-Iranian times.

In monotheism, the second phase of Vedic thought, Varuṇa emerges as chief of the gods of the natural and moral order. At the same time, the systematizing impulse of the Indian mind developed the notion of *Ṛta*, which not only contributed to the evolution of monotheism but laid the rudimentary basis for a scientific approach to medicine. *Ṛta* refers to "Fixed or settled order, law, rule . . . ." (Stutley & Stutley, 1977, p. 252) and has given rise to diverse though related meanings.

Epistemologically, it signifies truth; theologically, it means divine law; morally, it represents the good; ontologically, it is "the immanent dynamic order or inner balance of the cosmic manifestations themselves" (Stutley & Stutley, 1977, p. 252). Varuṇa is the guardian of *Ṛta*, and all the other gods are subsequent to its order and subject to its operation, as in the case of classical Greece. This notion posits immanent order in the universe, as distinguished from law externally imposed. The gods are not the creators of law but are its shining exemplars. Again, the seeds of this notion belong to an earlier period, for we encounter it in the Avesta as *asha* where it refers to that which is normal. Thus, in its simplest form, *Ṛta* is the universal "norm" that pervades all levels of existence, making for Truth, Beauty, and Goodness. Nothing lies outside its scope, and it provides the nexus whereby nature, humans, and gods participate in a common, harmonizing reality. In such a view, the physical, the moral, and the spiritual are organically brought together under an all-inclusive norm. By the same token, the notion of *Ṛta* eliminates the possibility of supernatural caprice and to that extent opens up a scientific approach to life.

Where the Vedic sense of *Ṛta* prevails, disease is *anṛta* for it contradicts established order. In the classical medical texts, the Vedic notion of *Ṛta* is taken up by the fundamental Hindu concept of dharma.

The Ṛg Veda also introduces us to the *bhiṣaj*, the Indian doctor who subsequently came to be known as the *vaidya*. He functioned as a healer through the utilization of a vast store of herbs. Since most diseases were attributed to demonic action, it is probable that the herbs were originally tied to the wrists or other parts of the body in order to stave off the demonic incursions.

We come now to the Atharva Veda, which is the source of Āyurveda. Caraka states that because both of their purposes are the same, namely, "for the sake of longevity," Āyurveda constitutes a part of the Atharva Veda.

The practice of medicine in the Atharva Veda entailed a good grasp of human anatomy, but this knowledge was limited to "the coarser anatomy of the human body, naming its various external subdivisions, and many of its internal organs" (Bolling, n.d., p. 763). It was vague in its understanding of the finer aspects of the circulatory system. Disease was attributed to and identified with a host of demons: the *piśācha* and *atrin*, who devoured flesh; the *kanva*, who destroyed embryos; and the *rakṣasas*, who caused insanity. Sometimes disease was explained as an act of divine retribution brought on by sin. At other times supernatural theories gave way to the more mundane explanation of disease as being caused by the activity of worms in various parts of the organism.

The Atharva Veda has a long list of diseases, but often the terms are too general and of uncertain meaning. In a few instances a clear identification can be made, as in the case of dropsy, which is known as *jalodara* or "water belly." Here, the symptoms described, including pain as a result of the puffing of the eyes and of the feet, are linked with the underlying cause; however, in most instances, symptoms are merely recorded without any indication of a knowledge of what is really causing the disease (Bolling, n.d., p. 763). Lacking the medical knowledge, gods or demons are held accountable for the disease, most frequently demons are blamed.

The remedies against disease (demons) are basically religio-magical. The hymns of the Atharva Veda comprise charms and imprecations, the full secrets of which are found in its ancillary text, the Kauśika Sūtra. Two remedial approaches are generally followed; propitiation and exorcism. In the first course, the demon is offered something pleasing to its own nature; in the second instance, it is confronted with something contrary and plainly offensive. This two-track approach became the basis for the division of medicine into homeopathy and allopathy (Bolling, n.d., p. 767).

The ceremonies of the Kauśika Sūtra are characteristically exorcistic. Demons are evicted from the patient through various methods, such as fumigation, laying on of hands, rubbing the body, and the pouring on of ceremonial water. The underlying basis of the diverse remedies found in the hymns and ceremonies are plainly symbolic magic. The following hymn, which is a charm against jaundice, is illustrative of this form of therapy.

> Unto the sun let them both go up—your heartburn and your yellowness; with the color of the red bull do we envelop you.
>
> With red colors do we envelop you for the sake of long life; so that this person may be free from harm and may become non-yellow.
>
> Those cows [or herbs] that are Rohinī [the Red One] as presiding divinity, as also cows which are red—their every form and every power—with them do we envelop you. Into the parrots do we put your yellowness, and into the yellow-green *ropaṇākā*-birds. Similarly into the turmeric [or yellow wagtail?] do we deposit your yellowness. (Atharva Veda, in De Bary, 1958, p. 18)

A common cause of death was by the bite of poisonous snakes; hence many hymns aim at the exorcism of serpents. The following hymn contains a charm to forbid snakes to enter the living quarters of the family.

Let not the serpent, O gods, slay us with our children and with our men. The closed jaw will not snap open, the open one shall not close. Homage to the divine folk [i.e., the serpents by way of exorcistic euphemism]. Homage be to the black serpent, homage to the one with stripes across its body, homage to the brown constrictor[?] homage to the divine folk.

I smite your teeth with tooth, I smite your two jaws with jaw; I smite your tongue with tongue; I smite your mouth, O Serpent, with mouth. (Atharva Veda, in De Bary, 1958, p. 18)

In the last verse, the exorcist shifts from euphemistic speech to symbolic action by striking the venomous parts of a symbolic serpent with the corresponding anatomy of, presumably, a dead snake (Atharva Veda, in De Bary, 1958, p. 18).

Though the treatment of disease was predominantly magical, other types of remedies are resorted to that have symbolical effects of their own, as in the ritual of pouring water through a reed to facilitate the passage of urine, when this is constricted by some nervous condition. Later, this symbolical device was developed into primitive technology whereby the urethra was probed in order to relieve urine retention. Similarly, the early practice of symbolically applying a burning torch to a snake bite, to terrify the demon, developed into a method of cauterization (Bolling, n.d., p. 767).

The materia medica of the Atharvans was a rich repository of natural elements drawn from water, earth, plants, trees, roots, animals, and various foods. In addition to the curative properties of these substances, much trust was placed in the strict observance of magical specifications in the preparation and administration of the remedies.

*   *   *   *   *

The previous section provided an overview of the medical notions found in the Vedic literature. The next step is to delineate the ideas that the classical medical texts incorporated from the traditional sources and to specify the notions that they rejected. We are helped in this task by the work of J. Filliozat, who has made a careful study of the relationship of the Āyurveda to the Veda. His findings are summarized here.

First, Āyurveda has substantially eliminated Vedic therapeutics. The ancient therapeutics was fundamentally of a religio-magical character, and the treatments failed to proceed along any scientific lines. On the other hand, Āyurveda has partially preserved the nosological nomenclature of the Veda and has drawn substantially from its physiological speculations and its anatomical notions (Filliozat, 1964).

In respect to Vedic anatomy, Filliozat points out that although many of the terms used are "only metaphorical designations," many of which have not survived, nevertheless, Vedic anatomy "possesses an extremely ample vocabulary." The texts describing the horse sacrifice supply a notable list of internal organs, as do the passages that establish similarities between human or animal anatomy and the various parts of the universe (which is conceived as the cosmic body of a human or animal). The Vedas also contain references to constitutive organic elements picked up by Āyurveda, such as the notions of *rasā* or organic sap; *ojas* or vital sap; and the notion of bile conceived of as liquid fire.

Similarly, with respect to physiology, Āyurveda has adopted several of the earlier Vedic concepts that postulate the existence of multiple breaths circulating inside the organism through a system of internal canals. According to Filliozat (1964, p. 187),

> Already in the veda the breaths have names which they will constantly have later on. When only two of them are named, they correspond either to inspiration and expiration to the breath of the antiro-superior part of the body and to that of the postero-inferior part. When three, four or five breaths sometimes are named, they correspond to specialised diverse animal spirits whose functions have been specified by classical medicine.

Thus, to a considerable extent Āyurveda has inherited Vedic anatomical conceptions and physiological speculations; however, contrary to some scholars, Filliozat maintains that the fundamental Āyurvedic theory of the three elements (*tridoṣa*) was not formed in the Vedic period. "In fact the notion of phlegm hardly prefigures in the *Ātharvaveda* which limits itself to mentioning an oedomatous affection whose name will be, later on, used to designate occasionally the phlegm itself" (Filliozat, 1964, p. 187). Only in the Śatapatha Brāhmaṇa, which belongs to the early part of the first millennium B.C.E., does the notion of phlegm emerge under the name, *śleṣman*. Filliozat (1964, p. 187) concludes:

> Indian medicine has, therefore, drawn on the Veda even for the principal elements of its general doctrines. Thereby Āyurveda is the legitimate heir to the Veda, but it has developed to a large extent the patrimony thus received. It has coordinated and systematised ancient ideas and it has constituted an immense treasure of observations and experience, both concerning the diseases and the means of curing them.

Filliozat's somewhat philological approach tends to overlook the psychology of Vedic medicine, a characteristic that is perpetuated into the classical period. One should not dismiss the imprecations, charms, and incantations found in the Vedas as mere magic, for often underlying the magic is a suggestive element that is possessed of therapeutic potency. For instance, the power of suggestion is clear in the steps taken to cure a person of jaundice (*hariman*—"yellowness"). First the demons of jaundice are conjured to leave the body of the patient in favor of a more suitable habitation, namely the yellow orb of the sun. Next, the patient is bound with an amulet made with the hide of a red bull, and a red potion is also spread on the patient's body to suggest the restoration of the system to its natural color. In addition to these external devices, the patient is made to drink the decoction of milk and butter in which the red amulet had previously been soaked. Since this amulet had been dedicated to the gods, it is internally invested with celestial qualities. Finally, the red potion that had been rubbed over the patient's body is washed down and allowed to descend upon green and yellow birds tied to his feet, thereby displacing the "yellowness" to a kindred source. Throughout the procedure, the patient is kept fully informed of each phase of the operation and is assured of the healing that is taking place.

Similarly, the suggestive element dominates when a vast array of healing herbs are invoked to effect a cure. The underlying notion is that each herb has a healing specialty and that in order to ensure a cure taking place, their combined forces must be brought to bear. The patient is made aware of the specific virtue of each herb, and their remedial effects are vividly described. Zimmer (1948, p. 9) highlights this suggestive aspect of early Indian medicine:

> The appeal to the patient's imagination in so addressing him, the conjuring up of the healing forces inherent in his body to assist the doctor in his efforts, all these practices again point to the magic or psycho-somatic character of this kind of treatment.
>
> Moreover, the accumulation of several means and drugs to be on the safe side (the persuasive power of charms playing a rather subsidiary role) and the stimulating of the patient's spontaneous forces for recovery, all these traits persist through the subsequent, somewhat more rational, periods of Indian medicine.

CLASSICAL INDIAN MEDICINE

The intermediary texts that built up the vast pyramid of Āyurvedic medicine over the centuries have not survived. At the apex of this structure are certain extant texts known as the *Bṛhattrayi* or "Great Trio." They comprise the Caraka saṃhitā, the Suśruta saṃhitā and the

Aṣṭāṅgahrdaya by Vāgbhata. The supreme authority is invested in the Caraka saṃhitā by Agniveśa. It declares:

> The methods of treatment prescribed by Agnivesa are meant both for the healthy (for the maintenance of their positive health and prevention of disease) and for the patients (for the cure of their ailments). Whatever is mentioned in this work is available elsewhere and things not mentioned here are not to be found anywhere else. (Sharma & Dash, 1976, p. xxii)

Caraka states that Āyurveda has eight branches of medical specialties: "1. Internal medicine, 2. Science of diseases specific to supra-clavicular region, viz. eye, ear, nose, mouth, throat etc., 3. Surgery, 4. Toxicology, 5. Science of demonic seizures (Psychology), 6. Pediatrics, 7. Science of rejuvenation and 8. Science of aphrodisiacs" (Sharma & Dash, 1976, p. xxii).

The Caraka saṃhitā is made up of 120 chapters with the following sections:

1. *Sūtrasthāna*, or the section on general principles, having 30 chapters;

2. *Nidānasthāna*, or the section on diagnosis of diseases, having eight chapters;

3. *Vimānasthāna*, or the section on specific determination of drugs etc., having eight chapters;

4. *Śārīrasthāna*, or the section on anatomy (including embryology), having eight chapters;

5. *Indriyasthāna*, or the section on prognostic signs, having 12 chapters;

6. *Cikitsāsthāna*, or the section on therapeutics, having 30 chapters;

7. *Kalpasthāna*, or the section on pharmaceuticals, having 12 chapters; and

8. *Siddhisthāna*, or the section on the successful administration of *panckarma* (five elimination therapies), having 12 chapters (Sharma & Dash, 1976).

The authorship of Āyurveda is given divine origins. According to the Caraka saṃhitā, Brahmā originally imparted the knowledge of Āyurveda, which was then transmitted to Daksa Prajāpati, to the Aśvins, to Indra, to Bharadvāja, to Ātreya Punarvasu, and thence to Agnivśa. Five other disciples studied Āyurveda at the feet of Ātreya, along with Agnivśa, namely: Bhela, Jatūkarna, Parāśare, Hārita, and Kṣārapāṇi—all of whom authored their own texts. Such recourse to legendary ancestry, with some smattering of historical data, is a common Indian device found in all areas of scientific, philosophic, and artistic endeavors, for the purpose of laying claim to antiquity and authority. For our purpose, the legends are only fanciful ways of establishing what we, on literary and theoretical grounds, can discern as an unbroken line of continuity in the transmission of medical data. For example, the theories of wind, of the breaths, and of the combustible nature of bile, and so on, provide a bridge between the Vedic saṃhitās and the manuals of classical medicine, thereby confirming the antiquity of Āyurveda put forth by the legends.

More than 43 Sanskrit commentaries written between the fourth century of the common era to the present time have more or less survived (Sharma & Dash, 1976). Of these, the *Āyurveda-dīpikā* by Cakrapāṇi (eleventh century) is considered the most eminent; therefore, it shall serve as the basis for our understanding of the Caraka saṃhitā. Our source is the *Caraka Saṃhitā* (text with English translation and critical exposition based on Cakrapāṇi Datta's *Āyurveda-dīpikā*) edited by R. K. Sharma and Bhagwan Dash (1976). With these introductory notes, we now turn to the *Caraka Saṃhitā* for an overview of the Āyurvedic approaches to health and healing.

Philosophy and Psychology

The development of medicine in India has gone hand in hand with the development of philosophy. The reason for this is that Indian philosophy is more than intellectual curiosity; it is the quest for the elimination of moral and physical suffering that characterizes all of human existence. The goal of philosophy is to liberate the human consciousness to its native level of being; and sound health is both the condition and creation of this philosophic end. As a result, various philosophies have flourished in India, and the one that has principally provided the basis for Āyurveda has been the Sāṁkhya philosophy of the great sage Kapila.

This is not the place to give an exposition of Sāṁkhya, but only to highlight the elements of the system that have a bearing on the presuppositions of Āyurveda. First, we highlight the Sāṁkhya theory of causation (*satkārya-vāda*). This theory postulates that an effect originally exists in its material cause prior to its appearance as an effect. Thus, the pot exists implicitly in the clay; the oil in the seed; and the curd in the milk. The logical consequence of the doctrine of *satkārya-vāda* is that *prakṛti* (ultimate ground) is the ultimate cause of all objects of the material world, including the human mind, intellect, body, and senses. Sāṁkhya is a dualistic system in which *prakṛti* is the material principle.

As the uncaused cause of all that is, *prakṛti* is eternal, subtle, and universally pervasive. Its existence as the ultimate ground of the world is inferred by various logical reasons.

Prakṛti is comprised of three elements: *sattva, rajas,* and *tamas,* which are inferred as existing in the ultimate cause by an examination of the ordinary objects of the world. They are the elements of pleasure, pain, and indifference, respectively, and are called *guṇas* because they serve the ends of *puruṣa,* the second ultimate principle. *Sattva guṇa* is the inherent power in people and things that makes for happiness, lightness, and illumination. *Rajas guṇa* is the power of mobility, which gives rise to experiences of pain. It is the driving force of *sattva* and *tamas,* which, by themselves, are motionless. *Tamas guṇa* is the power of indifference; it produces resistance, ignorance, and confusion. The *guṇas* are inherently opposed to one another, and yet cooperate in the functioning of all objects in the world. The degree to which one *guṇa* prevails over the other two, determines the nature of that person or thing. This does not imply a condition of stasis, for all things in the world are continuously in process due to the volatile character of the *guṇas;* however, a distinction is made between change in the states of cosmic dissolution and evolution. Before creation (*pralaya*), the *guṇas* change internally and homogeneously, and in the absence of combinations, cosmic equilibrium prevails (*samyavastha*). The creative process begins once the *guṇas* interact with one another; this heterogeneous transformation is known as *virupa-parinama.*

The second principle in this dualistic system is *puruṣa* or the Self. *Puruṣa* is the pure, eternal, all-pervading consciousness. In the individual, the self is a conscious spirit and is to be distinguished from the total body-mind complex. At all times it is the subject of knowledge—never the object.

Evolution commences when nonintelligent *prakṛti* comes into contact (*samyoga*) with inactive *puruṣa.* The contact serves mutual purposes, analogous to the cooperation of a blind man and lame man, trying to make their way out of a forest. The encounter shatters cosmic equilibrium, and the activated *guṇas* contend with each other for predominance, combining in varied strengths, and thereby producing different objects in the world. The first product of *prakṛti* is *mahat* or *buddhi.* In the macrosmos, it is cosmic intelligence (*mahat*); in the individual, it is intellect (*buddhi*). Intellect has closest affinity to the transcendent, and in its pure (*sattvika*) state enjoys health and happiness; but vitiated by *tamas,* it becomes the ignorant prey of sorrow and disease. The second product of *prakṛti* is ego (*ahaṅkāra*), the sense of "mineness." From the *sattvik* side of ego, evolve the five organs of perception, the five organs of action, and the mind (*manas*). From the *tamasik* side of ego, the five subtle elements are derived (*tanmatras*). The *rajas* side of ego supplies the energy for the transformation of *sattva* and *tamas* into their evolutes.

This sketch of Sāṁkhya should suffice to bring out important medical implications. First, there are the two ultimate principles, *puruṣa* and *prakṛti*, which, although opposite, nevertheless cooperate with one another in the act of creation. This cooperation among opposites is also evident in the functioning of the three modes of nature: *sattva* (purity), *rajas* (passion), and *tamas* (darkness). Just as in the case of a lamp, the ingredients of fire, oil, and wick, although possessed of mutually inhibiting properties, function together to produce light; so also the three diverse dispositions of nature harmonize to enable the human spirit to become enlightened and thereby achieve liberation. Thus, for Āyurveda, spirit and matter, soul and body, although different, are not alien, insofar as they can be brought together in a healing relationship with consequences that are mutually beneficial.

Secondly, by espousing the philosophy of cosmic evolution, Āyurveda conceives of man in the universe as a microcosm. All forms of matter, including human beings, are composed of five elements: Ether (space), Air, Fire, Water, and Earth. These elements are the products of energy springing forth from cosmic consciousness. Therefore, it is possible for all human beings to experience matter as energy. The parallelism between human nature and nature at large suggests that humans are in a systemic relationship with the creative forces of the universe and encompass powers that are only dimly known through the phenomenon of "miracles."

The Yoga system of Patañjali is closely allied with the Sāṁkhya system. Actually, the spiritual, mental, and physical values of Yoga have been tried and tested in India from the time of the Indus Valley civilization, and it is recognized through all of the subsequent literature. Its contribution in the present context is that while it agrees with Sāṁkhya that knowledge of the self's transcendence over the physical world (including the world of our own body, senses, mind, intellect, and ego) is what brings about liberation, such saving knowledge presupposes the purification of the mind and body. The way to this purification is through Yoga. Yoga helps one tune out the whole physical world in which one is normally enveloped and with which one is prone to identify; what remains is pure self-consciousness. The transcendent spirit is then totally isolated from physical reality and thereby comes into its own—free from all the pain, misery, and death that characterize physical existence. Before we explain the discipline whereby the self is able to distinguish itself from the psycho-physical organism, we need to understand certain fundamentals of Yoga psychology.

First, there is the self (*jīva*), the free spirit that is beyond all physical and psychical changes. This self is associated with the gross body (and particularly with the subtle body comprising the senses), the mind (*manas*), the ego, and the intellect.

The intellect, or *citta* (Sāṁkhya-*buddhi*), assumes the forms of various objects through which knowledge arises. For example, our knowledge of a chair is conveyed to us through a mental image of the chair, and that image is due to *citta's* assumption of the form of the chair. Because of this cognitive process, *citta* is in a state of constant change. These changes of *citta* are reflected upon the self due to their association. So it appears that the self (*puruṣa*) suffers change and is subject to disease, decay, and death. In fact, all pain and joy are happenings within the physical and psychical organisms of the individual that *puruṣa* transcends; but as long as the changes of *citta* occur, *puruṣa* will be identified with them.

The unequivocal way of ending this erroneous identification is first by restraining the activities of the body and *citta* and, finally, by eliminating them. This involves the transmutation of *citta* from its phenomenal state of activity to its original state of nonactivity. Here, precisely, lies the goal of Yoga, and this is what gives it its definition as the "elimination of mental modifications." To achieve this goal, one must climb five levels of the mental life (*cittabhumi*). At the fourth level (*ekarga*), the mind is freed from all disturbances and can engage in prolonged concentration. But the mental processes are not yet eliminated, and so one advances to the final level (*niruddha*). Here the mental processes are altogether arrested. The mind returns to its original tranquil state, and the self (*puruṣa*) abides in its own essence. This is true liberation. It marks the end of all pain and suffering. "Yoga is one of the spiritual paths that leads to the desired goal of a total extinction of all pain and misery through the realization of the self's distinction from the body, the mind and the individual ego" (Chatterjee & Datta, 1968, p. 301).

Building on this description of Yoga psychology, Yoga ethics provides practical methods of purification whereby the self discovers its distinction. The underlying thought is that unless a person is morally strong, he or she cannot undertake spiritual discipline. Moral integrity is necessary for the upward climb.

The Yogic discipline of purification has eight steps (*Astanga Yoga*). The first two, *Yama* and *Niyama,* are sensitive to the quality of life style. Inasmuch as the body and mind are in close union, for better or for worse, they are bound to have a mutual impact on one another.

The third step, *Āsana,* deals with postures. These are exercises intended to restore the body to high levels of energy due to Yoga's perceived correlation between one's capacity for concentration and one's state of health. Concentration is not just a matter of the mind, but of the body also. Disease is not only a physical liability, but also a mental and spiritual liability. Various postures are prescribed for every type of ailment. For example, in the case of the *vāta* type of constipation, the recommended *āsanas* are "Backward Bend," "Yoga Mudra," "Knee to Chest," "Shoulder Stand," and "Corpse." The *āsanas* for the *pitta* type of migraine headache are "Sheetali," "Shoulder Stand," and "Fish." The *āsanas* to be performed for sinus congestion are "Fish," "Boat," "Plough," "Bow," and "Breath of Fire" (Lad, 1984, p. 115).

The fourth step is *Prāṇāyāma,* or control of breath. This involves the suspension of breathing either in exhalation or inhalation. When this takes place, the capacity for concentration is enhanced. In *Prāṇāyāma,* the final purpose is mental, but this exercise also has therapeutic physical effects because the heart is strengthened through respiratory control. The result is similar to that of aerobic exercise, which strengthens the heart to the point that its beat is markedly reduced.

The next three steps are internal to Yoga, as compared with the five previous ones which were external aids. They are *Dhāraṇā, Dhyāna,* and *Samādhi.* These are techniques of concentration whereby one can control the mind without use of the body. They climax in the state of *Samādhi,* in which the subject is lost in the object of contemplation and is therefore not aware of it. *Samādhi* is a difficult state to achieve, requiring years of effort, but in the meantime the *yogin* develops enormous physical and psychic powers that keep the body vital, the mind tranquil, and ensure longevity.

Our brief discussion brings out a distinct correlation between Āyurveda and the science of Yoga. In its goal to isolate spirit from matter, Yoga relies on its mental and physical discipline. It is at this juncture that it makes alliance with Āyurveda, for it is only a fit body that can reach the spiritual goal. At the same time, the physical science of Āyurveda is given direction by the philosophical and psychological insights of Yoga. This mutuality explains why, traditionally, the student of Yoga is first initiated into the study of Āyurveda. For the rest of the yogi's life, he or she continues to rely upon Āyurveda to maintain stamina. Vasant Lad (1984, p. 113) aptly refers to Āyurveda and Yoga as "sister sciences," and explains why:

> Yoga is the science of union with the Ultimate Being. Āyurveda is the science of living, of daily life. When yogis perform certain postures and follow certain disciplines, they open up and move energies that have accumulated and stagnated in the energy centers. When stagnant, these energies create various ailments. Yogis may temporarily suffer physical and

psychological disorders because in the course of yogic cleansing of the mind, body and consciousness, disease-producing toxins are released. Employing Āyurvedic diagnoses and treatments, the yogis deal effectively with these disorders.

Physiology

Āyurvedic physiology is developed around the five theoretical conceptions of *Pancamāhabhūtas* (five eternal substances), *Tridoṣas* (three humors), *Sapta Dhatūs* (seven basic tissues), *Agnis* and the three *Malas* (excretions).

Pancamāhabhūtas.   In the course of evolution, as described by Sāṁkhya, there emerges from inert matter certain subtle materials (*tanmātrās*), which, although imperceptible, have definite characteristics. They are the "generic essences" of physical energy represented by sound, touch, color, taste, and smell. When these subtle essences begin to compound, gross matter manifests itself in variegated forms. The production of the five gross physical elements takes place in the following manner. First, the sound energy produces the Ether element (*ākāśa*), which has sound quality perceived by the ear. Second, the energy of Touch, combined with the movement of Ether, produces Air (*vāyu*), which has the qualities of sound and touch. Third, the energy of Color, combining with the energies of Sound and Touch, produce Fire, which has the qualities of sound, touch, and color. Fourth, the energy of Taste, in combination with the essences of sound, touch, and color, produce Water, which has the qualities of sound, touch, color, and taste. Fifth, the energy of Smell, combining with all of the above essences, produces Earth, which incorporates the qualities of sound, touch, color, taste, and smell. The subsequent evolution of the world, including the human constitution, is from these five elementary principles of Earth, Water, Air, Fire, and Ether. Of course, one should not attribute commonplace meanings to these elemental substances.

The five elements enter the body through food and become reconstituted in the physiology and anatomy of the individual. As with the rest of nature, the body is in a continuous state of transformation. Death is the final act by which the organism is returned to its original state.

The *Tridoṣas.*   The five elements of Ether, Air, Fire, Water, and Earth take form in the body as the *tridoṣas*, or humors. These three elements are wind (*vāta*), bile (*pitta*), and phlegm (*kapha*). *Vāta* is a product of Ether and Air. *Pitta* is produced from Fire and Water; and *kapha* from Earth and

Water. These three body elements, along with blood, sustain the body and regulate all organic and psychic functions. Without them, the body cannot exist. When they are in a state of dynamic equilibrium, the body enjoys health and well-being; but when there is a loss of balance, disease results. Each *doṣa* has three states: aggravation, diminution, and equilibrium. Āyurveda maintains that healing can only proceed upon a sound understanding of the *tridoṣas.*

Wind is the most important of the three humors. It is a combination of the two universal elements of Air and Ether (*ākash*). However, it is not to be confused with atmospheric air. *Vāta* refers to motion. "Bodily air, or *vāta,* may be characterized as the subtle energy that governs biological movements. This biological principle of movement engenders all subtle changes in the metabolism" (Lad, 1984, p. 115). *Vāta* is active in the processes of respiration, circulation, evacuation, and chiefly in the functions of the nervous system. It is principally located in the stomach, small intestines, chest, and in all passages, such as the ears, eyes, nose, throat, rectum, and generative organs. There are five kinds of Air, the most important of which is *Prāṇa vāyu,* or Vital Air. It supports life (*prāṇa*) and is situated in the chest. As long as *vāta* is in a state of equilibrium and is able to flow freely over the body to help it perform its vital functions, there is health; but when it is diminished, weakness sets in and diseases arise in the areas of digestion, respiration, circulation, and voice. Hypertension, paralysis, pain, and stiffness of the limbs, and cardiac dysfunction are common. *Vāta* is usually deranged by excessive physical strain, sleeplessness, and eating the wrong quantity and quality of food.

The second humor is *pitta,* or bile. It literally means heat and is comprised of the elements of Fire and Earth. It controls the enzymes and hormones and affects all chemical functions, including digestion and metabolism. Body temperature and the tonality of the skin and eyes come from *pitta,* as do emotional intensity and intellectual acuity. It can be disturbed in some 40 ways, causing high temperatures and the incidence of jaundice, urticaria, sleeplessness, sluggishness, and a craving for cooling foods. These derangements are often brought on by the harboring of hostile thoughts and feelings, fatigue, fasting, and eating incorrect foods. *Pitta* is found in organs such as the heart, liver, spleen, and skin, but its center is in the stomach and small intestines.

The third humor is *kapha,* or phlegm. It regulates the two other humors and is a combination of Ether and Water. It is chiefly located in the region of the head, chest, and stomach and is found in the moist parts of the anatomy. There are five kinds of phlegm that lubricate the moving parts of the body and provide moisture for the brain, eyes, and skin.

Kapha also aids in digestion by softening the food; it provides sexual energy; it sustains the entire physical organism; and it helps in such mental processes as memory retention. When *kapha* is morbidly diminished, the body loses its liquidity; vessels are hardened; thirst is sharpened; heat is increased; digestion is impaired; the joints are immobilized; and the individual becomes tardy and anorexic. Causes of these derangements include failure to exercise and faulty diet.

Like the mind, the *tridoṣas* permeate the entire organism, but a special division is ascribed to each one. *Kapha* lies above the navel; *pitta* is in the trunk, above the pelvic region; and *vāta,* is below the pelvis. The strength of each is regulated by the time of day. In the cool of the morning, phlegm predominates; in the heat of midday, the effects of bile are strongest; and in the evening, it is the wind that is most felt. The same principle applies to the changing seasons, each having a proneness to a particular *doṣa.* The human life cycle is explained in similar terms. In the growing years, *kapha,* which governs the anabolic process of the body, is most active; in maturity, when life takes on a certain stability, *pitta,* which controls the metabolic process, is at the fore; and in the advanced years, when the body begins to decline, *vāta,* governing the catabolic process, is most manifest. For each region of the body there is an elemental angularity that the physician must take into account in making diagnoses or prescribing remedies. The most fundamental particularity of all is the constitution of each individual. Typically, each person has a characteristic constitution—that of *vāta, pitta,* and *kapha.* This does not imply the singularity of any one factor, rather its prevalence in consort with the others. For example, a person of *vāta* constitution has a combination of all three *doṣas,* but it is *vāta* that dominates.

The Seven Elements.   The five proto-elements (*mahābhūtas*) that are responsible for the creation of the entire material world are also present in the seven elements, and, as in the case of the *tridoṣas,* one or two may predominate. These seven constructing elements are known as *dhātus,* meaning: "that which enters into formation of the basic structure of the body as a whole" (Dash & Junius, 1983, p. 27). Therefore, as "the basic tissue elements," the *dhātus* constitute the body and support and sustain it. Of special importance is their role in the body's immunological system. They comprise the body's fluids and its hard and soft parts. These seven elements are: plasma (*rasā*), blood (*rakta*), flesh (*māṁsa*), fat (*meda*), bone (*asthi*), marrow (*majjā*), and semen (*śukra*).

Rasā is the nutritional extract from digested food and provides nourishment for the entire organism. It enters into the blood and is transferred successively into the remaining elements. The blood (*rakta*) is responsible for oxygenating the system and conveying nutrients. Flesh (*māṁsa*) and muscle constitute the organs and supply the body with connective strength. Fat (*meda*) proceeds from flesh and is the lubricating element in all bodily parts. Bone (*asthi*) comes from fat and gives the body its skeletal structure. Marrow (*majjā*) fills the bones and, with the nerves, conveys sensory messages. Sperm (*śukra*) originates from marrow and is the reproductive element.

The seven elements are directly influenced by the *tridoṣas*. Therefore, to maintain them in a state of health, it is necessary to follow a good diet, exercise regularly, and thus keep *vāta*, *pitta*, and *kapha* in proper balance.

The essence of all of these elements is known as *ojas*, meaning power. It gives vitality to all of the tissues and is found throughout the body. In a healthy state, *ojas* gives firmness to the body, a shining color to the skin, and energizes the internal and external organs. In the event it is diminished by hunger, injury, exhaustion, or anxiety, the individual's complexion changes; he or she feels bloated and complains of fatigue and loss of strength. There are three degrees in the diminution of *ojas*; the last terminates in death.

The Agnis.   Health and healing in the Āyurvedic system is intimately connected to food and its proper digestion. This explains the pivotal function of the *agnis*. They act as enzymes in the digestion and absorption of food. There are 13 *agnis*, the principal one being located in the stomach and the gastrointestinal tract. The literal meaning of *agni* is fire, and *Jatharagni* is "the digestive fire in the stomach." Its task is to break down the intake of food. Next, there are the five *bhūtagnis* relative to the five elements. They are the "fire" in the liver. These enzymes "adapt the broken down food into a homologous chyle" and aid in the process whereby "the *mahābhūtic* composition of broken down food is now made into the same composition as that of the *mahābhūtas* of the body." There are also seven *dhātvagnis*, which are relative to the seven basic tissues (*dhātus*) of the body. These enzymes work on the "cooked" food, synthesizing the various tissue elements (Dash & Junius, 1983).

In the event that the digestive and metabolic functions of biologic fire are impeded, the unprocessed food accumulates in the intestines and proceeds to decompose. This undigested and unassimilated substance is known as *ama*. It is a major factor in the production of endogenous diseases. It blocks the digestive tracts, and when it is chemically transformed into toxins, it enters the bloodstream, causing injury to the internal organs.

The Three Malas.   These secretions (*malas*) that are counted among the constituents of the body include: urine (*mūtra*), feces (*shakrit*), and perspiration (*sweda*). The *malas* are waste products, following the process of digestion; but in the Āyurvedic system, these excretions are not exactly waste. For instance, prior to elimination, the solids in the intestinal tract give it support and retain nutrients that are slowly absorbed.

*   *   *   *   *   *

In summary, the human body is the evolutionary product of *prakṛti* (the ultimate ground) through contact with *puruṣa* (the primal self-conscious principle). In this respect it shares a common origin with all material, living, conscious, and unconscious entities. The normal state of the body is one in which all its elements function in balanced equilibrium, including the 11 *indriyas* (five sense organs, five organs of motion, and the mind); the *tridoṣas* (counterparts of the cosmic principles of air, radiant energy, and water); the 13 *agnis* (digestive "fires"); the three *malas* (excretions); and the seven *dhātus* (elementary materials, e.g., plasma, blood, marrow, etc.). In Āyurveda, balance is synonymous with health. Caraka states that the maintenance of equilibrium is health and, conversely, that the disturbance of the equilibrium of tissue elements is the disease. This brings us to the Āyurvedic practice of medicine with its twofold objective of the maintenance of health and the healing of disease.

The Practice of Medicine

Physicians.   Caraka clearly specifies the requirements of a physician. First, the young man desirous of entering the medical profession should select a suitable preceptor, one who is

> well grounded in scriptures; equipped with practical knowledge, wise, skillful, whose prescriptions are infallible, . . . who has all the necessary equipments for treatment, . . . who is acquainted with human nature, and the rationale of treatment, . . . who is free from vanity, envy and anger, . . . and is capable of expressing his views with clarity. (Sharma & Dash, 1976, vol. 2, p. 217)

Likewise, the preceptor should select a disciple with the following qualities:

> tranquility; generosity; aversion to mean acts; . . . liberal mindedness; birth in the family of a physician or having the disposition of a physician; . . . inquisitiveness for truth; physical perfection; modesty and

absence of ego; ability to understand the real meaning of things; . . . absence of addictions; . . . uninterrupted taste for the theory and practice of the science; . . . good-will for living beings. . . . (Sharma & Dash, 1976, vol. 2, pp. 218, 219)

As part of his initiation, the medical candidate swears to uphold the following code of professional ethics:

You should make efforts to cure the patient. You must never give way to any ill will towards your patients even at the cost of your life. You should never think of committing adultery and should not aspire for any property belonging to others. Your appearance and apparel should make you look modest. You should not take wine, commit sins or have association with those committing sinful acts. Your speech should be pleasant, pure, righteous, blissful, excellent, truthful, useful and moderate. Your behavior should be in conformity with the time and place, based on the recollections of the past experience. You should always make efforts for the upliftment of your knowledge and adoption of such methods as would give you good health. . . . Women, in the absence of their husbands and guardians, should not be treated by you. . . . You should enter the residence of the patient accompanied by a person who knows the place and who on his part, has obtained permission to enter there. While doing so you should be well clad, with your head bowed down, having a good memory, having concentration of mind, and acting with proper thinking. Having entered there, your speech, mind, intellect, and senses should be entirely devoted to nothing except the welfare of the patient and allied matters. Family customs (secrets) should not be disclosed by you to outsiders. Even having known that the patient's span of life has come to a close, you should not disclose this to the patient himself or to the son or father, etc. of the patient, because it may cause shock to the patient or to his relatives. Even though actually possessed of wisdom, you should not exhibit it to others. Many people get very much irritated to hear such self-praise even from a saint. (Sharma & Dash, 1976, vol. 2, pp. 223–224)

Disease.   Suśruta defines disease (*vyādhi*) as any condition that afflicts a human being with pain. Based on their origin, he classifies all diseases in a fourfold manner: (1) external (*agantuja*), (2) internal (*śārīra*), (3) mental (*mānasa*), and (4) natural (*svābhāvika*) (Ray, Gupta, & Roy, 1980, p. 48).

Suśruta further defines disease according to its threefold intensity: (1) curable (*sādhya*), (2) relievable (*yāpya*), and (3) incurable (*asādhya*). The curable disease may require some medication or surgery.

Factors responsible for the humoral derangements that cause disease are also placed in three divisions.

First, there are the internal factors (*ādhyātmika*), arising out of the body or the mind. These could have preconceptual hereditary causes that go back to defects within the spermatozoa or the ovum. The hereditary factors could also be postconceptual, arising, for example, during pregnancy. Improper life style or diet could also upset the body and produce disease. In addition to these internal bodily factors, internal mental factors produce psychosomatic conditions.

Second, there are external factors (*ādhibhautika*) that produce humoral derangements caused by the physical and material environment. For instance, one could fall into a hole in the ground or be bitten by a poisonous snake. Changes in the seasons also precipitate certain illnesses.

Third, the supernatural forces (*ādhidaivika*) impact upon the humors. The *ādhidaivika* diseases could be providential, such as "the acts of God," or they could be natural, such as hunger, thirst, senility, etc. In the case of the individual who follows a destructive life style, these natural factors are prematurely manifest (Ray, Gupta, & Roy, 1980).

Suśruta describes all diseases as passing through three phases: phase one anticipates the main disease; phase two marks the full manifestation of the disease; and phase three appears as a symptom that proceeds from the main disease (Ray, Gupta, & Roy, 1980).

Diagnosis.   Caraka emphasizes the importance of correct diagnosis of a disease:

> A physician should first of all diagnose the disease and then he should select proper medicine. Thereafter, he should administer the therapy applying the knowledge of the science of medicine (he has already gained). A physician who initiates treatment without proper diagnosis of the disease can accomplish the desired object only by chance; the fact that he is well-acquainted with the knowledge of application of medicine does not necessarily guarantee his success. On the other hand, the physician who is well-versed in diagnosing diseases, who is proficient in the administration of medicines and who knows about the dosage of the therapy that varies from place to place and season to season, is sure to accomplish the desired object. (Sharma & Dash, 1976)

Āyurveda lays down intricate guidelines for the diagnosis of a vast roster of diseases with reference to their etiology, symptoms, and prognosis.

Caraka has a threefold diagnostic methodology based on the three *pramanas* (sources of knowledge). These are *Śabda* (authoritative statements), *Pratyaksa* (direct observation), and *Anumana* (inference) (Sharma & Dash, 1976).

Authoritative instructions are the teachings of specialists "who know things in their entirety, without any doubts, and by virtue of their own realisation. One cannot be authoritative if he knows things only piece meal," or on the basis of memory, which is not reliable enough for the "science of medicine" (Sharma & Dash, 1976, p. 162). The research of such experts provides a tested repository of direct knowledge of the possible causes, symptoms, severity, duration, complications, recovery, and convalescence of specific diseases. An able physician must appropriate this bank of knowledge in order to become fully equipped to detect the possible causes and symptoms of every type of disease. The testimony of the patient also constitutes authoritative knowledge because it provides "information regarding the causitiveness, laxity or mediocre nature of the bowel, etc." (Sharma & Dash, 1976, p. 162).

Prior to the administration of drugs or any form of treatment, direct observation is necessary. The patient should be given a thorough examination.

> The dosage in which a therapy is to be administered depends upon the intensity of morbidity as well as the strength of the patient. A strong patient with a serious disease needs the therapy in a stronger dose. Mistakes like giving strong therapies to weak patients and vice versa can be avoided if patients are duly examined beforehand. Even if a weak person is suffering from a serious disease which requires a strong therapy for cure, he should not be given a strong therapy all of a sudden. Such a patient should be given strong therapy slowly and gradually, depending upon his strength and power of resistance gained. (Sharma & Dash, 1976, p. 262)

In order to ascertain the strength and intensity of the disease, the patient should be examined with

> reference to his *prakṛti* (physical constitution), *vikṛti* (morbidity), *sāra* (excellence of *dhātus*, or tissue elements), *saṃhanana* (compactness of organs), *pramāṇa* (measurement of the organs of the body), *sātmya* (homologation), *sattva* (psychic conditions), *āhāraśakti* (power of intake and digestion of food), *vāyāmaśakti* (power of performing exercise), and *vayas* (age). (Sharma & Dash, 1976, vol. 2, pp. 261, 262)

The clinical examination should be conducted with the full use of all five senses. Thus, with the ear the physician should hear the sounds of the digestive tract and changes in the voice; with the eye he should observe changes in body weight, form, vitality, and color; with the tongue he should taste (more often through inference); with touch he should feel changes in temperature and skin texture; and with smell he should detect odors, especially those that mark the imminence of death. The objective of this examination is to find out which of the *tridoṣas* is affected, and this knowledge is gathered by a detailed observation of the patient's tongue, face, lips, nose, eyes, nails, etc. Each of these organs bears definite signs identified with the derangement of *vāta, pitta,* or *kapha.* Pulse examination (*nāḍī-parīkṣa*) (later introduced through the Arabians or Persians) played a key role in diagnosis.

Once the physician has made the detailed clinical examination, both on the basis of his interrogation of the patient and direct observation, he is in a position to infer which particular *doṣa* is responsible for the patient's disease. Following the diagnosis, the physician makes his prognosis. If the disease is curable, he proceeds to the next step of treatment.

Treatment.   Āyurvedic therapy aims at correcting the imbalances and derangements of the bodily humors and restoring equilibrium. It does so by coordinating all of the material, mental, and spiritual resources of the whole person, recognizing that the essence of these potencies are manifestations of cosmic forces.

> At the *material level,* Āyurveda is concerned with the fundamental causes of illness, the development and function of the human organism, the identification of different diseases, toxic and pathological conditions, and also the properties, potencies, and physiological actions of the different substances which can be used as correctives by external or internal application. At the *mental level,* Āyurveda concerns itself with the removal of ignorance of the patient and with the prescription of a course of conduct (*ācāra*) for him, so that the ultimate causes of imbalances are removed as far as possible. It also provides a rational guidance for man, expounding the causes of life and death, health and illness, happiness and misery, and even success or failure in life. *But above all, the aim of Āyurveda is the attainment of the ultimate truth or salvation* by which the human mind realizes the identity of the individual soul with the Universal Soul (the Supreme Consciousness) and can thus rise above unhappiness, pain, and mortal destruction. (italics supplied) (Ray, Gupta, & Roy, 1980, p. 1)

Of course, the main preoccupation of the medical texts is with practical therapeutic methods, so that will be our focus.

Suśruta mentions five objectives and factors relative to therapeutics (Su. 1.27):

Puruṣa (the patient with a mind and body), for whom the treatment is intended;

Vyādhi (ailments, incidental to the actions of the three *doṣas* and blood);

Auṣadha (drugs, with specific physical properties, physiological actions, taste, potencies, and efficacy, etc.), the material aids in treatment;

Kriyā (cultivation, collection, selection, processing, compounding, administration, auxiliary processes, surgical method, etc.), the material aids in treatment;

Kāla (seasonal and climatic factors, the time and frequency of medication or surgical treatment) (Ray, Gupta, & Roy, 1980, p. 51)

All forms of treatment were to reflect the above considerations. Furthermore, Suśruta delineates four components for the treatment of all diseases. These are

Saṃśodhana (cleansing processes)—eliminative or radical treatment;

Saṃśamana (pacification and tranquilization of deranged bodily humors)—sedative or conservative treatment;

Āhāra (proper diet);

Ācāra (correct conduct, observance of hygienic rules, and prescribed medical diet)—regiminal treatment. (Su. 1.21)

We shall touch briefly on the two main methods of treatment in Āyurveda, namely, medications and surgery.

Āyurvedic medicines fall into two categories: those that rejuvenate, such as elixirs and aphrodisiacs, and those that heal diseases. Rejuvenating therapies were aimed at the development and maintenance of mental faculties, the senses, and physical vigors. Curative medicines were mainly derived from vegetable, animal, or mineral substances. Later, Indians learned the medicinal effects of mercury and opium from the Arabs.

Suśruta is chiefly concerned with surgery (*salya*). Surgical operations were of eight types: excision, incision, sacrification, puncturing, probing, extraction, drainage, and suturing. The operations most frequently performed were those of laparatomy, stone, and cataract.

Along with medicines and surgery as methods of treatment of diseases, Āyurveda gives great prominence to diet and to hygiene, as previously noted.

Caraka infers a correlation between diets and drinks with life from the actual experience of life. Those whose eating and drinking practices are wholesome live long; those whose practices are unwholesome die a premature death. A preliminary definition of "wholesome" and "unwholesome" states: "The food articles which maintain the equilibrium of bodily *dhātus* and help in eliminating the disturbance of their equilibrium are to be regarded as wholesome; otherwise they are unwholesome" (Sharma & Dash, 1976, p. 420). It is said that a self-controlled person "lives for hundred years free from diseases by the intake of wholesome food" (Sharma & Dash, 1976, p. 565). Food is basic for the attainment of all blessings, here and hereafter, for only a person having a healthy body has the strength to perform all activities necessary for happiness and salvation; and for the preservation of health, food is essential.

All varieties of food, both solid and liquid, are listed, giving their properties (heaviness, lightness), their composition (in terms of the five elements), their pharmacological and therapeutic effects (e.g., nourishing and invigorating), their taste (*rasā*), their potentiality (*virya*), their taste following the process of metabolism (*vipaka*), and specific action (*prabhava*). Departing from the religious literature, the consumption of meats is not principally forbidden. The best foods are rice, barley, wheat, beans, peas, lentils, and millet; the best water is rainwater collected in autumn. Fresh foods possess the highest quality. The manner in which foods are combined is equally important. For example, milk and meat do not mix. Together, they produce toxins that vitiate the *tridoṣas*. Hunger is the body's signal that the digestive enzymes are ready, marking the proper time to eat. Should drink be taken at this time, the "digestive fire" is reduced. Not only is there a time to eat and to drink; but the manner in which this is done is also noteworthy. To feel the full flavor of food, we must be aware of what we are eating. In the end, we are what we eat. And since the quality and quantity of food must be adapted to one's individual constitution, food must remain a personal matter.

Along with diet, various methods of personal hygiene are deemed essential for the maintenance of positive health. Collyrium applications are recommended for the care of the eyes; fragrant cigars are to be smoked "for the elimination of *doṣas* from the head"; oral hygiene, including teeth brushing, tongue scraping, gargles, chewing of fruits, fresh leaves, flower stalks and cinnamon extracts, is necessary to "strengthen the jaws, gums, and give depth of voice"; oiling of the head, nostrils, ears, skin, and full body massage will slacken "the onslaught of aging"; bathing is important to cleanse, remove fatigue, stimulate the libido, and to enhance *ojas*; wearing clean apparel adds to bodily charm, pleasure, and grace; using scents and garlands to stimulate the libido, produce charm with aroma, enhance longevity, and prevent inauspiciousness; wearing of gems and ornaments signifies prosperity, auspiciousness, longevity, grace, and prevents dangers from snakes and evil spirits; caring for hair and nails augment libido, longevity, cleanliness, and beauty; wearing footwear, carrying an umbrella, and using a walking stick offer protection against the elements, reptiles, and enemies.

It was also considered good hygiene not to suppress, or artificially to excite, the natural bodily urges, such as elimination, sleeping, sneezing, and the like.

In addition to physical hygiene, emphasis was also placed on mental hygiene. Negative emotions were to be substituted by positive ones, because feelings of fear, anger, and greed produce toxins that aggravate the bodily humors and weaken the internal organs.

CONTEMPORARY PERSPECTIVE

The question that emerges from our survey of this ancient medical tradition is: What contemporary values and insights does Āyurveda have for our contemporary situation? The question can be answered in many forms, but due to the limits of space, we shall discuss it in the most basic context of the meaning of health. So the question before us is: What is health?

The World Health Organization (WHO) defines health as a "state of complete physical, mental and social well-being, and not merely the absence of disease or infirmity." This definition is certainly an improvement over earlier definitions, which were informed by mechanistic models of the body rooted in Newtonian physics. It was not too long ago that our thinking about health was functionally concentrated upon different systems, such as the cardiovascular, respiratory, alimentary, and nervous systems, but the WHO definition shows a more integrated appreciation of human existence in its multidimensionality. D. B. Bisht (1985, p. 1), a participant in the WHO deliberations, summarizes the new definition this way:

> Illness is now considered to be physiologically and chemically grounded, but socially and culturally conditioned. Health is perceived as a multidimensional process involving the well-being of the whole person in the context of environment. The "perfect functioning" approach to health conceptualizes health, biologically, as a state in which every cell and every organ is functioning at optimum capacity and in perfect harmony with the rest of the body; psychologically, as a state in which the individual feels a sense of subjective well-being and of mastery over his environment; and socially, as a state in which the individual's capacities for participation in the social system are optimal.

How adequate is this definition of health? If the logic of this definition is to correlate the meaning of health with the full range of human potentialities, then the definition limits those potentialities to the physical, mental, and social dimensions of the person. There is no accounting for the spiritual dimension of life. True, it is difficult for science to try to define the spiritual, but is it scientific to ignore the phenomenon?

Among the differentia that qualitatively separate *homo sapiens* from animal forbears, is the perennial quest for meaning in life. This search proceeds from his perception of himself as a subject, distinct from all other entities. In religion, this self-awareness leads the seeker to aspects of life that transcend the boundaries of the body and the mind. In Āyurveda, the term *āyus* stands for the combination of the body, the sense organs, the mind, and soul. We are reminded:

> The body made of the five *māhabhūtas* (basic elements) serves as an abode of the enjoyments and sufferings of the soul. The sense organs are the eyes, etc.; the *sattva* is the mind, and the soul is the bearer of knowledge. All these combined with the virtue of the invisible past actions are designated as life. (Sharma & Dash, 1976, p. 26)

Three implications follow from this concept of *āyus:* (1) that spirituality represents a dimension of health, as do the body and the mind; (2) that spirituality, although super-psychic and super-somatic, is not isolated from the body-mind complex, but embraces and empowers every cell and fiber of the organism; and (3) that the relationship of spirituality to health is reciprocal—health promotes spirituality and spirituality promotes health.

If this concept of *āyus* is sound, then our definition of health should be extended beyond physical, psychological, and social well-being, to include spiritual well-being. The inclusion could revolutionize health care. A recent report on the life style of the people of Framingham, Massachusetts, illustrates our point.

Framingham is the home of the world-famous Framingham Heart Study—"the longest-running and most comprehensive study of its kind in medical history." Begun in 1948, for the past 40 years the townsfolk have participated in a program in which they are regularly examined for heart disease. "They give blood, blow into tubes, walk on treadmills, get their hearts checked with the latest gadgets and answer question after question about whether they've been sick, what they eat, how much they exercise and generally how they live their lives." As a result of the program, most people are well aware of the fact that in order to lessen their chances of dying from a heart attack or stroke, they should avoid smoking, eating fatty red meat, being overweight, and having high blood pressure and high levels of cholesterol. Knowing all this, one would assume that the people of Framingham would be pursuing healthy life styles and that few of them would be dying from heart attacks and strokes. But that conjecture would be wrong. According to Dr. William Kannel, former director of the study:

> I think basically they have the same problems that everyone else has. . . . I think its clear that simply identifying a problem does not make it go away. It takes more of a sustained effort at behavior modification. It isn't enough to tell somebody, "Your blood pressure is too high." It is very difficult to swim upstream against your culture. You say, "Yeah, I probably should change my diet," but then the TV comes on and says "Eat Twinkies and that will make all the girls come flocking," or "Smoke Winstons, it will make you a cowboy and glamorous."

The researchers have gathered invaluable data from this study, which now has an annual budget of $2 million, but in spite of scientific success there is human failure. For all their specialized care and scientific information, the people of Framingham have behaved as if they have had none of these advantages.

In the final analysis, it appears that health is a matter of self-perception. When the dimensions of health are expanded to include spirituality as a fourth dimension, the recognition of this factor vitalizes the other three levels. On the physical, mental, and social levels, spirituality promotes positive attitudes toward work, exercise, diet, personal habits, mental discipline, and social expression. Conversely, when this dimension is missing in the lives of people, they seem to lose the energizing power that comes from a sense of purpose and meaning in life. Gradually, we are becoming increasingly aware of the fact that this loss of meaning is often the root cause of so many of our psychosomatic disorders. The evidence keeps growing: the dimensionality of the spirit is etiologically related to health. This is not a call to abdicate medicine in favor of religion, for although Āyurveda values the primacy of the spirit, health is valued as an indispensable means to that goal. Health may not be everything, but everything without health is nothing.

References

Bisht, D. B. (1985). *The spiritual dimension of health.* New Delhi: Directorate General of Health Services, Government of India.

Bolling, G. M. (n.d.). Disease and medicine (Vedic). In J. Hastings (Ed.), *Encyclopedia of religion and ethics* (Vol. IV). New York: Scribners.

Bose, A. C. (1966). *Hymns of the Vedas.* Bombay: Asia Publishing House.

Chatterjee, S., & Datta, D. (1968). *An introduction to Indian philosophy.* Calcutta: Calcutta University Press.

Dash, B., & Junius, M. M. (1983). *A handbook of Āyurveda.* New Delhi: Concept Publishing Company.

De Bary, W. T. (Ed.). (1958). *Sources of Indian tradition* (Vol. 1). New York: Columbia University Press.

Filliozat, J. (1964). *The classical doctrine of Indian medicine.* New Delhi: Munshiram Manoharlal.

Kashikar, C. G. (1977). Preface to the second edition. In J. Jolly & C. G. Kashikar (Trans.), *Indian medicine.* New Delhi: Concept Publishing Company.

Lad, V. (1984). *Āyurveda: The science of self-healing.* Santa Fe, NM: Lotus Press.

Radhakrishnan, S., & Moore, C. (Eds.). (1967). *A source book in Indian philosophy.* Princeton: Princeton University Press.

Ray, P., Gupta, H., & Roy, M. (Eds.). (1980). *Suśruta sāṁhita: A scientific synopsis.* New Delhi: Indian National Academy of Science.

Sanyal, P. K. (1964). *History of medicine and pharmacy in India.* Calcutta: Amitava Sanyal.

Sharma, R. K., & Dash, B. (Eds.). (1976). Preface. *Caraka sāṁhita.* Varnanasi: Chowkhama Sanskrit Series Office.

Stutley, M., & Stutley, J. (Eds.). (1977). *Harper's dictionary of Hinduism.* New York: Harper & Row.

Zimmer, H. (1948). *Hindu medicine.* Baltimore: Johns Hopkins Press.

2

Yoga and Healing

SUNDAR RAMASWAMI

The practice of Yoga induces a primary sense of measure and proportion. Reduced to our own body, our first instrument, we learn to play it, drawing from its maximum resonance and harmony. With unflagging patience we refine and animate every cell as we return daily to the attack, unlocking and liberating capacities otherwise condemned to frustration and death.

Yehudi Menuhin, in the Foreword to *Iyengar*, 1980

Humanity's quest for the wellspring of health is as old as humankind itself. The ancient Druids—who were both magi and hierophants—the alchemists of premodern Europe, the mystics of medieval Christendom, not to mention the wise Greeks, all evidenced a consummate preoccupation with the techniques of human transformation. The search for a psychosomatic apparatus, so superbly healthy that it would serve as a fine instrument for accelerating human evolution, reached its zenith in India in the 3rd century B.C. Even as the Age of Pericles was drawing to a close in ancient Greece, Patanjali formulated his *Yoga Sutras*, describing a means for achieving supreme physical and mental health.

In Patanjali's scheme, humanity was poised for a final evolutionary step, the merging of individual personal consciousness with Godhead, the cosmic consciousness of which the person ego is but a speck. This liberation of self from its tempero-spatial existence was *moksha*, a condition that represented the apex of mental health. A superbly healthy body was a precondition for this to occur.

Yoga is not only ideally suited for optimum physical and mental health, but it also confers a sense of self-reliance, a sense of harmony with the laws of the universe, and an unfolding of latent potentialities as well as the capacities for healing and regeneration.

This chapter describes the various systems of yoga—Patanjali's Ashtanga Yoga, Kundalini Yoga, personality theory in yoga psychology, theory of learning and motivation in yoga, the varieties of mystic yogic experiences, the dangers on the yogic path, and the psychotherapeutic applications of yoga, including its role in stress disorders.

THE SYSTEMS OF YOGA

The word "yoga" is derived from the Sanskrit root *yuj*, meaning to yoke or bind. It means the yoking of the powers of body, mind, and soul to God, the union of personal will with the will of God. Yoga is one of the six orthodox systems of Indian philosophy, which include: (1) *Nyaya* (analysis), which was based on logic and was predominantly used in the debates with Buddhist teachers; (2) *Vaisheshika* (particular characteristics), which was a type of atomic philosophy; (3) *Sankhya* (enumeration), which was essentially atheistic and recognized the dualism between matter and soul; (4) *Yoga* (application), which was based on physical control of the body and implied that perfect control over the body and the senses led to knowledge of the ultimate reality; (5) *Mimamsa* (inquiry), which grew out of a feeling that the source of brahmanical strength—the *Vedas*—was being neglected, and whose supporters emphasized the ultimate law of the *Vedas* and refuted the challenge of post-Vedic thought; and (6) *Vedanta* (end of the *Vedas*), which emerged finally as the predominant system and gained wide acceptance in later times. *Vedanta* also claimed origin in the *Vedas* and posited the existence of the Absolute Soul in all things—the final purpose of existence being the union of the individual and the Absolute Soul after physical death (Thapar, 1966).

Yoga philosophy has its main source in the *Bhagavad Gita*, wherein Krishna explains to Arjuna the meaning of yoga as a deliverance from pain and sorrow. The *Gita* also gives other explanations of the word "yoga": *Karma Yoga* is the yoga of selfless action. It is pithily summarized as unceasing work in the name of the Lord with complete abandonment of desire. The practitioner is affected neither by success nor by failure.

The yoga of knowledge is *Jnana Yoga*. In the *Gita*, Krishna describes the nature of *atman* (self) to Arjuna. One who gains an understanding of the self through intuitive understanding is embarked on Jnana Yoga. *Bhakti Yoga* is for the emotional individual who seeks self-realization through devotion to and love of a personal God.

References to yoga abound in the *Upanishads*, the treatises composed by the forest philosophers from 700 B.C. onward. Yoga philosophy was systematized by Patanjali in his classical work, the *Yoga Sutras*, which consists of nearly 200 aphorisms. In his codification, Patanjali stresses control of the mind. According to Patanjali, the mind is the king of the senses and one who has conquered the passions, senses, thought, and reason is a king among all people, a *raja*. Hence, he is the *Raja Yogi.*

Patanjali, however, never alludes to Raja Yoga but calls his compendium Ashtanga Yoga, or the yoga of eight limbs. Swatmarama, the author of the *Hatha Yoga Pradipika* (*hatha* means force), called the same path Hatha Yoga because of the rigorous discipline it demanded (Iyengar, 1980).

It is widely held that Raja Yoga and Hatha Yoga are entirely different and in fact opposed to one another—Patanjali's *Yoga Sutras* deal with spiritual training and Swatmarama's Hatha Yoga stresses physical discipline.

> It is not so, for Hatha Yoga and Raja Yoga complement each other and form a single approach toward Liberation. As a mountaineer needs ladders, ropes and crampons as well as physical fitness and discipline to climb the icy peaks of the Himalayas, so does the Yoga aspirant need the acknowledge and discipline of the Hatha Yoga of Swatmarama to reach the heights of Raja Yoga dealt with by Patanjali. This path of Yoga is the fountain for the other three paths. It brings calmness and tranquillity and prepares the mind for absolute unqualified self-surrender to God, in which all these four paths merge into one. (Iyengar, 1980, pp. 7–8)

Consequently, the Ashtanga Yoga of Patanjali may be thought of as integrating Bhakti Yoga, Karma Yoga, Jnana Yoga, and Swatmarama's Hatha Yoga. It may be referred to as the science of Raja Yoga, since it implies a mastery over the self.

In the 5th century A.D., a new cult associated with female deities emerged in India. This fertility cult became the nucleus of a number of magical rites, which in a later form are called Tantrism. The mother image was accorded great veneration since life was created in the mother's womb. The emphasis was on *shakti*—the female creative energy—as essential to any action. The *kundalini*, according to Tantra, is a type of shakti that lies dormant in the human body. Its location is generally identified as being at the base of the spine. When *kundalini* is awakened, it ascends the spinal column to the crown of the head, giving rise to mystical experiences. The arousal of the *kundalini* is a process of purification that culminates in the ecstatic union of finite existence (*samsara*) with unconditional reality (*nirvana*). The *Hatha Yoga Pradipika* describes techniques for the arousal of *kundalini* energy. Two other texts devoted in their entirety to the awakening of *kundalini* are the *Satchakranirupana* (description of the six centers) and *Padukapanchaka* (fivefold footstool). These texts comprise *Kundalini Yoga*. In recent years, the *kundalini*, or serpent power, has attracted the attention of those interested in a unified planetary consciousness as well as the next step in the evolution of the human being (Ring, 1982).

THE YOGA OF PATANJALI

Before discussing Kundalini Yoga in greater detail, it would be instructive to delineate the eight limbs of Patanjali's Ashtanga Yoga.

1. *Yama* (moral commandments)
2. *Niyama* (self-purification)
3. *Asana* (posture)
4. *Pranayama* (rhythmic breath control)
5. *Pratyahara* (sense withdrawal)
6. *Dharana* (concentration)
7. *Dhyana* (meditation)
8. *Samadhi* (higher unitive consciousness)

Usually, the entire eightfold path is referred to as Raja Yoga; however, it is also common to refer to the first four steps as Hatha Yoga and the last four, which focus more on the mental realm, as Raja Yoga. Patanjali's system is pragmatic in that he includes a detailed discipline of external behavior in his attempts to take advantage of all available means to promote growth. *Yama* and *niyama* control the yogi's passions. *Asanas* keep the body and glands healthy and harmonious. These initial three phases are *bahiranga sadhana*, the outer quest. The next two stages, *pranayama* and *pratyahara*, teach the yogi to regulate the breathing and thereby control the mind. These two stages are known as *antaranga sadhana*, the inner quest.

With the completion of the aforementioned stages, the more gross aspects of one's being have been brought under control; behavior, body, energy, and senses have been mastered. The final phase of the work is achieved in three steps comprised of *dharana, dhyana,* and *samadhi.* This phase is referred to as *antaratma sadhana,* the quest of the soul.

KUNDALINI YOGA

I have already made a brief reference to the yoga of *kundalini shakti.* This yoga is effected by a process known as *Satchakrabheda,* the piercing of the Six Centers (*chakras*) or Lotuses (*padma*) of the body by *kundalini shakti,* which is often referred to as the Serpent since one of its names is *bhujangi,* or serpent. The term *"kundala"* means a coil or a bangle. *Kundalini shakti* is spoken of as a serpent because, like a snake, it lies coiled when at rest. References to *kundalini* are found in the *Upanishads,* but it is only with the advent of Tantrism in the 5th century that Kundalini Yoga gained an impetus as a means for attaining unitive consciousness.

A description of the *chakras* (literally, wheels), which are localized vortices of bioenergy situated along the vertebral column, is essential to an understanding of the operation of *kundalini.* There are points of convergence between Western anatomy and physiology and the Tantric nervous system. Nevertheless, there are aspects peculiar to Tantric occultism (Avalon, 1974). Writers of the yogic school use the term *"nadi"* for nerves. However, the *Yoga Nadis* are not ordinary nerves but subtler lines of direction along which the vital forces run. As in Western anatomy, the Tantric school divides the vertebral column into five regions: the coccygeal, sacral, lumbar, dorsal, and cervical. The spinal cord shows different characteristics in the five different regions. These five regions roughly correspond to the regions assigned to the governing control of the five lower *chakras,* namely, *muladhara, svahisthana, manipuara, anahata,* and *visuddha.* The vital force, *pranik,* is transmitted through the *nadis,* which are said to number in the thousands. According to Kundalini Yoga, it is only the grosser *nadis,* such as the physical nerves, arteries, and veins, that are known to modern medical science. Most of the *nadis* are invisible and exist in subtle forms serving as conduits for *prana* (also called *pranik,* the vital force). The yogic practice of *pranayama* (breath control) is said to purify the *nadis.* There are 14 principal *nadis,* of which the most important are *Ida, Pingala,* and *Susumna.* The *Susumna* is situated within the *merudanda,* or spinal column, and extends from the lowest *chakra* (i.e., the plexus *muladhara*) to the *Sahasrara Padma,* or thousand-petalled lotus at the crown of the head. The thousand energy pathways of this center are representative of the experience of overwhelming light and bliss that results when *kundalini* ascends through the *Susumna.*

The two outer *nadis,* the *Ida* (also known as *Sasi,* or Moon) and *Pingala* (also known as *Mihira,* or Sun), are thought to embody heating and cooling functions and are related to the left and right nostrils through which the yogi practices *pranayama.* The lowest *chakra,* the *muladhara,* is the meeting place of the three *nadis.* The distinction between the heating and cooling functions, the hot "Sun" and the cool "Moon," reflects positive and negative energy forces in the universe. In this view, *Ida* is the conduit of the lunar current, and *Pingala* is the conduit of the solar current.

The first center, *Muladhara Chakra,* lies midway between the genitals and the anus. It is regarded as associated with the earth element and the general distribution of *prana* in the body. The reader must bear in mind that the *chakra* is not meant to be present in the gross body at the place described, rather it is the subtle center of the gross region. The *Muladhara Chakra* or *Padma* (lotus) is described as having four petals. The *Svadhisthana Chakra* is the second lotus proceeding upward and has six petals. This *chakra* is located in the genital area. It is associated with the water element and sexuality (Sannella, 1987). The third *chakra, Manipura,* is located at the center of the navel and is a lotus of 10 petals. This and the other lotuses hang downward except when *kundalini* passes through as they turn upward. The *Anahata Chakra,* the fourth center, is located at the heart. The third and fourth *chakras* are associated with the fire and air elements or digestion and feelings. At the base of the throat is situated the *Visuddha Chakra,* which has 16 petals.

The *Ajna Chakra* is the first of the higher centers. It is located between the eyebrows and is commonly regarded as the "third eye" or the locus of the mind. It is also considered the seat of extrasensory powers. The final center in this sequence is *Sahasrara Chakra,* the thousand-petalled lotus at the top of the brain. It is often identified with the pineal gland. When *kundalini* reaches this center, the yogi attains the state of pure consciousness. This center is also regarded as the seat of *Shiva* and *Shakti,* the static (masculine) and dynamic (feminine) aspects of Reality, respectively.

How is *kundalini* aroused? What does this awakening hold? Knowledge of the human transmutative process was not confined to Hindu India. It was an essential part of the esoteric teachings of Tibetan Buddhism, Chinese Taoism, and the spirituality of certain American Indian tribes as well as the Bushmen of Africa. It was, however, only in Hindu India, of which Patanjali's *Yoga Sutras* represent the apogee, that the process was most carefully studied, dissected, and elaborated. Consequently, the awakening of the psychospiritual transmutative process is best understood in the light of the *kundalini-bodhana,* the awakening of the *kundalini.*

The awakening of the *kundalini* heralds one's entry into unknown dimensions of human existence. As Jung (1932) stated, "When you succeed in awakening the *kundalini,* so that it starts to move out of its mere potentiality, you necessarily start a world which is totally different from our world" (p. 110). The arousal of *kundalini* is a mighty process of purification. The Sanskrit scriptures mention that in its ascent *kundalini* encounters and "burns off" various kinds of impurities. There are three major blockages that *kundalini* pierces. They are located at the lowest center, the *Muladhara Chakra,* the heart center of *Anahata Chakra,* and the *Ajna Chakra,* located between the eyebrows. These blockages may be viewed as stress points.

> Thus, in its ascent, the *kundalini* causes the central nervous system to throw off stress. This is usually associated with the experience of pain. When the *kundalini* encounters these blocks, it works away at them until they are dissolved. This best demonstrates the self-directing behavior of the aroused *kundalini.* It appears to act of its own volition, spreading through the entire psychophysiological system to effect its transformation. (Sannella, 1987, p. 31)

When the blockage is dissipated, there is free flow of *kundalini shakti.*

Signs of *Kundalini* Arousal

It is useful to classify the signs and symptoms of the awakening of *kundalini* into four basic categories: motor, sensory, interpretive, and nonphysiological (Sannella, 1987). The automatic body motor movements are known to yoga as *kriyas* (spontaneous actions). These movements, which may be spasmodic or smooth, range from mere muscle twitching to prolonged trembling. Unusual breathing patterns (e.g., rapid or shallow breathing, breath retention, etc.) are also epiphenomena that accompany the *kundalini-bodhana.*

The sensory accompaniments of *kundalini* awakening are best described by Sannella (1987):

> The skin or the inside of the body may tingle, tickle, itch, or vibrate. Apt descriptions are a deep ecstatic tingle and orgasmic feelings. These sensations often start in the feet and legs or the pelvis and move up the back to the neck and the crown of the head and then down to the forehead, the face, the throat and the abdomen, where they terminate. (p. 95)

Extreme temperature changes, usually in the direction of extreme heat, occur frequently. Photistic (light) experiences are quite common.

Sometimes these lights illuminate specific areas of the body such as the inside of the skull. Tonal experiences consisting of internally heard sounds such as hissing and roaring are frequently reported in accounts of *kundalini* awakening. The *Yoga Sutras* refer to these sounds as *nada,* or the mystical sound *Om.* "Some of the effects of the *kundalini* event are as obvious to the subject as running into a wall. Pain is one of these" (Wolfe, 1978, p. 36). The pain is mostly centered around the head, the nape of the neck, and the spine. It is said to occur when *kundalini* encounters a blockage. McCleave (1978) has given a detailed account of headaches associated with *kundalini:* "Migraine may be a precursor to *kundalini* activity or an associated ailment. Cluster headaches, a form of particularly harsh headache that generally strikes males, might be explained by the cyclic nature of *kundalini"* (pp. 23–24).

The interpretive phenomena are mental processes that explain the event. They consist of extreme emotion such as joy or anxiety, trance states, feelings of alienation, distorted thinking, an active fantasy life, and so forth. The *kundalini* process, it seems, stirs up the unconscious, especially those elements an individual deeply longs to repress. Dissociation and a sense of detachment wherein the individual feels a spectator of his or her own thoughts, feelings, and sensations occur because of the ego's withdrawal from identification with active mental processes. There is also the danger that the individual undergoing the *kundalini* process may become egotistically identified with the transformation believing that he or she has been divinely chosen for some great mission.

A signal interpretive phenomenon is single seeing, best described by Swami Muktananda (1974): "My eyes gradually rolled up and became centered on the *akasha* (space) or *sahasrara* (crown of the head). . . . Now instead of seeing separately, they saw as one" (p. 132). The one-eyed Cyclops of Greek mythology may well exemplify this phenomenon. According to E. A. S. Butterworth (1970):

> I know of no possible explanation of the "eye" in the forehead of the Cyclops if it is not the *Ajna-chakra* of a form of yoga. Odysseus, as I suggest, in grinding out the "third eye," shows, in our *Odyssey,* his antagonism to any such view of man. (p. 175)

Alyce Green (1975) reports that her biofeedback subjects saw an inner vision of a single eye during deep relaxation.

The nonphysiological phenomena include out-of-body experiences (OBEs), which have been elegantly described by Kenneth Ring (1982). According to Ring, his subjects, who had survived a near-death experience (NDE), reported that they had visually clear OBEs. At the most minimal level, Ring's respondents reported either no sense of bodily connection or no awareness of the body. Some were aware of the body moving in some undefined nonphysical realm. Most commonly, an individual with an OBE would report that he or she was aware of seeing the body as though viewing it from outside. Elsewhere, Ring (1984) states that the NDE has little to do with death itself, but the experience of coming close to death triggers the transmutative process of *kundalini*. In this sense, the transformatory effects of the NDE are but the transformatory effects of *kundalini*.

It would be instructive to conclude this discussion of Kundalini Yoga by describing some *kundalini* experiences. Sannella (1987) describes the phenomena experienced by the 19th-century Carmelite nun St. Therese of Lisieux as a case of spontaneous *kundalini* awakening. Therese, a novice at a Carmelite convent, developed constant headaches when 10 years old:

> One evening, while preparing for bed, she began to shiver uncontrollably. These spells continued for a week and were uninfluenced by any treatment. The shivering was not accompanied by fever, and it disappeared as mysteriously as it had come. A few weeks later, however, she was stricken with a "strange melange of hallucinations, comas and convulsions." She appeared to be in delirium, crying out against unseen and terrifying creatures. She tossed violently in bed, hitting her head on the bedboards as if some strange force were assailing her. These "convulsions," which sometimes resembled the contortions of a gymnast, were occasionally so violent that she would be thrown out of bed. There were rotary or tumbling movements of her whole body that were quite beyond her normal flexibility. . . . St. Therese was attended regularly by a competent physician who was unable to help her and frankly admitted to being confused by her symptoms. He was, however, firm in his opinion that it was not hysteria. (pp. 39–40)

In retrospect, adds Sannella (1987), St. Therese's experiences are the symptoms of spontaneous *kundalini* arousal.

The case of St. Therese shows that *kundalini* phenomena are crosscultural. Underhill (1961), in her celebrated study of mysticism, has described the awakening of Richard Rolle of Hampole, the father of English mysticism. The heat experience of *kundalini* awakening is also commented upon in Sufi literature. Baneky Behari (1971) cites from Sufi sources:

> By troth I see, as the physician tries to touch my hand, his hand is burnt and patches and swellings immediately appear on it. Such is the heat of the

fire of separation. He alone knoweth my condition who hath endured such pain cheerfully when it fell to his lot. (p. 182)

The experience of light is beautifully described by Gopi Krishna (1971):

Whenever I turned my mental eye upon myself I invariably perceived a luminous glow within and outside my head in a state of constant vibration, as if a jet of an extremely subtle and brilliant substance rising through the spine spread itself out in the cranium, filling and surrounding it with an indescribable radiance. (p. 87)

An engaging account of the awakening of *kundalini* is provided by Mary Lutyens (1975) in her description of the "process" the celebrated Indian sage Jiddu Krishnamurti underwent in 1922–23 in Ojai, California:

Every evening about 6:30 to 8, Krishna has gone into a state of semi-consciousness when the ego seems to leave and the physical elemental is allowed enough consciousness to suffer, to talk and even transmit intelligently any piece of information that may be necessary. He complains of agonizing pain while he is in this state, centering mostly in the spine; so we have surmised that his *kundalini* is being awakened. (pp. 179–180)

Lutyens then goes on to describe the climax of the process by quoting from a letter Krishnamurti wrote to Lady Emily Lutyens, wife of New Delhi's architect:

Don't worry about me, because I think, this all has been arranged, so that I could go through it by myself. Probably the feminine influence was not wanted and They took care that I should not have it. Last 10 days, it has been really strenuous, my spine and neck have been going very strong and day before yesterday, the 27th, (February, 1923) I had an extraordinary evening. Whatever it is, the force or whatever one calls the bally thing, came up my spine, up to the nape of my neck, then it separated into two, one going to the right and the other to the left of my head till they met between the two eyes, just above my nose. There was a kind of flame and I saw the Lord and the Master. It was a tremendous night. Of course, the whole thing was painful in the extreme. (p. 202)

Once underway, the *kundalini* process may take years to reach its culmination. Krishnamurti's process was going on still in 1948.

Krishnaji had been suffering excruciating pain in his head and neck, his stomach was swollen, tears streamed down his face. He suddenly fell back on the bed and became intensely still. The traces of pain and fatigue were wiped away, as happens in death. Then life and an immensity began to enter the face. The face was greatly beautiful. It had no age, time had not touched it. . . . The body radiated light; a stillness and a vastness illumined the face. . . . After some time he saw us and said, "Did you see that face?" He did not expect an answer. He lay silently. Then, "The Buddha was here, you are blessed." (Jayakar, 1986, p. 129)

Years later, in 1961, the process was still going on. "The whole process has been going on all day—the pressure, the strain and the pain at the back of the head; woke up shouting several times, and even during the day there was involuntary groaning and shouting" (Krishnamurti, 1976, p. 23).

It reached its culmination in early 1980. Referring to himself in the third person, Krishnamurti writes:

All the time that K was in India until the end of January 1980 every night he would wake up with this sense of the absolute. . . . The whole universe is in it, measureless to man. When he returned to Ojai in February, 1980, after the body had somewhat rested, there was the perception that there was nothing beyond this. This is the ultimate, the beginning and the ending and the absolute . . . . The movement had reached the source of all energy. (Lutyens, 1983, pp. 237–238)

A case of *kundalini* awakening in America is described by Thomas Wolfe (1978). Wolfe practiced both *kundalini* meditation and biofeedback.

I was startled by a forceful thrusting and thumping about in my lower back, the Kanda region of classical *Kundalini* lore. . . . Soon my stomach got very hot and I began to sweat . . . a relentless heat—conflagration—had begun to move slowly over the surface of my entire head. (pp. 111–114)

Kundalini and Evolution

Ring (1984) has stated his belief that the NDE is but a reliable trigger for awakening the *kundalini*. Certainly, there are striking parallels between phenomena described by near-death experiencers and those that accompany the rising *kundalini*.

What then is the significance of the *kundalini*? Ring, like Gopi Krishna (1971), believes that *kundalini* is the mechanism that propels humanity's evolution. He states that the goal of the *kundalini*-mediated evolutionary process is to carry humankind toward a higher dimension of consciousness. The arousal of *kundalini* leads to a figurative death, an ego death that involves the transformation of the nervous system and the experience of divinity. To use St. Paul's phrase, the "old Adam" dies and a new cosmically conscious person is reborn. The activation of latent spiritual potentials by a *kundalini*-mediated transformation of the nervous system generates a new human being characterized by a noetic understanding of the universe.

Bentov (1977) has proposed a convincing but as yet unverified model of how the *kundalini* transformation occurs. According to Bentov (1977) and Motoyama (1981), the heart-aorta system produces an oscillation of about 7 Hz in the skeleton. The skull accelerates the brain up and down, producing acoustical plane waves reverberating through the brain at KHz frequencies. These acoustical plane waves are focused by the skull onto the ventricles, thus activating and driving standing waves within the third and lateral ventricles. Standing waves within the cerebral ventricles in the audio and supersonic ranges stimulate the sensory cortex mechanically, resulting in a stimulus traveling in a closed loop around each hemisphere. Such a traveling stimulus may be viewed as a current. As a result of these circular currents, each hemisphere produces a pulsating magnetic field; the two fields are of opposing polarities. This magnetic field, radiated by the head acting as an antenna, interacts with the electric and magnetic fields already in the environment. The head may be regarded then as simultaneously a transmitting and receiving antenna tuned to a particular one of several resonant frequencies of the brain. The resonant frequency of the brain would be modulated by environmental fields that would be fed back to the brain (Sannella, 1987). This, then, is a tentative model for the evolutionary transmutation of the nervous system.

Like Ring's near-death experiencers, those who have undergone the *kundalini*-mediated transformation show evidence of paranormal abilities (e.g., clairvoyance, telepathy, precognition, etc.). The awakening bestows not only psychic abilities but is also the fountainhead of creativity, genius, and compassion. Gopi Krishna, Muktananda, and others have remarked on the spiritual concomitants of the awakening: selflessness, compassion, absence of duality, loss of fear of death, and an indifference to material possessions. The many contemporary accounts of *kundalini* experiences seem to suggest that humanity is perhaps well on its way toward the next step in evolution.

THE YOGIC THEORY OF PERSONALITY

In yoga psychology, personality is a multilevel construct. The physical aspects of personality (*annamaya*) consist of the organism comprised of the vital organs, the glands, the brain, the nervous system, and the musculoskeletal system. The instinctual aspect (*pranayama*) consists of the various drives such as sex, hunger, thirst, and so forth. The mental aspect (*manomaya*) includes perception, memory, and sensation as well as clairvoyance and other such psychic abilities. The rational aspect of personality (*vijnanamaya*) is comprised of intellectual functions such as judgment, discrimination, and evaluation. The rational mind is also known as *buddhi.* Yoga psychology admits of an unconscious mind (*citta*) that is the repository of creativity, imagination, and the residual impressions of past experiences. The latter, in turn, give rise to dispositional tendencies known in yoga as the *samskaras.* The functioning of the personal ego is called *ahamkara.*

The Mind in Yoga

The mind is regarded as the "internal instrument." It has three main functions. First, the lower mind collects incoming sense impressions and coordinates them with motor responses. Because of being bombarded with numerous stimuli, this aspect of the mind is considered to be in constant flux. The lower mind, called *manas,* also registers memory traces.

The second function, *Ahamkara* (the ego function or I-ness), transforms the sensory impressions into a personal experience by relating them to one's individual identity (Rama, 1976). *Ahamkara* takes what comes in and relates it subjectively to a sense of I-ness. "When the sensory-motor mind functions, 'a rose is seen.' But when *ahamkara* adds its influence, 'I see a rose'" (Rama, 1976, p. 70).

The third major function of the mind is judgment. This function pertains to the evaluation of the situation and choosing a course of action. This is the function of *buddhi,* which is often referred to as the crown jewel of discrimination. The interplay between these three aspects of the mind produces normal, waking consciousness. Above these structures there is a suprasensory and supraintellectual level of personality that consists of pure spiritual intuition. This state is transcendental or fourth-dimensional consciousness and is called *turiya. Turiya* is unclouded cognition of the nontemporal Being. The individual, in the course of his or her personality growth through yoga and meditation, eventually attains this level of Being—a level of cognition when all the modifications of the psyche (*citta vritti*) are completely restrained or hushed into silence (Taimni, 1961).

According to Chaudhuri (1975), the development of personality from infancy to adulthood is characterized by the emergence of different aspects of the self. The infant identifies with the body even as he or she achieves object constancy. This is the material self or *anamaya purusha*. During the next stage of development, there is the identification with passions, impulses, and desires. This is the vital self or *pranamaya purusha*. The identification with one's mental nature as a sentient being is called *manomaya purusha*. It is also described as the aesthetic part of the personality. Next, the individual begins to perceive of himself or herself as a thinking, choosing, and deliberating being, the *vijnanamaya purusha*. The final stage of growth is a bold meditative breakthrough in consciousness leading to the discovery of the transcendental level of existence and the true self, *anandamaya purusha*.

In contemporary Western schools of psychology, especially in psychoanalytic circles, there is little hope of the human being ever being able to reach even an elementary consciousness of the self since, however much we may make conscious, there will always exist an indeterminate amount of unconscious material that belongs to the totality of the self. Full self-realization, therefore, is a never-to-be-attained ideal. Consequently, Western psychology contends that human sorrow can never be totally eliminated. For example, Jung (1969) believed that a turn away from the ego and toward the self would be a psychic catastrophe. The Western mind has viewed such a possibility as a threat of ego annihilation and of extinction of personal consciousness and has elected to stay identified with the subject-object mode of consciousness, thus keeping the transcendent consciousness as an object at a distance.

The aim of yoga psychology is to fully experience the Self, which is the center of pure consciousness. In this view, the assimilation of the ego by the Self, rather than being a psychic catastrophe, leads to a state of illumination.

To Western psychology, only the waking state is real. Yoga psychology, on the other hand, views the dream state and the stage of deep sleep as modes of consciousness just as valid or invalid, real or unreal, as the waking state. There are yogic methods for achieving a correlation between these different states, and the yogi who has attained to such a correlation is able to view dispassionately the different states of consciousness and attains to a fourth state of consciousness (*turiya*) that is realization of the real Self (Ajaya, 1983). The Self is variously called the *Purusha, Brahman, Atman,* or *Jiva* by different Hindu philosophical schools.

Mention must be made of two other structures that support and relate to *manas,* the mind. *Citta* (also *chitta*) has already been mentioned. It lies chiefly outside the sphere of awareness and, therefore, is the unconscious aspect of *manas.* It is also the memory bank and the storehouse of impressions, experience, memories, and repressed affect. According to

Swami Rama (1976), it is from *citta* that memories bubble up to appear on the screen of the lower mind. The mind in yoga is likened to a clear pool of water. Like a calm lake, it is lucid and clear until stirred up by mental modifications called *vrittis*. These are likened to the waves on a calm lake. *Vrittis* may arise due to sense impressions or from latent memory traces and may best be described as "thoughts." Patanjali, however, includes fantasies, perceptions, and the early stages of sleep in his description of the *vrittis*. His Ashtanga Yoga is a method of disentangling oneself from the *vrittis* and attaining to objective consciousness.

Mental Operations

The lower or sensorimotor mind merely collects information. It acts as a collecting device without the ability to evaluate the input (Rama, 1976). Judgment, evaluation, and discrimination are beyond the abilities of *manas*, the lower mind. It is *buddhi* that arrives at the proper decision.

> Such things as planning, desiring, memory, affection, gratitude, sexual impulses, shame, fear, love, attachment, hate, jealousy, anger and so forth are all phenomena which are properties of the lower mind. One is prompted to a particular act when a certain mental impulse springs onto the screen of *manas*. But it is *buddhi* which decides whether or not to give in to the impulse. (Rama, 1976, p. 78)

Manas, it has often been said, is a doubting faculty since it doubts the validity of every piece of information it receives. If *buddhi* is weak and not properly evolved, then one becomes a victim of impulses, circumstances, and sentimental reactions.

When *manas* is not actively receiving sense input, it is open to internal input from *citta*, which is the bed of the mental stream in which the mind operates. *Citta* is the unconscious of yoga psychology, although Patanjali himself uses the term somewhat loosely to include all mental functioning.

> In part it acts as a passive reservoir, receiving and storing impressions from all the impacts the world offers. Even before the more advanced, conscious aspects of the mind come into being, *chitta* is accumulating, like an immense lake bed, a huge pool of sensory impressions and data. All of the mind, *buddhi*, the capacity for decisions, *ahankara*, the sense of I-ness or identity and even *manas*, the sensory-motor mind, arise out of this basic consciousness called *chitta*. (Rama, 1976, p. 81)

Citta reacts to outside influences by resurrecting primitive urges or instinctual reactions like the id of Freudian psychology. When *citta* is not actively responding to outside stimuli, then it passively allows bubbles of memories, fantasies, and impressions to surface to the mind. To allow the yogi to observe his or her inner mental contents, Patanjali urges a voluntary sensory deprivation, which he calls *pratyahara* or sense withdrawal. It is in this context of reducing or filtering external sensory input that seeking a quiet place, closing one's eyes, and other such techniques are relevant. Thus, in the quiet, sense-deprived state of meditation, the unconscious slowly discloses its contents. This process has much in common with the analyst's couch where gazing at a blank ceiling and free associating serve to enable the unconscious to yield its treasures.

While this process is occurring, *ahamkara*, the sense of I-ness, appropriates aspects of the experiential field as "me" and "mine," thus successfully creating the subject-object split. In its rudimentary aspect, *ahamkara* maintains the integrity of the organism; in the infant, it helps individuation and makes survival possible. Later, it lends identity, stability, and continuity to the organism.

Like *ahamkara*, *buddhi* also develops in stages. In its rudimentary aspect, it acts as an organ of crude, perceptive discrimination. Subject to memories and emotions, it reacts by deciding that something is good or bad. At the next stage of development, *buddhi* is more mature and pragmatic, using reasoning to arrive at a purposeful and rational organization of actions. At its highest stage of development, *buddhi* concerns itself with a disinterested search for the pure Self (Aurobindo, 1971). In this aspect, *buddhi* reflects the transcendental laws of the universe and is in harmony with the unifying principles underlying sentient life. According to Aurobindo (1971), *buddhi* evolves gradually. But, according to Patanjali, *buddhi* is to be uncovered. It is a brilliant jewel, waiting to be cut and polished to reveal its true nature. *Buddhi* can either succumb to past impressions, habits, and emotions or can distance itself from the influence of memory traces and, by overcoming past programming, step outside the chain of causality. If *buddhi* succumbs to the influence of emotion and impulse, then evolution is halted. But if *buddhi* extricates itself from past programming, the evolutionary march continues.

> As *buddhi* becomes more evolved, it increasingly separates itself from the activities of *manas*. As it develops its capacity for making decisions that disregard the impulses and impressions flowing through *manas*, it becomes increasingly independent of them. As a result, a level of I-ness evolves from which one can witness mental events without being involved in them. Eventually there emerges a kind of vantage point which exists above and beyond the hectic activity of the train of thoughts. This provides a point of observation, then, from which the mental plane can be seen. (Rama, 1976, pp. 97–98)

This realm of pure, shining *buddhi* is *turiya*—the fourth level of consciousness—which is beyond the body and the mind. This is the stage of pure reason or intuition that is beyond the verbal, mental activity of the mind. The stages beyond *buddhi* are the purely reflective states attained in the higher stages of meditation. The lower of these stages gives rise to a global witness consciousness, which is pure Awareness. The final stage occurs when even a global awareness of the phenomenal world completely ceases, yielding to pure Consciousness without the contamination of objects. This is the realm of the Self (not to be identified with the ego-self of Western psychology) or *Purusha.* The practice of yoga is geared toward evolving to the realm of the Self that lies beyond the ordinary mental planes of conscious activity.

Memory

According to yoga psychology, past experiences leave memory traces, impressions, and images in the *manas* or lower mind. These traces are called *samskaras.* The *samskaras* bubble up to the surface of *manas* where they undergo a sort of filtration. The *samskaras* that result from experiences that have survival value and the ones that have made a vivid impression are easily accessed and recalled. On the other hand, painful experiences that are likely to contaminate the affective tone of the individual, if resurrected, are repressed. "This selection-rejection functioning of memory (*smriti*) is evidence of its origination from *maya,* the principle responsible for the practically useful mode of living" (Chaudhuri, 1975, p. 249).

In the higher reaches of meditation, there is said to occur a vast expansion of memory; thus, in the trance states before attaining *samadhi* (unitive consciousness), the individual would experience not only his or her immediate past but also previous lives. Such a recall, survey, and ultimate integration of the past are regarded as intrinsic to the process of self-realization.

LEARNING AND MOTIVATION IN YOGA PSYCHOLOGY

The yogic theory of learning rejects the notion of the individual as a stimulus-response organism. Yoga psychology concedes that in early childhood some sociocultural conditioning is necessary for the acquisition of survival skills as well as the dominant social mores. The individual also absorbs the cultural heritage of his or her society through social learning. Such learning includes knowledge of ethical norms, aesthetic forms, the spiritual aspirations considered as intrinsically worthwhile, and so forth. This knowledge is referred to as social law (*samaj dharma*).

Imitational learning is also involved in the development of *swadharma*, which is the law of caste roles. This knowledge involves an understanding of one's social position, caste role, and the rights and responsibilities that such a role implies (Chaudhuri, 1975).

In the early stages of individual development, yoga psychology stresses appreciation of the three basic tenets of life: law and order (*dharma*), wealth (*artha*), and biological drives such as hunger, thirst, and sex (*kama*). When these three values are satisfied, yoga stresses a fourth—self-realization (*moksha*).

The learning characterized in the fourth stage is a form of mastery learning under the tutelage of a guru (teacher). Chaudhuri (1975) eloquently captures the spirit of such learning:

> A mature spiritual guide (guru) sees to it that the disciple does not become emotionally fixated upon him. His main job is to help the disciple to discover the divine guru within the disciple's own unconscious psyche. As soon as the disciple learns to stand on his own feet, capable of treading the right path leading to the ultimate goal, the guru gracefully parts company, liberating the disciple from his last emotional bonds. (p. 254)

Chaudhuri (1975) recognizes the dangers of such a mode of learning. Guru-realization can substitute for self-realization in that an immature guru might unconsciously act in ways to keep his or her disciples under his or her hypnotic sway.

The process of learning reaches its culmination in the realization of the true Self. With enlightenment, the individual becomes a luminous center of Being (*lila sathi*)—a joyful avenue of manifestation of such values as peace, love, compassion, and creativity. After such a transmutation, the individual transcends conventional social morality and religious injunctions but nevertheless participates in the social process as a unique center of higher values.

> He is no more under any obligation or compulsion to act and serve in society. He is liberated from the conventional moral distinctions of good and evil, right and wrong. He sees through the relativity of all socioethical norms. In consequence, he perceives the game-character (*lila*-ness) of all life. But out of the fullness of his freedom and the spontaneity of his creative joy he participates in society and in world affairs with a view to playing his own distinctive role, however small, in the unfolding drama of human society, regardless of profit and loss, praise and blame, approbation

or vilification. His own true Self becomes his ultimate guru. (Chaudhuri, 1975, p. 255)

Yoga admits of three kinds of motivation: instinctive, cultural, and the spiritual or onto-aesthetic. Instinctual motives are classified as *rajas, tamas,* and *sattva.* The drive to overpower or dominate and the aggressive drive are called *rajasic.* The preoccupation with personal safety and security and the fear of bodily harm and death stem from the self-protective motive, the *tamasic.* The search for truth, freedom, and justice, and the altruistic impulse are the self-transcending motives, or *sattvic.*

Motives anchored in the dominant culture form the class of cultural motives. These include religiocultural ideas such as notions of good and evil, heaven and earth, and ethical injunctions. Choosing a particular profession, fighting for one's country, engaging in penances and ritualism are motives rooted in one's culture. Both instinctual and cultural motivations are bound to *samsara,* the wheel of life and death, since they are rooted in *maya* or illusion. When the individual transcends both instinctual and cultural motivations, he or she is propelled on the path of the egoless motive of self-realization. With *moksha* or liberation, the instinctual and cultural motives are reduced to cinder.

Liberated yogis return to the whirl of social action to dissipate their past *karma.* Such individuals are no longer interested in an emotional involvement with the world. Their motive is often described as the *lila* motivation of divine play, or onto-aesthetic motivation. This is best summed up by the immortal phrase, "I act, yet it is not I but Being that acts through me." It is this being motivation of the awakened person.

VARIETIES OF THE YOGIC EXPERIENCE

Chaudhuri (1975) has delineated several clearly distinguishable yogic experiences. In the initial stages of meditation, the individual is likely to encounter his or her identity as a stream of cognitions, emotions, and conative urges. This is the empirical self (*manomaya purusha*) that is subject to disturbance. As meditation proceeds, the meditator suddenly finds himself or herself as a witness to the stream of consciousness. He or she is the witness-consciousness (*saksi*), and this is the experience of *savikalpa samadhi.* In the next stage, the subject-object dichotomy disappears. The witness and the field of observation dissolve, and the Self is revealed as pure formless consciousness. This is the experience of *nirvikalpa samadhi.*

In the *Bhakti Yoga* (yoga of devotion) tradition, the repetition and remembrance of the Divine Name lead to a rapturous communion with the creative ground of existence. When this experience is intensified, the yogi experiences himself or herself within all things and beings in the world. Within the same Bhakti Yoga tradition, a further intensification of consciousness results in the mystic experience of Being as an eternal Thou. Being is perceived as the Divine Mother, the Beloved, or even an eternal child. Being may also be regarded as the Divine Lover with whom a mystic marriage is possible.

As the *kundalini shakti* reaches the crown *chakra,* Being-energy may be experienced as the dance of the goddess of destruction, *Kali,* bent on burning up the impurities of the organism. As the complex dance cleanses the nervous system, the yogi may experience the mystic fire, *Agni.*

In the Jnana Yoga tradition, the ultimate mystic experience is termed *Sat-Chit-Ananda,* Being-Consciousness-Bliss. This is the experience of Godhead as the indeterminable nontemporal ground of all determinate forms of existence. Another experience is the experience of Being as the Void. The ultimate substrate of the universe is experienced as absolute emptiness without determinants (*sunyata*). And in Kundalini Yoga the mystic experience is charged with coiled energy, and Being is experienced as *Shiva-Shakti* or Being-Energy.

It is appropriate now to turn to the many hazards that await the yogi embarked on the path of self-transcendence.

DANGERS ON THE YOGIC PATH

The foremost danger is that of an unhealthy introversion. As the meditator discovers the inner wellsprings of joy, there may occur a powerful urge to withdraw from society and lead a solitary asocial existence. Both meditation and the routine of life in an *ashram* (religious retreat) under the guidance of a guru may prompt regression to infantile modes of behaving, feeling, and thinking.

Such a regression may be reinforced by emotional fixation on the guru. The guru has the power to awaken the latent Being-energy of the disciple. With this power comes the danger of the disciple becoming dependent on the powerful, charismatic personality of the guru.

Still another unhealthy by-product of the yogic path is its lack of recognition of the roles of sex, the intellect, and the ego in healthy personality development. Yoga psychology sees these three components as excess baggage on the journey of enlightenment. Many gurus, consequently, have a pronounced negative attitude toward normal urges.

Thus, practices aimed at suppressing and controlling these functions abound in yoga. These may result in neurotic conditions when the spiritual quest goes awry.

The final danger on the path is spiritual hedonism. The *Samkhya* and *Vedantic* doctrines about the nonspirituality and unreality of the world provide ready rationalizations for those gurus who withdraw into the reclusive life of the Self. There can then occur a neurotic preoccupation with mystic bliss as the ultimate goal of life, the ultimate trip as it were. Such individuals may evidence a lofty disdain for urgent social concerns.

YOGA AND PSYCHOTHERAPY

It must be apparent to the reader by now that yoga is no mere mystical discipline, rather it is a supremely elegant system designed to promote optimal psychological and physical functioning. As such, it resembles what in the West is called "psychotherapy." Both psychotherapy and yoga are aimed at changing people's feelings about themselves; both alleviate anxiety and foster a measure of self-control and poise. But while the goals of most Western schools of psychotherapy are narrow—namely, to help the individual adjust to society—the goal of yoga is more radical: it is the maximization of joy and the complete unfolding of the human potential. The conventional therapist is often aligned with conventional social norms and interprets his or her work as "adjusting the individual and coaxing his unconscious drives into social respectability" (Watts, 1961, p. 20). The guru, on the other hand, fosters a radical transmutation of the psyche, a transformation that veritably heralds the birth of a new human being, altruistic, joyful, and centered in Being-consciousness. Therefore, it is not surprising that yoga techniques are increasingly being integrated into Western psychotherapy.

Psychophysiology of Yoga

Because of the rarity of the authentic mystical experience, most experimental studies of the effects of yoga draw heavily upon studies of meditation in normal subjects and yogis who may well be experiencing altered states of consciousness less profound than the highest yogic states. Nevertheless, there are areas of overlap in the accounts of mystics as well as experimental subjects: presumably the two experiences share similar characteristics.

Woolfolk (1975) has offered an excellent review of the psychophysiological effects of yogic meditation techniques. The scientific study of yoga actually began in 1935 when the French cardiologist Therese Brosse recorded the EKGs of yogis as they attempted to control their hearts. Brosse's recording of her subject, T. Krishnamacharya, showed he had been able to stop his heart completely. However, her experiment used but one electrode. When Mr. Krishnamacharya was studied again by the All-India Institute of Medical Sciences in 1961 (Wenger & Bagchi, 1961; Wenger, Bagchi, & Anand, 1961), more modern equipment was used. It was discovered that Mr. Krishnamacharya was able to "tilt" his heart in the chest cavity as a result of muscular contractions and that the change in the heart's position effectively eliminated the recording from lead 1—the lead that had been used in 1935 by Dr. Brosse. But the other electrodes continued to register the heart beat. The same experimenters also studied Ramanand Yogi, whose heart showed a cessation of pulsation under fluoroscopy when he attempted to stop it. When Ramanand Yogi was subjected to EKG studies, only a slight slowing was recorded. Based on these studies, Hoenig (1968) concluded that feats of yogic control did not appear to be promising as treatments for psychosomatic problems. On the other hand, Green (1971), in experiments with Swami Rama, showed that the swami was able to alter his EEG pattern and also create a temperature differential of 10 degrees Fahrenheit between the two sides of his palm. In another experiment at the Menninger Foundation, Swami Rama produced a state of atrial flutter during which the heart ceased to pump blood for 17 seconds.

What is one to make of these apparent conflicting results? Woolfolk's review (1975) cites several studies that attempt to reconcile the various differences. Anand, Chinna, and Singh (1961) and Wenger and Bagchi (1961) both have confirmed decreases in respiration and oxygen consumption among yogis. These researchers concluded that yogic meditation is most probably a state of deep relaxation of the autonomic nervous system. Benson, Greenwood, and Klemchuk (1975) reported decreased carbon dioxide production as well as lower blood lactate concentration in meditators. Goleman and Schwartz (1976), in their study of skin conductance and heart rate in meditators, found that in stressful situations meditation produces a psychophysiological response opposite to that seen in stress-related conditions. Banquet (1973) offered a detailed spectral analysis of EEG changes in meditation. The most pronounced finding was changes in the amplitude and frequency of alpha waves (8 to 13 Hz). Woolfolk's review (1975) concluded by suggesting that meditation seems to be associated with a slowing and increased synchronization of electrocortical rhythms and a slower rate of respiration. These changes are all in the direction of lowered arousal and suggest a diminishing of energy metabolism.

It is not surprising, therefore, to find that meditation is an excellent antidote to stress.

Yoga and the Stress Disorders

In 1969 Neal Miller convincingly demonstrated volitional control of kidney function, gastric changes, blood pressure, and so forth in experimental animals. Budzynski, Stoyva, and Adler (1970) demonstrated the relief of tension headache by use of biofeedback. Patel (1973, 1975), in a series of elegant studies done in England, reported lasting effects of biofeedback training in lower blood pressure when the biofeedback was combined with yogic practice. These results have been replicated by K. N. Udupa of the Indian Council of Medical Research. Udupa (1985) utilized the yogic practice of *Shirshasana* (a particular physical pose) to lower the blood pressure of hypertensive patients. Udupa's studies also indicate that yogic practices lead to a reduction of acetylcholine, an increase in catecholamine levels, a decrease in cholesterol, and an enhancement of endocrine functions. Udupa's work confirms the drop in blood pressure due to yogic practice found in earlier studies by Blackwell et al. (1976) and Pollock, Weber, Case, and Laragh (1977). In a similar vein, Benson, Steinart, Greenwood, Klemchuk, and Peterson (1975) confirmed the therapeutic efficiency of yogic practice in the treatment of cluster headaches. Finally, preliminary findings by Udupa (1985) suggest that yogic *asanas* may be of value in the treatment of bronchial asthma, functional cardiac disorders, and diabetes. It would be appropriate to conclude, then, that yogic practice induces a response that leads to the alleviation of major psychophysiological disorders.

Yoga and Personality Change

In one of the earliest studies of the effects of yogic practice on personality parameters, Orme-Johnson (1971) showed that the practitioners of transcendental meditation are less irritable than nonmeditators. Jung (1987) and Pazhayattil (1986) reported positive changes in self-esteem as the result of yoga practice. Nespor (1985) has successfully combined yoga with drug therapy in the treatment of chronic psychiatric patients. Cunningham (1981) presents the results of an attempt to use Kundalini Yoga with a psychiatric patient. Utilizing a meditation on the heart *chakra,* Cunningham's patient reported increased warmth and capacity for love and well-being. This study indicates that an expressive therapist may well be able to use imagery and *kundalini* arousal techniques in the healing process by assisting the patient in uncovering, releasing, and focusing the creative energy present within the individual.

A number of studies have focused on changes in body image as a result of yoga practice. As the reader can surmise, this approach has strong face validity since yoga is after all a form of body work. Engelman, Clance, and Imes (1982) showed that yoga practitioners changed significantly on self-cathexis and body cathexis. Yoga practice, which is essentially a nonverbal, intrapsychic form of therapy, was also effective in producing desired changes in feelings toward one's self and body. Clance, Mitchell, and Engelman (1980) report on increases in body cathexis and, consequently, on self-cathexis in children who practiced yoga.

The effects of yoga practice on self-concept have been investigated by several researchers. Gouger (1979) found positive changes in self-concept as a result of Hatha Yoga training in psychiatric outpatients. Rudolph (1981) founded positive changes in self-concept in female college students engaged in yoga practice. Edwards (1987) found that the practice of yoga resulted in positive changes in measures of negative personality characteristics such as depression, neuroticism, and anxiety.

These studies suggest that yoga, alone or in combination with other psychotherapeutic approaches, may play a useful role in mental health. Patanjali's Raja Yoga involves behavioral and psychophysical control, self-analysis, meditation, cognitive change, and change in consciousness. Balodhi (1986), at the National Institute of Mental Health and Neuro-Sciences in Bangalore, India, and Singh (1986), at the Benaras Hindu University, have reported on the successful use of yoga in patients hospitalized with anxiety and depression.

No investigation of yoga would be complete without a concomitant investigation of *pranayama* (breath control) and its effects. Studies in this area are sparse, however. Harrigan (1981) and Harvey (1983) studied the importance of breath in relation to achieving physiological self-control in behavioral therapies and in its relation to the emotional state in Gestalt and Reichian therapies. Subjects who learned yogic breathing exercises showed significant changes on several dimensions including increased vigor, decreased tension and fatigue, decreased depression and anxiety, and decreased frequency of somatic complaints. These results suggest that yogic breathing exercises positively affect mood and that they have clinical potential as a self-control technique for improving and stabilizing affective states.

The *Chakras* in Psychotherapy

Swami Rama (1976) has outlined the role of the *chakras* of Kundalini Yoga in psychotherapy. According to Rama, the meditation on each of the *chakras* can lead to new levels of psychosomatic integration. These syntheses are the result of an integration of two polarities, the *Ida* and the *Pingala,* or left and right aspects of the body.

Integration at the first *chakra* is the synthesis of the "good" and "bad" aspects of the self. This results in curtailment of the tendency to split off and project on to others the unacceptable aspects of oneself. The synthesis at the genital *chakra* is the reconciliation of the traits of masculinity and femininity, enabling the individual to incorporate aspects of both sexes into his or her personality. The synthesis at the navel *chakra* leads to the resolution of dominance and submission issues. The integration at the heart *chakra* confers qualities of empathy, sensitivity, and compassion. At the level of the throat *chakra,* integration leads to the ability to be creative and to re-create oneself or to grow and evolve.

The synthesis at the *ajna chakra* is considered very important. This is the integration of *ida* and *pingala* and results in the activation of *sushumna* and the third eye. The opening of the third eye confers extrasensory powers. The final synthesis at the crown *chakra* is the integration of the subject-object split and results in cosmic consciousness.

According to Rama (1976), Western psychotherapy, too, aims at raising consciousness from a lower *chakra* to a higher one, although therapy is not conceptualized in these terms. "The paranoid person is led toward contact-sensuality, ego-oriented persons toward concern for others, etc." (Rama, 1976, pp. 274–275).

Meditation on the different *chakras* may be prescribed for therapy of different disorders. According to Rama (1976), meditation on the solar plexus is effective for the relief of nightmares, meditation on the heart *chakra* helps develop emotional control, meditation on the sacral plexus helps cure psychogenic impotence and premature ejaculation, and so forth. These claims are intriguing and need further exploration.

The Yoga Therapist

The yoga therapist adopts a holistic orientation. He or she maintains an awareness of the interconnections between various facets of human functioning. The therapist helps the client become sensitive to his or her inner ecology. This may include sensitivity to breathing, diet, thought patterns, posture, areas of tension in the body, habits of relating to others and the world, and so on. The yoga therapist may include other professionals to complement his or her expertise.

Training in self-awareness and self-regulation of the body, diet, breath, habit patterns, emotions, states of mind, values, will, unconscious processes, desires, and relation to archetypal processes and to transcendent being—which are treated in isolation in various therapies—must be integrated in a truly synthetic approach to optimal functioning. If any area is left out, the therapy is incomplete. (Ajaya, 1983, p. 185)

Yoga therapy utilizes a multimodal approach. The therapist may meet clients individually or in groups; clients may include couples or families. The *ashram*, a residential retreat, serves as a form of milieu therapy that allows clients to work on inner healing for extended periods of time. While the yoga therapist might help the client resolve inner conflicts, develop ego-strength, and so on, the focus ultimately is on the spiritual concerns of the client. Consequently, yoga therapy emphasizes transcending limited identifications and cultivating awareness of the transcendent Self. These are concerns not often addressed in conventional Western therapeutic modalities.

Since yoga does not treat isolated symptoms, it breaks with the medical model. From this perspective, the yoga therapist is no expert and takes no responsibility for the patient.

The yoga therapist does not treat patients; instead he may teach, coach, guide or otherwise assist fellow players in the game of life. His method of teaching is not didactic, but consists of an ongoing dialogue with the client. He may provide guidance, but it is up to the client to practice the techniques of self-transformation. The client gradually learns to take responsibility in each aspect of his life—physical, interpersonal, mental, emotional, and spiritual. (Ajaya, 1983, p. 216)

Imitational learning, only recently studied in the West, has been of considerable importance in yoga therapy. The relationship between the guru and the disciple has always been paramount. The content of the teaching is regarded as less important than the context of the relationship in which it occurs. The guru models for the disciple the practices, behaviors, attitudes, and habits he or she wishes to inculcate in the disciple.

The use of paradoxical interventions, a recent innovation in Western psychotherapy, has always enjoyed a venerable tradition in Eastern disciplines. The Zen master uses *koans* or riddles to confound his disciples; the Hasidic and Sufi masters use wit and parable to shock their disciples into realization. This is true in yoga as well. Ajaya (1983) gives an example wherein a client, who resisted the therapist's injunctions, enjoyed relating descriptions of his inability to overcome his problems. The therapist joined with the client and began recording the client's detailed descriptions saying that he was writing a book on therapy failures and that his was an excellent case. Soon the client's complaints started diminishing, and he reported substantial improvement in his symptomatology.

The client then proceeded to give credit for his improvement to various people in his life. The therapist lamented that he was not being given enough credit and instructed the client to go around telling people how much the therapist had helped him. Soon the client started taking responsibility for the positive changes in his life.

According to yoga psychology, suffering can be a great teacher. It calls attention to areas of one's life that need attention and aspects of oneself that need to be changed. Yoga therapists, therefore, lay stress on helping their clients attend to situations that create sorrow instead of avoiding them. Pain provides a unique opportunity for growth by motivating a person to rectify imbalances within the individual and in his or her relationship to the world. This is not to say that yoga seeks out pain. The ultimate goal of yoga is to help mortals transcend the ephemeral world of sorrow. But yoga psychology holds that this cannot occur until one becomes aware of and then eliminates the cause of suffering, which is due to the identification with one's ego-self.

The Spiritual Dimension in Yoga Therapy

It must be clarified that yoga therapy is not aligned to any particular religion, god, or leader. Nevertheless, this therapeutic mode is rooted in the spiritual dimensions of life. The work on one's body-mind, on one's relationship to oneself and fellow beings, on inner conflicts, unconscious impulses, destructive habits, all have as their final culmination the realization of the Self beyond the ego-self, of the unity underlying the cosmos. While yoga may concentrate on the subject-object dimensions at first, it eventually helps the individual transcend the subject-object dichotomy.

With the ascent of the bioenergy known as *kundalini* to the fifth *chakra*, the ego-self surrenders to a universal center of love and wisdom. At the sixth *chakra*, the *ajna chakra*, there is a total detachment from individual perspective and one becomes a neutral observer of events.

And, at the seventh and final *chakra* at the crown of the head, there results a state of pure consciousness.

> The mind-created grid of time, space, and causation is transcended. All polarities are united and all forms dissolved. One awakens from the illusory world of distinctions and multiplicity. . . . At *sahasrara* there are no longer any melodramas or scenarios; even the realm of archetypes is left behind. Having reached this center, there is nothing more to be attained, nothing more to be known. One knows himself as the All in all; he realizes himself as the *atman* (Self) or unitary consciousness. (Ajaya, 1983, p. 319)

Conventional Western therapies have no inkling of the state of pure consciousness and hence offer no guidance for attaining to this mode of Being. Jungian psychology admits of the Self and regards dreams, myths, and spiritual traditions as symbolic expressions of the Self. However, even Jungian psychology offers no path to directly experience the Self, resting content to use its intimations in the service of the ego. In offering a direct, clear way to transcend the world of duality and experience pure consciousness, yoga therapy traverses far beyond the conventional practices of tinkering with one's personality with a view toward better adjustment to society. Yoga therapy, then, is both revolutionary and spiritual.

CONCLUDING REMARKS

Humankind has always had new frontiers to conquer. The famed silk route to China, the sea route to the magical Indies, the New World, the Wild West, and, more recently, outer space, have all cast their spell on the adventurous traveler. It now appears that a new frontier is emerging to beckon humanity on yet another mysterious quest. This time, however, the journey is an inner one, a compelling voyage of self-discovery and transformation that may be the boldest adventure of them all, for it may give birth to a noetic species.

The ancient science of yoga offers humanity a new vision—a being of pure consciousness in an ocean of bliss. The lower rungs of this evolutionary ladder, the first few miles of the journey, so to speak, seem akin to the approaches of Western psychology. They consist of behavioral self-adjustment, cognitive and affective changes, and peak experiences. The process brings about cleansing and healing of the organism. Such a healing is but a preparation of the organism to serve as a vehicle for the transformatory bioenergy latent within us. The adventure concludes with the birth of *Sat-Chit-Ananda*, the planetary mind that is Being-Consciousness-Bliss. Or has it only just begun?

References

Ajaya, S. (1983). *Psychotherapy east and west.* Honesdale, PA: Himalayan Institute.

Anand, B. K., Chinna, G. S., & Singh, B. (1961). Studies on Sri Ramanand Yogi during his stay in an airtight box. *Indian Journal of Medical Research, 49,* 82–89.

Aurobindo, S. (1971). *The synthesis of yoga.* Pondicherry: Sri Aurobindo Ashram.

Avalon, A. (1974). *The serpent power.* New York: Dover.

Balodhi, J. P. (1986). Perspective of Raja yoga in its application to mental health. *NIMHANS Journal, 4*(2), 133–138.

Banquet, J. P. (1973). Spectral analysis of the E.E.G. in meditation. *Electroencephalography and Clinical Neurophysiology, 35,* 143–151.

Behari, B. (1971). *Sufis, mystics and yogis of India.* Bombay: Bharatiya Vidya Bhavan.

Benson, H., Greenwood, M. M., & Klemchuk, H. (1975). The relaxation response: Psychophysiologic aspects and clinical applications. *International Journal of Psychiatry in Medicine, 6,* 87–98.

Benson, H., Steinart, R. F., Greenwood, M. M., Klemchuk, H. M., & Peterson, N. H. (1975). Continuous measurement of O_2 consumption and CO_2 elimination during a wakeful hypometabolic state. *Journal of Human Stress, 1*(1), 37–44.

Bentov, I. (1977). *Stalking the wild pendulum.* New York: Dutton.

Blackwell, B., Hanenson, I., Bloomfield, S., Magenheim, H., Gartside, P., Nidich, S., Robinson, A., & Zigler, R. (1976). Transcendental meditation in hypertension, individual response patterns. *Lancet, 1,* 223–226.

Budzynski, T., Stoyva, J., & Adler, C. (1970). Feedback-induced muscle relaxation: Application to tension headache. *Journal of Behavior Therapy and Experimental Psychiatry, 1,* 205–211.

Butterworth, E. A. S. (1970). *The tree at the navel of the earth.* Berlin: Walter de Gruyter.

Chaudhuri, H. (1975). Yoga psychology. In C. C. Tart (Ed.), *Transpersonal psychologies* (pp. 223–280). New York: Harper & Row.

Clance, P. R., Mitchell, M., & Engelman, S. R. (1980). Body cathexis in children as a function of awareness training and yoga. *Journal of Clinical Child Psychology, 9*(1), 82–85.

Cunningham, O. (1981). The relationship of psychic healing and insight-oriented treatment within an expressive framework. *Pratt Institute of Creative Arts Therapy Review, 2,* 15–24.

Edwards, L. R. (1987). Psychological change and spiritual growth through the practice of siddha yoga. *Dissertation Abstracts International, 48* (2–A), 340.

Engelman, S. R., Clance, P. R., & Imes, S. (1982). Self and body—cathexis change in therapy and yoga groups. *Journal of the American Society of Psychosomatic Dentistry and Medicine, 29*(3), 77–88.

Goleman, D. J., & Schwartz, G. (1976). Meditation as an intervention in stress reactivity. *Journal of Consulting and Clinical Psychology, 44,* 456–466.

Gouger, S. C. (1979). The effects of Hatha yoga on psychiatric outpatients. *Dissertation Abstracts International, 39*(11–B), 5554.

Green, A. (1975, July). Paper presented at the meeting of the Transpersonal Psychology Conference, Stanford University.

Green, E. (1971). Biofeedback for mind-body self-regulation: Healing and creativity. In J. Kamiya et al. (Eds.) *Biofeedback and self-control.* Chicago: Aldine.

Harrigan, J. M. (1981). A component analysis of yoga: The effects of diaphragmatic breathing and stretching postures on anxiety, personality and somatic/behavioral complaints. *Dissertation Abstracts International, 42* (4–A), 1489.

Harvey, J. R. (1983). The effect of yogic breathing exercises on mood. *Journal of the American Society of Psychosomatic Dentistry and Medicine, 30*(2), 39–48.

Hoenig, J. (1968). Medical research on yoga. *Confinia Psychiatrica, 2,* 88–89.

Iyengar, B. K. S. (1980). *The concise light on yoga* (Foreword by Y. Menuhin). London: Unwin.

Jayakar, P. (1986). *Krishnamurti: A biography.* San Francisco: Harper & Row.

Jung, A. R. (1987). Alternatives to psychotherapy. *Issues in Radical Therapy, 12*(4), 30–33.

Jung, C. G. (1932). *Kundalini yoga.* Unpublished manuscript.

Jung, C. G. (1969). *Collected works: Vol. 9, Part 2. Aion: Researches into the phenomenology of the self.* Princeton, NJ: Princeton University Press.

Krishna, G. (1971). *Kundalini.* Berkeley, CA: Shambhala.

Krishnamurti, J. (1976). *Krishnamurti's notebook.* San Francisco: Harper & Row.

Lutyens, M. (1975). *Krishnamurti: The years of awakening.* New York: Avon.

Lutyens, M. (1983). *Krishnamurti: The years of fulfillment.* New York: Avon.

McCleave, M. J. (1978, March). Kundalini, headaches and biofeedback. *New Age Magazine.*

Miller, N. (1969). Learning visceral and glandular responses. *Science, 163,* 434–445.

Motoyama, H. (1981). *Theories of the chakras: Bridge to higher consciousness.* Wheaton, IL: Quest Books.

Muktananda, S. (1974). *The play of consciousness.* Campbell, CA: Shree Guruder Ashram.

Nespor, K. (1985). The combination of psychiatric treatment and yoga. *International Journal of Psychosomatics, 32*(2), 24–27.

Orme-Johnson, D. W. (1971, August). *Transcendental meditation and autonomic lability.* Paper presented at the meeting of the First International Symposium on the Science of Creative Intelligence, Arcata, CA.

Patel, C. H. (1973). Yoga and biofeedback in the management of hypertension. *Lancet,* November, 1053–1055.

Patel, C. H. (1975). Twelve-month follow-up of yoga and biofeedback in the management of hypertension. *Lancet,* January, 62–67.

Pazhayattil, H. (1986). Western psychotherapy in relation to the classical Patanjali yoga: A phenomenological and clinical inquiry into consciousness change and therapeutic process in a combined East-West approach. *Dissertation Abstracts International, 46,* 4411–4412.

Pollock, A., Weber, M., Case, D., & Laragh, J. (1977). Limitations of transcendental meditation in the treatment of essential hypertension. *Lancet, 1,* 71–73.

Rama, S. (1976). *Yoga and psychotherapy.* Honesdale, PA: Himalayan Institute.

Ring, K. (1982). *Life at death.* New York: Quill.

Ring, K. (1984). *Heading toward omega.* New York: Quill.

Rudolph, S. G. (1981). The effect on the self-concept of female college students of participation in hatha yoga and effective interpersonal relationship development classes. *Dissertation Abstracts International, 42* (5A), 2039.

Sannella, L. (1987). *The kundalini experience.* Lower Lake, CA: Integral Publishing.

Singh, R. H. (1986). Evaluation of some Indian traditional methods of promotion of mental health. *Activitas Nervosa Superior, 28*(1), 67–69.

Taimni, I. K. (1961). *The science of yoga.* Wheaton, IL: Theosophical Publishing House.

Thapar, R. (1966). *A history of India* (Vol. 1). Middlesex, England: Penguin.

Udupa, K. N. (1985). *Stress and its management by yoga.* New Delhi: Motilal Banarsidass.

Underhill, E. (1961). *Mysticism.* New York: Dutton.

Watts, A. (1961). *Psychotherapy east and west.* New York: Pantheon.

Wenger, M. A., & Bagchi, B. K. (1961). Studies of autonomic functions in practitioners of yoga in India. *Behavioral Science, 6,* 312–323.

Wenger, M. A., Bagchi, B. K., & Anand, B. K. (1961). Experiments in India on voluntary control of the heart and pulse. *Circulation, 24,* 1319–1325.

Wolfe, W. T. (1978). *And the sun is up: Kundalini rises in the West.* Red Hook, NY: Academy Hill Press.

Woolfolk, R. L. (1975). Psychophysiological correlates of meditation. *Archives of General Psychiatry, 32,* 1326–1333.

3

Chinese Medicine: The Law of Five Elements

Donald M. Pachuta

In spring, hundreds of flowers; in autumn,
*   a harvest moon;*
In summer, a refreshing breeze; in winter,
*   snow will accompany you.*
If useless things do not hang in your mind,
Any season is a good season for you. [1]

Zen Flesh, Zen Bones
Compiled by P. Reps, 1957, p. 134

In this chapter we will examine an ancient system of healing. It is quite elaborate yet exquisitely simple. As we take this journey, it is useful to put the ancient Chinese system into perspective by comparing it with the origins of all healing traditions and by contrasting it to the Western system.

---

[1] Reprinted with permission from Charles E. Tuttle Company, Tokyo, Japan.

The origins of ancient Chinese medicine lie in the concepts of the Tao, Ch'i, and Yin/Yang. These three philosophical notions pervade all systems of Chinese medicine and most systems of Eastern healing that arose from them. There are a number of different systems that are called traditional Chinese medicine, but in this discussion, we shall explore only one of them in depth—the Law of Five Elements.

We will concentrate on two of the major cycles within the Law of Five Elements. The first of these is the Shen Cycle or the Cycle of the Spirit. It will demonstrate how the Chinese regarded officials, organs and functions, and the elements of Fire, Earth, Metal, Water, and Wood.[2] Students of psychology will discover how dreams and emotions fit into the Five Elements. The second major cycle, the K'o Cycle, provides a unique view of the relationships of emotions and the idea of emotional antidotes, which can be helpful in our daily lives as well as in psychotherapy. Finally we will investigate the diagnostic and therapeutic systems of ancient Chinese medicine.

EAST AND WEST: SIMILARITIES AND DIFFERENCES

All healing systems began in religion and philosophy and espoused mystical union with God or nature. In the great Chinese, Japanese, Korean, Indian, Tibetan, and other Eastern healing systems, this tradition remains intact after thousands of years. In Tibet, all of the medical books still are looked upon as sacred revelations of the Buddha. In contrast, modern Western medicine generally ignores its philosophical heritage, considers nature irrelevant, and avoids any spiritual identification.

In all cultures, the original healers were shamans or priests. Our Western traditions began with the Oracle at Delphi. In ancient Greece, the sick crowded the temple and the priests diagnosed them, often through the interpretation of dreams after hallucinogenic drugs. In ancient Hebrew and Egyptian cultures, healing also was done by priests and in temples. Even in the New Testament, in keeping with that tradition, Jesus tells some of the people who have been cured to show themselves to the priests or to bathe in the temple pool. The Greek tradition has persisted to some extent to the present time: Western physicians take the Hippocratic oath and swear by Apollo, the physician, and Asclepius, a god of healing. Also Western medicine has adopted the staff of Asclepius as its symbol: a single

---

[2]The officials and elements are capitalized to convey the broad notions ascribed to them in Chinese medicine. When referring to the narrower idea of an anatomical organ only they are not capitalized.

staff around which is a serpent coiled with its head pointed downward to indicate mastery over sickness.

An amazing similarity existed in the philosophy of Eastern and Western systems of healing in early times. We hear in the ancient Tao from China and in the Oracle at Delphi in Greece, the identical admonition: "know thyself." In the *Nei Ching*, the written text of ancient Chinese medicine, Ch'i Po said, "The most important requirement of the art of healing is that no mistakes or neglect occur" (Veith, 1972, p. 150). The first dictum of Hippocrates is: "Primum non nocere—First do no harm."

The teachings of Ch'i Po and Hippocrates became the founding traditions for Oriental and Western medicine, respectively. Both incorporated religion and philosophy, turned to nature, and created systems that lasted millenia. Ch'i Po and Hippocrates demonstrated general agreement in their philosophy of healing, in their perceptions of disease, and even in their descriptions of diseases. Both emphasized that perception is the fundamental tool of the physician. Both spoke of the internal and external causative factors of disease. They agreed that the internal factor, the spirit, is overwhelmingly important in both patient and practitioner. Hippocrates said, "Some patients though conscious that their condition is perilous, nonetheless recover solely through their contentment with the good graces of the physician" (Aphorisms). The similarities between the East and West persisted until the Judeo-Christian philosophy became predominant, and the differences became more pronounced due to Descartes's advocacy of a mind-body split. Of course, not all physicians abandoned the ancient Oriental system of medicine. For instance, several paintings of the fourteenth and fifteenth centuries depict European physicians taking pulses in the Chinese manner. Indeed, Sir William Osler, in this century urged his students to "feel the pulse with two hands and ten fingers" (Bean, 1950, p. 99).

With the inventions of the stethoscope, microscope, and thermometer, which ushered in the age of measurement in modern science, Western medicine discarded these exquisite tools of diagnosis of the total person at all levels of bodymindemotionspirit. In fact, more sophisticated technology is now causing the gradual abandonment of the stethoscope. Today it is rare to find a physician who can listen to the heart with a stethoscope and make an accurate diagnosis; whereas, this was the norm a generation ago. (See also Pachuta, 1981.)

The Eastern systems of healing have remained virtually unchanged. The Eastern way is circular. Oneness with the universe is a given, and one continually seeks balance and harmony within this oneness. Paradox is an illusion and can be mastered. Each individual is unique within the overall oneness. Sameness coexists with differences within and between all people. People are treated in the totality of bodymindemotionspirit. (The Chinese consider emotion part of mind and say bodymindspirit. I add emotion since our Western behavioral sciences focus on it as separate from mind and spirit.) All things, all people, and all systems can assist healing and have a place. A disease may have an external cause, but all diseases have an internal cause and involve to some degree an illness of the spirit. Thus, the patient has a primary responsibility, and the health care practitioner can only assist him or her in becoming well. The basic energy is treated; all else flows from it. In the Eastern systems, centeredness and wholeness of the practitioner are crucial, and love is essential to the cure.

In contrast, the Western healing systems are linear and emphasize differences. We have great difficulty in tolerating paradox. We stress the division of the person into body and mind, and the spirit is generally irrelevant to Western scientific medicine. The practice of medicine consists of the treatment of symptoms rather than of the whole person. To most physicians, only external sources of disease matter, and they pay little or no attention to the internal sources of illness. Therefore, the patient has little or no responsibility, and the practitioner is put on a pedestal. The state of being of such a practitioner is not relevant; for, it is the external medicine or the external technique that effects the cure. A pill exists or must be found for every ill. Love is completely ignored.

Ancient Chinese medicine was always a system of preventive medicine. In contrast, Western medicine, until very recently, had focused on the treatment of illness and paid little attention to prevention.

Finally, the Eastern systems of healing differ radically from the Western ones in their regard for their healing heritage. The Eastern systems display a deep reverence for their heritage. For the most part, we have lost that reverence in the West. Healing professionals must realize that every time they pick up a prescription pad or an acupuncture needle, they touch thousands of years of traditions and somehow share in the divine. We would do well to remember the words of Albert Einstein:

> The most beautiful and profound emotion we can experience is the emotion of the mystical. It is the power of all true science. He to whom this emotion is a stranger, who can no longer wonder and stand in awe, is as good as dead. To know what is impenetrable to us really exists, manifesting itself to us as the highest wisdom and the most radiant beauty . . . this knowledge, this feeling is at the center of all true religiousness and spirituality. (Pachuta, 1987, p. 4)

ANCIENT CHINESE MEDICINE

Tao

The philosophical origins of all the Chinese systems of medicine, regardless of differences in detail, lie in ancient traditions that are about 5,000 years old. The notions of Tao, Ch'i, and Yin/Yang play a dominant role for they run through all of the ancient and modern Chinese and other Oriental systems.

The ancient Chinese *Tao Te Ching* by Lao Tzu espouses a profound Way of Life. The word *Tao* (pronounced "dow") translates as *Way* and much more. The Tao is a way the universe unfolds—a way of nature, a way of the seasons, planting and harvest—it is a way of virtue, a way of heaven, a way of life, and a way of death. The Tao pervades every aspect of life and being. In later Taoist schools, Tao ultimately means something very much akin to God. Tao always remains cosmic and eternal. It is the oneness. The goal of life was to flow with the Tao, as individuals, families, groups, and society.

> When the Tao is present in the universe,
> The horses haul manure.
> When the Tao is absent from the universe,
> War horses are bred outside the city.[3]
>
> Lao Tzu (Feng & English, 1972, p. 46)

Ch'i—The Universal Energy

The Ch'i Energy, the one universal energy, the cosmic life force, is the most fundamental concept of the entire Chinese system of medicine. It is the vital life force, the flux, the flow. It is the energy of the heavens and the earth, the energy within and without. It is the vital life force that flows through us, and it does so in a very orderly and logical fashion on pathways called meridians.

Ironically, Western medicine, which so values order, generally denies the existence of an orderly flow of energy through us. But perhaps the greatest Western scientist, Albert Einstein, held the idea of a universal energy. He said that the different energies held by physicists were not separate but part of one single energy. Finally, in the last several years,

---

[3]From *Tao Te Ching* by Lao Tzu. Translated by Gia-Fu Feng and Jane English. Copyright © 1972 by Gia-Fu Feng and Jane English. Reprinted by permission of Alfred A. Knopf, Inc.

all notions of separate energies have crumbled, and his idea has been accepted.

The Ch'i flows in an orderly way. Balance and harmony of this energy means health. Imbalance or disharmony of the flow of Ch'i results in illness. This idea illustrates a fundamental Eastern notion: namely, that it is not possible to be sick in body without being sick in mind, emotion, and spirit. You cannot possibly have a sickness of the body, or the mind, or the emotions, or the spirit only; illness resides in the entire person, in the unity of bodymindemotionspirit. The spirit is the aspect that needs to be corrected first; only then can the other aspects be brought into balance or harmony.

The diagnostic system in Chinese medicine consists of an evaluation of the state of balance of this Ch'i energy, this life force. This assessment takes place not only in the whole person as bodymindspirit but also in each specific organ, function, or official. The therapeutic system aims to bring the organs, functions, and officials back into balance at all levels of bodymindspirit. It should be noted that Ch'i is universal energy that includes the divine. The fundamental notion of all Chinese philosophy and medicine is the profound oneness of all things and of all people with nature, with the universe, and with the divine.

Yin/Yang

The notion of Yin/Yang has pervaded discussions about the nature of the universe since ancient times. It is one of the underlying and unifying principles of many traditions. The Yin and Yang (see Figure 3.1) represent the fundamental dualities, opposites, and polarities of the universe; yet, they also represent the unity of the circle and the Tao. This duality within unity often presents a problem for Western students of philosophy and medicine. The circle represents the whole universe and contains all aspects of the universe, including opposites: Yin/Yang, white/black, female/male, night/day, earth/heaven, death/life, and so on. It is the unity containing the duality. They are opposite, yet contained within the

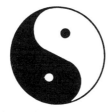

FIGURE 3.1.   Yin/Yang.

same circle. They are different yet the same. The Yin contains the Yang and the Yang contains the Yin.

Yin/Yang is not only outside of us in the universe but also within us, because we are part of the universe. It is our duality and polarity. It is our female/male, regardless of our genetic sex. It is our good/evil, darkness/light, rest/activity, softness/hardness, inside/outside, front/back, top/bottom, death/life, earth/heaven, and so on. Yet it is also our unity, our integration of all these things into a whole; it is a circle never ending and complete.

To the Western mind, things are black *and* white or black *or* white. But in the Eastern way, things are black/white. In the Judeo-Christian tradition, all opposites are warring forces. The chief battle is good against evil. One must triumph, and we must be sure that it is good. In the Eastern way, the inseparable Yin and Yang gently wrestle with each other. Nothing in the universe is one or the other. Everything contains Yin/Yang. They are part of the same reality. They are merely opposite polarities of the same magnet, and it is impossible to have one without the other.

Westerners have great difficulty with this concept. We hold that light battles with darkness, life with death, good with evil, positive with negative. As Alan Watts said (1975, p. 20):

> Thus, the ideal to cultivate the former and be rid of the latter flourishes throughout much of the world. To the traditional way of Chinese thinking, this is as incomprehensible as electric currents without both positive and negative poles. For polarity is the principle that plus/minus, north/south (and indeed all parts of opposites) are different aspects of the same system. The disappearance of either one of them would be the disappearance of the entire system.

As Lao Tzu said:

> Under heaven all can see beauty as beauty only because there is ugliness.
> All can know good as good only because there is evil.
>
> Therefore having and not having arise together.
> Difficult and easy complement each other.
> Long and short contrast each other;
> High and low rest upon each other;
> Voice and sound harmonize each other;
> Front and back follow one another.[4] (Feng & English, 1972, p. 2)

---

[4]From *Tao Te Ching* by Lao Tzu. Translated by Gia-Fu Feng and Jane English. Copyright © 1972 by Gia-Fu Feng and Jane English. Reprinted by permission of Alfred A. Knopf, Inc.

Many things are paradoxical, but Westerners try to ignore the paradoxes because they are confusing. The Eastern philosophies, religions, and healing systems confront them directly. Judaism was once very Eastern and mystical but changed after it became a state religion. Ecclesiastes could have been written by Lao Tzu.

To everything there is a season,
and a time to every purpose under the Heavens: . . .

A time to plant, and a time to pluck up that which is planted; . . .

A time to weep, and a time to laugh;
a time to mourn, and a time to dance; . . .

a time to embrace, and a time to refrain from embracing; . . .

a time to keep, and a time to cast away:

a time to keep silence, and a time to speak.

Ecclesiastes, 3:1–7

TRADITIONAL CHINESE MEDICINE: LAW OF FIVE ELEMENTS

Many modern systems arise from the ancient Chinese philosophy. Many of these involve numbers from 1 to 12. For example, one system is based on three heaters or coolers, and another is founded on eight principles or conditions. Regardless of variation, all arise in and remain faithful to ancient tradition, including Tao, Ch'i, and Yin/Yang.

We shall examine the tradition called Five Elements, Energies, or Phases based on the ancient Tao, Ch'i, and Yin/Yang. It encompasses all aspects of being; and it offers a spectacular map of the universe and of how we, bodymindspirit, belong to it and function in it. It also provides the background for several elaborate systems of healing.

Much of the Five Element information can be found in the *Nei Ching,* translated as *The Yellow Emperor's Classic of Internal Medicine.* This book was probably written between 200 and 600 B.C., although the oral tradition was thousands of years old, and it contains references to ancient writing, which are now lost. Unfortunately, much is lost in the translation from Chinese to English. The original Chinese is exquisite. One need only read any work by Claude Larre to gain a profound appreciation of this fact. Furthermore, words resemble only the shadow of reality: the Chinese are convinced that reality is lived and that discourse is an inherently imperfect way of conveying that which is lived. Jack R. Worsley, founder and president of the College of Traditional Chinese

Acupuncture, U.K., developed the chart "Law of Five Elements" (see Figure 3.2). He has done more than anyone to bring a complex Eastern system of philosophy and healing to the West. (See also Porkert, 1974; Worsley, 1973, 1982.)

Lesson

As we begin to examine the Five Elements, the following lesson is illuminating (see *Journal of Traditional Acupuncture, 5:* 2, 1981, p. 61).

In ancient times a young couple approached an old master and asked, "Please, master, speak to us of marriage and the place of love in our union."

And the master said, "See that marriage is a union manifesting the Five Energies of nature held within us, and that love is only but one of those energies."

"Then please, master, speak to us of the Energies in nature that are held within us."

And the master said:

"The Fire Energy is like the sun, always warming the mind/body/spirit, bathing your relationship with love; experience this manifestation of nature within you as the urge to love, and express that love to your partner.

The Earth Energy is like the soil, always giving to the mind/body/spirit, providing your relationship with nourishment; experience this manifestation of nature within you as the urge to nurture, and express that nurturing to your partner.

The Metal Energy is like the gem, always sustaining to the mind/body/spirit, entrusting your relationship with strength; experience this manifestation of nature within you as the urge to be strong, and express that strength to your partner.

The Water Energy is like the spring, always refreshing to the mind/body/spirit, forming your relationship in change; experience this manifestation of nature within you as the urge to change, and express that change to your partner.

The Wood Energy is like the tree, always supportive to the mind/body/spirit, seeding your relationship in growth; experience this manifestation of nature within you as the urge to grow, and express that growth to your partner.

You are the Laws of Nature.

You are Love.

You are Nourishment.

You are Strength.

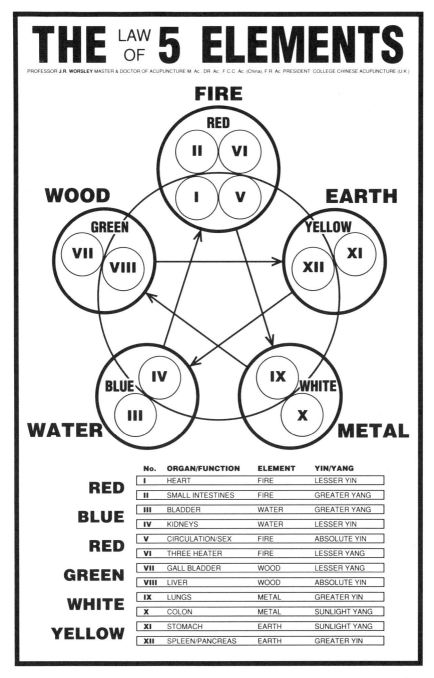

FIGURE 3.2. The law of the 5 elements. (Reprinted with permission from J. R. Worsley.)

You are Change.

You are Growth.

And know that the Energies will move and be moved, seeking their balance between the forces of control and creativity. And so your relationship will seek those balances also."

And with that, the master turned and gently walked away.

Although we rarely look at ourselves in this manner, the Chinese hold that each of us reflects the laws of Nature, Love, Nourishment, Strength, Change, and Growth and that we are at one with the universe and the eternal Tao. Many concepts, especially the elements and officials that are all encompassing, frequently raise disbelief in the student from the West. It is useful to willingly suspend our disbelief in approaching this system.

LAW OF MOTHER/CHILD—THE SHEN CYCLE

One of the broadest principles underlying all Eastern systems is that they are a map of nature. Thus, they aid us in recognizing how we are in or out of harmony with nature. One of the fundamental differences in Eastern and Western philosophy is that in the East man is one with nature, with the seasons, the trees, the water, the wind, and so on. Man is no exception to the rules and laws of nature. In the West, on the other hand, we have isolated and alienated ourselves from nature. The Hebrew scriptures say, "To everything there is a season." Yet Westerners resist being part of nature. We are always in a hurry. When we are in the season of winter, none of us can instantly make it spring. Yet we try. We lack the patience of the Orient. There it would be considered absurd to hate winter or rainy days or any of nature's manifestations.

Figure 3.2 shows five circles and smaller circles within those. The entire universe is a circle containing the Yin/Yang and all opposites. The clockwise flow of the circles forms the Shen or Spirit Cycle.

In the *Nei Ching,* the Emperor asked Ch'i Po, "What is meant by Shen, the Spirit?" Ch'i Po answered: ". . . The spirit cannot be heard with the ear. The eye must be brilliant of perception and the heart must be open and attentive, and then the spirit is suddenly revealed through ones' own consciousness. It cannot be expressed through the mouth; only the heart can express all that can be looked upon" (Connelly, 1979, p. 34). Ch'i Po further stated: "The utmost in the art of healing can be achieved when there is unity. . . . When the minds of people are closed and wisdom is locked out, they remain tied to disease. . . . It becomes apparent that those who have attained spirit and energy are flourishing and prosperous, while those perish who lose their spirit and energy" (Connelly, 1979, p. iv). In other words, healthy people flow with the Tao, through the Shen and all other cycles. The unhealthy resist and fight the natural flow.

As the seasons beget each other, they enunciate one of the laws of the Five Elements—the law of mother/child. The red circle, fire, flows to the yellow circle, earth: out of the ashes of fire comes earth. The Chinese knew about the "big bang" theory even then. Earth is the mother of metal—the white circle—for metals come from the earth. Metal is the mother of water—the blue circle—for metals melt into liquid and water condenses on metal. In the modern Chinese version, all elements of the periodic table are on the metal element, and the hydrogen and oxygen of water arise from the metal element. Water nurtures and gives rise to wood, the green circle. Wood, in turn, creates fire.

This law of mother/child in nature continues with the seasons. Fire is summer which mothers earth, late summer, or the season of harvest. Earth, in turn, mothers metal or autumn. The latter spawns water or winter, and this produces wood or spring. Wood begets fire, which is summer.

The Officials

The Chinese had developed a system of astronomy that mapped the heavens in a way that Western science has found acceptable. Also, their system of mapping the earth is still in use today. Between the heavens and the earth stands man. A fitting image might be that of a person standing on top of a hill with arms outstretched to the heavens.

The ancient seers also mapped out an orderly flow of Ch'i energy in man. They looked upon it as a system of internal government. Within this system, there are 12 organs or functions (the small circles within the five elements in Figure 3.2), and each of the 12 organs or functions acts as an official in this internal government. Table 3.1 lists each of the 12 organs or functions and the corresponding official. These have been given Roman numerals in order to aid study by Westerners.

The Ch'i energy that controls each official flows through the body on a defined anatomical pathway. Besides these 12 organs, several other meridian systems carry the Ch'i energy throughout the body.

The purpose of all the officials is to maintain order, balance, and harmony within the government. Thus, the Heart, the Supreme Master or Controller, is the emperor of the kingdom. This official is everything that the word "Heart" evokes. It means "soul, spirit, love, joy"; it encompasses all notions of heart held throughout history, at all levels of

TABLE 3.1.   THE LAW OF FIVE ELEMENTS (THE OFFICIALS)

Number	Organ/Function	Element	Official
I	Heart	Fire	Supreme Master
II	Small intestine	Fire	Separator of the Pure from the Impure
III	Bladder	Water	Official of the Eliminator of Liquid Waste
IV	Kidneys	Water	The Storehouse of the Vital Essence
V	Circulation/sex (pericardium)	Fire	The Heart Protector
VI	Three heater	Fire	The Official of Heating and Cooling
VII	Gallbladder	Wood	The Official of Decision Making and Judgments
VIII	Liver	Wood	The Official of Planning
IX	Lungs	Metal	The Official That Receives Ch'i from the Heavens—the Official of Rhythmic Order
X	Colon	Metal	The Great Eliminator; the Drainer of the Dregs
XI	Stomach	Earth	The Official of Rotting and Ripening and Assimilation
XII	Spleen/pancreas	Earth	The Official of the Distribution and the Transporter of Energy

bodymindemotionspirit, and at all levels of the universe. In addition, the Ch'i energy that controls the Heart flows along a pathway called the heart meridian, which has numerous points along the way.

The Small Intestine is the Official called the Separator of the Pure from the Impure. It is a mystery how the Chinese could know the function of the anatomical small intestine without the benefit of modern technology or even autopsies. The officials are believed to function at all levels of bodymindemotionspirit. Thus, the Separator of the Pure from the Impure does not merely separate the physically pure from the impure, it also separates the mentally pure from the impure, the emotionally pure from the impure, and the spiritually pure from the impure.

The ancient Chinese separated the stomach, small intestine, and colon, without benefit of autopsy or scientific study. The Colon, the Great Eliminator, eliminates physical waste, mental waste, emotional waste, and spiritual waste from the internal government. The notion goes far beyond a mere anatomical organ.

Circulation/Sex, the Heart Protector, controls far more than simply the circulation of the blood and the function of the anatomical sexual organs. This official is concerned with the circulation of the individual among other people, allowing them to have intimate relationships knowing that the Heart is protected from harm. The notion of the anatomical pericardium probably was added much later, and the original concept involved a function rather than a specific anatomical organ.

Correspondences and Associations

Table 3.2 shows some of the correspondences and associations of each of the elements. It gives us an idea of the complexities and the all-inclusive concept of an element. For example, in addition to the tables each element has correspondences with a specific meat, a fruit, a vegetable, a grain, etc. Of interest to psychologists are the dream correspondences. We should emphasize here that in Chinese Medicine discussed later there are no psychologists distinct from healers of the body. Our Western split of body, mind, emotion, and spirit totally contradicts all of the Chinese notions. There is only one practitioner who treats the person in the totality of bodymindemotionspirit, whether with acupuncture needles, herbs, moxa (heat to acupuncture points), mantra therapy, or lessons in a Way of Life. All of these come from the ancient Chinese system. There are no psychotherapists in Oriental medicine, only teachers. The only exception to the totality of treatment is "barefoot doctor" acupuncture, designed for first aid. This can be learned in 8 to 12 weeks and contrasts with the exquisite system that treats the total bodymindspirit.

Fire.   Fire is associated with the season of summer, the climate heat, the direction south. It encompasses the organs and functions of Heart, Small Intestine, Circulation/Sex, and the Three Heater (this has no Western anatomical counterpart but may well fit the endocrine system). Fire supports and fortifies the circulation and blood vessels. Its sense organ is the tongue, and its secretion is perspiration. Its time of day is from 11:00 A.M. to 3:00 P.M., the time of the Heart and Small Intestine, as

TABLE 3.2.   THE LAW OF FIVE ELEMENTS (CORRESPONDENCES AND ASSOCIATIONS)

	Fire	Earth	Metal	Water	Wood
Color	Red	Yellow	White	Blue	Green
Season	Summer	Late summer	Autumn	Winter	Spring
Climate	Heat	Humidity	Dryness	Cold	Wind
Direction	South	Center	West	North	East
Organs	Heart small intestine circulation/sex three heater	Stomach spleen/ pancreas	Lungs colon	Bladder kidneys	Gallbladder liver
Fortifies	Blood vessels	Muscles	Skin/hair	Bones	Ligaments
Sense organ	Tongue	Mouth	Nose	Ears	Eyes
Secretion	Perspiration	Saliva	Mucous	Spittle	Tears
Time of day	11 A.M.–3 P.M. 7 P.M.–11 P.M.	7 A.M.–11 A.M.	3 A.M.–7 A.M.	3 P.M.–7 P.M.	11 P.M.–3 A.M.
Emotion	Joy	Sympathy/ empathy	Grief	Fear	Anger
Sound	Laughing	Singing	Weeping	Groaning	Shouting
Odor	Scorched	Fragrant	Rotten	Putrid	Rancid
Taste	Bitter	Sweet	Pungent	Salty	Sour
Power	Mature	Decrease	Balance	Emphasize	Birth
Life aspect	The spirit	Ideas/ opinions	Lower spirit	Willpower	Spiritual faculties

well as from 7:00 to 11:00 P.M., the time of the Heart Protector and Three Heater. Fire includes the emotion joy, the sound of laughter, the odor scorched, and the taste bitter. All the elements contain a power and a life aspect. Fire is associated with the power to mature and its life aspect is the spirit.

Earth.   The color yellow, late summer, humidity, the direction center, the organs Stomach and Spleen/Pancreas belong to Earth. It fortifies muscles. Its sense organ is the mouth, and its secretion is saliva. The time of the Stomach is from 7 to 9 A.M., and the time of the Spleen/Pancreas is from 9 to 11 A.M. Earth encompasses the emotion empathy, the singing voice, a fragrant odor, and a sweet taste. Its power is to decrease. Westerners have been trained to usually view decrease negatively; yet, decrease is a part of balance. If the fires and expansion of summer did not decrease, the planet would burn up. The life aspect of Earth incorporates ideas and opinions. Beyond all this, Earth is the Divine Mother.

Metal.   The color white, the season autumn, the climate dryness, the direction west, and the organs Lungs (skin) and Colon reside in Metal. It fortifies skin and hair. Its sense organ is the nose, and its secretion is mucous. The time of the Lungs is from 3 to 5 A.M., and the time of the Colon is from 5 to 7 A.M. Metal contains the emotion grief, the sound of weeping, a rotten smell, and a pungent taste. The power of Metal balances. Its life aspect harbors the lower spirit. Also Metal includes the Father, the Creator, the Heavens, and the Air.

Water.   Water is associated with the color blue, winter, cold, north, the Bladder, and the Kidneys. It fortifies bones. Its sense organs are the ears, and its secretion is spittle. The time of the Bladder is from to 3 to 5 P.M., and the time of the Kidneys is from 5 to 7 P.M. Water includes the emotion fear, the sound of a groaning voice, a putrid odor, and a salty taste. Its power emphasizes, and its life aspect is willpower. Beyond this, Water has many spiritual points on its meridians. It contains the primordial stuff of the universe, its very essence; and hence it represents utmost power. The ancient Chinese placed the nervous system in the sea of bone marrow, under the control of Water. Also they put blood in the sea of bone marrow (they knew that marrow made blood) under the control of the Kidneys. Only centuries later was it "proven" that the kidneys control the bones and secrete a hormone that controls the making of red blood cells.

Wood.   Wood is associated with the color green, spring, wind, east, the Gallbladder, and the Liver. It fortifies ligaments and tendons. It is our eyes and our tears. The time of day of the Gallbladder is from 11 P.M. to 1 A.M., and the time of the Liver is from 1 to 3 A.M. Anger, a shouting voice, a rancid odor, and a sour taste are associated with Wood. Its power is birth, and its life aspect is spiritual faculties. Wood encompasses creativity and spiritual vision.

*   *   *   *   *

We have a hard time accepting the organs as mother of each other. How can the Liver or Gallbladder be the mother of the Heart (see Table 3.3)? Western "scientific" research maintains that there is no relationship between gallbladder disease and heart disease. Yet, I saw three young women die of heart attacks after having had their gallbladders removed, although they had no known underlying disease. It encourages me to know that others know this connection. An acquaintance who had had two previous heart attacks was hospitalized with a gallbladder attack. Both the surgeon and the cardiologist told her that they would not touch her gallbladder until she had resolved the anger at her husband (perhaps the cause of the attack). Whenever I see a patient who needs gallbladder surgery, I always assist them in dealing with their anger prior to the surgery.

Times of Day.   Table 3.2 shows the times of day. This is the circadian and biological rhythm that indicates when the energy of a particular official peaks in the course of the day. Even Western science is actually finding that chemotherapy is less toxic at certain times of the day than at others.

The Gallbladder is the official of Decision Making, and the Liver is the official of Planning. Their peak time is from 11 P.M. to 3 A.M. Hence, people avoid making decisions while they are awake. We intuitively recognize the wisdom of this approach, and many of us choose to "sleep on" a matter of major consequence. From 3 to 5 A.M. is the time of the Lungs, the Heavens, the Father, Creation, and the Spirit; and from time immemorial, in all cultures, this has been the time of meditation.

From 5 to 7 A.M. is the time of the Colon. You eliminate first, then you take in. This principle operates at all levels. You must eliminate your judgments and prejudices in order to take in new ideas. The time from 7 to 9 A.M. belongs to the Stomach, and the time from 9 to 11 A.M. belongs to the Spleen/Pancreas.

The energy of the Heart peaks between 11 A.M. and 1 P.M. and that of the Small Intestine peaks between 1 and 3 P.M. From 3 to 5 P.M. is the time of the Bladder. From 5 to 7 P.M. is the time of the Kidneys. From 7 to 9 P.M. is the time of the Heart Protector. From 9 to 11 P.M. is the time of the Three Heater.

We all have our own time of day when we are at our best depending on our level of balance and harmony. Most people have a problem around 3 P.M. This is the time of the Bladder, the official of the Storehouse of Energy. In this culture, we tend to draw heavily on our general storehouse of energies, and hence we become tired. Some people avoid this by drinking water at 2:30 or 2:45 P.M. and honoring the Water element.

Emotions.   The Law of Five Elements, and indeed all Eastern systems, consists of cycles and rhythms. As part of nature and the universe, people feel the organs, functions, and emotions of the season they are experiencing. Each time I speak before a group, I ask how many people in the audience have suddenly and unexpectedly felt the emotion of that season. Usually 90 percent of the audience has had such an experience in

TABLE 3.3.   THE LAW OF FIVE ELEMENTS (THE SHEN AND K'O CYCLES)

Heart		(Fire)	*Small Intestine*		(Fire)
Circulation/Sex		(Fire)	*Three Heater*		(Fire)
Child of	Liver	(Wood)	Child of	Gallbladder	(Wood)
Controlled by	Bladder/kidneys	(Water)	Controlled by	Bladder/kidneys	(Water)
Mother of	Spleen/pancreas	(Earth)	Mother of	Stomach	(Earth)
Controller of	Lung/colon	(Metal)	Controller of	Lung/colon	(Metal)
Stomach		(Earth)	*Spleen/Pancreas*		(Earth)
Child of	Small intestine/Three heater	(Fire)	Child of	Heart, circulation/sex	(Fire)
Controlled by	Gallbladder/liver	(Wood)	Controlled by	Gallbladder/liver	(Wood)
Mother of	Colon	(Metal)	Mother of	Lung	(Metal)
Controller of	Bladder/kidneys	(Water)	Controller of	Bladder/kidneys	(Water)
Lung		(Metal)	*Colon*		(Metal)
Child of	Spleen/pancreas	(Earth)	Child of	Stomach	(Earth)
Controlled by	Heart, small intestine, circulation/sex, three heater	(Fire)	Controlled by	Heart, small intestine, circulation/sex, three heater	(Fire)
Mother of	Kidneys	(Water)	Mother of	Bladder	(Water)
Controller of	Gallbladder/liver	(Wood)	Controller of	Gallbladder/liver	(Wood)
Bladder		Water	*Kidneys*		(Water)
Child of	Colon	(Metal)	Child of	Lung	(Metal)
Controlled by	Stomach, spleen/pancreas	(Earth)	Controlled by	Stomach, spleen/pancreas	(Earth)
Mother of	Gallbladder	(Wood)	Mother of	Liver	(Wood)
Controller of	Heart, small intestine, circulation/sex, three heater	(Fire)	Controller of	Heart, small intestine, circulation/sex, three heater	(Fire)
Gallbladder		(Wood)	*Liver*		(Wood)
Child of	Bladder	(Water)	Child of	Kidneys	(Water)
Controlled by	Lung/colon	(Metal)	Controlled by	Lung/colon	(Metal)
Mother of	Small intestine, three heater	(Fire)	Mother of	Heart, circulation/sex	(Fire)
Controller of	Stomach, spleen/pancreas	(Earth)	Controller of	Stomach, spleen/pancreas	(Earth)

the preceding two or three weeks. Naturally, we experience all the emotions to some degree in all the seasons. Some days of autumn feel like summer, winter, or spring. But the emotion of the season predominates. Also the organ associated with a season is more susceptible during this time. On the worse winter-in-summer day that I have ever seen, the temperature dropped 50 degrees for a record low, and I saw more urinary tract infections and kidney/bladder disease that day than on any day of my life. More stomach complaints arise in late summer. More lung, skin, or colon problems appear in autumn. Indeed, many of the seasonal variations of illnesses known to Western medicine can be predicted by this ancient system.

Let us now examine the various emotions within the Shen Cycle. Fire is the emotion joy. Joy is the mother of the emotion of the Earth, sympathy or empathy. In the holy Indian scripture, *Bhagavad Gita*, empathy is the statement, "When a person responds to the joys and sorrows of others as if they were his own, he has attained the highest state of spiritual union" (6:32). Empathy, in turn, is the mother of grief, the emotion of Metal. Grief is the mother of fear, the emotion of Water. Fear is the mother of anger, the emotion of Wood. And although many people question this, anger is the mother of joy. For example, one minute a child may be screaming at you in anger, and the next he may be bouncing on your lap, joyous as can be. If you ask about his anger, he may not even remember it. He has passed from anger to joy in accordance with nature's law of mother/child. Also arguments are often followed by the joy of reconciliation. Anger thus leads to the heart.

Western medicine is now recognizing the role of anger in illness. Suppression of anger creates a lot of disease. Fire contains the cardiovascular system and the small intestine, the site of most ulcers. When anger is suppressed and blocked, it cannot feed the Fire and flow into joy and serious problems arise in the fire. The heart, blood vessels, and small intestine do not receive the Wood energy, and disease sets in. Cardiovascular diseases kill more people than the other top five causes of death combined. Most people who work with cancer patients know that they have a lot of repressed anger, often manifested as frustration, bitterness, hatred, or envy. These feelings play a major role in the development of cancer as well as in its outcome.

Suppressed anger is endemic in our society. Anger is the forbidden emotion because we hold it as sinful. Sometimes it is appropriate to be sad, or afraid, or in need of sympathy, but it is never appropriate to be angry. We are encouraged from birth to repress anger rather than to appropriately express it. This defies all the natural laws and thwarts all efforts to maintain balance and harmony. To rid yourself of anger, often a simple communication of it will suffice. A lot of patients say, "Well, I don't hold anything in—I don't have to worry about it. I just blow my top and it's gone." Blowing your top is pathological. You should not have to blow your top. You should not suppress the anger until it reaches a boiling point and leads to an explosion.

LAW OF MASTERY—THE K'O CYCLE

The arrows in Figure 3.2 illustrate a second major cycle, the K'o Cycle. Understanding this is important to all areas of Chinese medicine but particularly to the areas of emotions, thoughts, and behavior. The K'o Cycle is the cycle of mastery or control. As Table 3.3 indicates, Water is the controller of Fire; for Water puts out Fire. Fire controls (burns) Metal. Metal controls (cuts) Wood. Wood controls Earth; for, if we cut down all trees, we shall have floods, which will wash the Earth away. Earth controls (dams) Water.

Emotions and the Cycles

One important lesson of the Chinese approach is that there are a limited number of emotions. Knowing this prevents people from becoming overwhelmed. You can feel joy or the lack of joy, sympathy or the lack of sympathy, grief or the lack of grief, fear or the lack of fear, anger or the lack of anger.

Every autumn I receive a number of similar calls. The caller says, "I'm depressed." I answer, "No you're not. You are John or Mary or Mike." Then he or she says, "Okay, I'm sad." I respond with, "No, you're not sad. You are John or Mary or Mike." Next he or she says, "I feel depressed." I tell the caller that depression is a sophisticated intellectual concept. To "feel" depressed is impossible. It is not a feeling. Then finally the caller says, "Okay, I feel sad." I say, "Ah, ha! Wonderful. Welcome to the human race. The whole universe feels sad. It's autumn, the trees are sad. The leaves are dying, the acorns are falling, the insects are dying. The whole universe is sad. Why should you be any different?" This conversation often helps a great deal in relieving alienation from the self and from nature. Also, feeling sad is far less overwhelming than "feeling" or "being" depressed and thus easier to manage.

Time and again, I hear, "I'm frustrated." No, you *are* not frustrated, and you cannot possibly *feel* frustrated. Frustration, like depression, is a sophisticated intellectual concept that contains no emotion. The feeling behind frustration is anger. Frustration is a major pathogenic force in physical and mental illness, because we suppress the anger, intellectualize it as frustration, and it eats away inside us. As Figure 3.2 indicates, anger is mothered by fear and controlled by grief. Hence, whenever you are angry, it would be useful to ask, "What am I afraid of? What am I sad about?" For instance, if you feel annoyed by having to wait in traffic, if you feel angry at the "bum" who cut you off, ask yourself those questions. You may discover that you are afraid that you will feel embarrassed at being late and that people will think ill of you. Also you may feel sad due to the anticipated loss of prestige and self-esteem. As you find the cause of the anger, it will dissipate.

Since anger is generated by fear, it follows that the most violent anger is indicative of the greatest fear. Paranoia is an abnormal fear, fear of something that is not real. Paranoia is the diagnosis that the psychiatry ward staff perhaps fear most, for they know that those patients are prone to violence. This is an acknowledgment in Western psychiatry of the concept that fear is the mother of anger.

The next big issue is guilt. Most people will not say, "I am guilty." That is too heavy. Instead, they say, "I feel guilty." No one feels guilty, because guilt is an intellectual notion. If you look into your self, you will discover that it is a very powerful force and that much of your life is run by guilt. The emotion under guilt is fear, the fear of retribution.

You can change your life with these three things: know that you never are or feel depressed, that you never are or feel frustrated, and that you never feel guilty. On the other hand, it is fine to feel sad, angry, or afraid. Welcome to the human race.

Often when we experience or feel something, we do not express it. We run it through the mind and suppress it. Eventually our mind begins to determine how we feel. Our concepts determine our emotions. This process often begins in childhood, when parents tell us how we feel. Being as we are is far easier than trying to be how we are not. It takes no effort and no energy to feel sad when we feel sad or to feel angry when we feel angry. Yet we spend a great deal of energy trying to be unlike ourselves. For example, if we begin to "feel" a little depressed, we waste all our energy trying not to be depressed or blaming ourselves for being depressed, since we believe that we should not be depressed. It is more natural to feel and experience the sadness, and then it quickly goes away. At the very least, it does not interfere with our functioning. To live fully and to be the master of your own emotions is to feel angry when you feel angry, sad when you feel sad, afraid when you feel afraid, and so on. Mastery is being how you are.

Emotional Antidotes of the K'o Cycle

Empathy/Fear. The K'o Cycle is written in our hearts. We all know it at some level, but many of us do not function by it. Mastery of the emotions involves knowing the K'o Cycle of control. The controlling emotion is the antidote of the emotion it controls. Fear is controlled by empathy, not by love or joy as is often thought. You can tell someone who is afraid that you love him or her, and it does absolutely no good. But if you tell the person that you understand, the fear lessens. If you tell a child who just fell down, "Mommy loves you," it does not help. But if you look the child in the eye and say, "Hey, that must really hurt," he or she stops cold, looks up at you, and says, "Yes, it does hurt." The child experiences that you know the feeling. I treated a man who was beaten and robbed. He had received a lot of love from others, but he still had numerous symptoms. When I empathized with his fear, he fully recovered. Empathy is the antidote.

Joy/Sorrow.   We often use empathy as the antidote for sadness with very disappointing results. When we say to a friend whose mother has just died, "I know how you feel," the reaction is, "You can't possibly know how I feel. This is my experience, not yours." Yet if we put our hand on the friend's shoulder and tell him that we care, the grief starts to subside. The antidote for grief is love and joy. Joy is a major preventer and cure of depression.

Anger/Sympathy.   Anger is the antidote for sympathy. There are people who are grand victims, and they carry a sign that says, "Give me sympathy." On their back, they have another sign that says, "I am a doormat, step on me." These people are sympathy sponges that will soak up every ounce of your energy and still not be satisfied. They usually evoke an angry reaction.

I saw a woman in the emergency room who was receiving intravenous medication to treat her asthma. She was not responding to any of the drugs, because she was wailing on and on about how nobody understood her. I walked in on this scene and I said, "Stop it, enough. Shut up." The residents thought my bedside manner left something to be desired. I said to her, "Your job is to stop wheezing. It is not to lie here and moan. Your problems will not be solved in this emergency room. The only thing that will be decided here is whether we take you out of here in a box or we move you up to a bed. Your job is to stop wheezing, and we are giving you the best medicines to help you do the job." Even as I said this, you could hear the wheezing subside. This patient never had another emergency room visit. When she began to wheeze, she would call me, and I helped her get in touch with her own anger; the wheezing always stopped.

The best way to obtain sympathy is to ask for it. Simply say to a friend, "Jean, I need some sympathy. How about it?" If she agrees, you have your sympathy. Or she may say, "I'm tired; I can't give you any right now, wait until later. Let's have a drink first and relax." All sympathy needs can be met this way.

Grief/Anger. Some say sadness is a quiet anger. That is an interesting observation because grief is the antidote for and controller of anger. If you react to anger with sadness, it helps to express it: "It makes me sad seeing you angry." Very often this response will dissipate the anger. When I was a junior medical student, I was asked to draw blood from a man who had just beaten up six police officers. As I entered the room, he screamed at me, "What do you want?" He was a giant of a man, and I trembled as I explained. He became even angrier and refused to cooperate. I looked up at him and said, "You know, it really makes me sad to see you like this." Immediately he went from violent to peaceful, and I had no problem carrying out my assignment. The expression of grief did it. Of course, it cannot be phony. Often we use sympathy to try to deal with anger, but generally it does not work.

SYSTEMS OF DIAGNOSIS AND THERAPY

The Law of Five Elements chart is not only a map of the universe, nature, and ourselves, but also an exquisite diagnostic system. The Chinese used all of the correspondences and associations (Table 3.2), including color, the sound of the voice, the predominant emotion, the smell, as well as the pulses on the wrist, and dreams to diagnose imbalance, predisposition to imbalance, and the type and extent of imbalance.

The art of diagnosis aims to evaluate the state of balance and harmony of the Ch'i, the Life Force, the Universal Energy. We already noted that excesses or deficiencies indicate lack of balance. Statements such as "I prefer summer," "I like green," "I enjoy liver," "I don't especially care for liver," "I am not fond of blue," may indicate balance. Those who say, "I can't stand summer," "I despise blue," "I detest red," "I can't live without eating liver several times a week," are manifesting excesses and show a lack of balance or harmony in an element.

In the diagnostic system, the law of mother/child must be borne in mind. According to it, if the mother becomes sick, she cannot nurture the child, and it, in turn, becomes ill. Thus, an imbalance in a particular element may be due to the imbalance in the mother of that element.

An imbalance in the flow of Ch'i that controls Wood may result in disease in the liver or gallbladder, in a craving or avoidance of sour tastes, in abnormal anger and resentment, and in acute and chronic back pain. However, the imbalance also may cause the child—Fire—to scream, so that the person may have symptoms in the heart, circulation, sexual organs, endocrine system, and so on.

Imbalance in the flow of Ch'i energy that controls Water may show up as kidney disease; a craving for salt or avoidance of it; excess fear; lack of willpower, drive, or resolve; sexual inadequacy; and problems with cold. A person can even have pain radiating on a meridian pathway that makes no sense to Western doctors. Such pain is then diagnosed as psychosomatic. But the problem is readily made clear by a practitioner skilled in Chinese medicine. (See also Pachuta, Branson, & Measures, 1973.)

Color

A person in a state of disharmony is predominantly colored with one or more of the following five colors, regardless of skin color. Green is the color of anger (Wood). We are all familiar with the expression, "Green with envy." Envy is an intellectualization of anger. In England they say, "You look livery." The liver and gallbladder are on the green circle and are associated with anger. We say, "He has a lot of gall." That comes from a place of anger. Red is the color of joy (Fire); yellow is the color of empathy (Earth); white is the color of grief (Metal); blue is the color of fear (Water). With training and by letting go of your barriers, it is not hard to see these colors. The color, of course, is associated with all the other correspondences of that element.

Sound

The sound of anger is shouting. Some people's voices grate your eardrums even when they are speaking softly; others seem to be yelling all the time. The sound of joy is laughing. A laughing voice contains a "ha, ha, ha" regardless of the content. A laughing voice generally indicates an imbalance in the Fire element. Of course, it may also point to a problem in the mother of Fire (Wood). The singing voice of Earth, or sympathy, often brings out anger in the listener, because it sings all the time, regardless of the content. The voice of Metal, or sadness, is a weeping voice or crying. Some people sound as if they are weeping even at times of great joy. The voice of Water, or fear, is a groaning voice. Some people groan all the time, even if they win the lottery.

Taste

Each of the elements has an associated taste. The taste of Wood is sour; the taste of Fire is bitter; the taste of Earth is sweet; the taste of

Metal is pungent; and the taste of Water is salty. A craving or aversion for a particular taste can indicate an imbalance in an element. It is interesting that the ancient Chinese associated the Earth element with the spleen/pancreas and a sweet taste, even though they did not know about diabetes.

Odor

Odor also provides much diagnostic information. The odor of Fire is scorched or burnt; the odor of Earth is fragrant; the odor of Metal is rotten; the odor of Water is putrid; and the odor of Wood is rancid. For instance, a patient I saw with acute abdominal pain emitted an odor like perfume, which helped me diagnose an infarct in his spleen, an Earth organ. Another patient smelled distinctly like burned pipe tobacco (Fire). He had chronic hepatitis. The liver is associated with the Wood element, which is the mother of Fire. This is an example of the child screaming when the mother is ill.

Pulses

Each of the 12 officials has a pulse. These pulses, six on each wrist, tell a skilled practitioner a great deal. After watching a famous practitioner take a pulse, a cardiologist said, "I, who have taken a hundred thousand pulses, realized that I had never even taken one."

In the Western system, a person who has a pulse of plus three might be considered to be better off than the one who has minus three. In the Chinese system, the two conditions are equally undesirable, for zero represents balance and harmony.

Dreams

Imbalance also can be revealed in dreams, either by the predominance or absence of a particular element or of correspondences of that element. Dreams of flames, burning, or searching for fire can reveal an imbalance in the Fire element. Dreams associated with the Earth element could involve an excess or lack of food, the predominance or absence of the color yellow, a fragrant odor, a sweet taste, and so on. Since Earth is associated with assimilation and connection, dreams of disconnection or lack of association with others also could indicate an imbalance in the Earth element. Dreams associated with Metal could contain metal objects, the color white, weeping, a rotten odor, a pungent taste, or flying through the air. Dreams associated with the Water element could involve ships, the color blue, fear, groaning, a salty taste, or a putrid odor. Dreams of Wood could focus on plants, forests, the color green, anger, a sour taste, and a rancid smell. In the interpretation of dreams, we must always keep in mind the law of mother/child. For instance, a dream of fire may indicate an imbalance in the Wood element, and so on.

The Chinese system of healing includes a variety of therapies, such as traditional acupuncture, mantra therapy, herbal therapy, and even behavioral therapy. These are no therapists, only teachers of a Way of Life for the whole bodymindemotionspirit, and all therapies, no matter how different, are directed at altering an unbalanced Ch'i.

Causative Factors

The Chinese propose seven external and seven internal causative factors of disease. The number 7 is somewhat mystical. The seven external causative factors of disease are cold, heat, humidity, fire, dryness, dampness, and wind. Originally there were only five internal causative factors. These were the five emotions: excess or lack of joy, sympathy, grief, fear, and anger. Later the Chinese added two additional factors: anxiety and constitutional or hereditary factors.

CONCLUDING REMARKS

The people who know the most about the Chinese system say that they know little and will never master it in one lifetime. It is awe inspiring by its breadth; it provides an exquisitely beautiful map of nature and the universe. Yet it also is reassuring by indicating man's place in this all-encompassing scheme. Lao Tzu provides us with a wonderful summary of the Tao:

Empty yourself of everything.
Let the mind rest in peace.
The ten thousand things rise and fall while the Self watches their return.
They grow and flourish and then return to the source.
Returning to the source is stillness, which is the way of nature.
The way of nature is unchanging.
Knowing constancy is insight.
Not knowing constancy leads to disaster.
Knowing constancy, the mind is open.
With an open mind, you will be open-hearted.
Being open-hearted, you will act royally.
Being royal, you will attain the divine.

Being divine, you will be at one with the Tao.
Being at one with the Tao is eternal.
And though the body dies, the Tao will never pass away.[5]

(Feng & English, 1972, pl 16)

References

Bean, W. B. (Ed.) (1950). *Sir William Osler, aphorism from his bedside teachings and writings.* New York: Henry Schuman.

Easwaran, E. (Trans.) (1985). *Bhagavad Gita.* Petaluma, CA: Nilgini Press.

Connelly, D. M. (1979). *Traditional acupuncture: The law of the five elements.* Columbia, MD: The Centre for Traditional Acupuncture.

Feng, G. F., & English, J. (Trans.) (1972). *Lao Tsu: Tao Te Ching.* New York: Vintage Books.

Larre, C., Schatz, J., & de la Vallee, E. R. (1979). *Survey of traditional Chinese medicine.* Sarah Elizabeth Stang (Trans.). Columbia, MD: Traditional Acupuncture Foundation.

Pachuta, D. M. (1981). The integration of east and west. *Journal of Traditional Acupuncture, 7:1,* 29–34.

Pachuta, D. M. (1987). *The life you save may be your own.* Baltimore: Institute for Learning Mastery Press.

Pachuta, D. M., Branson, B. M., & Measures, J. (1983). Acupuncture and other adjunct therapy in the treatment of acquired immunodeficiency syndrome. *Journal of Traditional Acupuncture, 7:2,* pp. 27–30.

Porkert, M. (1974). *Theoretical foundations of Chinese medicine: Systems of correspondence.* Cambridge, MA: The MIT Press.

Reps, P. (1957). *Zen Flesh, Zen Bones.* Rutland, VT: Tuttle.

Veith, I., (Trans.) (1972). *Nei Ching: The Yellow Emperor's Classic of Internal Medicine.* Berkeley, CA: University of California Press.

Watts, A. (1975). *Tao, the watercourse way.* New York: Pantheon Books.

Worsley, J. R. (1973). *Is acupuncture for you?* New York: Harper & Row.

Worsley, J. R. (1982). *Traditional Chinese acupuncture. vol. 1. Meridian and points.* Tisbury, Wiltshire, England: Element Books.

---

[5]From *Tao Te Ching* by Lao Tzu. Translated by Gia-Fu Feng and Jane English. Copyright © 1972 by Gia-Fu Feng and Jane English. Reprinted by permission of Alfred A. Knopf, Inc.

4

Buddhist Psychology: Implications for Healing

SUNDAR RAMASWAMI
ANEES A. SHEIKH

Such was the Buddha's impact that people sometimes felt he must be something more than human. "Are you a god?" they asked. "No." "Are you an angel?" "No." "A saint?" "No." "Then what are you?" they asked. "I am awake," replied the Buddha.

Smith, 1958; Walsh, 1983

Gautama Siddhartha, who after his enlightenment was hailed as the Buddha, was born more than 500 years before Christ. It was a time when Confucius was sharing his wisdom in China and a new age was dawning in Greece. Humanity was poised to invent its first philosophy. Thales of Miletus, Pythagoras of Samos, and Alcmaeon of Groton were laying the foundations of Western civilization even as the Buddha was preparing to enlighten India.

Siddhartha was nurtured in a Hindu family; consequently, it is not surprising that Buddhism retains many Hindu concepts. Yet, the Buddha dramatically altered the world view of his day, representing an evolutionary ideal that people could attain through their own efforts. The "eightfold path" of Buddhist thought may be considered a series of ethical techniques for the psychological maturation of human beings and consists of the following: right views, right resolve, right speech, right action, right livelihood, right effort, right mindfulness, and right concentration.

Joy Manne-Lewis (1986) has analyzed the constructs pertaining to the attainment of enlightenment by the Buddha and refers to them as the "axioms of the psychology of enlightenment." They are:

1. There exists a state of Enlightenment.
2. Enlightenment is attainable by a person.
3. There is a method for the attainment of Enlightenment.
4. There are discrete, ordered stages leading to Enlightenment.
5. Enlightenment is both a cognitive and an affective state.

The aim is the cultivation of certain mental qualities that characterize the highest levels of enlightenment—qualities that are extolled by all the great religious and consciousness disciplines. In Buddhist psychology, some of these qualities are called the 10 *paramitas* or perfections. "The ten *paramitas* might be thought of as involving five overlapping categories: effort (determination and energy), ethics (ethicality and truthfulness), nonattachment (renunciation, patience, and equanimity), service to others (generosity and living kindness), and wisdom" (Walsh, 1983, p. 219). This goal is best understood in the context of the psychological formulations of Buddhism.

This chapter confines itself to those psychological constructs advanced by the *Theravada (Hinayana)* school of Buddhism, a school regarded as being closer to the original teachings of the Buddha. It is beyond the scope of this chapter to examine the postulations of the other major school, *Mahayana* Buddhism. The psychological inquiries of *Theravada* Buddhism are contained both in the discourses of the Buddha and its elaboration by later commentators. The discourses, collectively called *Sutta Pitaka*, consist of several *nikayas*, or sayings (e.g., *Arguttara Nikaya*, Gradual Sayings). The elaboration of the original discourses by later Buddhist commentators is called the *Abhidhamma*, literally, beyond the original teaching.

THE BUDDHIST CONCEPT OF SELF

There is no contrast, in Buddhism and other religions, more significant than that of their notions of self. Western concepts of self can be traced back either to Plato or Aristotle and their Christian interpreters, St. Augustine and St. Thomas Aquinas. Both the Platonic-Augustinian tradition and the Aristotelian-Thomistic tradition affirm the existence of an individual soul. The Vedic literature of ancient India, too, posited an individual soul that was transported to heaven after death by the fire god, Agni, who consumed the physical body at cremation. Later, the Upanishadic philosophers proclaimed that the individual soul or *Atman* was in its essence identical with *Brahman*, the ground of all existence, the eternal substrate of the universe.

In a radical departure from the prevailing Hindu view of self, the Buddha denied the existence of a permanent soul or self. He proclaimed that the notion of self is false and that there is no individual or abiding self apart from a cluster of factors.

> What is called "soul" or "thing" is a mere name—a name for a complex of constituents. The concept of a soul as the substrate of the changing states of consciousness, or of a thing as the bearer of attributes is a myth. There is no unity holding together the states or the attributes. (Mahadevan, 1974, p. 122)

According to the Buddha, the person is made up of five factors or *skandhas:* material form (body), perception, sensation, consciousness, and mental acts (ideas, volitional action, etc.). The person does exist in a conventional sense: the "I" is a useful linguistic device to refer to the ever-changing physical and mental elements that constitute the individual. But in an absolute sense, in the sense of a permanent substance created by God, surviving death, uniting with God, or going to hell or heaven, the "I" is an illusion. Thus, when one says, "This is my house," one inserts a fictitious self into the actuality of one's experience. Psychopathology results when this fictitious "I" claims for itself bits and pieces of the universe (Conze, 1975).

> Life is a continuous being without a beginning or an end. . . . There is no static moment when the becoming attains to beinghood. No sooner than we conceive it by the attributes of name and form than it has changed to something else. How do we come to think of things, rather than of processes in this absolute flux? By shutting our eyes to the successive events. It is an artificial attitude that makes sections in the stream of change, and calls them things. Identity of objects is an unreality. (Radhakrishnan, 1951, p. 369)

The combination of mental and material qualities—the *skandhas*— makes up the individual. It is this psychophysical complex that gives rise to individuality. The physical and mental elements that constitute the individual are forever changing and are extinguished only when desire for existence is extinguished. The *skandhas* are an ever-changing bundle from moment to moment and from birth to birth. The only continuous thread is *bhava*, or continuity of consciousness over time.

There are only mental states: thoughts, emotions, memories, sensations, and perceptions. There is no "I" behind them; yet, without them there is no sense of "I." The "I" derives its existence from these mental states. The "I," says Rahula (1962, p. 65), is "like the smell of a flower: it is neither the smell of the petals, nor of the colour, nor of the pollen, but the smell of the flower."

Individuality is merely the result of the basic unifying tendency of life. Every living being tends to organize a unity, to create a center, a core. This center, by organizing and assimilating various elements, maintains the structure of the individual. This tendency to create a center is called *ahamkara* or the *principium indivuationis*. It is this principle that calls itself "I" and confers self-consciousness. But this central principle soon exceeds its legitimate functions and constructs a separate, permanent ego that is in contrast to the rest of the world. It is this split that is the cause of conflict (Govinda, 1961). This self-consciousness, which is the result of the illusion of a separate ego, fetters the individual like a bird in a cage. To Buddhism, the illusion of a separate self is original sin. It is the cause of evil, of death, and of all the sorrows to which mortals are heir.

The separate ego regards itself as subject and views everything else as objects—it is the "knower" in contrast to objects that are known. What is the relationship of this self to various mental states? Mental states are regarded as objects by the self, which looks at them from a distance, from the outside. According to Buddhism, this division of mental contents into a subjective self and objective mental states is a great error. All mental states are subjective and not objects of a subject, since the self is but a series of mental states.

If they are only mental states, how does Buddhism account for personality? Bhattacharya (1963, p. 220) suggests that although Buddhism denies a definite, self-contained self it does concede an indefinite self. He described this indefinite self as a series of items that is nothing *over and above* the items, and yet it is not absolutely identical with them. The self is the series of mental states; this series is not identical to the items that make up the series nor is it totally different from them. According to Bhattacharya (1963, p. 221), personality can "as much center round such indefinite self as round a self that is definite." This notion of indefinite self is vital to the doctrines of *karma* and rebirth.

CONCEPT OF PERSONALITY

In Buddhism, personality does not refer to entities such as the "ego" or the "unconscious" but to a complex aggregate of processes. It is from the continuous flow of these processes that the semblance of personality arises. The person is comprised of five aggregates of *skandhas:* matter, feeling, perception, mental formation, and consciousness.

The Aggregate of Matter (Rupa khandha)

The primary qualities of matter are considered to be solidity, fluidity, heat (fire element), and motion (air element). There are also the following derived qualities: eye, ear, nose, tongue, body, visible form, sound, odor, flavor, femininity, masculinity, life faculty, heart basis, bodily intimation, verbal intimation, space element, lightness of matter, malleability, wieldiness of matter, growth, continuity, aging of matter, impermanence of matter, and physical nutriment. The first five derived qualities (eye, ear, nose, tongue, and body) are regarded as internal qualities; the remaining are regarded as external.

The Aggregate of Feeling (Vedanakhandha)

Vedana is that which is felt. Buddhaghosa (1976) grouped *vedana* in several ways. Basically, all feelings can be classified as pleasant, painful, or neutral. This threefold classification becomes fivefold with the added differentiation of bodily or mental feelings: bodily pleasurable, bodily painful, mentally pleasurable (joy), mentally painful (grief), and feelings of indifference (equanimity). Feelings of joy and equanimity are associated with the *jhanas*—that is, the higher states of consciousness—which will be described later. Bodily pain (*kayika dukka*) is produced as a result of bodily contact, and grief (*domanassa*) is a mental pain produced through mental contact.

The Buddha distinguished between sensory pleasures and the feelings of rapture that are a by-product of meditation:

Here, Ananda, a monk, aloof from pleasures of the senses, aloof from unskilled states of mind, enters and abides in the first meditation that is accompanied by initial thought and discursive thought, is born of aloofness and is rapturous and joyful. This, Ananda, is the other happiness that is more excellent and exquisite than that happiness. (*Middle Length Sayings,* 1954–1959, vol. II, p. 67)

Sense pleasures are regarded as "gross" in that they lead to attachment and lust. The pleasure felt in the *jhanic* states is a higher pleasure since it is free of attachment.

The Buddha recognized that painful feelings can be internally generated from bile and phlegm, bodily humors, and changes in seasons. These painful feelings, as well as the pain of physical illness, cannot be avoided even by an *arahat* (a Buddhist saint). But an *arahat's* pain is only physical with no emotional overtones: he or she maintains his or her equanimity and does not show aversion.

> If a monk sees a delightful object with the eye, he does not hanker for it, does not thrill thereat, does not develop lust for it. His body is unmoved, his mind is unmoved, inwardly well established and released. If he sees a repulsive object with the eye, he is not shocked thereat, his mind is not unsettled or depressed or resentful because of that. (*Samyutta Nikaya*, 1884–1904, vol. V, p. 74)

The Aggregate of Perception (Sanna)

Perception is divided into the same three types as is the aggregate of feeling—that is, pleasurable, painful, and neutral. Since there cannot be a state of consciousness divorced from perception, perception has 89 divisions—the same number as consciousness (Buddhaghosa, 1976). Perception is further divided into sensuous and nonsensuous perception.

Perception (*sanna*) is one of the four mental aggregates of the person. The exact translation of the term *sanna* presents some difficulties, for in the Buddhist texts it means different things in different contexts. In the early texts, *sanna* was used to refer to consciousness and was roughly synonymous with *vinnana*. *Sanna* also was described as a faculty of discrimination that distinguished between various perceptual events. Again, there is little difference between *sanna* and *vinnana* (Rhys-Davids, 1978). In the *Nikayas, sanna* is said to occur after *vinnana*, which means that *vinnana* may be interpreted as *perception* and *sanna* may be regarded as a later activity that distinguishes the perception by selective attention.

The Aggregate of Mental Formations (Sankharas)

The *sankharas* or mental formations encompass volitional and conational activities. The term *sankhara* has been translated as habit, craving, effort, and volitions leading to *karma* formations. Johannsson (1979) distinguished four meanings: perceived things, mental contents, activities, and dynamic processes. In the *Samyutta Nikaya* (1884–1904), certain kinds of possessions, such as palaces, elephants, chariots, and jewels are referred to as *sankhara*. The *Samyutta Nikaya* also refers to functions such as speech, thought, reasoning, and ideations as *sankharas*. Certain kinds of erroneous beliefs also are called *sankharas*. The *Majjhima Nikaya* (1948–1951) classified *sankhara* into three categories: breathing as body-*sankhara*; thought, reasoning, and speech as speech-*sankhara*; and ideations as mind-*sankhara*.

According to the Buddha, volitional acts can be expressed through three doorways—body, speech, or mind. Hence, the classification of *sankharas* as bodily formations (*kaya-sankhara*), verbal formations (*vaci-sankhara*), and mental formations (*mano-sankhara*) finds support from several scholars (de Silva, 1979; Dhammaratana, 1964).

The *Samyutta Nikaya* also defined *sankhara* as will or intention, and the *Anguttara Nikaya* (1885–1900) described *sankhara* as *karma* or action. Johannsson (1979) said that this analysis defines *sankhara* as an intentional act pertaining to any of the six sensory modalities.

Sankharas form a link in the chain of Interdependent Origination and are conditioned ultimately by ignorance. Since Buddhism aims at the destruction of ignorance, its aim also is to eradicate the *sankharas*. For example, in the first *jhana*, the *sankhara* of speech ceases; in the fourth, the *sankhara* of body stops; and later, the *sankharas* of ideation and sensation fade (Johannsson, 1979).

The *arahat*, the awakened one, is supposedly free of all *sankharas*. However, since he or she continues to exist, the *sankharas* remain as one of the *skandhas*. Therefore, it may be more accurate to say that the *arahat* does not generate *sankharas* leading to *karmic* effects.

The Aggregate of Consciousness (Vinnana)

Vinnana, or consciousness, makes up the third link in the chain of Dependent Origination and is one of the five personality factors. *Namarupa*—name and form—is supposedly conditioned by consciousness. *Vinnana* plays a crucial role in the process of rebirth. The *Digha Nikaya* (1890–1911) described the descent of consciousness as a descent into the mother's womb. In the *Anguttara Nikaya* (1885–1900) it was likened to a seed "which will grow if it is planted into the field of action (*kamma*) and is watered by craving (*tanha*)" (Johannsson, 1979, p. 57). However, it would be erroneous to conclude that the descent into the womb implies the postmortem survival of consciousness. At death, *vinnana* transmits *karma* to a new being and provides the impulse for the development of a new consciousness, and the "old" *vinnana* disintegrates.

BHAVANGA: THE BUDDHIST UNCONSCIOUS

The word *bhavanga* first made its appearance in the *Milindapanha* (Basu, 1978). In answer to the king's questions on the sleep state, Nagasena stated that in deep sleep the mind goes into *bhavanga*, although the bodily processes continue to function.

In the *Nikayas*, mind was regarded as empirical consciousness. This empirical consciousness was active during the wakeful state and could be transcended in the higher states of consciousness. But what happens to the mind in dream and sleep states? The rival Brahmanical school had its own explanation. According to the Upanishads, in deep sleep the soul returns to *Brahman*, the state of Pure Consciousness, and is temporarily absorbed in *Brahman*. The wakeful state is, therefore, a return from *Brahman*.

To the Buddhists *bhavanga* came to mean both a factor and a cause of existence. It is the cause of "the unbroken continuity of the individual in various existences" (Sarathchandra, 1958, pp. 80–81). Buddhaghosa (1976) likened *bhavanga* to the perennial flow of a river, and Sarathchandra (1958, p. 80) described it as the "unbroken flow of unconscious life within the individual mind."

Buddhist psychologists then proceeded to use *bhavanga* to explain intuition, the relationship between *jhana* (higher consciouness) and ordinary empirical consciousness, postmortem survival, and the states of sleep, trance, and dream. Nyanatiloka (1950, 1971) said that impressions and experiences are stored in *bhavanga*, from which they occasionally approach the threshold of full consciousness. Thus, *bhavanga* explains memory, *karma*, and rebirth.

Buddhaghosa (1976) suggested a link between the *bhavanga* of an individual at the time of his or her death and his or her *bhavanga* at the time of rebirth, thus establishing continuity between lives. At rebirth, consciousness is said to receive the dying thoughts; thus, one's consciousness and the moral tone of one's life are affected by one's previous life. There are three kinds of dying thoughts: *karma*, *karma-nimitta*, and *gatinimitta*.

Karma, as we have seen, is the motive force of one's good and bad actions. According to Sarathchandra (1958), this motive force revives in the dying person memories of his or her good and bad actions; all these memories are distilled into the last thought. *Karma-nimitta* refers to the physical object that was involved in the performance of a moral act. For example, if the dying person had donated funds for the building of a hospital, then at the instant of death the image of the hospital would arise in his or her mind, thereby guaranteeing a befitting rebirth. *Gatinimitta* refers to the indication (in the form of a mental image) of a person's future fate perceived by that person at the moment of death. These elaborate explanations serve to emphasize the continuity of *bhavanga* from one life to another.

Mind in its vacant condition is *vithimutta* (thought-free). In its active condition, it was known as *vithicitta*. *Bhavanga* is the natural, pristine condition of the mind; when this condition is interrupted by thought, cognitive processes begin.

Anasuya

Anasuya is an unconscious impulse, a dormant disposition, or a latent tendency. *Anasuyas* are tenacious by nature; they have embedded themselves in the unconscious and are the foundation of our baser reactions (e.g., anger and greed). According to de Silva (1973), the anasuyas are irrational and impulsive:

1. The *anasuya* of craving (*kamaroga*)
2. The *anasuya* of anger (*patigha*)
3. The *anasuya* of conceit (*mana*)
4. The *anasuya* of ignorance (*avijja*)

The *anasuyas* differ in their strengths; some are easier to eradicate than others. Certain *anasuyas* go together—for example, the *anasuyas* of *roga* (greed) and *patigha* (anger).

Buddhist psychology regards these latent tendencies to be present at birth. The *Majjhima Nikaya* (1948–1951) said that the *anasuyas* of *byapadanusuya* (a leaning of malevolence), *silabbataparamasanasuya* (a leaning to rites and customs), *vicikicchanasuya* (a tendency to perplexity), and *sakkayadittanasuya* (a tendency to love one's body) are latent in the newborn infant.

The *anasuyas*, Buddhist psychology holds, have evolved through numerous previous lives and serve to explain certain personality traits. According to de Silva (1973), the *kamaroga anasuya* (craving) is similar to the libido theory, the *patigha anasuya* (anger) resembles the death instinct, and the *anasuyas* of *mana* (conceit), *dittha* (wrong opinion), and *bhavaraga* (craving for existence) are similar to the ego instinct.

The *anasuyas* pass through three stages before they can have an impact on behavior (Buddhaghosa, 1976). The first stage is *Anasuyabhumi*, or a latency period, during which the *anasuyas* lie dormant in *bhavanga*

(Sayadaw, 1961). In the second stage, *Paariyutthana-bhumi,* the *anasuyas* manifest themselves as thought processes. In the third stage, *Vitikamma-bhumi,* the *anasuyas* become overpowering and lead to sinful transgressions. Thus, the *anasuyas* exert a powerful influence on our behavior, an influence of which we are unconscious.

The *anasuyas* can be overcome through the practice of meditation. Every higher *jhana* progressively eliminates the *anasuyas,* and the mind of the *arahat* is completely free of the *anasuyas.*

Asava

De Silva (1973) compared the *asavas* to the Freudian id. There are four *asavas:* sensuality, lust for life, speculation, and ignorance. The word *asava* literally means "flowing toward," and it has been translated as "canker" or "influx." The term canker suggests "that which frets, corrodes, corrupts or consumes slowly and secretly" (de Silva, 1973, pp. 61–62). The *asavas* are also regarded as intoxicants that diminish the power of reason. The various meanings given to the *asavas* suggest that they represent the primitive, untrammeled side of human beings.

THE BUDDHIST AND FREUDIAN UNCONSCIOUS

According to Brunswick (1959), the true psychoanalytic meaning of the unconscious is dispositional. De Silva (1973) asserted that to Freud unconscious tendencies are but a special case of latent dispositions. These views suggest that the Buddhist unconscious, with its dispositions and latent tendencies (the *anasuyas*), is similar to the concept of Freud.

The Freudian unconscious is accessible only through special techniques, such as deep hypnosis or free association. In Buddhist psychology, too, the unconscious can be known only through special methods, such as telepathy or extrasensory perception acquired through meditational practices.

The Freudian unconscious has life and death instincts and the libido for its contents. They are comparable to the threefold drives of Buddhist psychology—*kama-tanha* (drive for sensuous gratification), *bhava-tanha* (drive for self-preservation), and *vighava-tanha* (the aggressive drive).

Unlike the Freudian unconscious, the unconscious in Buddhism contains both bad and good dispositions. De Silva (1973), proposes that the *sankharas,* which he regards as unconscious contents, consists of both good and bad dispositions. As we have already noted, the *sankharas* influence behavior not only in this life, but also determine the course of one's next life.

COGNITION

In Buddhist psychology, the entire process of perception takes 17 thought-moments and includes the following stages: perception of sense-object, vibration of life-continuum, awareness, receiving or assimilation, investigating or discriminating, determining, and, finally, complete apperception or cognition. The process takes 17 thought-moments only if the sensory stimuli are powerful. If the sensory stimuli are weak, the process may take 15 moments, because *javana* (full cognition) is absent.

A similar process occurs when a mental object comes within the sensory field of the mind, since the latter was considered a sixth sense organ. The mind was regarded as a sense organ sensitive to ideas, memories, imaginings, and thoughts.

Sarathchandra (1958) translated the stage of *javana* as cognition. Thus, cognition is the final step in the perceptual process. However, the earlier steps in the perceptual process all involve cognitive activity.

The Buddhist cognitive terms include *vitakka* (thinking) and *vicara* (reasoning). Two types of *vitakka* are distinguished: (1) *kama vitakka, byapadia vitakka,* and *vihimsa vitakka* (thoughts of love, of aggression, and of harming) and (2) *nekkhamma vitakka, abyapada vitakka, avihimsa vitakka* (thoughts of renunciation, of nonaggression, and of not harming). The former are *akusala* (unwholesome), and the latter are *kusala* (wholesome).

Thinking is also analyzed according to the sense modalities involved: *rupa vitakka* (visual thought), *sada vitakka* (auditory thought), *gandha vitakka* (olfactory thought), *rasa vitakka* (gustatory thought), *photthabba vitakka* (tactual thought), and *dhamma vitakka* (ideational thought). *Vitakka* is also regarded as speech activity, since speech follows thought (Johannsson, 1979). Also, thought and intention go together. Thus, in the *Nikayas, vitakka* is closely allied to *sankappa* (intention). *Vitakka* can lead to *chanda* (ambition), *tanha* (craving), or *papanca,* which is the "tendency to produce associations, wishful dreams and analytic thought" (Johannsson, 1979, p. 195).

The term *paccavakkhati* is used to denote introspection, while *sati* and *sampajana* refer to mindfulness and mental composure, respectively. In meditation, all types of thought gradually cease. To attain the first *samadhi* (concentration), all unwholesome thoughts should be discarded.

If this is difficult, the meditator should actively cultivate good thoughts. In the fourth level of *samadhi*, discursive thinking ceases.

As mentioned earlier, Buddhism regards extrasensory perception as a valid means of knowing. The Pali word for extrasensory perception is *dassana*. Two kinds of *dassanas* are mentioned: *vimutti-nana dassana*, or knowledge and insight of salvation, and *yathabhuta-nana dassana*, or knowledge of things as they are (de Silva, 1979).

Panna, or wisdom, is the highest type of cognition in Buddhist psychology. The Doctrine of Interdependent Origin, which explains the cause of sorrow by spanning one's past life, current life, and a future rebirth, rests on ignorance that can be eliminated by developing *panna*. *Sati* (mindfulness), *dhamma* (literally, *law*), *viriya* (energy), *piti* (bliss), *passaddhi* (tranquility), *samadhi* (concentration), and *upekkha* (equanimity) are the elements that foster *panna*.

Panna is regarded as an intellectual tool that penetrates ignorance. *Panna* is understanding *par excellence*. It is *panna* that enables one to understand the Doctrine of Interdependent Origin, the Four Noble Truths, and the facts of *anatta*, *anicca*, and *dukkha*. Johannsson (1979) made it clear that *panna* is not mere knowledge. "Knowledge is then not enough; more important is it to examine and understand. *Panna* refers to a conscious, especially visual clarification of facts, laws and doctrines. To understand it is to see relations and connections" (p. 198).

In the *Anguttara Nikaya* (1885–1900), *panna* is described as one of the four lamps, the other three being the sun, the moon, and fire.

CONSCIOUSNESS

According to Buddhism, consciousness is a relationship between the subject (*arammanika*) and an object (*arammana*). The interaction between the two produces a resultant consciousness that is a product of a number of variables of both subject and object (Rao, 1978). Based on the characteristics of the resultant consciousness, 89 states of consciousness were delineated by the early Buddhist psychologists.

From the point of view of *Nirvana*, two modes of consciousness were identified: directed consciousness and undirected consciousness.

> Directed consciousness is that which, in recognition of the goal, has entered the stream and is wholly bent upon freedom, which means that the decisive reversal of attitude has ensured. Undirected consciousness, on the contrary, allows itself to be driven hither and thither by instinct-born motives and external impressions. (Govinda, 1974, p. 80)

These two modes are labeled worldly or mundane consciousness, and *Nirvana* is considered supramundane. *Nirvana*, which entails extinction of desire, is ultimate reality. It is regarded as the highest good or perfection and positive bliss. It is the cessation of all mental constrictions, the absence of ignorance, the ending of sorrow. *Nirvana* is emptiness in the sense that it is empty of "self." It is freedom from craving, time, duality, and becoming.

From the point of view of objects, consciousness is designated as the material and the immaterial, or the limited and the unlimited. These two divisions distinguish between objects perceivable through the senses and objects perceivable only through the mind.

The subject is said to live on one of four realms of existence—three planes of consciousness and one transcendental plane. These planes of existence are not to be sought in the mysteries of space, for they are found in one's own mind. The sensual plane is the domain of form bound by craving (*kamadhatu*); the immaterial plane is the domain of the formless (*arupadhatu*) and is free of craving. The fine material plane is the domain of pure form (*rupadhatu*). The objects in this plane possess shape and form; therefore, they cannot belong to the realm of the formless. However, these objects cannot belong to the realm of sensuous craving, since they are free from craving and ego entanglement. The domain of pure form is one of intuitive contemplation of form (Govinda, 1974).

In the sensuous domain (*kamadhatu*), a tension is said to exist between the subject and the object. In the other two planes, the objects of consciousness are freed of ego entanglement. There is no "I" involvement in these two planes. Thus, we have three planes of consciousness: consciousness that dwells in the realm of sensuous craving, consciousness that dwells in the realm of pure form, and consciousness that dwells in the realm of the formless (Govinda, 1974).

The fourth and last plane is the supramundane or transcendental plane. It is called *lokuttara* (literally, "beyond worlds"). This is the plane that is associated with *Nirvana*.

According to Dhammaratana (1964), consciousness is threefold according to its ethical nature: wholesome, unwholesome, and indeterminate. Every type of consciousness is said to be motivated by the mental attitude of the individual, this attitude is regarded as the "root cause" that conditions consciousness. Passive states of consciousness that result from sensory impressions are regarded as not conditioned by root causes and hence are morally neutral (indeterminate). Whether a type of consciousness is moral (wholesome) or immoral (unwholesome) is dependent on whether it is conducive to the goal of *Nirvana*. Also, only *Nirvana* can bring about radical and permanent changes in one's mental make-up. The *arahat's* mind is completely free of unhealthy mental factors.

It should be noted that in the Buddhist view of the nature of consciousness is essentially open and unconditioned.

> This open, receptive awareness is essentially free from habitual fixations and narrow self-limiting concerns. It fully reflects and resonates the world, the process of *what is* at every moment. . . . Mind represents an open space for unconditioned presence in the world, a unique source of new meaning, creativity, spontaneity, freedom, peace and compassion. (Welwood, 1979, p. 4)

MENTAL HEALTH IN BUDDHIST PSYCHOLOGY

The Buddha is often called the Supreme Healer. He embodied the qualities of the ideal physician—serene detachment and selfless compassion—moreover, he devoted his life to the alleviation of human sorrow (Birnbaum, 1979).

According to the *Abhidhamma*, physical illness is often the consequence of unhealthy mental states. Inner poisons, such as lust and anger, cause physiological imbalances in bile and phlegm that activate disease states. This view is amazingly contemporary: the increasing recognition of the role that the mind plays in setting off disease states has spawned several new areas of inquiry, such as behavioral medicine and psychoneuroimmunology.

On several occasions, the Buddha prescribed meditation exercises to his disciples to combat physical illness. It may be recalled that in the Buddhist view, meditation is the royal road to optimal health. If mental "currents" can be set right through meditation, healing is bound to follow (Birnbaum, 1979).

How does meditation heal? By eliminating emotional toxins, such as anger and lust, meditation brings about psychological and, therefore, physiological harmony. Lack of sense control, lack of restraint, and lack of right knowledge are often at the roots of illness; they are the most important cognitive and motivational components in mental illness (de Silva, 1979). Meditation relieves the distress of such mental illnesses.

The criterion of mental health in the *Abhidhamma* is equally simple: healthy mental factors must be present and unhealthy mental factors must be absent. Conversely, mental disorder is caused by the presence of unhealthy factors and the absence of healthy ones. Every mental disorder, the *Abhidhamma* asserts, results from particular combinations of unhealthy factors. These factors already have been discussed, but a brief recapitulation may be helpful. Every mental state is composed of mental factors that are *kusala* (wholesome) or *akusala* (unwholesome). Each state is made up of a specific subset of factors that flavor and define that state. Each state determines the particular mix of factors of the succeeding mental state. In addition to the healthy and unhealthy factors, seven perceptual-affective elements are present in every mental state. Apperception (*phassa*) is awareness of an external object. Perception (*sanna*) refers to its recognition as a sense object. Volition (*cetana*) always accompanies apperception. The feeling tone aroused by the sense object is *vedana*. The focusing of awareness is *ekaggata*, and it is followed by directing attention to the sense object (*manasikara*). *Jivitindriya*, or psychic energy, fuels the other six factors.

The various healthy and unhealthy factors operate within the matrix of these seven elements. Of the various unhealthy factors, the major perceptual one is delusion (*moha*). Delusion is said to cloud the mind and to result in misperception. It directly leads to false view (*ditthi*), which is miscategorization. The chief false view is the assumption of a permanent ego-self. Unhealthy factors that are cognitive include shamelessness (*ahirika*) and remorselessness (*anottappa*). The majority of unhealthy factors are affective. Agitation (*uddhacca*) and worry (*kukkucca*) are two important affective factors. Greed (*lobha*), avarice (*macchariya*), and envy (*issa*) are a set of unhealthy factors that form a cluster relating to clinging (Hall & Lindzey, 1978).

Every unhealthy factor is opposed by a healthy factor.

> The key principle in the *Abhidhamma* program for achieving mental health is the reciprocal inhibition of unhealthy mental factors by healthy ones. Just as in systematic desensitization, where tension is supplanted by its physiologic opposite relaxation, healthy mental states are antagonistic to unhealthy ones, inhibiting them. (Goleman, 1976, p. 43)

The most important healthy factor is insight (*panna*), which is the opposite of delusion. Insight is the clear perception of "what is." Mindfulness (*sati*) is the clear comprehension of an object. When these two healthy factors are present, they eliminate every unhealthy factor and introduce other healthy factors. The cognitive factors, modesty (*hiri*) and discretion (*ottappa*), occur when there is thought of an evil act. They are accompanied by rectitude (*cittujjukata*) and confidence (*saddha*), which is certitude based on right knowledge and perception. Nonattachment (*alobha*), nonaversion (*adosa*), impartiality (*tatramajjhata*), and composure (*passadhi*) oppose the unhealthy cluster of greed, avarice, aversion, and envy (Hall & Lindzey, 1978).

A final group of healthy factors has both psychological and physiological effects: buoyancy (*ahuta*), pliancy (*muduta*), adaptability (*kammannata*), and proficiency (*pagunnata*). They lend flexibility and ease and allow the individual to perform at the peak of his or her skills.

Healthy and unhealthy factors tend to arise in groups and are mutually inhibiting. A single healthy factor (e.g., insight) can inhibit all the unhealthy ones; occasionally, a single unhealthy factor (e.g., delusion) can suppress all the healthy factors. The presence of even a single unhealthy factor brands that mental state as unhealthy.

Biological and situational factors, one's *karma*, and the psychological status of the previous mental state, all act to determine one's mental state. These factors combine in different ways; and the hierarchy of how the factors combine present determines one's thinking and action. If a certain combination of factors occurs frequently, it becomes a personality trait.

The normal individual's mental states are a mix of healthy and unhealthy factors. Occasionally, a person experiences a wholly unhealthy or wholly healthy mental state, but very few constantly experience only healthy states. The singular goal of Buddhist psychology is to increase the presence of healthy mental states and eliminate unhealthy ones altogether.

The practicing Buddhist "embarks on a multilevel program for attaining a plateau of purely healthy mental states. He must undergo a coordinated effort of behavioral and affective self-control, combined with self-regulation of perceptual and cognitive processes, particularly attention" (Goleman, 1976, p. 44). The basic method is meditation, which thoroughly restructures attentional habits; the end product is the *arahat*.

The Arahat: The Ideal
Personality of Buddhism

The *arahat*, a prototypical saint, is the embodiment of supreme mental health. The word *arahat* comes from two words: *ari*, which means "foe," and *han*, which means "to kill." An *arahat* is a slayer of the foe—that is, a slayer of turbulent passions. In Gandhara art (a school of Buddhist art), the *arahat* is shown as dignified and serene. In various Buddhist scriptures, this individual is described as a person

who has greatly lived, who has done what had to be done, who has shed, the burden, who has won his aim, who is no longer bound to "becoming," who is set free, having rightly come to know. He has shed all attachment to I and mine, is secluded, zealous and earnest, inwardly free, fully controlled, master of himself, self-restrained, dispassionate and austere. (Conze, 1975, pp. 93–94)

The *arahat* has liberated himself or herself from pride, conceit, hatred, and selfishness and is full of wisdom and compassion. He or she finally is emancipated from the fetters of sensory existence and enters the deathless state, *Nirvana*. This person is an individual in whom sensual desires and ignorance have dried up.

Some scholars derive the word *arahat* from *arhati*, which means "worthy of." The *arahat* has conquered the self and hence is the conqueror of the universe and worthy of homage or adoration. The *arahat* is beyond good and evil in the sense that his or her conduct is the spontaneous expression of an emancipated mind and not the product of a calculated adherence to social rules (Sangharakshita, 1980). The egolessness of the personality results in actions that are truly selfless. The *arahat* is incapable of greed, anger, or egoism. The *arahat's* sense of inner poise and tranquility, egolessness and detachment from passions, and skillful response to the challenges of the moment are reminiscent of the state of "flow" that has been described by Csikzentmihalyi (1975).

The experience of *Nirvana* radically and permanently alters the *arahat's* personality traits. Johannsson (1970) described the *arahat* as a person who is free of sense desires, anxiety, anger, resentments, or fears of any sort; who is without dogmatism; who calmly accepts loss, disgrace, pain, or blame; who has no experience of suffering; who has no need for approval, pleasure, or praise; who desires nothing beyond the necessities; who displays openness, impartiality, compassion, and loving kindness toward others; who possesses quick and accurate perception; who demonstrates alertness and calm delight in all experiences no matter how ordinary; and who displays equanimity in all circumstances and skill in taking action. "From the perspective of most Western personality theories the *arahat* must seem too good to exist; he or she lacks many characteristics they assume intrinstic to human nature" (Hall & Lindzey, 1978, p. 373).

What happens to the *arahat* after death? Rahula (1962) compared the *arahat* to a fire gone out when the supply of wood has been consumed or to a flame extinguished when the oil has been used.

BUDDHISM AND PSYCHOTHERAPY

In Buddhism, psychology cannot easily be separated from psychotherapy. The study of humans had as its proper object the transformation of humans. Meditation was a tool not only for exploring the mind but for transforming the mind, for achieving a state of optimal psychological functioning. As such, it resembles what in the West is called "psychotherapy." Both psychotherapy and Buddhist meditative techniques are aimed at changing people's feelings about themselves; both alleviate anxiety and guilt, and both foster a measure of self-control and inner poise. But, the goals of most of the Western schools of psychotherapy are narrow—that is, to help the individual adjust to society. "In the process it may be viewed as desirable for the individual to fulfill himself, but the criterion of success is usually socially oriented, for example, having friends, attaining good family relationships, holding a productive job and so on" (Corsini, 1979, p. 500). The therapist is often aligned with conventional social norms and interprets his or her work as "adjusting the individual and coaxing his 'unconscious drives' into social respectability" (Watts, 1961, p. 20).

The therapeutic goal of Buddhist psychology is more radical: it is the maximization of human happiness and the unfolding of the human potential. The fullest expression of human capacities as well as the individual's awakening to his or her higher possibilities are also the goals of the human potential (HP) movement. The HP movement reflects the conviction among many psychotherapists that the human being uses only a fraction of his or her capacities. These practitioners also believe that a broad spectrum of techniques exists to assist people in expressing their fullest potential (Corsini, 1979).

The HP therapist uses a variety of methods, from behavior therapy to acupuncture. What is remarkable in this diversity is the cross-fertilization that occurs between different modalities. Of interest to us is the use of yoga, meditation, *mantra* recital, and other Eastern devices. Several meditative techniques are used by the HP practitioner to change the client's self-image (Corsini, 1979).

While the HP therapist attempts to alter the client's self-image, Buddhist psychology attempts to correct the seminal error of a human being: the belief in an abiding self and the separation of the "me" and the "other." This division leads to emotional and cognitive dissonance (Carpenter, 1977). Human beings can overcome this split by turning inward and achieving insight (Kondo, 1952).

One major similarity between the guru and the therapist lies in their attempts to alter the individual's relationship to himself or herself and to society. In Eastern psychology, this goal is achieved in two steps: (1) "personal restoration," that is, disentanglement from various forms of social conditioning, and (2) "social rehabilitation," or developing sane ways of relating to other people and social institutions (Murase & Johnson, 1975).

Two psychotherapeutic modalities based on Buddhism (*Sanshi-mompo* and Naikan therapy) highlight the personal restoration and social rehabilitation that Murase and Johnson (1975) mentioned.

Sanshi-mompo is a type of therapy in the Zen tradition, in which a master "gives help and aid in an interview through the medium of language to a person so that he may develop his ability to the maximum and adjust more properly to his circumstances" (Koga & Akishige, 1973, p. 71). This self-actualization involves relinquishing one's self-attachment or, in psychotherapeutic terms, surrendering a neurotic view of the world and self. It also involves an adaptive response—what Koga and Akishige called "not being attached to anything or influenced by anything" (p. 71).

Naikan therapy is another contribution of the meditative tradition to psychotherapy. Murase and Johnson (1975) called it a "specialized form of self-reflection" (p. 62). One of the goals of Naikan therapy is the assumption of personal responsibility for selfish and irrational behavior. This emphasis on personal responsibility is similar to a crucial concept in reality, therapy (Glasser, 1965). In Naikan meditation sessions, which last from 4:30 A.M. until 7 P.M., the client is instructed to meditate on his or her personal responsibility to significant others and to the world around. Naikan counselors provide the themes on which to meditate. For a further discussion of Naikan therapy, see Chapter 7, "On Being Natural: Two Japanese Approaches to Healing."

These two psychotherapeutic modalities, *Sanshi-mompo* and Naikan therapy, illustrate how Buddhism has been used in psychotherapy in the East. Meditation, the principal psychotherapeutic tool of Buddhism, also can enrich traditional Western psychotherapy in several ways: (1) by offering insight into self-defeating behaviors by focusing on them and exaggerating them; (2) by severing the tight grip of thinking on behavior by retraining attention; and (3) by producing an integrated hypothalamic response that decreases sympathetic activity. For a detailed discussion of the topic of meditation, see Chapter 15, "Meditation East and West." The rest of this chapter will discuss Buddhism in relation to several major Western therapeutic systems.

Buddhism and Behavior Therapy

Several affinities exist between Buddhism and behavior therapy. Behaviorism minimizes theory building, preferring operationalism. Likewise, the Buddha considered metaphysical speculations futile and believed his ideas to be testable in the crucible of experience. Both behavior modification and Buddhism emphasize self-control; both have the avowed intention of helping the individual control and modify bodily processes in order to enhance well-being (Mikulas, 1978).

But differences between the two should not be minimized. Unlike behaviorism, Buddhism considers introspection a valid tool of self-knowledge. While behaviorism stresses the value of counterconditioning in undoing neurotic behavior, Buddhism stresses insight.

Mikulas (1978) related the Four Noble Truths of Buddhism to behavior therapy. The first truth states that life is full of sorrow. The Pali word *dukkha*—loosely translated as "sorrow"—is teeming with nuances: anxiety, alienation, distress, discontent, and so on. Much of human dissatisfaction stems from the gap between the ideal self and the actual self, from the discrepancy between what is and what should be. The greater the gap, the greater the discontent.

The second truth states that attachment is the source of suffering. From the point of view of psychotherapy, one may conceptualize this attachment as clinging to ideals, concepts, and models. Such an attachment defines the individual and is the source of the ego (Mikulas, 1978). The technique of mindfulness is a self-monitoring procedure in which the practitioner merely notes his or her mental contents, whether they be ideas, desires, or memories. By neither pursuing nor rejecting these, the client learns to let go of the powerful sway of "assumptions, beliefs and/or self-statements which are putting the client at variance with his or her world or goals" (Mikulas, 1978, p. 62).

The third truth states that suffering ends when an individual is freed from craving and attachment; and the fourth truth outlines the method of ending attachment as taught by the Buddha. The elimination of attachments has many similarities with behavioral techniques whereby the client learns to relax, to detect anxiety-inducing cues, and to apply strategies of counterconditioning (Suinn & Richardson, 1971). In fact, behavioral self-management and the Buddhist practice of eliminating attachments can be effectively combined. The client is first put into a state of deep relaxation by means of meditation and deep muscular relaxation. Now, the client identifies/recalls specific anxiety-producing cues as well as disturbing attachments. He or she then turns attention inward and becomes aware of thoughts and feelings acutely. These mental contents may be seen as a "desensitization hierarchy," thus, a global and natural desensitization may occur.

Hendricks (1975) believed that meditative exercises act as "discrimination training" to desensitize emotionally laden thoughts. "In the process of continually returning one's attention to the meditative stimuli (namely *mandala, mantra, koan,* or breath) the client learns to discriminate thought from other stimuli" (Carpenter, 1977, p. 399). Both "good" and "evil" thoughts are experienced as just "thoughts," and clients learn not to identify themselves with their thoughts. Consequently, they cease to derive their lasting personality traits from their thinking.

The transcendental meditation (TM) technique may also be regarded as inducing relaxation through reciprocal inhibition in psychotherapy. Wolpe (1958) described a procedure to reduce anxiety by counterconditioning through relaxation. The client is first put into a state of deep muscle relaxation; graded anxiety-producing stimuli are then repeatedly paired with this relaxed state until the link between these stimuli and anxiety is abolished.

Wolpe has used hypnosis and progressive relaxation (Jacobson, 1938) successfully to induce relaxation. Block (1977) argued that the use of TM as a relaxation inducer has certain advantages not found in other methods. According to Block, TM as an anxiety inhibitor permits treatment of a substantially broader spectrum of disorders. Traditional psychotherapy may be used in the early stages of therapy to lay the proper foundation for TM. First, clients should be trained to focus their attention on their problems and anxieties. This would help them recognize their style of dealing with them (e.g., denial and avoidance). An understanding of their habitual and automatic responses makes subsequent use of TM doubly effective. After clients have achieved a state of deep relaxation using TM, they can deliberately imagine the painful stimuli. Therapists also can construct a hierarchy of anxiety-provoking mental pictures, and clients ascend this hierarchy step by step.

Block (1977) suggested several other benefits that may accrue as a result of regular TM practice. The relaxation induced by TM tends to extend to other aspects of one's life: TM may confer the "hardiness" so invaluable in meeting the petty aggravations of life. The everyday annoyances of life probably contribute more to illness than major life-changes do.

The general reduction in anxiety that accompanies the practice of TM also helps in the development of therapeutic insight (West, 1975). TM has several advantages over other relaxation techniques. Relaxation is more quickly induced by means of TM, making possible a more selective desensitization (Block, 1977). TM does not require elaborate equipment (unlike biofeedback, for example), pharmacological agents (e.g., tranquilizers), or special settings. Hence, the client can use TM for counterconditioning in actual life situations. TM also fosters independence in that a therapist is not needed.

Buddhism and Cognitive Therapy

Psychiatrists, psychologists, and other mental health professionals work to relieve suffering. According to Ponce (1987), Buddhism offers clear and succinct diagnostic, etiologic, prescriptive, and prognostic statements. The diagnosis: suffering is life. Everything about our daily life—the way we relate to others, the way we think, behave, an so on— leads to suffering. The etiology of the disease is ignorance (*avidya*)— ignorance of how things really are and ignorance of the nature of self. Desire, aggression, and delusion are the symptoms of the disease, and they must be replaced by detachment, the only healthy relationship to a world that is constantly changing. The treatment is the eightfold path that leads to *Nirvana*, the "blowing out" of the symptoms.

The basic tenet of cognitive therapy is the notion that unhappiness and symptoms of mental illness are due to erroneous views of reality. Therefore, the task of the cognitive therapist is to vigorously challenge the individual's maladaptive assumptions and beliefs. Ponce (1987) identifies the three major areas of concern: the individual's core assumptions about the nature of the world, about the nature of the self, and about the relationship between the two. Cognitive therapists focus mainly on two of these assumptions, neglecting the notion of the self. The aim of therapy is, what Ponce calls, a "paradigm shift" in the way of perceiving the world.

Meditation can be used as a cognitive therapeutic technique whereby the individual practices being a detached observer of a process where thoughts and images enter the mind and disappear, feelings and sensations come and go, in a continuous flow. (Parry & Jones, 1986). This process is likely to lead to a shift toward primary process thinking, a mode of thinking essential for the cohesive integration of a sense of self. In summary, the cure is right knowledge or recognizing things as they really are.

Buddhism and Psychoanalysis

Psychoanalysis is a passive form of therapy. Techniques for inducing altered states of consciousness (e.g., meditation) are also passive. But while psychoanalysis stresses verbalization in order to gain insight, meditation focuses attention inward in a nonverbal, nonconceptual manner. Psychoanalysis remains a predominantly rational and intellectual, albeit introspective, technique for self-understanding. Carrington and Ephron (1975) suggested that a combination of psychoanalysis and meditation techniques may "more effectively reach nonverbal, nonconceptual areas" (p. 44). They have explored a number of ways in which the two systems may profitably interact.

Psychoanalysts can well utilize some meditative techniques as an adjunct to traditional therapy. The release of constricted creative energies and the increase in physical energy (less need for sleep, increased physical endurance, etc.) that accompany the practice of meditation have "frequently been reflected in the psychoanalytic hour by an increase in the productiveness of a patient's free association" (Carrington & Ephron, 1975, p. 47).

Patients also are markedly less self-critical following the practice of meditation; they exhibit fewer paranoid ideations and show greater tolerance for guilt-inducing material. The spontaneity and receptivity resulting from a less critical super-ego may enhance therapeutic prospects. The authors also stated that feelings of joy, sadness, or anger, which are frequently reported by meditating patients, indicate affective readiness. Consequently, the immediate postmeditation period may be particularly efficacious for analytic therapy.

According to Carrington and Ephron, meditation may increase the individual's sense of separate identity. "The experiencing of a new and convincing sense of 'self' during meditation appears to form a base of self-awareness which may be built upon to advantage in the psychoanalytic treatment" (Carrington & Ephron, 1975, p. 49). However, meditation is intended to ultimately reveal the illusion of selfhood, hence, Carrington and Ephron's assertion seems questionable.

Meditation has been used to uncover repressed material, to make the unconscious conscious, and to disarm "the ego against instinctual demands" (Freud, 1936, p. 146). Thus, it is a useful device to induce primary-process thinking and to abort defense mechanisms.

Meditation also may serve to enhance and heighten therapeutic skills and hence may be of value in the training of mental health professionals. Carrington and Ephron (1975) enumerated the changes in their professional work as a result of taking up meditation:

1. An increased receptivity to their own perceptions of unconscious conflicts
2. Better insight into dreams and other primary-process material
3. Increased sensitivity to clients' conflicts
4. Increased ability to handle clients' negative transference reactions

A more comprehensive survey of the relationship between psychoanalysis and Buddhism (of the Zen variety) is offered by Erich Fromm (1970). According to Fromm, there is currently a spiritual crisis in Western culture. This is "the automatization of man, his alienation from himself, from his fellow man and from nature. Man has followed rationalism to the point where rationalism has transformed itself into utter irrationality" (Fromm, 1970, pp. 78–79). Human beings, Fromm eloquently asserted, suffer from an inability to experience affect. Both Zen Buddhism and psychoanalysis are ways out of this crisis. According to Suzuki, Fromm, and de Martino (1970):

> Zen in its essence is the art of seeing into the nature of one's being, and it points the way from bondage to freedom. . . . We can say that Zen liberates all the energies properly and naturally stored in each of us, which are in ordinary circumstances cramped and distorted so that they find no adequate channel for activity. . . . It is the object of Zen, therefore, to save us from going crazy or being crippled. This is what I mean by freedom, giving free play to all the creative and benevolent impulses inherently lying in our hearts. (p. 122)

According to Fromm (1970), this description of the goals of Zen Buddhism is also a description of the aims of psychoanalysis. Freud was not merely concerned with a "cure" for mental illness. His ultimate aims were insight into self, liberation from the tyranny of the unconscious (and hence from neurotic symptoms and inhibitions), knowledge of reality (and thus liberation of energy and happiness). To Freud, the relationship between analyst and client is firmly grounded in love of truth.

Fromm (1970) identified one other principle in psychoanalysis that is similar to Buddhism—that is, the principle that knowledge leads to transformation. Freud's primary concern was the human being's psychic evolution, and he recognized that self-knowledge can bring this about. According to Fromm (1970), this psychic growth consists in overcoming alienation—"to be fully born, to develop one's awareness, one's reason, one's capacity to love, to such a point that one transcends one's own egocentric involvement, and arrives at a new harmony, at a new oneness with the world" (p. 87). This process is accompanied by the disappearance of narcissism and the dawning of well-being. Human beings become open, responsive, awake, empty.

How does psychoanalysis accomplish its goal? In Freud's language, it is done by transforming id into ego or making the unconscious conscious. In Freud's view, the conscious and the unconscious were different parts of the personality, each with its particular contents. Freud's unconscious contains an individual's vices; Jung's unconscious holds an individual's wisdom. Another way of looking at the conscious and the unconscious, a way pertinent to this discussion, is to characterize them as states of awareness and unawareness. This raises the question, what makes for unawareness? According to Fromm (1970), every society by its own practice of living and by the mode of relatedness, of feeling and perceiving, develops a system of categories which determines the forms of awareness. This system works, as it were, like a socially conditioned filter; experience cannot enter awareness unless it can penetrate this filter. (p. 99)

Language and logic are two aspects of this filter. The third aspect relates to the content of experience: every society suppresses certain thoughts and feelings from being thought or felt.

But what does it mean to become aware, to make the unconscious conscious? In Freud's narrow view, it meant calling into awareness repressed impulses and instinctual desires. In Fromm's view, the average individual is only half awake; he or she is conscious of fictions but has the potential to become conscious of the reality behind the fiction. Consequently, to make the unconscious conscious means to wake up, to know reality. This is what Buddhism means by "enlightenment."

Enlightenment often has been described as the art of seeing into one's nature (Suzuki, 1956). With enlightenment

all your mental activities will now be working in a different key, which will be more satisfying, more peaceful, more full of joy than anything you ever experienced before. The tone of life will be altered. . . . The spring flower will look prettier, and the mountain stream runs cooler and more transparent. (Suzuki, 1949, pp. 97–98)

With enlightenment, human beings become totally attuned to reality, more responsive, and more awake. In the language of the neoanalysts, they achieve a completely "productive orientation." They relate to the world not exploitatively but creatively (Suzuki et al., 1970). Both Buddhism and psychoanalysis are ethical in nature. Covetousness is contrary to Buddhist precepts, and freedom from greed is a necessary condition for salvation. In psychoanalysis, libidinal evolution proceeds from the oral receptive to the genital or from the greedy to the productive and fully functioning orientation.

Both Buddhism and psychoanalysis proclaim the individual's self-sufficiency and emancipation from authority. In Zen, a guide is considered helpful at first, but eventually the cord between master and disciple is severed. "Be a refuge unto yourself," said the Buddha. While psychoanalysts concede that initially a mentor may be necessary, they have devised methods (e.g., working through transference) to deal with the dependency this relationship might foster. The attitudes of the Buddhist teacher and the analyst toward their pupils are remarkably similar. Both act as mirrors, both are compassionate yet sentimental, and, above all, both are aware that in reality no one can save another.

In Buddhist tradition and in psychoanalysis, the liberated being is described as awake. According to psychoanalysis, the individual is repressed and consequently experiences, not objects and people, but words. Becoming conscious of the unconscious involves freeing oneself from alienated and parataxic experience. "It means to wake up, to shed illusions, fictions and lies, to see reality as it is" (Suzuki et al., 1970, p. 129).

It must be emphasized that although Buddhism and psychoanalysis share the same goal, their techniques of realizing it are quite different and embedded in vastly different philosophical positions. Buddhism is thoroughly Indian and owes some of its ideas to Hinduism; psychoanalysis is Western and traces its lineage to Greek wisdom and Hebrew ethics. Nevertheless, a knowledge of Buddhist psychology, and particularly meditation, will be a valuable aid for psychoanalysts. Buddhism can clarify and quicken the processes of analytic therapy.

Buddhism and Gestalt Therapy

Gestalt therapy is an ahistoric, existential therapy developed by Frederick (Fritz) Perls (1893–1970). It focuses on the here and now, on the immediate ongoing awareness of one's experiencing. Also it stresses personal responsibility and the unity of the person; its therapeutic approach restores awareness and heals the split within the self.

Both Gestalt therapy and Buddhism, particularly Zen, stress present-oriented living. For Perls, nothing exists except the "now." Since the past is "gone and the future has not yet arrived, only the present is significant. One of the main contributions of the Gestalt approach is its emphasis on the here-and-now and on learning to appreciate and experience fully the present moment" (Corey, 1977, p. 73). Polster and Polster (1973) proclaimed that power is in the present. To stray from the present detracts from living fully. Most people waste their energies lamenting the past or preparing to live. According to Gestalt theory, anxiety is the gap between the now and the later. In Buddhism, too, the present is all. When asked to describe enlightenment, a Zen master remarked, "I eat when I am hungry and sleep when I am tired. That is all there is to it."

In both Buddhism and Gestalt therapy, awareness is the primary therapeutic tool. Awareness is the ability to attend to what is. Clients in Gestalt therapy are asked to describe their moment-to-moment awareness of thoughts, feelings, and sensations. Elaborating on the Buddha's "Discourse on Mindfulness," Nyanaponika Thera said, "Bare Attention is the clear and single-minded awareness of what actually happens *to* us and *in* us, at the successive moments of perception" (Nyanaponika, 1962, p. 30). Buddhism recognizes four basic objects of mindfulness: body, feeling, state of mind, and mental contents. Thus, as in Gestalt therapy, the objects of awareness encompass the entire spectrum of the individual's experiencing, extending from his or her body and its functions, to feelings, and to the contents and processes of thought and perception. In fact, Perls (cited in Fagan & Shepherd, 1970) said that the task of all deep religions and of good therapy is the same: an awakening of sensory experience.

Perls (1969) rejected the Freudian view of the unconscious. He maintained that the unconscious—a storehouse of repression, a servant to the pleasure principle—belongs to the vast domain of the conscious. He did not deny the physiological unconscious. We are unconscious, for example, of the way cells divide and grow, of digestion, and of synaptic transmission; however, this unconscious is a "far cry from Freud's seething cauldron. It is a marvel of efficiency, order, balance" (Schoen, 1978, p. 104). Basically, Gestalt therapists assert that the conscious mind is its own enemy. It is the source of mental illness, but it also has the potential to work its own cure.

The Buddha, too, saw the human mind as the fountainhead of sorrow. It is the conscious mind that clings to the false idea of a separate self. The way out of this impasse is also through the conscious mind—that is, by altering it. Insight, which he prescribed as the sovereign remedy for the sickness, is again within the province of the conscious mind.

The Buddha invited the individual to solve his or her problems the only way they can be solved—by and for himself or herself. No savior, no god, no ideology, no sacred book, no Buddha can save the individual. In Gestalt therapy, too, the central assumption is that individuals can themselves cope effectively with their problems.

Buddhism and Existentialism

The Buddha, like Kierkegaard, recognized the sensual aspect of life. The desire for sensuous gratification, *kama-tanha,* is a powerful force in human affairs. It is propelled by *kama-raga* (passions) and the *anasuyas* (latent tendencies). Furthermore, in their endless quest for pleasure, human beings seek variety. The *Samyutta Nikaya* (1884–1904) said that humans search for variety and find delight "in this and that, here and there" (vol. V, p. 421). Like Kierkegaard, the Buddha asserted that pleasures must end in sorrow. The Buddhist critique of pleasure is based on the concept of *dukkha.* The word *dukkha,* while commonly translated as "sorrow," also refers to the despair and the meaningless of life.

Buddhist theory is more elaborate and systematic than Kierkegaard's concept. It consists of the five precepts, the ten good actions, and the eightfold path. The first two codes ensure a harmonious family and social life. The eightfold path is a systematic program for attaining *Nirvana*. Thus, while the existentialist refuses to codify ethics, the Buddhist offers a ready-made set of rules for ethical conduct (Tachibana, 1975).

Concerning religious life, both Kierkegaard and the Buddha condemned mere attachment to rites and rituals. Both rejected metaphysical speculation and emphasized the importance of self-knowledge and choice (de Silva, 1974). Nevertheless, while existentialists are scornful of reason, the Buddha recognized the importance of reason.

Several important differences emerge from a study of religious concepts of Kierkegaard and Buddhism. Neither God, nor sin, nor guilt, nor self-mortification and repentance have any place in Buddhism. The path to salvation is through self-knowledge and insight. On the other hand, notions of a Savior, of sin, of guilt, and of repentance occupy a prominent place in the writings of Kierkegaard.

Both the Buddha and the existentialists focused on the tragedy of life. The Buddha renounced the worldly life as a result of becoming aware of sickness, old age, and death. He proclaimed that life was inherently sorrowful, since it eventually ends in death. The existentialists, too, propose that life is meaningless since it ultimately ends in death. The recognition of the inevitability of death prompted both the Buddha and the existential philosophers to use death as a gateway to a richer life. Meditation on death occupies an important place in both Buddhism and existentialism. The Buddha recommended the meditation on death as a corrective for persons in whom greed and attachment predominate: the constant recollection of death would lead to a lesser attachment to worldly concerns and, consequently, to a more harmonious life. Of greater importance is the fact that awareness of death is bound to remind us that we are caught in the wheel of birth and death, that death will surely be followed by a rebirth and a redeath. Consequently, the meditation on death will serve to encourage us to redouble our efforts to achieve *Nirvana* in this life. Rollo May (1961) proposed that by realizing that death awaits us, we can make every moment count. The knowledge that we are finite lends urgency to the present. We only have a limited amount of time to actualize our possibilities. The complete acceptance of death without fear, denial, or morbidity will lead to a richer life.

In Buddhism, the concept of *dukkha* includes a kind of anxiety that is strikingly similar to Kierkegaard's (1944) angst. Existential anxiety is part of the fabric of human existence. It results not only from the awareness of freedom and responsibility, but also from the awareness of eventual nonexistence. In Buddhism (de Silva, 1974), there is anxiety regarding the nonexistent; this anxiety is divided into subjective and objective anxiety. Anxiety over the loss of a personal possession is called objective anxiety concerning the nonexistent. When a person who believes in an everlasting soul hears a discourse of the Buddha denying its existence, he or she succumbs to a subjective anxiety concerning the nonexistent.

The word "alienation," according to de Silva (1974), connotes a sense of otherness, strangeness, foreignness, difference, etc. This sense of strangeness of 'dissociation' has at least three basic facets: dissociation from others, oneself and the world at large" (p. 61). He suggested that the partial or complete domination of the personality by a particular drive may be called self-alienation, for, under such conditions, one is denied access to aspects of one's personality. The Buddha identified greed as the cause of self-alienation: greed (*lobha*) leads to attachments and obsessions that eventually come to dominate the personality. Alienation from others is a direct consequence of egoism or the craving for self-preservation (*bhava-tanha*). "In an acquisitive society that nourishes the egoistic proclivities of man, with the emphasis on the accumulation of wealth, property and status symbols, human relationships become mechanical" (de Silva, 1974, p. 68). The increasing industrialization of the world has resulted in our alienation from nature.

The concept of alienation has received considerable attention from the existentialists. They argued against the alienation of humans by technology and bureaucracy. When humans allow themselves to be dominated by others or by their environment, they become alienated and succumb to an inauthentic existence (Hall & Lindzey, 1978). The way to overcome alienation is to lead an authentic life. Authentic existence consists of living up to the full range of one's possibilities.

Two major differences between Buddhism and existentialism must be mentioned. While Buddhism analyzes human existence strictly in terms of cause and effect, existentialism denies cause-effect relationships in human existence.

Existentialists might be said to be aware of the first Noble Truth of Buddhas, namely that all life is suffering, but not to see a way out; so they struggle continuously to confront life and reconcile it with these apparent inevitabilities. However, the Buddha went further. In the remaining of these noble truths, he pointed the way out of this dilemma, a way that leads directly to the transpersonal realm beyond the ego and existential levels." (Walsh & Vaughan, 1983, p. 26)

CONCLUDING REMARKS

The psychology of Buddhism rests on the notions of the absence of a separate self, impermanence of all things, and the fact of sorrow. Human beings suffer because of self-delusion, striving to possess that which inevitably must crumble, and because of desire. The Buddha did not stop with a mere diagnosis. He proclaimed that the cure is to reach a higher state of being, wherein self-knowledge has eradicated delusion, attachment, and desire. Buddhist psychology asserts that not only all psychological pain is caused by false knowledge and covetousness, but also that physical illness can be traced to these factors. In viewing physical and mental disease states holistically, Buddhism is far ahead of the times. Only recently has the scientific world acknowledged the interrelation of body and mind.

As we have seen, a therapy based on Buddhist principles is likely to utilize cognitive restructuring, behavioral techniques, and insight-oriented methods to effect a complete healing. Such a cure would necessarily involve a radical change in consciousness, an awakening to an enlightened state where fear and desire do not exist. An organism free of fear and desire would be a fully functioning, superbly healthy, and truly intelligent form of life. It is this wonderful gift of life that Buddhism has to offer.

References

Basu, R. N. (1978). *A critical study of the Milindapanha.* Calcutta: Firma KLM Private.

Bhattacharya, K. (1963). The concept of self in Buddhism. *Philosophy Today, 7,* 216–223.

Birnbaum, R. (1979). *The healing Buddha.* Boulder, CO: Shambhala Publications.

Block, B. (1977). Transcendental meditation as a reciprocal inhibitor in psychotherapy. *Journal of Contemporary Psychotherapy, 9*(1), 78–82.

Brunswick, E. F. (1959). Meaning of psychoanalytic concepts and confirmation of psychoanalytic theories. In M. Levitt (Ed.), *Readings in psychoanalytic psychology.* New York: Appleton-Century-Crofts.

Buddhaghosa, B. (1976). *The path of purification (Visuddhimagga)* (Vols. 1–2) (B. Nyanamoli, Trans.). Berkeley, CA: Shambhala.

Carpenter, T. J. (1977). Meditation, esoteric traditions—Contributions to psychotherapy. *American Journal of Psychotherapy, 31*(3), 394–404.

Carrington, P., & Ephron, H. S. (1975). Meditation and psychoanalysis. *Journal of the American Academy of Psychoanalysis, 3*(1), 43–57.

Conze, E. (1975). *Buddhism: Its essence and development.* New York: Harper & Row.

Corey, G. (1977). *Theory and practice of counseling and psychotherapy.* Monterey, CA: Brooks/Cole.

Corsini, R. J. (1979). *Current psychotherapies.* Itasca, IL: F. E. Peacock.

Csikzentmihalyi, M. (1975). Play and intrinsic rewards. *Journal of Humanistic Psychology, 15*(3), 41–63.

de Silva, M. W. P. (1973). *Buddhist and Freudian psychology.* Columbo, Sri Lanka: Lake House Investments.

de Silva, M. W. P. (1974). *Tangles and webs.* Columbo, Sri Lanka: Lake House Investments.

de Silva, M. W. P. (1979). *An introduction to Buddhist psychology.* New York: Harper & Row.

Dhammaratana, U. (1964). *Guide through Visuddhimagga.* Varanasi, India: Tara Printing Works.

Fagen, J., & Shepherd, I. (1970). *Gestalt therapy now.* New York: Harper Colophon.

Freer, L. (Ed.). *Samyutta Nikaya* (Vols. 1–6). (1884–1904). London: Pali Text Society.

Freud, S. (1936). *The problem of anxiety.* New York: Norton.

Fromm, E. (1970). Psychoanalysis and Zen Buddhism. In D. T. Suzuki, E. Fromm, & R. de Martino (Eds.), *Zen Buddhism and psychoanalysis.* New York: Harper & Row.

Glasser, W. (1965). *Reality therapy.* New York: Harper & Row.

Goleman, D. (1976). Meditation and consciousness: An Asian approach to mental health. *American Journal of Psychotherapy, 30*(1), 41–54.

Govinda, L. A. (1961). *The psychological attitude of early Buddhist philosophy.* London: Rider & Co.

Govinda, L. A. (1974). *The psychological attitude of early Buddhist philosophy.* New York: Samuel Weiser.

Hall, C. S., & Lindzey, G. (1978). *Theories of personality* (3rd ed.). New York: Wiley.

Hendricks, C. G. (1975). Meditation as discrimination training: A theoretical note. *Journal of Transpersonal Psychology, 7,* 144.

Horner, I. B. (Trans.). (1954–1959) *Middle length sayings* (Vols. 1–30). London: Pali Text Society.

Jacobson, E. (1938). *Progressive relaxation.* Chicago: University of Chicago Press.

Johannsson, R. E. A. (1970). *The psychology of nirvana.* New York: Anchor.

Johannsson, R. E. A. (1979). *The dynamic psychology of early Buddhism.* London: Curzon Press.

Kierkegaard, S. (1944). *The concept of dread* (W. Lowrie, Trans.). Princeton, NJ: Princeton University Press.

Koga, Y., & Akishige, Y. (1973). Psychological study on Zen and counseling. In Y. Akishige (Ed.), *Psychological studies on Zen.* Tokyo: Zen Institute of Komazawa University.

Kondo, A. (1952). Intuition in Zen Buddhism. *American Journal of Psychoanalysis, 12,* 10.

Mahadevan, T. M. P. (1974). *Invitation to Indian philosophy.* New York: Humanities Press.

Manne-Lewis, J. (1986). Buddhist psychology: A paradigm for the psychology of enlightenment. In G. Claxton (Ed.), *Beyond therapy.* London: Wisdom Publications.

May, R. (Ed.). (1961). *Existential psychology.* New York: Random House.

Mikulas, W. (1978). Four noble truths of Buddhism related to behavior therapy. *Psychological Record, 28,* 59–67.

Morris, H., & Hardy, H. (Eds.). (1885–1900) *Anguttara Nikaya* (Vols. 1–4). London: Pali Text Society.

Murase, T., & Johnson, F. (1975). Naikan, Morita and western psychotherapy. In G. R. Patterson (Ed.), *Behavior change.* Chicago: Aldine.

Narada, M. (1968). *A manual of Abhidhamma.* Kandy, Ceylon: Buddhist Publication Society.

Nyanaponika, T. (1962). *The heart of Buddhist meditation.* London: Rider.

Nyanatiloka, M. (1950). *Buddhist dictionary.* Columbo, Sri Lanka: Island Heritage Publication, Ferwin & Co.

Nyanatiloka, M. (1971). *Guide through the Abhidhamma-pitaka.* Kandy, Ceylon: Buddhist Publication Society.

Parry, S. J., & Jones, R. G. A. (1986). Beyond illusion in the psychotherapeutic enterprise. In G. Claxton (Ed.), *Beyond therapy,* London: Wisdom Publications.

Perls, F. (1969). *Gestalt therapy verbatim.* Moab, UT: Real People Press.

Polster, E., & Polster, M. (1973). *Gestalt therapy integrated.* New York: Brunner/Mazel.

Ponce, D. E. (1987). *Buddhism, system theory and cognitive psychotherapy.* Paper presented at the Third International Conference, Buddhism and Christianity: Toward the Human Future, Berkeley, CA.

Radhakrishnan, S. (1951). *Indian philosophy* (Vol. 1). New York: Macmillan.

Rahula, W. (1962). *What the Buddha taught.* New York: Grove Press.

Rao, K. R. (1978). Psychology of transcendence: A study in early Buddhistic psychology. *Journal of Indian Psychology, 1*(1), 1–21.

Rhys-Davids, C. A. F. (1978). *The birth of Indian psychology and its development in Buddhism.* New Delhi: Oriental Books Reprint Corporation.

Rhys-Davids, T. W., & Carpenter, J. E. (Eds.). (1890–1911) *Digha-Nikaya* (Vols. 1–3). London: Pali Text Society.

Sangharakshita, B. (1980). *A survey of Buddhism.* Boulder, CO: Shambhala.

Sarathchandra, E. R. (1958). *Buddhist psychology of perception.* Columbo, Sri Lanka: Ceylon University Press.

Sayadaw, L. (1961). *Manual of insight.* Kandy, Ceylon: Wheel Publications.

Schoen, S. (1978). Gestalt therapy and the teachings of Buddhism. *Gestalt Journal, 1*(1), 103–115.

Smith, H. (1958). *The religions of man.* New York: Harper & Row.

Suinn, R. M., & Richardson, F. (1971). Anxiety management training: A nonspecific behavior therapy program for anxiety control. *Behavior Therapy, 2,* 498–510.

Suzuki, D. T. (1949). *Introduction to Zen Buddhism.* London: Rider.

Suzuki, D. T. (1956). *Zen Buddhism.* Garden City, NY: Anchor Books, Doubleday.

Suzuki, D. T., Fromm, E., & de Martino, R. (Eds.). (1970). *Zen Buddhism and psychoanalysis.* New York: Harper & Row.

Tachibana, S. (1975). *The ethics of Buddhism.* London: Curzon Press.

Trenkner, V., R. Chalmers, & C. A. F. Rhys-Davids (Eds.). (1948–1951) *Majjhima Nikaya* (Vols. 1–30). London: Pali Text Society.

Walsh, R. (1983). The ten perfections: Qualities of the fully enlightened individual as described in Buddhist psychology. In R. Walsh & D. H. Shapiro (Eds.), *Beyond health and normality.* New York: Van Nostrand Reinhold.

Walsh, R. N., & Vaughan, F. (1983). Towards an integrative psychology of wellbeing. In R. Boorstein (Ed.), *Transpersonal psychotherapy.* Palo Alto, CA: Science and Behavior Books.

Watts, A. (1961). *Psychotherapy east and west.* New York: Pantheon.

Welwood, J. (1979). *The meeting of the ways.* New York: Schocken.

West, L. J. (1975). Transcendental meditation and other nonprofessional therapies. In A. M. Freedman, H. I. Kaplan, & B. J. Sadock (Eds.), *Comprehensive textbook of psychiatry* (Vol. 1). Baltimore: Williams & Wilkins.

Wolpe, J. (1958). *Psychotherapy by reciprocal inhibition.* Stanford, CA: Stanford University Press.

5

Mind, Disease, and Health in Tibetan Medicine[1]

MARK EPSTEIN
LOBSANG RAPGAY

First open this heap of skin with your intellect,
Then separate the flesh from the network of bones with the
*   scalpel of discriminating awareness.*
Having opened the bones also look at the marrow
And see for yourself
Whether there is anything solid.

sGam. po. pa., 1971

INTRODUCTION

For the past 10 centuries a vast reservoir of medical and psychological knowledge has accumulated in Tibet, long isolated atop the great

---

[1]An earlier version of this paper was published in *ReVision* (Epstein & Topgay, 1982). It is included here with permission.

Central Asian plateau. Its valleys have nurtured such a variety of medicinal plants that early Indian traders came to refer to the country as the "land of the healing herbs." Its monasteries have cultivated the illuminating spiritual and psychological insights of Tantric Buddhism, and its medical practitioners have preserved a unique synthesis of several of the world's oldest and most influential healing traditions. It is one of the paradoxes of history that Tibet's rich and diverse culture did not become available to Westerners until many Tibetans fled their homeland in the wake of the Chinese invasion of the mid 1950s. Western researchers have since been impressed by the clarity, complexity, and sophistication of the Tibetan mind and heritage.

In order to begin to appreciate the Tibetan understanding of mental health, one must first accept the fundamental belief in a vital force or energy that is assumed by all traditional Asian philosophical, religious, and medical systems to pervade the human organism. Termed *prana* in Sanskrit and "ch'i" (Kao, 1979) by the Chinese, this life force is said to move in channels throughout the body, underlying the psychological process. This energy is said to dissolve in death, to be blocked or disrupted in disease, and to be channeled or controlled in the practice of meditation. It is the core concept of Tibetan medicine, psychiatry, and Tantric meditation (Clifford, 1984).

Both *prana* and *ch'i* have come to be equated with such phenomena as breath, air, wind, or creative life force; yet, it would be more accurate to say that these are only aspects of a more universal energy. "All forces of the universe, like those of the human mind, from the highest consciousness to the depths of the subconscious, are modifications of 'prana.' The word 'prana' can therefore not be equated with the physical breath, though breathing ('prana' in the narrower sense) is one of the many functions in which this universal and primordial force manifests itself" (Govinda, 1960, p. 137). Breathing is a means of extracting this energy from the environment (Evans-Wentz, 1958, p. 126), and thus control of the breathing process in meditation is one means of affecting the movement of prana.

Traditionally, *prana* is described according to three aspects—(1) the underlying energy itself, (2) the channels in which it moves, and (3) the movements or currents within those channels. The underlying energy is conceptualized as the life source, often symbolized by semen, which is the "'seed' of all forms the being takes" (Rao, 1979, p. 53). It permeates all things and yet is in itself not definable. "But in its own essential and inalienable nature, it is 'zero,' 'naught.' It lacks the dimensions of existence, and is thus not grasped" (Rao, 1979, p. 13).

The channels in which this energy moves are termed *nadis* in Sanskrit and *tsas* in Tibetan. These pathways make up a kind of psychic nervous system whose anatomy is well known to all practitioners of Tantric meditation. The Chinese also postulate the existence of energy channels in the body through which the ch'i moves, and they refer to these channels as "meridians."

The movement of this energy within the channels of the human organism is termed *vayu* in Sanskrit and *rlung* in Tibetan. The word *"vayu"* is "derived from the root 'va,' 'to breathe' or 'to blow,' (which) refers to the motive power of 'prana.' These 'vayu' . . . control the bodily functions; and thus each has its own place and duty. Health, essential for the yogin, depends upon keeping each vital-air normal, or in its own channel of operation" (Evans-Wentz, 1958, p. 132).

The Tibetan tradition has probed, explored, and described the complex patterns of this energy as profoundly as any. Both medical and religious texts lay strong emphasis on these currents of psychic energy, and much of Tibetan psychiatry and medicine is concerned with the manifestations and treatments of disruptions or blocks in the flow of *prana*. In fact, when Tibetan medicine is examined with an eye to descriptions of mind and mental disorders, it becomes clear that what is being discussed is how these currents of *prana* function in health and disease. Tibetan medical texts are filled with descriptions of the manifestations of dysfunction of the *pranic* flow, and Tantric religious texts voluminously elucidate the reorganization of these currents that occurs in death or in meditation. An understanding of the Tibetan approach to mind is not possible without an appreciation of the character of these *pranic* currents.

SYSTEMS OF PSYCHOLOGY

Tibetan concepts of personality derive from two major branches of the Buddhist texts: the Tantric teachings on the nature of mind (particularly those termed "Highest Yoga Tantra"), and the sutra system of Abhidharma. The Tantric teachings emphasize the spiritual and emotional aspects of mind, with particular reference to subtle states of consciousness that are manifested during death, intermediate state, and birth, and that are specifically cultivated in advanced meditation practices (Lati & Hopkins, 1979).

The *Abhidharma* is a system of psychological theory derived from the moment-to-moment observation of the workings of the human mind in meditation. It describes the composition of the mind as a constellation of wholesome, afflictive, and neutral mental factors of perceptual, cognitive, and affective qualities, and goes on to analyze the radical restructuring of mental contents that occurs through the practice of meditation. Of the three types of mental factors, the afflictive factors (e.g., greed, hatred, pride, envy, lack of insight) are seen as the ultimate underlying causes of both physical and mental diseases, and it is only through the practice of meditation that these afflictive factors can be rooted out and destroyed (Goleman & Epstein, 1980). Three afflictive mental factors in particular are singled out as the roots of all unwholesome states of mind: (1) desire or attachment (grasping after pleasant objects or experiences); (2) hatred, anger, or aversion (pushing away or avoiding unpleasant objects or experiences); and (3) ignorance or confusion (not clearly understanding the nature of a given object or experience).

Mental health is defined as a mind freed from the influence of the afflictive mental factors, and that is the goal of the process of meditation. For those who have not realized this goal, a certain amount of mental disharmony is inevitable. In dealing with problems of mental disturbance, Tibetan medicine recognizes the imperfection of the unenlightened mind and does not seek to accomplish the impossible. Therefore, certain "less-than enlightened" mental states and disorders are described and treated by Tibetan medicine, and mental influences are readily accepted as contributing factors in the etiology of disease.

In terms of psychopathology, the classification of nervous and mental diseases occurs within the major medical texts. Psychiatry, in the Tibetan view, is one aspect of the medical system as a whole. Concepts of etiology, methods of diagnosis, and means of treatment are similarly applied to diseases of both body and mind. Medical practitioners are trained to recognize and treat mental disorders as well as physical ones; there is no distinct class of specialists in the treatment of psychopathology within the medical profession.

FUNDAMENTALS OF TIBETAN MEDICINE

History

According to historical sources, Tibet first opened its doors to the cultural and religious influences of the societies surrounding it in the seventh century A.D. The Tibetan alphabet was adopted from the Sanskrit during the reign of King Srong-btsan-sgam-po (627–649), and the first translations of Indian and Chinese Buddhist texts began. The process of investigation, translation, and preservation of Buddhist teachings continued into the 13th century, at which time it was curtailed due to both the Moslem invasion of India and the ascendance of Genghis Khan in China. The centuries of cultural transmission brought medical theories and practices to the Tibetan people along with religious teachings. Some of the most famous early translators and religious leaders also were accomplished masters of medical theory.

The origins of Tibetan medicine may be traced to a medical conference organized by King Srong-btsan-sgam-po, who invited doctors from India, China, and Persia to his court. Each translated a text into Tibetan and then collaborated on a text growing out of their mutual discussions. The Persian doctor, Galenos (whose name may reflect the Greek origin of his teachings), remained in Tibet to serve as the king's physician (Rechung, 1973). An even larger international conference took place during the reign of King Khri-srong-lde-btsan (800–815), and was attended by representatives from India, Kashmir, China, Persia, Nepal, Afghanistan, and Sinkiang. Again, each attendant translated at least one text of their tradition. Discussions and debates were held at Samye, and several Tibetan youths were chosen to master the accumulated medical knowledge. Among them was one of the most celebrated of Tibetan physicians, gYu-thog-Yon-tan mGon-po (786–911). This time, the Chinese representative remained in Tibet to serve as the royal physician (Finckh, 1975; Rechung, 1973).

The most fundamental of the Tibetan medical texts is the four-part, 156-chapter *rGyud-bshi*. The *rGyud-bshi*, whose full title translates as the "The Four Secret Oral Tantras on the Eight Branches of the Medical Tradition," is a reworking of a Sanskrit text, the *Amrta Astanga Guhyopadesa Tantra*, which is thought to have been complied in the fourth century A.D. (Tsarong, 1979). The original Sanskrit work is lost, and there remains not even a reference to it in the Indian medical tradition (Dash, 1976).

The *rGyud-bshi* remains the most popular, widely studied, and frequently commented upon Tibetan medical text. It is divided into four parts: (1) the Root Treatise, which contains an overview of the eight disease groups (bodily diseases, childhood diseases, female diseases, nervous diseases, wounds, poisoning, diseases of the elderly, and infertility); (2) the Explanatory Treatise, which further classifies the range of diagnosis, treatment, and disease; (3) the Treatise of Instruction, which describes each disease in detail and includes a section on nervous and mental disease; and (4) the Final Treatise, which describes methods of diagnosis (e.g., questioning, examination of pulse, examination of urine) and methods of therapy (e.g., diet, behavioral modification, herbal medicines, and moxabustion) (Finckh, 1980). Translations of the early sections of the *rGyud-bshi* are available (Donden & Kelsang, 1977; Tsarong, 1979), but translations of the more detailed later sections have not been completed. In addition to this fundamental text, scores of other medical texts are available in untranslated form (catalogued by Tibetan Medical Center, Dharamsala, India).

Concepts

Tibetan medicine is fundamentally concerned with maintaining the balance of the three *nyes-pa* (pronounced "nyay-bas")—literally the three "defects," "faults," or "forms of punishment." These *nyes-pa* have a dualistic function: when kept in balance they maintain physical and mental health; but when they are disturbed—that is, increased or decreased—they act as causes of disease. The *nyes-pa* are said to be essential for life and for the continuance of the mind-body complex; and yet they must always be regarded as potential causers of harm. Consistent with the Buddhist view that existence itself contains the seed of suffering, the *nyes-pa* represent essential bodily processes that in themselves become "forms of punishment."

The three *nyes-pa* are *rlung* (pronounced "loong"), *mKhris-pa* (pronounced "tri-pa"), and *Bhad-kan* (pronounced "bay-gan"). The common translations of "wind," "bile," and "phlegm" are helpful in that they roughly indicate the general qualities of the three *nyes-pa*, but the translations may be harmful in that they tend to create impressions among Westerners that are not present for the Tibetans. The three *nyes-pa* represent physical processes whose harmonious interaction is necessary for life, from the cellular to the organismic level.

Prana is described as being in continuous flux; this movement of *prana* is called *rlung*, which has the qualities of roughness, lightness, coldness, mobility, compactness, and subtleness. The *rlung* consists of *pranic* currents, and it is most prominent in those bodily processes characterized by motion or flow (e.g., the nervous, vascular, or muscular systems). The *mKhris-pa* is said to possess the qualities of heat, greasiness, sharpness, lightness, purging, and moistness. It is most prominent in bodily processes characterized by heat generation or energy production (e.g., digestion and metabolism). *Bhad-kan* has the qualities of greasiness, coolness, heaviness, bluntness, softness, firmness, and adhesiveness. It is most apparent in bodily processes characterized by cooling, lubrication, and energy conservation (e.g., thermoregulation, synovial fluid or mucus production, some digestion, and sleep). According to Tibetan medicine, when a given *nyes-pa* is disturbed, those bodily processes most characteristic of that *nyes-pa* tend to reflect the disturbance (Touw, 1980).

Tibetan medicine ultimately attributes imbalances in any of the three *nyes-pa* to psychological causes. The three *nyes-pa* owe their existence to the three afflictive mental factors that are the roots of all unwholesome states of mind and that in Buddhist theory, are the basis of birth in cyclical existence.

> The very fact that one takes birth is a reflection of the fact that we are subject to disease. We take birth due to the fact that we have ignorance— this being the distant cause of all disorders; thus, that we have taken birth is itself a reflection of the fact that we are subject to disorders due to ignorance—a failure to understand how things really are. Because of this misapprehension of the nature of things other types of negative states of mind are generated. For instance, due to ignorance we generate close-mindedness, a type of ignorance which makes us fail to recognize faults, negativities, or shortcomings we have. Consequently, the other four types of negative minds—desire, hatred, pride, and jealousy—are produced. These give rise to physical manifestations in the form of the three hu-mours. The nature or characteristics of desire actually correspond to wind, vital currents; due to this correspondence, desire produces wind disorders. Hatred is like fire, or tremendous energy; from it energy or bile disorders arise. From close-mindedness, which is deep, heavy, dull, and cloudy, phlegm disorders are produced. The characteristics of the phlegm . . . correspond to the heaviness of close-mindedness. (Donden & Hop-kins, 1974)

Thus, the psychological theory of the *Abhidharma* is tied to the medi-cal theories of the three *nyes-pa*, and disease states are seen as crystal-lizations of dominant stages of mind.

MIND, CONSCIOUSNESS, AND *RLUNG*

In order to understand mental illness from the Tibetan point of view, an understanding of the nature, properties, and functions of *rlung* is essential. In fact, according to Tibetan medical theory, the intrinsic, natural functioning of the mind depends on the balance of *pranic* cur-rents. Mind not only has the light, fluctuating nature of *rlung*, but con-sciousness itself depends on *rlung* to successfully ascertain its object of awareness.

According to Buddhist psychological theory, each moment of aware-ness is dependent upon the simultaneous arising of three factors: (1) an object of one of the five senses or the mind, (2) the sense or mind faculty, and (3) a specific consciousness directed at one of the five senses or at the mind that has the function of "knowing" the perception. Thus, for example, a moment of visual awareness depends upon the visual object, the eye-sensing faculty, and consciousness of the sensation; a moment of mental awareness depends upon the mental object (thoughts or emotions that are categorized under the rubric of "mental factors"), the mind that generates the thought, and the faculty of consciousness directed at the mental event.

Tibetan medical theory asserts that *rlung* serves as the medium for consciousness, facilitating its actions and enabling it to move from object to object. "The way that rlung acts as the basis or mount of consciousness is exemplified by a horse serving as a mount for a rider" (Lati & Hopkins, 1979, p. 32). In this sense, consciousness is carried by the currents of *rlung* as it changes its object moment to moment. Without the medium of *rlung*, this change in objects could not occur.

Tibetan theory holds that mind, consciousness, and *rlung* can all be described along a continuum of corporeality, from the grossest and most physical to the subtlest and most ethereal. Mind, for instance, is described in terms of the gross faculties of physical sensation, the subtle faculties of thought and emotion, and the very subtle mind that continues into the intermediate state, serving as the foundation for the next birth. *Rlung* is categorized along the same continuum, from physical to subtle to very subtle. Examples of this will be given below.

Five major subdivisions of *rlung* are distinguished on the basis of their location, their area of circulation, and their function. These major subdivisions represent the distinctive *pranic* currents that support the psychophysical organism.

1. *Life-sustaining current*—From the point of view of mental disorders, this current is the most relevant. Its source is located variously at the crown of the head or in the heart, but in all cases it is said to circulate between head and chest. It enables swallowing of food, respiration, spitting out of saliva, and sneezing. It also "provides clarity to one's mind and to the sensory organs and . . . provides the physical basis for life to lodge itself. Literally, 'it provides the physical basis for the mind'" (Donden, 1980). The life-sustaining current itself can be broken down into five secondary currents, each of which serves as the basis for one of the five sense consciousnesses associated with sight, hearing, smell, taste, and touch. These secondary forms serve as "aids in the apprehension of objects by the five sense consciousnesses" (Lati & Hopkins, 1979, p. 66). On a subtler level, the life-sustaining current serves as the basis for conceptual mental consciousness (Lati & Hopkins, 1979), and on a very subtle level, it is this aspect of *prana* that supports the very subtle mind that passes from one life through the intermediate (*bardo*) state to the next life.

2. *Ascending current*—This current is located at the chest but circulates through the nose, tongue, and throat regions. It functions to promote body tone, and, in a similar fashion, it aids mental tone by helping memory, "enabling one to reflect on what one has previously experienced" (Donden, 1980). It also supports speech and swallowing.

3. *Pervasive (diffusive) current*—Located variously at the heart or crown of the head, this current is nevertheless found in every part of the body, especially in the joints. It serves to help flexion and extension of the limbs, muscular action, physical growth, and the smooth performance of bodily functions in general, including the thinking process.

4. *Metabolic (fire-accompanying) current*—Located at the stomach, it circulates in all hollow parts of the body, including the nerve and blood vessels. After decomposition and initial digestion of solid foodstuffs, it aids the overall process of digestion by enabling absorption of particularized matter.

5. *Descending current*—Located in the pelvic region, it circulates through the gastrointestinal tract, the large intestine, the bladder, and the genitals. It controls the mechanism of semen production, of ovulation and menstruation, of childbirth, and of collection and discharge of excretory matter.

Thus, *rlung* is said to serve as the basis for nerve, skeletal muscle, smooth muscle, and vascular transport activity as well as much of the hormonal and membrane transport activity. On a more subtle level, it serves as the foundation for mental and sense consciousness. As such, *rlung* encompasses the mind but is not limited to it. Indeed, mind is not seen as separate from body; mind is inseparably linked to the body through the medium of *rlung*. Thus, mental disturbance is said to be reflected in an alteration of the flow of *rlung*; likewise, disturbance of *rlung* anywhere within the organism is said to produce correlative mental or emotional disturbances.

RLUNG IN DEATH AND MEDITATION

Nowhere is the theory of *rlung* more important than with regard to the death experience. According to the teachings of Highest Yoga Tantra, the process of dying may be described in terms of the sequential dissolution of the various aspects of *rlung*. "Upon the serial collapse of the ability of these [*pranic* currents] to serve as bases of consciousness, the events of death—internal and external—unfold" (Lati & Hopkins, 1979, p. 13). In death, all the *pranic* currents of the body ultimately dissolve into the very subtle life-sustaining current that then serves as the basis for the consciousness of the intermediate state (*bardo*) between physical death and rebirth. Practitioners of the Highest Yoga Tantra seek, through meditation, to consciously mirror the death experience by deliberately bringing about the same dissolution of vital currents that occurs at death (Chang, 1963; Lati & Hopkins, 1979). This difficult process involves gaining mastery over the currents of *prana*, mimicking the many alterations of consciousness that Tantric theory describes as occurring at death. "Psychologically, due to the fact that consciousness of varying grossness and subtlety depends on the [*pranic* currents] like a rider on a horse, their dissolving or loss of ability to serve as bases of consciousness induces radical changes in conscious experience" (Lati & Hopkins, 1979, p. 15). By bringing about these experiences in meditation, familiarity with the process of death is said to be gained. Perfection of this Yoga thus allows mastery over death, the transformation of the very subtle life-sustaining *prana* into the basis of the "metaphoric clear light" and "illusory body," and subsequent freedom from rebirth (Lati & Hopkins, 1979, pp. 71–72). These descriptions lie at the heart of such works as *The Tibetan Book of the Dead* and account for much of the theory behind advanced Tantric meditation practices.

RLUNG DISEASE

Mental disorders are described in two major sections of the Tibetan medical Tantras: the general category of *rlung* disease and the category of "madness" (*smyo*). In order to appreciate the Tibetan conception of mental disturbance, it is necessary to understand in some depth the Tibetan conceptualization of the nature, etiology, and symptoms of *rlung* disorders.

Etiology

According to Tibetan medicine, the disorders of the flow of *prana* are numerous, and each disorder can vary in degree of severity. Initial disorders are said to arise from disturbances in the flow of *prana* through its natural channels. Repeated aggravation, however, leads to an increase of *rlung* beyond its normal range. But at this point, *rlung* is still confined to its natural channels. The two processes of initial disturbance and aggravated increase are usually inseparable; together they result in alterations of the functions of those organ systems that are predominantly *rlung* in nature. With continued disturbance and aggravation, *rlung* increases beyond a critical point overflowing its natural channels and disrupting the other two *nyes-pa* and the bodily processes dependent on them. In a similar way, if one of the other *nyes-pa* is disturbed and aggravated, it will also overflow and affect the circulation of *rlung*, causing symptoms of decreased *rlung* to appear. General causes of *rlung* imbalance are said to include: improper diet or behavior patterns, seasonal factors, improper medications, poisons, external forces or spirits, and the fruition of negative actions (Donden, 1980). Some of these causes (e.g., the dietary, seasonal, behavioral, and toxic factors) are ascertainable through questioning or reasoning; some (e.g., the influence of external forces) are deducible through examination; and others (e.g., the fruition of negative actions) are assumed when all other causes are absent.

Certain behavioral factors are said to serve as pathological agents in the formation, augmentation, and disruption of *rlung*. They represent extremes of mental and physical behavior that directly influence the circulation of *rlung* in the body, with both physical and mental ramifications. These factors include:

1. Poor diet (e.g., excessive bitter, light, or coarse foods, such as coffee, cucumber, strong tea, or pork)
2. Excessive sexual intercourse
3. Insufficient food or prolonged fasting
4. Insomnia
5. Physical, oral, or mental strain or exertion on an empty stomach
6. Obsessive thoughts ("thinking about something for a long time without actually doing something about it" [Donden, 1980])
7. Hemorrhage
8. Excessive vomiting or diarrhea
9. Exposure to cold (e.g., breezes)
10. Lack of appetite
11. Excessive joy or sadness
12. Depression (especially as a result of frustrated desire)
13. Malnutrition (insufficient protein)
14. Straining in passing excreta, forceful retention of excreta, excessive, forceful sneezing or spitting

Rlung Disorders

Categories. There are said to be a total of 63 different *rlung* disorders, each describable in terms of the symptom complexes that comprise it. Of these 63, 48 fall into the general category of disorders severe enough to affect a particular organ system directly, and 15 fall into a specific category of disturbances in the function and balance of the five subdivisions of *rlung* described earlier.

The diseases in the general category are summarized in terms of their effects on skull, heart, lung, liver, stomach, large intestine, kidneys, or the whole of the body. Long-standing overflow of *rlung* from its natural pathways produces disorders characterized primarily by neurological symptoms (e.g., muscular rigidity, spasms, emaciation, swelling/distension, contracture of limbs, aching pain, loss of sensory function, numbness and tingling, and coma).

Diseases in the specific category are summarized in terms of the manifestations of disturbance of each of the five major *pranic* currents. Specific symptom complexes reflect disturbance of specific *pranic* currents in ways that will be detailed shortly.

Symptoms.   It is clear that the spectrum of disorders of *pranic* flow encompasses much more than just mental disturbance. Tibetan medical texts contain detailed descriptions of the symptom complexes that characterize the physical deterioration that results from *rlung* disturbance. Contained in these lists are a host of what Western health professionals have come to call "non-specific complaints." The individual, suffering from one or more of these symptoms, feels that something is wrong, but the Western physician is often unable to make a definite diagnosis. While acknowledging that behavioral and dietary factors may be etiological agents, the Tibetan physician does not dismiss these symptoms as "psychosomatic"—to the Tibetan physician they reflect a disturbance in the flow of the body's *prana*. An explanation exists within the Tibetan system for these complaints, and patients are treated accordingly.

Symptoms of *rlung* disturbance follow (Donden & Kelsang, 1977). The constellation of signs and symptoms may seem nebulous, but according to Tibetan medicine they are primary indicators of *pranic* disturbance:

Pulse is empty and adrift, disappears when pressed
Urine is clear and watery with no transformation on cooling
Restlessness
Sighing
An unsteady, flighty mind
Giddiness
Tinnitus (ringing in the ears)

Tongue is dry, red, and rough with astringent taste even when no food has been eaten

Erratic and diffuse pains

Coldness and shivering

Diffuse pain on movement in all parts of the body

Lassitude

Muscle cramping inhibiting flexion/extension

Feeling as if flesh has separated from skin and bones have separated at joints

Sensation of broken bones

Sensation of eyes and other organs bulging out

Sensation of limbs being bound

Goosebumps

Insomnia

Yawning, trembling, desire to stretch

Anger

Impression of pelvic region (bones and joints) being pounded

Backache, pain in chest and jaw bones

Pain in *rlung* focal points (first, sixth, seventh vertebrae) especially when pressed

Dry heaves

Distended stomach

Abdominal noises

Symptoms of aggravated increase of *rlung* (Donden & Kelsang, 1977) include dryness of the body, attraction to warmth, trembling, bulging of the abdomen, constipation, talkativeness, dizziness, decreased strength, sleeplessness, and diminished clarity of the senses. Symptoms of decreased *rlung* include low energy, little speech, physical discomfort, unclear memory and attention, coldness, poor digestion, heaviness, lassitude, oversleeping, difficulty in breathing, excess saliva and mucus, and looseness of the limbs.

To the Tibetan physician, the presence of any of these mental and physical symptoms is immediately suggestive of a *rlung* disorder. Confirmation is obtained through the analysis of the pulse and the urine and through questioning for the presence of pathological agents listed previously.

At certain times, the given constellation of symptoms, physical signs, and personal history indicates a specific disturbance of one of the five major currents: life-sustaining, ascending, pervasive, metabolic, or descending. We will now examine some of these specific disturbances.

Disturbance of the Life-sustaining *Rlung.*   Most common anxieties, minor depressions, and uncontrollable surfacings of emotion as well as giddiness or breathlessness are attributed to primary disturbance and aggravation of the balance of the life-sustaining *pranic* current called *sok-rlung.* When the life-sustaining current is more seriously affected—that is, through invasion of its channels by other increased currents—violent or hysterical behavior may appear. In extreme cases, psychosis may result.

The causes of disturbed *sok-rlung* are said to include mental strain of any kind, a diet excessively low in protein, fasting or hunger for long periods, physical exertion exacerbating any of the above, and straining in passing excreta. Disturbance is more likely to occur when external circumstances are very much in flux. In short, Tibetans conceive of most anxieties and depressions in terms of a disturbance in *sok-rlung,* in the life-sustaining *pranic* current that provides the physical basis for the mind. Since the mind is said to rest on the life-sustaining current, a disturbance in that current similarly disturbs the mind and creates pain.

Meditation-induced *Sok-rlung.*[2]   One area in which the Tibetan culture can undisputedly claim expertise is in the theory and practice of meditation. A specific kind of *sok-rlung* disorder is said to be associated with meditation: it is a complication of improper meditation practice and is widely referred to simply as *"sok-rlung."* Tibetan physicians, lamas, and meditation instructors are well versed in the predisposing causes, symptoms, and treatments of this disorder. As Westerners become increasingly fascinated with meditation, a recognition of this disorder may prove to be necessary.

According to Tibetans, this type of *sok-rlung* is more likely to arise in meditators who are improperly instructed in methods designed to concentrate the mind. If the meditation object is not suitable for the individual, if the developed concentration is tarnished by negative states of mind or not balanced with sufficient mindfulness, and if the mind is not concentrated with the proper effortlessness, *sok-rlung* may develop. The last condition

---

[2] This section on meditation-induced *sok-rlung* was compiled after interviews in the spring of 1981 with Dr. Yeshe Donden, Dharamsala, India; Ven. Lobsong Gyatso, Principal, The Buddhist School of Dialectics, Dharamsala, India; Ven. Kalu Rinpoche, Sonada, India; H. H. Gyalwa Karmapa, Rumtek Monastery, Sikkim.

is perhaps the most important. If strain develops in the mind's attempt to concentrate itself on the object of meditation, if the mind is forced into submission rather than being gently guided into one-pointedness, if the mind squeezes and tightens in its attempt at concentration, then the mind is said to "rise up" in its attempt to find the object. As the mind rises up, the *pranic* current on which it is mounted rises with it, producing the symptoms and signs of *sok-rlung*. This same rise in *sok-rlung* also will occur when obsessive inner thoughts about progress in meditation arise in a mind already concentrated to the degree that external sensory inputs no longer occur.

The result of this disturbance of *sok-rlung* is said to be a kind of manic state in which the mind races. Instead of becoming calm through the practice of meditation, the mind reacts to the forceful attempt to subdue it and becomes unable to settle on any object. The individual becomes anxious, restless, often dramatically emotional, and insensitive to the guidance of teachers due to the mind's inability to concentrate effectively on another's words.

A sensitive teacher can best note the disturbance of *sok-rlung* at an early stage by engaging in slow, quiet conversation with the individual and observing the way his or her mind and speech jump from subject to subject, often before one thought is completely finished. The person's pallor, appearance of the eyes, restlessness, and reluctance to answer questions also provide valuable clues to the presence of this disorder. Physically, the neck, shoulders, and upper back often ache.

Changing the meditation object or careful instruction in the method of meditation may be sufficient to correct this disorder in its early stage. In more advanced cases, a halt to all efforts at meditation is recommended; an ample diet of nutritious, high-protein food is prescribed; and the affected individual is instructed to relax, to avoid worrisome thoughts, and not to spend too much time alone. Disturbance of the life-sustaining current is recognized as one hazard of meditation practice, affecting beginners as well as those with developed powers of concentration, and efforts are made to recognize the signs of the disorder as soon as they appear.

Other *Rlung* Disorders.   While most mental disturbances, according to Tibetan medicine, are reflective of disordered life-sustaining *rlung*, disruptions of the balance of the other four major *pranic* currents also occur, with psychophysiological manifestations. These disruptions may be limited to one individual current or may occur in conjunction with or as a side effect of disturbed life-sustaining *rlung*.

For example, the balance of the ascending current can be disrupted through causes as diverse as the suppression of vomit, the lifting of heavy objects, or excessive emotionalism, especially weeping. Manifestations include difficulty in swallowing, fatigue, malaise, and difficulties with memory. Pervasive *rlung* is disrupted through overactivity, physical stress, restlessness, resting in damp places, shock, fright, depression, or phobic behavior. Symptoms include general wasting, insomnia, and decreased mental functioning as evidenced by prolonged staring and gaping, fainting, excessive verbal activity, and unsubstantiated fears.

Metabolic *rlung* disturbances can be aggravated by indigestible food or daytime sleeping and can result in indigestion, lack of appetite, vomiting, or abdominal hyperactivity. Descending *rlung* can be aggravated by straining at passing excreta or by increase in bile. Its disturbance produces constipation, bad breath, and pain in the pelvic region.

A fully developed case of clinical depression, with its complex of weight loss, anorexia, constipation, inability to concentrate, and insomnia, could represent imbalance of at least four of the five major *pranic* currents. The life-sustaining *rlung* disorder is reflected in the depressive mood state; pervasive *rlung* disorder is manifested in the substandard mental functioning, insomnia, and general wasting; metabolic *rlung* disorder could contribute to loss of appetite; and descending *rlung* disorder could play a role in constipation. It is rare, in fact, for a long-standing disturbance of the life-sustaining current not to influence the balance of the other currents (Y. Donden, personal communication, March 1981).

Therapeutics

According to Tibetan medicine, there are four types of treatment for *rlung* disorders: diet, behavior, medications, and secondary therapeutics (e.g., massage, moxabustion, or enemas). Although some disorders can be remedied merely by dietary and behavioral manipulations, most require medications compounded from a vast array of natural, predominantly herbal, sources. Other disorders are also helped by the secondary measures, especially by massage with oils.

General dietary guidelines for *rlung* disorders include high-protein intake, especially from meat, soups made from bones, hot milk, cooked dough of grains, seed oil, brown sugar, garlic, and onion. Behavioral guidelines include abstinence from the pathogenic factors detailed previously; a congenial, warm, not too light or bright environment, preferably on the ground floor; warm clothing; pleasant friendly speech; the company of congenial, amiable friends; and a comfortable room and bed to induce undisturbed sleep.

A variety of herbal compounds, containing from 8 to 35 ingredients, are used to treat *rlung* disorders after accurate diagnosis is made through questioning and through analysis of pulse and urine.

MADNESS[3]

General Features

Although several authors (Ardussi & Epstein, 1978; Burang, 1957) make reference to the Tibetan conception of madness (*smyon-pa;* pronounced "nyon-ba"), none appear to have had access to the fundamental medical works on the subject. Tibetan medicine depends heavily on Tantric theory for the description and explanation of madness. According to Tantra, in madness, it is the life-sustaining current that is primarily affected—especially in its subtle form as the basis for mental consciousness. In the Tantric descriptions, the site of the life-sustaining current is the heart. In the area of the heart lie the primary channels that contain the life-sustaining current, which in turn supports or serves as the mount for the mind of conceptual mental consciousness. Psychosis is said to result when the space or channel containing the subtle life-sustaining *prana* is forcefully entered by another energy, usually a spirit but sometimes merely another increased *nyes-pa*, disturbing the relationship between *pranic* flow and mind.

As with other disorders, certain factors are said to encourage the development of madness. Depression, mental discomfort, mental exertion, a weak heart, poor diet, and behavioral patterns, such as excessive use of drugs or alcohol, are listed as predisposing causes. In addition, in the pathogenesis of madness, the interference of harmful spirits is said to act as a "condition" for its development. This condition acts as a helping agent, the immediate external factor that precipitates the changes in consciousness, but it cannot act without the predisposing causes. Thus, cause and condition act together to disrupt the *pranic* currents that support the mind.

The mechanics of this disruption are described in some detail in the religious Tantras that are quoted in medical texts. The heart center is conceived as an eight-petaled lotus in whose center lies the "king of channels." The heart center is the site of the very subtle *rlung* that serves as the basis for the consciousness of the intermediate (*bardo*) state. This channel is thought to be as tiny as the width of a hair in a horse's tail. Surrounding this channel are the four major channel pathways going in four different directions, plus two more pathways, one above the heart

---

[3]The following material is based on a translation of Chapter 78 of Part III of *rGyud-bshi* made with commentaries by Dr. Yeshe Donden, Dharamsala, India to the authors.

center and one below. These six channels, or "six collections of consciousnesses," represent the locations of the five divisions of the life-sustaining current that support the sense consciousnesses and the pathway of the subtle life-sustaining current that supports the mind of conceptual mental consciousness. Their locations are as follows:

East (anterior): Ear consciousness—blackish color
West (posterior): Nose consciousness—yellowish color
North (lateral): Taste consciousness—whitish color
South (lateral): Eye consciousness—reddish color
Superior (above): Body consciousness—greenish color
Inferior (below): Mental consciousness—bluish color

The invasion by spirit or *nyes-pa* is said to occur through the anterior channel, through the current that supports ear consciousness. It proceeds through the anterior channel to the inferior channel, site of the support of mental consciousness. This invasion creates a blockage in the inferior site, occluding or reversing the current of *prana* upon which the mind rests. Thus, control over the functioning of mental processes is lost; loss of memory and hysterical behavior precede full-fledged psychosis.

Mind, memory, and mental consciousness are thus disturbed. The capacity to sense the pleasant or unpleasant feelings that normally accompany all sense awareness is lost. The ability to feel happy or sad and to understand the nature and causes of suffering is lost. "One becomes like a chariot without a driver and nowhere does one find any consciousness which is under one's control" (Y. Donden, personal communication, March 1981).

Although this process is sometimes said to be caused by a spirit "robbing" the subtle life-sustaining current, this is not in fact the case. Rather, the spirit forcefully enters the site of the life-sustaining current, delocalizes it, and begins to function itself in that space. This is akin to two people living together in one room; when one becomes more powerful, the other loses control, and struggle becomes commonplace. No longer does the affected person's mind bear its original nature; however, the individual has not totally lost his or her mind either. The sensory organs and consciousnesses "function in total dependence on the objects they come in contact with" (Y. Donden, personal communication, March 1981), often rendering the individual incapacitated in his or her own environment and causing him or her to react in a stimulus-bound fashion without the benefits of rational judgments or memories.

Seven types of madness are distinguished:

1. Madness with primary disturbance of *rlung*—The affected individual is thinly built, is temperamental and emotionally labile, has reddish sclera and is worse after eating (i.e., while digesting food).

2. Madness with primary disturbance of *mKhris-pa*—The affected individual is frequently angry, desires cool food, has yellowish sclera and urine, and has vision disturbed by images of fire or stars.

3. Madness with primary disturbance of *Bhad-kan*—The individual is quiet, anorexic, withdrawn, drowsy, physically moist with excess mucus and saliva.

4. Madness with complex disturbance of all three *nyes-pa*—The individual shows symptoms and signs of the three types listed above.

5. Madness primarily characterized by depression—Often it is precipitated by separation from possessions or family. The individual is self-centered (often punishing himself or herself for no reason), and becomes easily aggressive or delerious with no control over body, speech, or mind. At these times, he or she often may be overheard muttering meaningless words. In quieter moments, the individual excessively ponders emotional losses, has a withdrawn attitude, and suffers from insomnia.

6. Madness primarily due to toxic causes, that is, to external or internal poisons invading the body—The individual is characterized by pallor, weakness, wasting, and delerium.

7. Madness primarily due to harmful spirit—These cases are characterized by a sudden change in personality. The individual acquires the temperament and behavior patterns of one of 60 types of harmful spirits known to Tantric demonologists. Even in the above six cases, the influence of spirits cannot be discounted.

Spirit Influences

As can be seen from the preceding discussion, Tibetan healers regard spirit possession as an activating condition of psychosis. In the Tibetan view, there are many different kinds of possession, some deliberate, healthy, and functional, and some inadvertent and dysfunctional.

Of the six realms of Tibetan cosmology—humans, animals, hungry ghosts (pretas), hell beings, jealous gods, and gods (devas)—it is primarily the hungry ghosts that cause psychosis. These beings are motivated by all of the afflictive emotions (e.g., hatred, desire, and ignorance), are able to travel as fast as thoughts, and are sometimes attracted to humans predisposed to their influence. The deliberate forms of spirit possession are found, for example, in those sought by the Tibetan oracle. Such an individual "acts as a mouthpiece for the gods or spirits who possess him and speak through him, very often without his own knowledge of what is being said, answering directly the questions of those who consult him" (Prince Peter of Greece and Denmark, 1978).

According to Tibetans, the first line of therapy for disorders presumed to be caused by spirits is religious. The services of a lama or similarly trained doctor are employed, and ceremonies designed to "throw off" the harmful influences are performed. In many of the Tantric rituals employed in such cases, the doctor or lama assumes the role of *vajracarya* or hierophant, becoming "a kind of funnel for sacred life force to pour into the profane world" (Wayman, 1968, p. 175) through his evocation of and identification with various aspects of the enlightened mind (Stablein, 1973, 1978; Wayman, 1973). As a preventive measure, the affected individual will then undertake certain spiritual practices designed to ward off further harmful influences. The cultivation of charity and other wholesome actions is also thought beneficial for affected individuals— the force of the merit accompanying such actions is thought to help subdue the negative influence.

CONCLUDING REMARKS

One of the great strengths of Tibetan medicine, and one of the reasons that it may more easily come to benefit the West than other traditional systems, is the voluminous literature describing every aspect of the practice—from classification of disease, to diagnosis, treatment, and pharmacology. Analysis of traditional texts about mental health and illness reveal the incredible clarity of this medical system that is particularly attuned to the infinite variety of physical, mental, emotional, and spiritual symptoms, none of which are slighted or ignored. As befits a culture in which the spiritual dimension is inextricably linked to the material one, the "psychic anatomy" is as precisely described as the physical. Nevertheless, Tibetan medicine does not claim ultimate success; it rests on a philosophical premise succinctly put forth by a contemporary Tibetan physician: "The root is beginningless ignorance. Due to its force we are caught in cyclic existence, in the round of repeated birth, aging, sickness, and death. Ignorance is with us like our own shadow; thus, even if we think that there is no reason to be ill, even if we think we are in very good health, actually we have had the basic cause of illness since beginningless time" (Donden, 1986, p. 26).

References

Ardussi, J., & Epstein, L. (1978). The saintly madman in Tibet. In J. F. Fisher (Ed.), *Himalayan anthropology.* The Hague: Morton.

Burang, T. (1957, 1974). *Tibetan art of healing.* London: Watkins.

Chang, G. (1963, 1977). *Teachings of Tibetan yoga.* Secaucus, NJ: Citadel Press.

Clifford, T. (1984). *Tibetan Buddhist medicine and psychiatry: The diamond healing.* York Beach, ME: Samuel Weiser.

Dash, V. (1976). *Tibetan medicine.* Dharamsala, India: Library of Tibetan Works and Archives.

Donden, Y. (1977). *The ambrosia heart tantra, vol. 1: The secret oral teaching on the eight branches of the science of healing* (J. Kelsang, Trans.). Dharamsala, India: Library of Tibetan Works and Archives.

Donden, Y. (1980). *Introductory lectures on Tibetan medicine* (S. Topgay, J. Kelsang, & J. Hopkins, Trans.). Unpublished manuscript.

Donden, Y. (1986). *Health through balance: An introduction to Tibetan medicine* (J. Hopkins, Ed. and Trans.). Ithaca, NY: Snow Lion.

Donden, Y., & Hopkins, J. (1974). *Tibetan medicine.* (J. Hopkins, Ed. and Trans.) Lectures.

Epstein, M., & Topgay, S. (1982). Mind and mental disorders in Tibetan medicine. *Revision, 5*(1), 67–79.

Evans-Wentz, W. Y. (1958). *Tibetan yoga and secret doctrines.* London: Oxford University Press.

Finckh, E. (1975, 1978). *Foundations of Tibetan medicine* (Vol. 1). London: Watkins.

Finckh, E. (1980). Tibetan medicine—theory and practice. In M. Aris & A. San Suu Kyi (Eds.), *Tibetan studies in honor of Hugh Richardson.* New Delhi: Vikas Publishing.

Goleman, D., & Epstein, M. (1980). Meditation and wellbeing: An eastern model of psychological health. *ReVision, 3*(2), 73–85.

Govinda, L. A. (1960). *Foundations of Tibetan mysticism.* New York: Samuel Weiser.

Kao, J. (1979). *Three millennia of Chinese psychiatry.* New York: Institute for Advanced Research in Asian Science and Medicine.

Lati, R., & Hopkins, J. (1979). *Death, intermediate state and rebirth in Tibetan Buddhism.* New York: Gabriel Press.

Prince Peter of Greece and Denmark. (1978). Tibetan oracles. In J. F. Fisher (Ed.), *Himalayan anthropology.* The Hague: Morton.

Rao, S. K. (1979). *Tibetan meditation.* New Delhi: Arnold-Heinemann.

Rechung Rinpoche. (1973, 1976). *Tibetan medicine.* Berkeley, CA: University of California Press.

sGam. po. pa. (1972). *Jewel ornament of liberation.* (Translated and annotated by Herbert Gunther). Berkeley, Shambhala.

Stablein, W. (1973). A medical-cultural system among the Tibetan and Newar Buddhists: Ceremonial medicine. *Kailash: A journal of Himalayan studies,* 1(3), 193–203.

Stablein, W. (1978). A descriptive analysis of the content of Nepalese Buddhist "Pujas" as a medical-cultural system with reference to Tibetan parallels. In J. F. Fisher (Ed.), *Himalayan anthropology.* The Hague: Morton.

Touw, M. (1980). 300 turn of the century Ayurvedic botanical remedies. Unpublished manuscript, Arnold Arboretum, Harvard University.

Tsarong, T. (1979). Concepts in traditional Tibetan medicine: Pathophysiology, diagnosis, and treatment. *Acupuncture & Electro-Therapeutic Research, International Journal, 4,* 149–158.

Wayman, A. (1968). The religious meaning of possession states. In R. Prince (Ed.), *Trance and possession states.* Montreal: R. M. Bucke Memorial Society.

Wayman, A. (1973). Buddhist tantric medicine theory on behalf of oneself and others. *Kailash: A journal of Himalayan studies.* 1(2), 153–158.

6

Sufism: The Way to Universal Self

A. REZA ARASTEH[1]
ANEES A. SHEIKH

Shibli was asked: "Who guided you in the Path?"
He said: "A dog. One day I saw him, almost dead with thirst,
standing by the water's edge.
"Every time he looked at his reflection in the water he was
frightened, and withdrew, because he thought it was another
dog.
"Finally, such was his necessity, he cast away fear and leapt
into the water, at which the 'other dog' vanished.
"The dog found that the obstacle, which was himself, the
barrier between him and what he sought, melted away.
"In this same way my own obstacle vanished, when I knew
that it was what I took to be my own self. And my Way was
first shown to me by the behaviour of a dog."

Haschmi, 1973, p. 129

---

[1]Section I of this chapter is written by the two authors; however, Dr. Arasteh is the sole author of Section II. Parts of this chapter are revised versions of portions of the first author's previously published works for which he holds the copyright (Arasteh, 1964, 1973, 1980, 1984).

This chapter consists of two complementary parts. Section I presents the nature and the psychological significance of Sufism. Section II discusses the therapeutic aspects of Sufism in relation to Western psychotherapy and healing. While Western ideas of health are sociohistorically bound, Sufism relates human health to psychocosmology.

I. SUFISM: NATURE AND PSYCHOLOGICAL SIGNIFICANCE

Mysticism can be viewed as the inward dimension of all religions. Originally, the term "mysticism" was used in reference to the mystery cults of the Greeks. For them, mystics were a select group who had knowledge of the divine. They shared in this knowledge not due to their own efforts, but because they were blessed with an innate capacity for it. The mystics were expected to keep silent about this knowledge, since most people lacked the capacity to understand it.

However, over the years, the term "mysticism" has taken on a much broader meaning. It involves a feeling shared by all human beings: a longing for the Ultimate Source, Perfect Goodness, Eternal Wisdom, Supreme Beauty, Divine Love, or God (Smith, 1973). This feeling is not only universal but also eternal. Picton defines mysticism as "the spiritual realization of a grander and boundless Unity, that humbles all self-assertion by dissolving it in a wider glory" (see Smith, 1973, p. 2). The mystic longs to pass from the finite to the infinite, from the realm of appearances to reality, and finally to merge with Being.

Mystics claim that the soul is capable of achieving this goal, and they base their assertion on certain postulates (Smith, 1973):

1. Knowledge of the highest order can be gained not by intelligence but only by the spiritual faculty of intuition.
2. All human beings carry within their soul a divine spark that longs to be united with the Eternal Flame.
3. No one can achieve direct knowledge of God without purification from the self. Selfishness and sensuality obstruct a clear vision of God.
4. Love is the soul's guiding light in the ascent to God; for only love can free the soul from the chains of selfishness and sensuality.

Sufism: The Mysticism of Islam

Sufism is the mystical or inward aspect of Islam. Stoddart (1985) likens Islam's outward dimension or "exoterism" (*sharia*) to the circumference of a circle, and the inner truth or "esoterism" (*haqiqa*) to the circle's center. The line from the circumference to the center represents the spiritual path (*tariqa*) that proceeds from observance of rituals to inner conviction, from belief to vision. Actually, the Arabic word "*sufi,*" like the Sanskrit word "*yogi,*" refers only to someone who has reached the goal; however, it is commonly applied also to those struggling toward it (Stoddart, 1985).

The Rise of Sufism. Within 25 years of the prophet Mohammed's death, most of the virtues that he had nurtured in his flock had fallen into disuse, and a decadent, heartless society emerged. Like many other significant spiritual movements, Sufism represents a rebellion against the prevailing condition. The Sufis' goal was to achieve a renaissance of the human spirit that would enable people to live simple, harmonious, and happy lives. They aspired to teach their contemporaries that egoism and the inevitably ensuing strife are folly and that the essence of the universe is spiritual (Fatemi, Fatemi, & Fatemi, 1976). Another dream of the Sufis, as expressed by Rumi, was "not to foster but rather to heal the schism between minds" evident in the disputes of the numerous Muslim, Jewish, and Christian sects (see Fatemi et al., 1976, p. 15). This goal of reconciliation clearly forms a part of the Sufi dogmas:

1. There is only one God.
2. There are as many ways to reach Truth (God) as there are people on this earth, but all ways entail the annihilation of the ego and selfless service to mankind.
3. The cardinal law is the law of reciprocity. We can live in harmony with our fellow human beings only if we possess a keen sense of justice, and the latter thrives only in a mind that has rid itself of selfishness and arrogance. The world can be a harmonious place only if justice is the dominant power.
4. Human brotherhood unites all people in the fatherhood of God.
5. Love is the underlying principle of morality. It springs from self-denial and expresses itself in service to others. It can reconcile all differences and heal all wounds.
6. The cardinal truth is self-knowledge; for, knowledge of self ripens into knowledge of God (Fatemi et al., 1976; Khan, 1979).

A Psychological Frame of Reference for Sufism. The Western psychological frame of reference, a product of Western culture, is inadequate for interpreting Sufism; however, Jung's analytical psychology explains it better than any other school. In fact, so-called "scientific" psychology and Freudian psychoanalysis perhaps are useful only for interpreting the nature of the fragmented person. The inadequacy of scientific psychology stems from its obsession with trying to be an "objective" science, and Freudian psychology suffers from its founder's limited concept of human beings. Evidence of these inadequacies can be found by a historical analysis of various schools. Early psychologists started the scientific study of human beings from the wrong assumption; instead of beginning from the basic difference that sets us apart from animals—that is, our ability for creative vision—they began with the common denominators of animal-human behavior. Later, Freud made a similar error; before having a clear concept of human beings, he investigated mental illness and its cure. Had Freud been a philosopher turning his attention to medicine, instead of being a physician turning to philosophy, his theories would have taken a different form. Furthermore, had he been acquainted with other cultures, he would have made fewer mistakes (Arasteh, 1965).

In psychology, as in all the sciences, we possess only partial truth. Truth is like a gigantic diamond that fell to earth aeons ago and broke into pieces. The pieces were scattered all over the earth, but when the natives in a particular region found a piece, they mistook it for the whole diamond. Furthermore, even if we were to bring all the pieces of the diamond of truth together, we still would have only a fragmented diamond. In order to have validity, our collection of fragments of truth about human beings must encompass the range of their development. We propose the following four successive stages of growth as frames of reference for systems of psychology:

1. During the initial stage of growth, the child's expression is dominated by biological forces. A psychobiological approach is most useful here.

2. The second stage appears as soon as socialization is rooted. We must realize that the biological force is manifested through psychocultural forces. This calls for a new theory and technique—that of psychocultural analysis.

3. The third stage begins with the objectivization of the ego and the awareness of single reality. Experiential analysis, emphasizing experience and insight, is most relevant here. At its peak, this stage will be transformed into cosmopsychology.

4. At this stage of cosmopsychology, the person's insight is harmonized with the pulsation of the universe—that is, the ordinary

experience belongs to the stage of "I-ness" (ego world), which at the experiential level becomes "he-ness," and a deeper perception arises from the world of "oneness."

Space is lacking to discuss the various inclusive systems or stages of human growth, but it suffices to reiterate that the Sufi's path of individuation begins at the experiential level and proceeds to insight into cosmopsychology. The Sufi point of view entails repudiation of the long-acknowledged belief that human beings are social animals and recognition that we are religio-psychological beings who began life in the unconscious union with nature. In the process of evolution, we separated from nature, experienced pain, time, and space; or, if you wish, we were cast from Paradise, and since then we have been seeking a new union. Psychologically, we are evolving in terms of innumerable phases of relatedness and unrelatedness, and cultural renaissances, and we will ultimately reunite with the cosmos in a conscious existence state. In other words, there is a *koan* (as in Zen Buddhism) that we try to decipher, there is a treasure (as in Sufism) that we try to discover, or there is a Messiah (as in Christianity) that we try to emulate. There are innumerable degrees of awareness, each engulfing the one before it, until "not-being" reaches the shore of being.

Before we discuss the nature of Sufism, we must differentiate between the experience, which is the union of the subject-object, and the behavior as interpreted by Western psychologists. Undoubtedly, in healthy individuals, experience and behavior overlap and inner and outer expression are the same; but in many cases, behavior is the rationalization or inhibitor of experience—it is a cover. Experience has an organic and illuminatory nature, whereas, behavior is characterized by conditioning. It is experience, not behavior, that produces change and, at the same time, strengthens one's sensitivity. It is said that all the conditioning of Pavlov's dog was undone by one night's flood in the cellar where the dog was kept. In fact, those who prepare to take the path of Sufism must first "uncondition" themselves.

The Nature of Sufism. Numerous scholars have attempted to determine the meaning of the word "Sufi." Some have argued that the term originates from "*safa*"—referring to the Sufi's purity of heart; others claim that "*saff*" means "of the first rank or vanguard"; and still others insist that the term "Sufi" refers to their wool garments. Furthermore, because some Sufis stayed in caves, they became known as "*shikaftis,*" which means "of the cavern"; those who subsisted on little food were called "paupers"; others were better known for their ardor, and sometimes they were called "illuminati," intuitionists, or "sincere ones." However, it is apparent that these terms reflect merely external qualities. Sufism is an art of rebirth, a process of regaining one's naturalness, a way out of automation, and a vehicle for creative vision. It is the process of awareness of the world of multireality and the perception of single reality. It is loyalty to life and cosmic laws, harmonization with true nature. It is liberation from the cultural self and relatedness to the cosmic self.

In essence, Sufism is an inner experience that leads to identification with one's object of desire, the so-called beloved, or if you prefer, the ideal-ego. In the history of Sufism, the object of desire has passed through an evolutionary process. The early Sufis were seeking the true qualities of a Muslim as stated in the Koran (Lings, 1975; Shah, 1970). The Sufis of the ninth century, beginning with Ali Abu Mansur al-Hallaj (who was crucified because he claimed he was creative truth) and culminating with Attar, chose the image of Allah (One) as their object of desire. Still later, other Sufis (e.g., Rumi and Hafiz) identified with the process of creative unconscious, identified as love (Arasteh, 1980).

The process of this identification was manifested in the I-thou relationship. "Thou" can be any object of desire, and "I" can be any person at any stage who is incited by the proper object of desire. In the process of union of I and thou, the essential point is the inner motivation of the seeker. The heart must be motivated from within. The thou, the object of desire, must be worthy enough. In Sufi literature, the purity of heart—the most essential of all—and the intention are often compared to a clear mirror.

A story from Rumi's *Mathnawi* (see Arasteh, 1980) illustrates this point beautifully. At one time a group of Greek and a group of Chinese artists were claiming to be the best artists. The king, a patron of art, put them to a test. He housed them in separate rooms, one opening into the other. The Greeks requested all kinds of paints and started to paint a beautiful picture, while the Chinese asked for nothing except tools with which to remove the rust and discoloration of the wall. They spent their time cleaning and polishing the wall until it shone like a mirror. After some time, the king visited the artists. When the Greeks drew aside the curtain, the king saw a picture so beautiful that it robbed him of his wits. When he entered the room of the Chinese, they drew aside their curtain; the reflection of the Greek painting on their mirror-like wall was so overwhelmingly beautiful that it robbed him of his sight. The polished wall symbolizes the heart of the Sufis, which when freed from the rust of greed, possessiveness, and prejudice, reflects inner and outer reality and grasps truth spontaneously and so quickly that interpretation and search are not needed (Shafii, 1985). As Rumi says, "When the psyche is in darkness one needs the light of reason to see his or her way through life, but when the psyche is illuminated no one needs reason's candle" (see Arasteh, 1980, p. 48).

If one's mirror has become cloudy, through socialization, competition, or professional recognition, one needs more cleansing than even an illiterate but natural person. If one's state is alienated through anger, hate, greed, envy, or jealousy, one needs to exert greater effort to attain inner freedom than does an honest craftsman. If one has become embedded in various rigid cultural patterns, especially forms of religion, one must undergo a greater struggle within oneself than the one who recognizes the experience of the founders of religion as more essential than the rules and regulations of the church.

In any case, when the seekers fall into the path, they notice their object of desire, and their bent is total concentration for union with the object of desire. This process is expressed in terms of the lover-beloved relationship, and its goal is a state of *qurb* (intimacy) with the beloved. However, there are a few pitfalls along the way, the most serious of which in the I-thou relationship is that the I knowingly or unknowingly enters the process of union in order to obtain the object of desire for himself or herself rather than for its own sake—that is, the I wants to manipulate and utilize something. The experience of the I-thou relationship never proceeds in this way. Utmost sincerity is a stringent requirement. The question arises, "How do we know that we are sincere in such a procedure and in such an act of devotion?" Although the act is its own proof, the Sufis also follow signs and symbols and watch over the rise and fall of their desires; in addition they analyze such desires and look into motives.

The Sufis have developed various exercises for drawing the total attention of the lover toward the beloved. One is a five-step dance that reveals the total outlook of the Sufis toward the process of the I-thou relationship. The dance starts with meditation, intense concentration on oneself in order to empty oneself, resensitize oneself, and gain one's state of naturalness. However, this is not enough. The Sufis know that the regaining of naturalness must occur through action. The dance serves this purpose.

The dancer takes steps and moves closed palms toward the chests (first act); then he or she takes another step, opens the palms, and moves the hands toward the ground, symbolizing release from the self (second act). Next, he or she raises the hands toward heaven to symbolize the nature of God and the fact that everything comes from Him (the third act). Then the dancer moves the hands over the head in such a way that the palms face the sky to symbolize that human beings do not know the nature of God (fourth act). Finally the dancer points the fingers of the right hand toward his or her object of desire, to illustrate that all that exists is thou. The Sufis perform this dance with intense concentration on their object of desire.

When I becomes thou, duality turns into unity resulting in an *"An"*—an opportune moment, new state, new feeling, and a situation in which one becomes aware of one's previous states and can communicate symbolically, holistically, and through experiential media. But how? By thinking? No. By conversation? No. By instruction? No. Then what is the anatomy of this mechanism of the I-thou relationship? Our knowledge of creative individuals in all fields tells us that this mechanism of I-thou relationship has its own fundamental qualities. It is a vehicle based upon the whole person rather than upon sense perception, action-reaction, stimulus-response, thinking, or logic. It has its own psychological dimension; but its laws and psychical mechanisms have merely been touched upon. Basically, the Sufi had to go through three stages to transcend into the state of individuation. These were designated as: (1) illumination of name (the cultural self), (2) illumination of qualities, and (3) illumination of essence. However, before the novice qualified to take these steps, he or she had to be purified through a long period of exercises, both inner and outer, best described as a process of rebirth and the way to individuation.

Sufism: The Way to Individuation

Sufism as a way of individuation can be summarized in two interrelated psychological steps: (1) disintegration (*Fana*) from a self-intellect, a partial soul, and a social self and (2) reintegration (*Baqa*) as the universal self—that is, activation of one's totality. According to the Sufis, we have inherited forces that can either lower us to a bestial state or can elevate us. In an evolutionary sense, this contradiction arose with the development of reason. At this stage, the faculty of reasoning finds itself challenged by our animal tendencies; out of these contradictions we must either go beyond reason to attain the state of certainty (*nafs e mutma'ana*) or fall downward into impulses (*nafs e amareh*). Indeed, so contradictory is our nature that we can rarely harmonize these discordant elements. Disharmony appears most often between (1) *nafs e amareh* (the force within us that commands regressive and evil acts) and reason; (2) reason and *nafs e mutma'ana* (which confirms certainty); and (3) intuition and reason in the final state of personality growth. All the Sufis describe *nafs e amareh*, or simply *nafs*, as being artful, cunning, motivated by evil, and passion producing. In the form of lust, it robs the mind of intelligence and the heart of reverence. It is the mother-idol that compels us to seek material aims in life and deprives us of growth.

In a social sense, *nafs* manifests itself in seekers of power—those who exchange their genuine human character for power and become slaves of it. The power of *nafs* develops such a craving in the mind that its victims constantly refine their skills in the art of guile and treachery and willingly commit inhumane actions to attain their goals. All their humane qualities are consumed by the evils ones, and they become a tool of power, wealth, and carnal desires.

In the conflict between reason and *nafs e amareh*, reason may triumph by satisfying *nafs*, by preoccupation with various fields, or by gaining the power derived from a virtuous life. If reason is relatively free from the trap of *nafs*, it may become totally preoccupied with the human situation. This would result in a partial or specialized human being, one who is busy with only one area of life and ignores the real self. Rumi (1952) explains in one of his discourses:

> Scholars argue heatedly about their specialities while ignoring their own selves—that which affects them the most. The scholar judges on the legality of this and that, but in relation to his own self he knows nothing about its legality or purity. (p. 82)

The individual tries to use logic in every human situation and to relate himself or herself to something that will bring harmony to the situation. But because this object of relationship is not genuine, the solution is temporary. Rumi (1952) describes this situation in *Fihi ma Fihi:*

> Everyone in this world has his own interest, whether women, wealth, knowledge or something else. Each believes that his comfort and joy rests in that one pursuit. Yet when he goes in search of that object he does not find satisfaction in it and returns. After a while he declares that he was not really seeking joy and mercy; he seeks anew but is disappointed again; so he continues on and on. (p. 106)

Rumi further declares that the intellectual self, proud of its knowledge, tends to become conceited and thus deviates from the real self. Nevertheless, the Sufis appreciate the individual's great potentialities, declaring that man is a mighty volume within which all things are recorded. If we let reason grow, it makes us aware of our potentialities and of the existence of an integrated state, and it helps us set the basic purpose of life, that is, union with all. Yet at this point, we may realize that reason is insufficient for handling our existential problem.

In this state of perplexity, a diversity arises between intellect and the real self, reason and intuition, I and not-I. Although the not-I exists in a very real sense, it may first appear veiled to us. Some people find it self-evident, others obscure; some experience it as an intimate part of themselves, to others it is inaccessible. When the mind is receptive, it may appear suddenly without the individual's realization, only to disappear a moment later.

The extent to which the self-intellect resists the voice of the real self will vary from one individual to another. One may become ambivalent and retreat to self-intellect again, another may hear the voice but ignore it, while still another may attend to it and become aware of his or her own state of being. Awareness cannot be attained from knowledge transmitted by others. We must be our own awakeners; we must ourselves conceive the idea of self-seeking. A secret voice (Hafiz's "real conscience") may tell us as it told Hafiz: "If you are a man come forth and pass on. Whatever else hinders you (name, fame, or desire) bypass it. Seek the truth" (Arasteh, 1962, p. 160).

After we have attained a state of awareness, we know intuitively that what we are is not what we can become. We have a glimpse of a better state of self-security, but the conventional veils deprive us of its advantages. In this state we may become aware of tension; this anxiety, which lacks any existential basis, compels us to retreat. A dominant ego nurtured by everyday society can easily drown out a dim inner voice and inhibit the rise of a universal self. This is true especially if we are under the pressure of social forces contradictory to the universal self or if we still associate with a group far removed from universality. But if we are lucky, we may be in a state of psychological disharmony. The voice of our true conscience now can challenge the social self. Our potential personality stands up to our I, questions it, and criticizes it. We begin to analyze ourself and to become more interested in ultimate certainty than in such temporary satisfactions as possessing wealth and fame. We recognize that we have one heart and are potentially one entity and are not able to split into several parts. Thus we fall into a state of quest, the object of which consists of becoming a real self, a perfect and universal person. It means union with all, becoming God-like, and being only the Truth.

Initially, we cannot perceive this state, because throughout our life, up to the point of awareness, mental blocks have hindered this perception. Therefore, the Sufis picture our task to consist of removing these barriers and becoming a mirror of the universe. The seekers encounter a difficult mental path; for in every act of search and reflection, they face the possibility of falling into an illusion and losing the proper mind set.

Selecting a Guide.   So perilous is the task that the Sufis emphatically advise the seekers to enlist the help of a guide (*Pir*), one who has undergone the experience and knows the road. Sufis assert that this guide is necessary because no person possesses the real touchstone to measure his or her own behavior, actions, and feelings. Also, every person reacts to passion and, in some way, admires his or her own actions. The difficulty arises from our inability to objectively measure our own vices. Thus, for both behavioral and mental change, we must have a constant associate who makes us aware of our status and guides us to transcend ourselves.

Such a guide can appreciate and understand the novice's waves of thought and guide him or her symbolically. Rumi (1952) advises seekers not to stray from the guide: "Take refuge in the shadow of the guide that you may escape from the enemy (*nafs*) that opposes in secret" (p. 117). In selecting the guide, the seeker should evaluate the companion according to his or her purpose and objective, not on the basis of race or nationality:

> Do not look at his figure and colour; look at his purpose and intention,
>
> If he is black (yet) he is in accord with you; call him white, for his complexion is the same as yours. (p. 120)

The guide cannot teach through instruction but only can set up a situation in which the inspired novice experiences what he or she should. Of course, he or she can experience only those situations that come close to his or her mental state.

> Soul receives from soul that knowledge, therefore not by book or from tongue,
>
> If knowledge of mysteries comes after emptiness of mind, that is illumination of heart. (Rumi, 1952, p. 121)

Traditionally, Sufi seekers traveled extensively on foot and visited various *khaneqas* (monasteries) in order to find their guide. They believed that at the sight of their master a heart-to-heart communication would take place. Although this master-novice relationship suggests formality and authoritarianism in its behavioral aspects, in mystical reality it is not so at all. Two souls are constantly communicating: one gives and directs, the other receives and makes progress. It is not that the novice is obedient to an order but that he or she is receptive to evolutionary changes. The more the seeker transcends, the less guidance he or she needs from the guide. This guidance promotes a rebirth; the guide serves only as a transfer in this path.

The nature of mystical experience also explains the receptive relationship between the master's soul and that of the seeker. The master perceives the invisible current of events, like a receptive radio with a strong antenna; whereas, the novice, like a small radio with a limited range of receptivity, must keep perception within narrow bounds and never concentrate on what is beyond his or her capacity. When a guide accepts a seeker, the latter must never question the leader. He or she must not criticize or judge the guide by his or her own standards. The novice must not be weakhearted or enraged by every blow that actually polishes the mirror of the heart (Ritter, 1955).

But what happens after one has decided to go through the process of rebirth? Traditionally, the individual passes through several behavioral stages (*moqams*) and a parallel set of reflexive internal modes (*hals*). The *moqam* is a required discipline achieved through exercise and daily practice; whereas, the *hal* is a subjective state of mind, dependent on sensations and not under the control of volition. Like James's "stream of consciousness," the *hal* is not static or rigid. It is like the flash of lightning that appears and disappears, or like snowflakes that fall on a river and vanish in a moment, becoming part of the current.

In traditional Sufism, the behavioral stages begin with "awareness"—that is, a final rebirth or the beginning of a new sign of living. Awareness may come to a person suddenly, or it may develop gradually. Yet awareness is not enough. The seeker must cease unsuitable past behavior: he or she must experience repentance (*tubeh*), decide to reform, and finally cleanse the self of enmity and cruelty. Now, the aspirant is in a position to select for himself or herself a "pole" leader, or a *dalil-e-rah* (the light of the path). After repentance, the novice goes through a stage of avoiding doubtful and uncertain acts (*vara*). The next stage focuses on piety (*zohd*); the novice concentrates on certain values and internal serenity. The following stage relates to patience (*sabr*) and is considered half the task and the key to joy. At every turn and at every level, the aspirant is faced with a situation, either favorable or unfavorable, that demands patience. The stage of trust (*tavakul*) is difficult to attain, for the individual must have trust without recourse to prayer. Satisfaction (*reza*) is the final stage, a culmination of all the past stages; it is positive and tranquil.

Accompanying these stages are somewhat parallel modes (*hals*) relating to the state of mind. These include: the state of observation of one's psyche (*muraqaba*), which entails the ability to measure one's behavior according to the object of the search; the state of nearness (*qurb*), which suggests that one is making progress toward the goal; the state of intense longing for divine unity (*showq*); the state of unconditional love for all (*mehr*); the state of hope of getting nearer (*omid*); the state of intimacy (*uns*); the state of contemplation on the unitary experience (*mushahida*); the state of securing the self (*itminan*), and finally the state of unification and certainty (*yaqin*) (Arasteh, 1980).

In summary, the seeker faces two major tasks: (1) to dissolve his or her present status (*Fana*)—that is, disintegration—and (2) to reintegrate again (*Baqa*). Disintegration refers to the passing away of the conventional self; reintegration means rebirth in the cosmic self. *Fana* means liberation from self-intellect, from the "I"; *Baqa* is the process of becoming "I," of bringing to light the secrets of the total personality. In a practical sense, it means cleansing one's own consciousness of what Rumi calls fictions, idols, and untruths and purifying the heart of greed, envy, jealousy, grief, and anger so that it regains its original quality of being a mirror reflecting the reality within it (Shabistari, 1880).

The process of rebirth is more difficult for some than for others. A pious person has less difficulty than one who previously lacked concern for purity in action. This is so because the former has a touchstone against which to measure his or her behavior; whereas, the latter lacks such a measure. Purity in action means living genuinely and depends on values that underlie the nature of universal man.

Through these behavioral and mental steps, the Sufis seek to uncover the passion that drives us to seek wealth and power—that is, they are more concerned with the motive than with the action itself. Thus, they emphasize removing undesirable thoughts in consciousness and controlling the passions arising out of *nafs*. As a first step in this direction, the guide tells the seeker to concentrate more and more on every single act and on the motives behind it. The seeker of the path of self-realization is instructed, "Behold the image of the end in the mirror of the beginning." To uncover the origin of action requires meditation, which in turn produces a more transcendental state of mind and prepares the individual for the experience of union. *Sama* (whirling dances) were adopted to actualize these peak experiences.

The more serious seekers, under the close supervision of their guides, then seek to empty their consciousness of unreal materials. They observe the contents of their psyches, watch over every mental state, analyze each experience, and perceive its imperfection. This intense concentration usually produces psychic tension or, more specifically, rapture. The more able Sufis also adopted intentional alienation (Shabistari, 1880). They customarily left social life and traveled alone, visiting prominent Sufis. This detachment from society provided the seekers with an excellent opportunity for becoming aware of what they once had thought perfect and of knowledge based on sense perception. At the same time, their immediate experiences enriched their being by activating insight, fostering love, and developing discernment in their approach to the state of emptiness (Nicholson, 1921).

In actuality, the serious Sufis gradually tore off the veils of consciousness one by one and ultimately attained their final state—that of nothingness—a state that is explained in this popular story: At one of the great court banquets, where everyone sat according to his rank awaiting the appearance of the king, a shabbily dressed man entered the hall and took a seat above everyone else. His boldness angered the prime minister, who demanded that he identify himself and reveal if he were a vizier. The stranger replied that he ranked above a vizier. The astonished prime minister then asked if he were a prime minister. The visitor claimed that he outranked a prime minister too. When asked if he were the king himself, he answered that he ranked over him too. "Then you must be the Prophet," declared the prime minister. The man asserted that he was above a prophet. The prime minister shouted angrily "Are you then God?" The man calmly replied, "I am above that too." Contemptuously, the prime minister asserted, "There is nothing above God." In reply the man said, "Now you know my identity. That *nothing* is me." This story illustrates how the Sufis sought to lose all labels, knowledge, and concepts, and how they strived to become empty and remain in an empty state, to attain a zero point so that they could become related to any state of being and achieve everythingness (Arasteh, 1964).

After the seekers have unfolded unconsciousness, they receive direct knowledge. Increasing insight leads to deeper knowledge of the life process. Like flashes of lightning, a succession of insights illuminates their minds and increases their vision. Now universal trust appears; imagination, perplexity, fantasy, and suspicion disappear entirely. They become the mirror of all. All that remains is to become all truth. They grasp truth intuitively and so quickly that interpretation cannot occur; thus, they have a direct relationship with evolutionary events. The illuminated ones brush aside the words, then the thoughts, that cover the surface of this intuitive current. They may seem unconscious, although they experience a dreamlike awareness:

> Even so a hundred thousand "states" came and went back to the Unseen, O trusted one.
>
> Every day's "state" is not like (that of) the day before: (they are passing) as a river that has no obstacle in its course.
>
> Each day's joy is a different kind, each day's thought makes a different impression. (Rumi, 1926, p. 220)

Dreams play an important role in the process of unification. Indeed, a number of well-known Sufis entered this path after repeatedly hearing a voice in their dreams. The inquiring nature of their psyches spurred them on to rebirth. Rumi views reality as a dream-like world; and it is in dreams that one leaves oneself and enters into another self, or, in his words: "In sleep you go from yourself to yourself (p. 202)." The unconscious becomes active in dreams; the cosmic self fully awakens. Rumi (1926) views conventional life as a state of sleeping:

> Your life in this world is like a sleeper who dreams he has gone to sleep.
>
> He thinks "Now I am asleep," unaware that he is already in a second sleep.
>
> Like a blind man afraid of falling into a pit, his self in sleep moves into the state of unconsciousness and thus reveals itself in dreams. (p. 131)

True sleep becomes wakefulness when accompanied by wisdom. The dream states of true sleep reveals the signs of the path and the selection of the guide. Due to this vision, the heart awakens and telepathic knowledge first appears between two hearts. Then every expression symbolizes a moment of life—an act of the state of union (Arasteh, 1964).

Thus, the Sufis analyze the filters of language, logic, and culture until they become aware of the reality of form and what exists beneath in order to attain oneness with all. By this reverse process, the seekers undergo an intense inner experience and discover that the materialistic and mystical essences of creation are the same. They feel the state of nonindividuality and perceive that there is nothing but motion. This positive energy is responsible for the interaction between particles; it is the factor that has caused evolution to proceed from plant, to animal, then to human beings. In passing from one state to the next, human beings have forgotten the previous ones, except that they have a feeling of relatedness toward them. It is this active force, namely "love," that interrelates the whole universe. Following this inner experience, the seekers recognize that the basis of evolution is not conflict, but rather the positive force of love. They discover that lover and beloved come from love.

To reiterate, individuals who have undergone this inner experience gain an understanding of the total situation. United with all, they then travel backward in time and reproduce their previous state whenever they are related to a similar situation. They have embraced all of life beyond good and evil. They have experienced qualities of every type of life—ordinary human existence and intellectual life. They have felt themselves variously as famous, as ambitious, and as religious people, and they have passed beyond all of them, finally deciphering their true selves. They have become images of their community, humankind, and the rest of the world. They accept them all, they feel related to all of them, and, in essence, they are all of them. Their Psychie becomes like a mirror, illuminating images. Thus, they can predict and possibly read by telepathy the thoughts of others; they exhibit certain powers, which to ordinary people seem extraordinary. Ultimately, these humble universal individuals experience "An," the creative movement, the true process of life.

Some Psychotherapeutic Results.   In brief, *An* is the moment of conception, the instant of birth and rebirth, and the experience of joy and originality, which the sufis have gained in their state of individuation. Its mechanism of growth is a dynamic relation between subject and object: initially the subject depends on the object of desire; then there is an instant of union, followed by the object's dependence on the subject; and finally each experiences union independently within the universe.

In this sense, the nature and process of *An* is similar to human creativity: a long period of mental effort, tension, patience, and struggle within the group precedes a relaxed state in which something new is created. Original production is possible only if the creator first perceives the vision, becomes faithful to it, notices its distance from his or her own reality, and then, even in spite of adverse public opinion, attempts to materialize it through unification with it.

It seems that in primitive men or in the uncontaminated child, the creative image or the means of experiencing *An*, exists before *thinking* becomes the instrument of reason and judgment. *An* exists before *concept* is born. However, the course of human history has kept us from retaining this pure quality. Only by assimilating the group's accumulated cultural experience and later leaving it, is it possible to become creative and experience *An* again. This concept can be utilized in education, child rearing, and therapy. However, its greatest contribution lies is psychotherapeutic training, especially through the master-disciple relationship—namely, the master's total commitment to care and the disciple's devotion. This relationship is possible only if one has an intense creative passion for turning a fragmented person into a whole individual.

A further contribution of *An* philosophy to Western psychotherapy deals with the vision of human nature as an entity. Thus, any therapy must emphasize conditions that will contribute to the restoration of a unitary experience and result in a spontaneous cure. For instance, a preverbal child in the care of a mother who cannot understand his or her nonverbal signs becomes irritable and perhaps neurotic, but as soon as the child learns to speak, a spontaneous cure is possible.

Consequently, we can conclude that with the acceptance of the principle of *An*, therapy as a technique takes on a new form. It is seen as a continual experiential exchange between therapist and patient until the situation is ripe for the spontaneous healing experience. In such a relationship, both therapist and patient are active. The major difference is that the therapist notices the succession of signs, interprets them, and enlightens the course of events, whereas, the patient remains unaware of this situation. Thus, the *An* experience and spontaneous therapy derived from it contradict several traditional Freudian analytical approaches: it makes a passive analyst active; it encourages a patient to become expressive rather than talkative; it transcends the mere symptom. Rather than make the patient self-conscious and aware of the negative aspect of the unconscious, the therapist will direct him or her to a new state—a new disintegration or a new integration, a new separation or relatedness directed toward a decrease in the hold of past traditions, good and bad, toward the rise of naturalness, sensitivity, receptivity, understanding the utilitarian service of thought, reason, and concept, and toward differentiating this quality from the prevailing dominant role of impulse and ego.

Furthermore, according to the experiential philosophy of *An*, no cure can result from becoming conscious of the neurosis of our time. In fact, the awareness of the neurosis is a hindrance to us. In order to regain our original unitary state, we must either create a new force that can defeat the social experiences, or we must erase them entirely from our psyche. The division of the psyche into id, ego, and superego deviates from the experiential psychotherapy of *An*. Actually, what is essential is our totality, on the one hand, and real experience on the other. The therapist-patient relationship must follow a plan so that these two qualities become active again. The most direct path to achieving this goal is through various nonverbal mechanisms, such as creative experience, songs, music, writing, crafts, art, and relating these products to the emotional experience of the patient in such a way that the chain of events creates a new experience of awareness and leads to a deeper realization of the totality of the person. The Sufis were activists, and their minds always developed new symbols. They advise us that the best remedy for a restless mind is physical activity for regaining bodily grace, and the best cure for a restless body is meditation. In other words, the control of the response to the demand of the psyche or of the body is essential for cure.

Finally, the Sufis accept the idea of transference but not as a projection of the parent-child relationship; rather, they perceive the identification with a realistic state of the master as an attempt by the seeker to receive the grace and blessing of the next state. In this sense the experiential therapy of *An* is oriented toward the future rather than the past. In this light, Ernest G. Schachtel's (1959) meaningful essay on amnesia in childhood deserves further interpretation. Indeed, the role of amnesia is of great importance in experiential therapy; great Eastern sages often failed to record their childhood experiences, because they considered them unimportant. To them the end is significant; this should be seen in the mirror of the being, so that the motive and effort match the goal.

Inner Evolution: An Allegory

It seems befitting to conclude the first section of this chapter with an allegory, *Mantiqul Tair (The Conference of the Birds)*, by a famous Sufi writer, Farid ud-din Attar (1967).

In his allegory, a flock of birds, resembling a group of travelers, passes through seven purifying stages of inner evolution before finally becoming one with the object of their search—God. The allegory opens as all the birds (seekers) assemble to seek a worthy leader. The saintly Hoopoe claims he knows a true leader, the legendary God-like Simurgh (Roc), who lives in the mountains of Qaf. Although Simurgh's home is nearly inaccessible, the Hoopoe offers to guide them there, for he feels that life acquires meaning only if one reaches Him.

However, when the Hoopoe describes the difficulties involved in reaching the Simurgh, the other birds find excuses for not undertaking the journey; to each one the Hoopoe points out his or her error. The lady-like nightingale declares that the rose carries the secret of love. If she is separated from the rose, she will surely die; the journey to the Simurgh would overtax her strength. The Hoopoe calls her a slave of untrue love. He advises her to seek self-protection and to forsake the passing love that a rose offers.

The parrot, in her green dress of everlastingness, insists that she is seeking the fountain of life, not Simurgh. The Hoopoe advises her to seek further growth and a better state of mind.

The pretentious peacock, who had sinned and been expelled from paradise, desires only to return there and nothing more. The Hoopoe comments that she has selected the wrong object of desire, for truth dwells in the heart.

The duck, in his holy robes, compulsively performs his ablutions again and again and lacks any desire for Simurgh. The self-satisfied partridge is so busy searching for jewels in the mountains that his heart burns from the pebbles that he has greedily swallowed. The Hoopoe tells him that his love of jewels has hardened his heart.

The haughty Homa steps forward boasting that whomever his shadow falls on becomes king. He smugly asks, "Does a maker of kings and giver of thrones need to seek the Simurgh?" The Hoopoe tells him, "You are a slave of pride satisfied with a bone. Even though you enthrone kings, you will lose their loyalty when misfortune strikes them" (p. 33).

Like an obedient statesman, the hawk protests, "Although the king has blinded me, he sets me on his hand and trains me to perform my duties correctly. I'm content with the morsels that I get from his hand. So why should I go to the Simurgh without being called?" (p. 34). The Hoopoe explains that a king's court is like fire, from which one must keep away.

The heron gives as his excuse his passion for the sea; the owl wants to remain in the serenity of the ruins; and the sparrow claims he is too feebleminded. In answer, the Hoopoe addresses all the birds, "You indulge in self-pity, identify yourselves with transitory things, and have no stake in the things that are enduring. You are all shadows of the Simurgh, but why is it that you have no love for Him? Prostrate yourselves and seek Him. You are perplexed, and you can only remedy the situation by striving and searching for the Simurgh, from whom this world came into being" (p. 34).

The birds finally agree to search for the Simurgh, but before beginning their journey, the Hoopoe describes the seven valleys, resembling the Sufi path to perfection, through which they must pass: Quest, Love, Understanding, Independence and Detachment, Pure Unity, Astonishment, and finally Poverty and Nothingness. The Hoopoe relates that in the Valley of Quest they will encounter difficult situations that will threaten to distract them from their goal. It may take a great deal of effort and time to overcome these obstacles. Gradually, they will give up all possessions, and they will devote themselves to the object of their desire. Finally nothing will matter except the pursuit of the goal; dogma, belief and disbelief all will cease to exist.

The Hoopoe tells his listeners that the Valley of Love will prepare them for understanding. True love results from perceiving the value of the object of desire. A metaphor aptly describes the manifestation of love. As soon as the individual realizes his or her origin, he or she becomes like a fish thrown on the back by the waves, struggling to get back into the water. Love provides insight and the strength to identify with the object of desire, for love knows no afterthought. With the growth of love, good and evil cease to exist.

The insight gained by love will bring them to the Valley of Understanding, a valley that has no beginning or end. There they must persist even though the knowledge gained is temporary. Gradually, each traveler will understand the truth according to his or her own receptiveness.

Each one will realize his or her potentiality, and each will see the whole of creation by insight into an atom. As they gain understanding of the relatedness of things, they will ponder on their secret. Many travelers have lost their way here; the traveler must have an intense desire to become as one ought to be, if he or she is to cross this difficult valley.

As they gain understanding, they will become detached and enter the Valley of Independence. Here they must become independent, materially and spiritually; they must rid themselves of the desire to possess and the wish to discover. Here they will feel that the world is a mere speck in the universe where nothing new or old has value. One can act or not act, but one still must ponder on the origin of existence.

In the Valley of Unity, everything is broken into pieces; everything loses its temporal and conventional meaning. Ultimately, they will find that the evolution of the universe and growth have come from the same source, that plurality has sprung from unity. Although the individual may see many forms, they are all one, just as oneness appears in number. Yet they must search further still, for that which they seek is beyond unity and number. The eternity of past and future vanishes as one ceases to speak of it. As they discover the invisible source of the visible world and the visible becomes nothing, then nothing is left to contemplate.

The Valley of Astonishment follows. In this valley they will experience sadness. Each breath will be a bitter sigh, and each sigh will become a sword. The ones who already have achieved unity will forget all, including themselves; they will fall into the state of bewilderment. Now they will be certain that they know nothing; they will be unaware of themselves; they will be in love but without knowing with whom. Their heart will be full and empty of love at the same time.

Bewilderment will give way to deprivation, an indescribable state characterized by muteness. Now, the ray of enlightenment will dispel the shadows that surround their being. They will find the secret of creation and many other secrets. They will grasp the beauty of Simurgh; for they will no longer exist separately.

Like the Hoopoe, the birds now also yearned for unity. Ultimately, some died in the excitement of perceiving this unified state. The rest wandered for years and experienced many hardships. Finally, 30 birds (*Si-murgh* literally means 30 birds) reached their destination. They approached the door of that being who exists beyond human reason and knowledge; they sat there in despair and waited. At last a voice announced that Simurgh would have nothing to do with a group that could only lament. The birds became anxious, but persisted. Now they had passed the final test, the veil of reason of the soul drew completely aside, and they discovered that Simurgh, the invisible leader, was themselves—

the *Si-murgh* (30 birds)—and that they themselves were the reflection of the essence. At first this discovery of self-transformation, this process of identification with their object of desire, astonished them, for they did not know if they were themselves or if they had actually become Simurgh. But gradually the unit of subject with object and illumination within them persisted. Attar says "And if they looked at both together, both were Simurgh, neither more nor less. This one was that, and that one this; the like of this hath no one heard in the world" (p. 140).

II. EXISTENTIAL HEALING: THE SUFI CONTRIBUTION

Therapeutic principles inherent in the Sufi system are of great significance for the present as well as the future course of psychology. One significant contribution of the Sufi psychocosmological system lies in the area of existential healing—that is, attaining a state where our system functions harmoniously with the universe.

While Freud emphasized the adjustment to social reality, Fromm, Suzuki, and Martino (1958) found social reality itself questionable and, in fact, called the social ills a crisis of our time. They defined this general malady as follows:

> It is the crisis which has been described as "malaise," "ennui," "mal du siècle," deadening of life, the automatization of man, his alienation from himself, from his fellowmen and from nature. Man has followed rationalism to the point where rationalism has transformed itself into utter irrationality. (pp. 78–79)

This state of civilization that Fromm et al. keenly observed occurred in the final rational state of Islamic civilization in the 17th century. Insight into that culture tells us that Sufism appeared to redefine the place of reason and theological rituals in an individual's life.

In an interesting paper, Jerome Frank (1979) redefines mental health:

> Since mental health is a rather meticulous concept, let me start by describing what I consider to be its essential features. Most of us would agree that, at the minimum, these include a sense that life has meaning, a feeling of personal security, the capacity to utilize opportunities for enjoyment and to accept and surmount, the inevitable suffering, life brings. If one can utilize suffering as an occasion for personal growth, so much the better. Especially important in these uncertain times are the capacity to establish and maintain mutually supportive relationships with others and to adapt to changing circumstances without becoming insecure. (p. 397)

If we see individuals as social beings, that is, as fragmented beings, Professor Frank's definition will be the healing measure. But real persons are cosmic beings; the person is life itself. Life is not separate from them as are their garments. The individual is the opportunity and the unfolding being, the meaning and the purpose, seeking to unfold himself or herself. The qualities that Professor Frank adds to individuals are not separate from them. Only intellectual persons feel that their mind and body are apart from each other. Artists, craftsmen, children, and even healthy, simple, illiterate men and women feel themselves as a whole. It is due to this observation that we define a human being as a potential biological harmonious system that can become a potential psychocultural harmonious system, or finally a potential psychocosmological harmonious system. The harmonious system at every stage of growth signifies health. It is in the final state of life—that is, after our inner evolution—that health becomes a constant, while in the rational and psychocultural state, it is a relative phenomenon and changes according to sociopsychological dynamic forces.

It was the transformation of the state of anxiety and the neurosis of sociorational man that promoted Sufism. In this sense, Sufism is the art of rebirth that turns the ever-changing mind to wisdom and produces an existential answer. In other words, the goal of the Sufi-master is attainment of a state of life without anxiety, a state of great inner joy and creativity. Such transcendental growth cannot be dictated by social forces or by competition with others, but by competition with one's self.

Case of Al-Ghazzali.   No one experienced this self-transforming, existential healing better than Abu-Hamid Muhammad Ibn Muhammad, known as Al-Ghazzali, who died 1111 A.D. Just as Kierkegaard considers Martin Luther to be the most significant patient for Christendom, in my opinion Al-Ghazzali is the most significant patient for Islamic society, with one difference—that is, Martin Luther failed to heal himself through Christian mysticism. However, Al-Ghazzali, with the help of the existential healing quality of Sufism, regained his naturalness and became creative; he cleared the path for Mowlana Jalal-al-din Muhammad Balkhi, known as Rumi, and other mystics.

Al-Ghazzali's father was a Sufi practitioner but illiterate. He had a great desire that his children receive a good education. Therefore, before his untimely death, he entrusted his two small sons to a Sufi friend who saw to it that the boys received a solid basic education. As a young man, Al-Ghazzali had already achieved renown in theology and Islamic philosophy. At about 30 years of age, he was appointed by the great Saljugh Vizier Nezamul-Mulk to the post of professor at the University of Baghdad. By the time he left Baghdad in search of meaning, at the age of 39, he had written 70 books.

He relates that from adolescence until past the age of 50, when he wrote his confession, he had lived in a vast ocean of knowledge, receiving all currents, penetrating its dark areas, and challenging its dangers. He had studied each sect and school in order to "disentangle truth from error and orthodoxy from heresy" (Al-Ghazzali, n.d., p. 13). His observations convinced him that the power of the environment determines a child's religion. But Al-Ghazzali soon freed himself, he confesses: "No sooner had I emerged from boyhood than I had already broken the fetters of tradition and freed myself from hereditary beliefs" (p. 14).

But at the age of 39, the contradictory forces that were activated within him by his search for truth, led him to doubt his knowledge. He relates: "The search after truth being the aim which I propose to myself. I ought in the first place to ascertain what are the bases of certitude" (p. 14). He came to believe that what is impregnable to sense perception cannot be accepted with certitude. Then he turned toward intellectual notions such as, "affirmation and negation cannot coexist together" (p. 17); but these intellectual notions raised the possibility of a power above reason, which, if it appeared, would convict reason of falsehood just as reason refuted sense perception. He also argued that if such a power is not apparent, it does not mean that it does not exist. His awareness of the state of dreams and the reality of ecstasy (i.e., the state of union involving the suspension of sense perceptions, which produces visions beyond the realm of intellect) made him uncertain of reason, and he looked for a way to escape from his uncertainty. In order to disentangle this knot, proof was necessary. But proof must be based on primary assumptions, and it was precisely these that he doubted.

Al-Ghazzali relates that for 2 months he was anxious and skeptical. A 2-year period of ambivalence followed, which he spent reviewing his knowledge of scholastic theology and philosophy and studying Sufis who had claimed to have gained knowledge in ecstasy. He then spent a year meditating on these systems in order to fully understand them: "I turned them over and over in my mind till they were thoroughly clear of all obscurity" (p. 26).

Although he concluded that theology has a pragmatic value for healing certain minds, he did not find it to be the remedy for his own malady. In his search for truth in philosophy (including science and mathematics), he discerned the relationship between faith and science and differentiated between genuine thinkers and amateurs. But again he did not find a remedy for his state of being. Finally, when he turned to Sufism, he found its principles easy to learn but difficult to practice. "I acquired a thorough knowledge of their research, and I learned all that was possible to learn of their methods by study and oral teaching. It became clear to me . . . that Sufism consists in experience rather than in definitions and that what I was lacking belonged to this domain, not of instruction, but of ecstasy initiation" (pp. 47–48).

At this point, Al-Ghazzali's inner turmoil became intense, for his fame, pride, honor, wealth, and knowledge stood in opposition to his awareness that certainty could only result from a comprehensive transformation of the moral being. He describes his anguish as follows:

> Still a prey to uncertainty, one day I decided to leave Baghdad and to give up everything. The next day I gave up my resolution. I advanced one step and immediately relapsed. In the morning I was sincerely resolved only to occupy myself with the future life; in the evening a crowd of carnal thoughts assailed and dispersed my resolutions. On the one side the world kept me bound to my post in the chain of covetousness, on the other side the voice of religion cried to me, "Up! Up! Thy life is nearing its end; and thou hast a long journey to make. All the pretended knowledge is naught but falsehood and fantasy. If thou dost not break thy chains today, when will thou break them? If thou dost not think of thy salvation when wilt thou think of it?" Then my resolve was strengthened; I wished to give up all and flee but the Temper, returning to the attack, said: "You are suffering from a transitory feeling, don't give way to it, for it will soon pass. If you obey it, if you give up this fine position, this honorable past exempt from trouble and rivalry, this seal of authority safe from attack, you will regret it later without being able to recover it."

> Thus I remained, torn asunder by the opposite forces of earthly passions and religious aspirations, for about six months from the month of Rajab of the year A.D. 1096. At the close of them my will yielded and I gave myself up to destiny. God caused an impediment to chain my tongue and prevented me from lecturing. Vainly I desired, in the interest of my pupils, to go on with my teaching, but my mouth became dumb. The silence to which I was condemned cast me into a violent despair, my stomach became weak, I lost all appetite, I could neither swallow a morsel of bread nor drink a drop of water.

> The enfeeblement of my physical powers was such that the doctors (physicians), despairing of saving me, said, "The mischief is in the *heart*, and has communicated itself to the whole organism; there is no hope unless the cause of his grievous sadness be arrested." (pp. 50–51)

It is evident that he was suffering from a depression due to an existential search and not due to ordinary causes. Life had become meaningless. Al-Ghazzali was suffering from what I have termed an *"existential moratorium,"* in contrast to Erikson's psychosocial moratorium. The psychosocial moratorium removes sociohistorical symptoms, and at best, helps a youth to become a copy of adults. But an anxious search in the period of an existential moratorium solves the individual's life orientation once and for all. It provides a monolithic system, a holistic psychology that, by its own nature, encompasses a great healing force.

Al-Ghazzali finally gathered his inner "courage to be" and detached himself from his position, honor, wealth, and even family. He secured his family and retained enough for "a pious living." He devoted himself to his own self-transformation and to experiencing the art of rebirth as advocated by Sufism. He traveled in the Middle East from Syria to Mecca; after his rebirth, he finally settled in Khorasan, where he was reunited with his family and lived creatively. His process of rebirth encompassed 10 years, and he reports this about those years:

> During my successive periods of meditation there were revealed to me things impossible to recount. All that I shall say for the edification of the reader is this I learned from a sure source that the Sufis are the pioneers on the path of God (during Al-Ghazzali's time attributes of God were a source of transfer of personality). There is nothing more beautiful than their life, no more praiseworthy than their rule of conduct, nor purer than their morality. The intelligence of thinkers, the wisdom of philosophers, the knowledge of the most learned doctors of law would in vain combine their efforts in order to modify or improve their doctrine and morals, it would be impossible. With the Sufis, repose and movement, exterior and interior, are illumined with the light which proceeds from the *Central Radiance of Inspiration*. (pp. 54–55)

Thus, we conclude that much healing takes place if an anxious person follows his or her inspiration. But the inner experience is difficult to describe; Al-Ghazzali says only this: "What I experience I shall not try to say. Call me happy, but ask me no more" (p. 56). However, Al-Ghazzali recommends *zekr* as an aid in moving from social reality to existential reality. *Zekr* is the repetition of the 99 names or attributes of God (see Table 6.1); *zekr* must be performed with sincerity and total concentration.

Zekr must begin with a psychophysical state of readiness. Then one chooses one of the attributes of God, or just the word "Allah," representing all of creation; now one begins to chant. One must concentrate on the heart and practice chanting without interruption. After a while, the lips become dry and one cannot utter the word again, but the registered motion continues in *heart*. It is at this moment that the gate of inspiration and enlightenment opens. One is ready now for receiving the Creator's blessings. The light of truth, the flash of creativity, the gem of wisdom, the new experiences then take place.

TABLE 6.1.   THE 99 NAMES AND ATTRIBUTES OF ALLAH

Number	Name	Attribute
1	AR-RHMAAN	The Beneficient
2	AR-RAHEEM	The Merciful
3	AL-MALIK	The Sovereign Lord
4	AL-QUDDOOS	The Holy
5	AS-SALAAM	The Source of Peace
6	AL-MOMIN	The Guardian of Faith
7	AL-MUHAIMIN	The Protector
8	AL-AZEEZ	The Mighty
9	AL-JABBAAR	The Compeller
10	AL-MUTA KABBIR	The Majestic
11	AL-KHAALIQ	The Creator
12	AL-BAARI	The Evolver
13	AL-MUSAWWIR	The Fashioner
14	AL-GHAFFAAR	The Forgiver
15	AL-QAHHAAR	The Subduer
16	AL-WAHHAAB	The Bestower
17	AR-RAZZAAQ	The Provider
18	AL-FATTAAH	The Opener
19	AL ALEEM	The All-knowing
20	AL-QAABID	The Constrictor
21	AL-BAASIT	The Expander
22	AL-KHAAFID	The Abaser
23	AR-RAAFE	The Exalter
24	AL-MUIZZ	The Honorer
25	AL-MUZILL	The Dishonorer
26	AS-SAMI'L	The All-hearing
27	AL-BASEER	The All-seeing
28	AL-HAKAM	The Judge
29	AL-ADL	The Just
30	AL-LATEEF	The Subtle
31	AL-KHABEER	The Aware
32	AL-HALEEM	The Clement
33	AL-AZEEM	The Magnificient
34	AS-SABOOR	The Patient
35	AR-RASHEED	The Guide to the Right Path
36	AL-WAARITH	The Supreme Inheritor
37	AL-BAAQL	The Everlasting
38	AL-BADEE'I	The Incomparable
39	AL-HAADI	The Guide
40	AN-NOOR	The Light
41	AN-NAAFI	The Propitious
42	AD-DAAR	The Distresser

TABLE 6.1. THE 99 NAMES AND ATTRIBUTES OF ALLAH *(Continued)*

Number	Name	Attribute
43	AL-MANI	The Preventer
44	AL-MUGHANI	The Enricher
45	AL-GHANEE	The Self-sufficient
46	AL-JAAME	The Gatherer
47	AL-MUQSIT	The Equitable
48	ZUL-JALAALI-WAL-IKRAAM	The Lord of Majesty and Bounty
49	MAALIK-UL-MULK	The Owner of Sovereignty
50	AR-RAOOF	The Compassionate
51	AL-AFUWW	The Pardoner
52	AL-MUNTAQIM	The Avenger
53	AL-TAWWAB	The Acceptor of Repentence
54	AL-BARR	The Source of All Goodness
55	AL-MUTA'AAL	The Most Exalted
56	AL-WAALI	The Governor
57	AL-BAATIN	The Hidden
58	AZ-ZAAHIR	The Manifest
59	AL-AAKHIR	The Last
60	AL-AWWAL	The First
61	AL-MUAKHIR	The Delayer
62	AL-MUQADDIM	The Expediter
63	AL-MUQTADIR	The Powerful
64	AL-QAADIR	The Able
65	AS-SAMAD	The Eternal
66	AL-AHAD	The One
67	AL-WAAHID	The Unique
68	AL-MAAJID	The Noble
69	AL WAAJID	The Finder
70	AL-GHAFOOR	The Forgiving
71	ASH-SHAKOOR	The Appreciative
72	AL-ALEE	The Most High
73	AL-KABEER	The Great
74	AL-HAFEEZ	The Preserver
75	AL-MUQEET	The Sustainer
76	AL-HASEEB	The Reckoner
77	AL JALEEL	The Sublime
78	AL-KAREEM	The Generous
79	AR-RAQEEB	The Watchful
80	AL-MUJEEB	The Responsive
81	AL-WAASI	The All-embracing
82	AL-HAKEEM	The Wise
83	AL-WADOOD	The Loving
84	AL-MAJEED	The Glorious

TABLE 6.1.   THE 99 NAMES AND ATTRIBUTES OF ALLAH *(Continued)*

Number	Name	Attribute
85	AL-BAA'ITH	The Resurrector
86	ASH-SHAHEED	The Witness
87	AL-HADQ	The Truth
88	AL-WAKEEL	The Trustee
89	AL-QAWEE	The Strong
90	AL-MATEEN	The Firm
91	AL-WALEE	The Protecting Friend
92	AL-HAMEED	The Praiseworthy
93	AL-MUHSEE	The Reckoner
94	AL-MUBDI	The Originator
95	AL-MU'EED	The Restorer
96	AL-MUHYEE	The Giver of Life
97	AL-MUMEET	The Creator of Death
98	AL-HAYY	The Alive
99	AL-QAYYOOM	The Self-subsisting

It should be noted that the rule of *zekr* required that it be practiced only when the seeker's state of the psyche demanded it. Often a guide had to be present. At all times, the Sufi had to differentiate between spiritual ecstasy and a natural impulsive force within him or her.

In summary, Al-Ghazzali's experience teaches us that health and healing require that one eliminate passions and unhealthy impressions on the psyche. This can be done by abstinence, patience, reexamination of social experience, renunciation of mental blocks, reintegration of the genuine moral self, and a great deal of practice. Finally one can attain total harmony and experience life in contentment, creativity, and relatedness to all.

After Al-Ghazzali had resettled in Khorasan, he wrote his major works: *The Revivification of Religious Science, Alchemy of Happiness, Fear and Hope and Others.* The late professor D. B. McDonald (1909) pays Al-Ghazzali this tribute:

The greatest, certainly the most sympathetic figure in the history of Islam, and the only teacher of the after generation ever put by a Muslim on the level with the four great humans . . . Islam has never outgrown him, has never fully understood him. In the renaissance of Islam which is now rising to view, his time will come, and the new life will proceed from a renewed study of his works. (p. 124)

A Case from Rumi. For a deeper understanding of the method and practices of existential healing we must turn to Mowlana Jalal-al-din Muhummad Balkhi, known as Rumi, who died in 1273. The insight of this Persian mystic into the interplay of natural and cultural forces within us is, in my opinion, much more profound than that of all Western analysts, including Freud and Jung.

In the following case, he demonstrates his impressive talent as a clinician. In his story, *Mathnawi*, Rumi highlights the individual's inner conflict as the source of all maladies. The main characters are the King, who symbolizes partial intellect and ungratified wishes; a beautiful maiden, who is the object of gratification; a young goldsmith, who represents worldly love and possession; an ordinary physician, who is the symbol of knowledge and intellect; and a spiritual physician, who is the real Sufi.

While hunting, the King saw a beautiful maiden. He fell in love with her and moved her to his palace. But soon the girl became ill. The King, full of sorrow, summoned all the physicians to cure her. The physicians boasted that they had drugs that would cure any malady, and the King replied that he would give his treasury as a reward to the one who healed her (i.e., he would sacrifice wealth for *nafs* and gratification). The physicians did all they could, but the maiden grew more ill (impotence of the ego intellect in the face of the existential search). The King became increasingly sad. In his deepest sorrow he cried out from the depth of his soul and fell into unconsciousness.

In this state, he heard a voice telling him that a spiritual physician would arrive and would cure his beloved. The King awakened and the spiritual physician appeared. The King warmly embraced him and led him to the bedside of the sick girl. The spiritual physician gave a remarkable description of the symptoms, made an accurate diagnosis of the illness, outlined the inadequacies of the ordinary physicians, and suggested an effective treatment:

> The (spiritual) physician observed the color of her face, (felt) her pulse, and (inspected) her urine; he heard both the symptoms and the (secondary) causes of her malady.
>
> He said, "None of the remedies which they have applied build up (health): They (the false physicians) have wrought destruction. They were ignorant of the inward state. I seek refuge with God from that which they invent."
>
> He saw the pain, and the secret became open to him, but he concealed it and did not tell the King.
>
> Her pain was not from black or yellow bile: The smell of every firewood appears from the smoke.

From her sore grief he perceived that she was heart-sore; well in body, but stricken in heart.

Being in love is made manifest by soreness of heart; there is no sickness like heart-sickness.

The Lover's ailment is separate from all other ailments; Love is the astrolabe of the mysteries of God. (Rumi, 1926, p. 10)

Rumi (1926) explains the art of healing of the spiritual physician:

Very gently He (the spiritual physician) said to her, "Where is thy native town? For the treatment suitable to the people of each town is separate.
And in that town who is related to thee? With what has thou kinship and affinity?"
He (the spiritual physician) laid his hand on her pulse and put questions,
One by one, about the injustice of Heaven. . . .
He inquired of the girl concerning her friends, by way of narrative.
And she disclosed to the physician (many) circumstances touching her name and (former) masters and fellow-townsmen.

He listened to her story (while) he continued to observe her pulse and its beating:

So that at whosoever's name her pulse should begin to throb, (he might know that) that person is the object of her soul's desire in the world.

He counted up the friends in her native town; then he mentioned another town by name.
He said, "When you went forth from your own town, in which town did you live mostly?"

She mentioned the name of a certain town and from that too she passed on (to speak of another, and meanwhile) there was no change in the color of her face or her pulse.

Masters and towns, one by one, she told of and about dwelling-place and bread and salt.
She told stories of many a town and many a house (and still) he asked about Samargand, the (city) sweet as candy.
(Thereat) her pulse jumped and her face went red and pale (by turns), for she had been parted from a man of Samargand, a goldsmith.

When the (spiritual) physician found out this secret from the sick (girl), he discerned the source of that grief and woe.

He said, "Which is his quarter in passing (through the town)?"

"Sari-i pul (Bridge head)," she replied, "and Ghatafor Street."
Said he: "I know what your illness is and I will at once display the arts of magic in delivering you" (that is, "I will perform miracles on your behalf").

"Be glad and care-free and have no fear, for I will do to you that which rain does to the meadow.

I will be anxious for you, be not anxious:
I am kinder to you than a hundred fathers.

Beware! Tell not this secret to anyone, not though the King should make much inquiry from you.

When your heart becomes the grave of your secret, that desire of yours will be gained more quickly." (p. 13)

After finding the cause of the illness, the King sent for the goldsmith and wed him to the maiden. She was soon cured, but then she discovered that her love had been for the sake of possession and that such a love is a disgrace. The spiritual physician guided the girl to overcome physical love, and gradually she related to eternity and gained her permanent health.

CONCLUDING REMARKS

It should be noted that all great men in Persian culture, whether they were philosophers, scientists, literary men, or statesmen turned to Sufism. They did so because they came to the awareness that man's nature is infinite, love is infinite, but reason is finite. Thus, they made reason serve love, and love serve humanity.

They recognized that knowledge can lead to only a restricted understanding, and it does not take the individual to the limit of one's potential, it does not satisfy one's yearning. Only love can enrich one's insight and unfold one's potentialities (Khan, 1982). In the human situation, love is the antidote to all human ills (e.g., greed, rivalry, jealousy, and hatred). True love does not stand in opposition to these, as is generally thought, but absorbs them.

Rumi describes this transforming power of love:

Hail O love, that bringest us good gain
Thou that art the physician of all ills,
The remedy of our pride and vain glory,
Our Plato and our Galen! (Rumi, 1926, p. 2)

Through love thorns become roses, and
Through love vinegar becomes sweet wine
Through love the stake becomes a throne
Through love the reverse of fortune seems good fortune,
Through love a prison seems a rose bower,
Through love a grate full of ashes seems a garden
Through love a burning fire is a pleasing light.

(Rumi, 1881, p. 79)

If persons would give love a chance, it would dissolve all prejudice, whether religious, racial, or social. Love can heal our troubled world and bring us closer to God. Rumi writes:

Lo, for I to myself am unknown, now in God's Name
    what must I do?
I adore not the cross nor the crescent. I am not a
    Christian nor a Jew.
East nor West, land nor sea is my home. I have kin not
    with angel nor gnome.
I am wrought not of fire nor of foam, I am shaped not of
    dust nor of dew.
Not in this world nor that world I dwell, not in Paradise
    neither in Hell;
Not from Eden and Paradise I fell, not from Adam my
    lineage I drew.
In a place beyond uttermost place, in a tract without
    shadow or trace,
Soul and body transcending I live in the soul of my
    loved one anew.

(Fatemi et al., 1976, p. 106)

Once the individual has looked upon the beloved or God, he or she becomes aware that the divine presence permeates all the world, rendering every aspect of it sacred. Another great Sufi teacher, Baba Kuhi of Shiraz, who lived during the 11th century, beautifully expresses this experience:

In the market, in the cloister—only God I saw.
In the valley and on the mountain—only God I saw.
Him I have seen beside me oft in tribulation;
In favour and in fortune—only God I saw.

In prayer and fasting, in praise and contemplation,
In the religion of the prophet—only God I saw.
Qualities nor causes—only God I saw.
I opened mine eyes and by the light of his face around me
In all the eye discovered—only God I saw.
Like a candle I was melting with his fire:
Amidst the flames outflashing—only God I saw
Myself with mine own eyes I saw most clearly,
But when I looked with God's eyes—only God I saw.
I passed away into nothingness, I vanished.
And lo, I was the all-living—only God I saw.

                                                    (Fatemi, 1973, p. 57)

References

Al-Ghazzali, H. M. (n.d.). *The confessions of Al-Ghazzali*. (C. Field, Trans.). Lahore, Pakistan: Ashraf Press.

Arasteh, A. R. (1962). *Succession of identities: Outer and inner metamorphoses*. Paper presented at the George Washington University, Department of Psychology.

Arasteh, A. R. (1964). *Man and society in Iran*. Leiden, Netherlands: E. J. Brill.

Arasteh, A. R. (1965). *Final integration in the adult personality*. Leiden, Netherlands: E. J. Brill.

Arasteh, A. R. (1973). Psychology of the Sufi way to individuation. In L. F. R. Williams (Ed.), *Sufi studies: East and west*. New York: Dutton.

Arasteh, A. R. (1980). *Growth to selfhood: Sufi contribution*. London: Routledge & Kagan Paul.

Arasteh, A. R. (1984). *Anxious search: The way to the universal self*. Bethesda, MD: Institute of Perspective Analysis.

Attar, F. D. (1967). *Mantiqul Tair [The conference of the birds]*. (C. S. Nott, Trans.). London: Routledge & Kagan Paul.

Erikson, E. (1958). *Young man Luther: Study of psychoanalysis and history*. New York: Norton.

Fatemi, N. S. (1973). A message and method of love, harmony, and brotherhood. In L. F. R. Williams (Ed.), *Sufi studies: East and west*. New York: Dutton.

Fatemi, N. S., Fatemi, F. S., & Fatemi, F. S. (1976). *Sufism: Message of brotherhood, harmony and hope*. New York: Barnes.

Frank, J. D. (1979). Mental health in a fragmented society: The shattered crystal ball. *American Journal of Orthopsychiatry*, July, 397–408.

Fromm, E. S., Suzuki, D. T., & Martino, R. (1958). *Psychoanalysis and Zen Buddhism*. New York: Basic Books.

Haschmi, M. Y. (1973). Spirituality, science and psychology in the Sufi way. In L. F. R. Williams (Ed.), *Sufi studies: East and west*. New York: Dutton.

Khan, I. (1979). *The inner life.* Geneva: International Headquarters of the Sufi Movement.

Khan, V. I. (1982). *Introducing spirituality in counseling and therapy.* Lebanon Springs, NY: Omega Press.

Lings, M. (1975). *What is Sufism?* Los Angeles: University of California Press.

McDonald, D. B. (1909). *The religious life and attitude in Islam.* Chicago: University of Chicago Press.

Nicholson, R. A. (1921). *Studies in Islamic mysticism.* Cambridge: Cambridge University Press.

Ritter, H. (1955). *Das Meerer der Seele.* Leiden, Netherlands: E. J. Brill.

Rumi, M. J. M. (1881). *Mathnawi* (translations of some selected pieces of the *Mathnawi* by E. H. Whinfeld). London: Trubrin Oriental Series.

Rumi, M. J. M. (1926). *Mathnawi* (R. A. Nicholson, Trans.). London: Luzac.

Rumi, M. J. M. (1952). *Fihi ma Fihi.* (*Discourses,* ed. by Firunzanfar). Tehran: University of Tehran Press.

Schachtel, E. G. (1959). *Metamorphosis.* New York: Basic Books.

Shabistari, M. (1880). *Gulshane Raz [The mystic rose garden]* (E. H. Whinfield, Trans.). London: Truber & Co.

Shafii, M. (1985). *Freedom from the self.* New York: Human Sciences Press.

Shah, I. (1970). *The way of the Sufi.* New York: Dutton.

Smith, M. (1973). *Studies in early mysticism in the near and middle east.* Amsterdam: Philo Press.

Stoddart, W. (1985). *Sufism.* New York: Paragon House.

7

On Being Natural: Two Japanese Approaches to Healing

DAVID K. REYNOLDS

"I have come empty-handed," said the student.
"Lay it down then!" said the teacher.
"But I have brought nothing with me; what can I lay down?"
"Then keep on carrying it!"

Chao-chou

Let's consider for a moment the quality of being ordinary. We fear that we *aren't* ordinary enough—that we are neurotic or overly shy or timid or suffering more than most people. We fear that we *are* too ordinary—that we aren't superior, that we don't live up to our potential, that we fail to show our best qualities to others. These fears are, of

This chapter is intentionally written in a more personalized style than is usually found in an academic publication. The two therapeutic lifeways described in this chapter make their appeal to students (not "patients") on an intimate, personal level. I hope to convey some of the natural appeal of their approach by use of this somewhat informal style.

course, perfectly ordinary. We worry about the peculiarity of fears that are perfectly ordinary. What makes Woody Allen funny is that we see our own self-doubts and anxieties reflected in his exaggerated performance of the ordinary.

Zen Buddhists say that everyone is already a Buddha; we simply fail to recognize it. This chapter describes the ways we are already ordinary, natural, just fine as we are—even though we may not be aware of our present perfection.

NATURAL QUALITIES OF WATER

Water is a symbol of the natural. By just naturally doing its thing, by just going about its water business in a water-like way, it accomplishes all sorts of feats. Not the least of its accomplishments is its ability to provide us with analogies that help make sense of human psychology and provide advice for successful living.

Most of my recent books have water in the title: *Playing Ball on Running Water; Even in Summer the Ice Doesn't Melt; Water Bears No Scars;* and *Flowing Bridges, Quiet Waters* (Reynolds, 1984a, 1986, 1987). The titles are taken from Zen koans or Zen-inspired poetry. Respectively, they refer in part to action in everchanging time, the chill stiffness of neurosis, the purposeful now-centeredness of water, and the subjective nature of situational changes.

The Eastern approaches to mental health, which form what we in the West call "constructive living," are Morita therapy and Naikan therapy. They aim at helping us be natural (Reynolds, 1980). Some people believe that modern technology and other aspects of modern life have alienated us from nature. What does it mean to become natural again?

Let's examine the natural behavior of water. First, water accepts the reality of the situation it is in. It doesn't say, "Now I'm in a glass; but I want to be in the ocean, so I'll sulk and daydream and not act like proper water." Only people do that. Water reflects whatever reality brings it.

> Tozan came to see Zen master Zenne of Kassan, and asked:
> "How are things?"
>
> "Just as they are." (Shibayama, 1970, p. 206)

In warm times water becomes warm, in cold times it becomes cold. It doesn't say, "I wish I were cool today. I shouldn't get this hot." It doesn't pretend it is warm when it is really cold. It simply accepts the reality of its temperature and goes about flowing toward the lowest ground.

People deny reality. They fight against real feelings caused by real circumstances. They build mental worlds of shoulds, oughts, and might-have-beens. Real changes begin with real appraisal and acceptance of what is. Only then is realistic action possible.

Water flows around obstacles. It doesn't stop on its way down a riverbed to try to fight with the big rocks that oppose it. It just heads toward its goal and eventually wears down its opposition. Whether the obstacles wear down quickly or not, water manages to get where it aims to go without any long-term distraction. People tend to get distracted by feelings (e.g., by anxiety before college exams) and shift away from their original purposes (e.g., by trying to resolve the anxiety instead of continuing to study for the exams).

Water is wonderfully flexible. It fills the circumstances it is in. It takes the natural amount of time to get where it is going. It moves at a natural pace—now rushing quickly, now flowing slowly, depending on the circumstances. Some people seem to be rushing around all the time, trying to force time to fit their desires. Other people never seem to stir themselves to fast action.

What is so outstanding about these qualities? They are just the ordinary qualities of water. This chapter is about being ordinary and natural human beings in much the same way and about the trouble we get ourselves into when we don't accept reality in the way that water does.

CONSTRUCTIVE LIVING

Constructive living is a joining of two psychotherapies and their associated lifeways with origins in Japan (Reynolds, 1984b). The two systems of dealing with human suffering and human existence are usually called Morita therapy and Naikan therapy. Both were developed in this century, but their roots extend back for hundreds of years into the history of East Asia. Morita was a professor of psychiatry at Jikei University School of Medicine in Tokyo. Yoshimoto was a successful businessman who retired to become a lay priest in Nara. Morita's method has its origins in Zen Buddhist psychology (not Zen Buddhist religion), and Yoshimoto's Naikan has its origins in Jodo Shinshu Buddhist psychology. Neither therapy requires that one believe in Buddhism or have faith in anything other than one's own experience. They work as well for Christians and Moslems and Jews as for Buddhists. Both are built on the naturalistic observations of humans and on careful introspection by their founders. I think that as you read about constructive living you will find that it isn't so very mystical or Oriental, rather it is practical and human and, well, realistic.

MORITA THERAPY

Feelings are an important part of human life. There are feelings we like (e.g., confidence, love, happiness, and satisfaction) and feelings we don't like (e.g., loneliness, depression, fear, and timidity). It isn't surprising that we try to generate certain feelings and eliminate others. The problem with feelings, however, is that we cannot control them directly by our wills. We cannot sit down and concentrate and make our shyness go away. We cannot force ourselves to stop feeling lonely on a Saturday night or to fall in love or out of love with someone. It just cannot be done. We cannot make ourselves stop feeling nervous before an exam, or anxious before asking someone out on a date, or tense before a job interview. Feelings are natural consequences of who we are and the situations we are in, just like clouds are natural consequences of temperatures and pressures and humidity. Feelings are natural and are just as uncontrollable as the weather.

Now, no one tries to fight with rain or fog. You never see anyone going outside waving a sword or a karate blow at rainclouds. And no ordinary humans try by their wills to make fog go away. No one ignores the weather, but we have all learned to dim our headlights in the fog and stay inside during hurricanes. And we do what we can reasonably do while waiting for bad weather to pass.

Feelings are just like that. The best way to handle unpleasant feelings is to recognize them (don't try to ignore them or pretend they aren't there), to accept them (you can't control them directly, so don't try to fight something you can't defeat), and to go about your business. Rain or fog may not stop you from going to school or to work, but you will take the weather into consideration while driving. In the same way, anxiety need not stop you from studying or asking for a raise in pay, though you'll take it into consideration when selecting a place and time to study or a proper moment to approach your boss. In time, unpleasant feelings pass, just like snowstorms. Grief, for example, never sustains its intensity forever. It fades little by little over time unless something comes along to restimulate it, then it fades again. Feelings are as changeable as the weather.

Feelings are natural phenomena, uncontrollable directly by our will; they come and go like weather. However, there is a clear distinction between feelings and behavior. Behavior (e.g., preparing for an interview or dealing with a difficult client) is controllable. Just as we can choose to go on a picnic even on a windy day, we can choose to dress properly for an interview (behavior) even though we cannot choose to get rid of our anxiety (feeling) about it. We can ask someone out on a date (behavior) while feeling shy. We can total up the check at a restaurant (behavior) even though we cannot avoid our unpleasant feelings about making others wait while we do so. This distinction between directly controllable behavior and directly uncontrollable feelings is a key feature of Moritist thought.

If we have no direct control over something, we cannot be held responsible for it. Who is responsible for an earthquake? We aren't responsible for having angry, spiteful, depressed, sexy, grumpy, greedy, or any other kind of feelings. Again, feelings are natural. On the other hand, we are responsible for what we do, our behavior, no matter what we are feeling. Although there are some exceptions (e.g., stuttering, sexual impotence, and trembling), for the most part behavior is controllable by our will, so we are responsible for that aspect of our lives all the time. To be sure, we find it convenient to try to escape from our responsibility for our actions by blaming our feelings. "I was so angry I couldn't help hitting him." "I was too distraught to thank her." "I feel the need for drugs is so strong that I steal to get them." But these feeling-based excuses don't hold water. Similarly, blaming parents, society, spouses, or children for our destructive behavior is to seek to avoid the responsibility that is solely ours no matter what past experiences we may have suffered through.

One of the interesting things about human beings is that what we do (our behavior) often influences how we feel. We never have direct control over our natural feelings, but sometimes we can influence our feelings by our actions. For example, if you don't feel like going on a job interview one morning, it is a waste of time to try to make yourself want to do so. It is natural to feel some hesitation about putting yourself on the line for someone else to decide whether you are worthy of hiring or not. There is no need to make yourself enjoy job interviews. However, if you get out of bed, get dressed for the interview, and go, you may find that while you're dressing, reading over your résumé, and driving to the appointment a sort of excitement and interest in what will happen arises. Sometimes this doesn't happen, but in either case, the interview gets done. Successfully completing a few job interviews and, having jobs offered to you as a result, may make job hunting even pleasurable. But lying in bed, putting off getting up, and failing to show up for the job interview never gives you a chance to succeed, it never gives you a chance to feel anything but uncomfortable about job interviews. The more we allow feelings to govern us, the more they spread to govern even larger areas of our lives. We can use our behavior to give ourselves the chance to succeed at accomplishing our goals. That success often produces confidence and other satisfying feelings.

Pleasant feelings fade over time just as unpleasant ones do, unless something happens to restimulate those feelings. Romantic love fades in a lot of marriages. Respect for others, school spirit, and patriotic feelings can be expected to fade unless restimulated somehow. That's what pep rallies, national anthems, and romantic dinners are all about. As you carry out these behaviors, certain feelings are likely to be stimulated or restimulated. If you want to keep love in your relationship, you must keep showing love to your partner. As you behave in thoughtful, loving ways you are increasing the chances of sustaining feelings of love for him or her. Romance in a marriage is sustained by gifts, dinners by candlelight, and other romantic behaviors.

But even this focus on influencing feelings indirectly through behavior is a bit unnatural. Sometimes you seem to do everything right, you plan the proper behaviors to generate certain feelings, and the feelings don't turn out as expected. A better strategy for living is to be purpose focused instead of feeling focused. Let the feelings take care of themselves while you go about accomplishing your goals through your behavior. As the emphasis in your life turns more toward using controllable behavior to achieve your goals, life steadies and becomes more satisfying. A purpose-oriented approach is more likely to be successful than a feeling-oriented approach simply because the latter isn't a game you can win with any consistency. You can't make good feelings last forever, and you can't make bad feelings go away at will. (Technically, it isn't proper to use words like "good" and "bad" when referring to feelings; like seasons, they have no moral qualities.)

If feelings are natural phenomena, isn't it strange that there are psychotherapies that try to make fears or guilt or depression go away? There are psychotherapies and self-growth methods that aim at producing happiness, confidence, and good feelings. I cannot see how such therapies can deliver on their promises. No one is happy or confident all the time; feelings keep changing. A more suitable goal for therapy or for human life in general seems to be to notice and accept these changes in feelings while steadily moving toward our goals—like water does.

Morita therapy holds that all humans are overly sensitive to their own faults and limits to some degree. Especially when we are ill or under stress we may become fixated on some mental or physical disturbance. We exaggerate the ringing in our ears, our stiff shoulders, our fear of flying, or our discomfort about eating in restaurants. To alleviate these problems you should not ignore them or fight them, but you must learn to accept them and develop proper, constructive behavior. Regardless of what is troubling us, it is important to accept the troubled feelings and get on about living. Of course, if there is something practical and concrete we can do to alleviate the cause of the problem (e.g., seeing a physician to rule out illness), that is included in the category of proper, constructive behavior. In general, the stronger we desire something, the more we want to succeed, and the greater our anxiety about failure. Our worries and fears are reminders of the strength of our positive desires. They are also reminders of our needs to be cautious, to prepare materials to avoid the embarrassment of lack of preparation, to work hard, to practice perfecting our skills, to develop our ability to persist and endure, to attack the environmental circumstances that caused them, and so forth. Our anxieties are indispensable in spite of the discomfort that accompanies them. To try to do away with them would be foolish. Morita therapy is not really a psychotherapeutic method for getting rid of "symptoms." It is more an educational method for outgrowing our self-imposed limitations. Through Moritist methods we learn to accept the naturalness of ourselves.

In their advanced stages Morita students accept themselves as part of the natural situation in which they are embedded. This is not some passive conformity, but a dynamic recognition that we exist as situationally embedded aspects of reality. We take on our identities from the circumstances in which we find ourselves. We are rather like the cursors on the computer screen of reality. The loss of self-centeredness, in more than one sense of the word, is an ultimate goal for some students of this method. However, relief from the obsessive pressure of phobias, anxieties, and psychosomatic difficulties is sufficient for many students.

Currently, there are more than 5,000 members of the Seikatsu no Hakkenkai Moritist organization in Japan. There are nearly fifty practitioners of Morita therapy in the United States, Canada, West Germany, and the People's Republic of China. A growing literature exists in English with seven books in print and several more in press and numerous articles and book chapters on the subject. Morita's collected works fill seven large volumes. From this rich source material adaptations are made to fit the needs of modern Japanese and non-Japanese students. Morita therapy is growing inside and outside Japan as never before (Fujita, 1966; Ishiyama, 1986a, 1986b, 1987; Iwai & Reynolds, 1970; Kondo, 1953; Kora & Ohara, 1973; Kora, 1965, Morita, 1983; Ohara & Reynolds, 1968; Reynolds, 1976, 1981a; Reynolds & Kiefer, 1977; Reynolds & Yamamoto, 1972, 1973; Suzuki & Suzuki, 1977, 1981).

What we have considered here so far has come from the thought of the Japanese psychiatrist, Morita Shoma (or Morita Masatake as he preferred to call himself). Now let's examine the contribution to constructive living made by the lay priest Yoshimoto Ishin and his Naikan (Murase, 1974; Reynolds, 1977, 1981b, 1983; Takeuchi, 1965).

NAIKAN

One of the factors that seems to influence how we feel is our attitude toward the world. If we are constantly concerned with getting our share and with making sure we aren't left out, if we are extremely self-focused and self-conscious, then we are likely to have a lot of miserable feelings. The world just never seems to send us green lights and lottery prizes and kind words when we want them—and we want them nearly all the time.

Have you ever stopped to think about how much of you is truly yours? Your name was given to you by your parents. So was your body. The words you use were taught to you by parents, peers, and teachers. Your body has grown and is sustained by food that people you don't even know produced and processed for you. The clothes you wear were created and sewn by others, bought with money given to you by someone else. Even the ideas you have seem to bubble to the surface of your mind, coming out of nowhere and passing along to be replaced by other thoughts from nowhere. There's nothing that is truly yours; it is all borrowed. Of course, it is the same for all of us.

You may say, of course, that you bought your clothes with your own money. But who gave you the money? Who taught you to do the work you do to earn the money? Who hired you? Who gave you the basic educational skills to learn your trade? The point is that when we trace back our achievements far enough, inevitably we see the fruits of others' efforts on our behalf. We have done nothing on our own.

Strange, then, that we should have the notion that we are "self-made." We believe that we got where we are by our own efforts. With just a little bit of reflection we can see that such notions of having come this far on our own are laughable. Deeper reflection allows us to see in even greater detail how we have been and continue to be supported on all sides in all sorts of ways by people and things and energies.

One result of sorting out the specific, concrete ways in which the world supports us (just as you are supporting me now by loaning me your eyes to read this chapter) is a feeling of gratitude. I don't deserve all this help from you, from this paper, from the electricity that powers this word processor (and even from the people who worked to generate this electricity), from the editor and publisher of this book, from the manufacturers of the printer's ink, from book designers, and from the people who taught me these lifeways. But, through Naikan, we can come to notice and appreciate how we are nurtured by the world. Before I underwent a week of Naikan training in Japan, I thought all this was my due. I took it for granted, and still I drift back into that attitude sometimes. But whether I recognize it or not, whether I accept it or not, whether I feel gratitude or not, whether I try to return the favors or not, reality keeps on being what it is. It keeps on giving to me, not in some abstract sense, but concretely, through Jim and Frank and Lynn and this keyboard and so forth.

The natural responses to realizing how we are supported by the world are (1) the desire to repay and (2) a sort of guilt when we see that we haven't been doing much repaying right along. Starting with our parents, our attitude shifts from how little we have received from them and how much more they owe us to one of how much we have received from them and how important it is to start working on giving back something to them. I'm not suggesting that all parents are perfect and that they have done a perfect job in raising us. But I am asserting that there were some adults in our lives who fed and clothed us and nurtured us when we were small. They did it whether they were in the mood or not, over and over again, whether we showed them gratitude or not—or we wouldn't have survived to be here today.

The gratitude and desire to repay apply to the people in your life today, as well, and to objects in your world. What have you done for your shoes lately, for your car, for electricity, for your toothbrush, for your stereo set? If you take a moment to consider what they have done for you, it seems not quite so odd to think of what you might do for them in return.

I've never met a suffering neurotic person who was filled with gratitude. Isn't that something? Gratitude and neurotic suffering seem to be antagonistic. If there is anything characteristic of neurosis it is a self-centeredness. Gratitude, on the other hand, is other centered. It carries with it the desire to serve others in repayment, even if it causes some inconvenience to oneself.

The most joyful people I have known have all been people who gave themselves away to others. The most miserable people I have known have all been concerned with looking out for themselves. Look at those around you. Isn't this true in your experience?

THE PRACTICE OF CONSTRUCTIVE LIVING

How does one go about practicing Morita and Naikan therapies? Both methods have what might be called inpatient and outpatient styles. The inpatient styles are only occasionally practiced in countries other than Japan. The outpatient styles have been modified somewhat for Westerners. Interestingly, however, the modified outpatient styles for Westerners have been reintroduced in Japan where they strongly influence the practice of these therapies there.

Inpatient Morita Therapy

Inpatient Morita therapy begins with a week of isolated bedrest. Within the Moritist hospital the patient is not permitted to read or write or converse or smoke or engage in any distraction other than eating three meals a day and taking care of other natural body functions. There is no escape from the waves of doubt, boredom, anxiety, regret, and the like that pass through the mind (more accurately, they *are* the mind in that setting). Past failures are reviewed mentally along with future potential troubles. Despite the suffering, time passes and the patient survives. Feelings and thoughts well up and fade. The patient learns some measure of acceptance of these mental phenomena.

Subsequent stages of inpatient Morita therapy offer the patient scaled tasks including weeding the garden, writing a journal of activities, participating in group sports, household chores, errands off the hospital grounds, and, finally, return to everyday life outside the hospital. Constructive activity at first provides a distraction from rumination about neurotic misery. In time, reality's tasks are carried out simply because they need to be done whether the symptoms are present or not. In fact, the subjective experience of symptoms declines over time; but that decline is merely a pleasant by-product of being able to do what needs doing while suffering or not.

The entire period of hospitalization varies considerably from place to place and patient to patient. Perhaps two or three months is the mean these days, although Morita himself began inpatient treatment in the 1920s with a period of one month.

Outpatient Morita Therapy

Outpatient Morita therapy involves teaching the student the principles of living (rather as they have been described here) and inviting the student to compare these concepts with his or her own experience. Whether the principles are fully understood or not assignments are made to give the student increasing experiential knowledge about the lifeway. For example, the student may be advised to get up at a particular time whether he or she feels like it or not. The student may be told to make the bed, prepare breakfast, and eat it regardless of anxieties or dreadful anticipation of what might happen during the day. The student may be asked to observe and report on detailed behaviors such as which foot touched the floor first when arising from bed, what was done with the toothpaste cap while brushing the teeth, and so forth. The focus is on attending to the activities rather than dwelling on complaints about mental anguish.

Reading assignments are given. Other techniques include keeping a Morita journal that separates behaviors and feelings, discussing fables that illustrate psychological truths, and completing homework tasks of various sorts. Moritist maxims help the client to keep the life principles in mind throughout the day. More detailed descriptions of assignments and other techniques are to be found in works by Reynolds (1984a, 1984b, 1986, 1987) and Ishiyama (1987).

Inpatient Naikan Therapy

Inpatient Naikan involves a week of intensive reflection on the following three themes: (1) what was received from some person, (2) what was done in return for that person, and (3) what troubles and worries were caused that person. The Naikan client spends each day from early morning until night in isolated reflection on these themes. At first the mother or mother surrogate is the object of reflection. What did my mother do for me during grammar school? What did I do in return for her? What troubles did I cause her? After a period of time, perhaps an hour or two, the therapist comes to listen to the Naikan client's accounting of what was recalled. The therapist listens gratefully, without comment or interpretation. Then, during the next period of Naikan meditation, the same three themes will be considered regarding the mother during the client's junior high school period. Again the therapist comes to listen. The pattern progresses in approximately three-year intervals until the present or until the mother died. Then the client begins again with the grammar school period working on the recollections of the father. Working from the past to the present, the client reflects on other significant persons in his or her life.

The method is simple, but it has a very powerful emotional impact on the clients. In effect, they measure themselves by their own standards of reciprocity and find themselves wanting. There is no escape into the excuse that they are being tested by someone else's standards (e.g., some religious code). Common results of inpatient Naikan include guilt, gratitude, a sense of having been loved in spite of one's failings, and the desire to repay others.

After the week is over, clients are encouraged to continue Naikan during shorter periods each day. Each morning the client is to continue reflecting about others in the past just as he or she did during the hospital period. In the evening the client is advised to reflect about that day—what was received from others during the day, what was returned to them, and what troubles the client caused others during the day.

Outpatient Naikan Therapy

Outpatient Naikan may take the form of daily Naikan reflection as described in the previous paragraph. The student may be asked to keep a journal of Naikan recollections and to bring the journal to the weekly outpatient sessions. Related assignments include saying "thank you" a minimum of ten times each day, particularly to a person with whom the student is currently on bad terms. Quarreling spouses are likely to receive assignments to bring gifts to each other and to perform services for each other in secret. To be sure, there is resistance to such assignments. The students may complain that they feel no gratitude toward their spouse and so cannot say "thank you." They may hold that the spouse doesn't deserve their words of gratitude, gifts, and services. At such times they are reminded of the difference between feelings (e.g., gratitude), which are uncontrollable and for which they have no responsibility, and behaviors (e.g., thanking and giving gifts), which remain in their control.

Another outpatient Naikan assignment is to ask the student to clean out a drawer. The items are removed from the drawer, and the drawer is cleaned. As the items are returned to the drawer one by one, each item is thanked for some specific service it performed for the student. We are served not only by people but also by the energies and objects in our world. Conservation of the resources in our world becomes a natural consequence of the grateful recognition of the services they perform for us.

COMMON FEATURES

Clearly, both Morita and Naikan therapies are directive and follow an educational model rather than a medical model of dealing with human suffering. Understanding the principles of the lifeway of constructive living is an important element in achieving some release from unnecessary misery. The students' efforts to change their behaviors are seen to be important in constructive living.

Both elements of constructive living are concerned with reality. Whether you believe it or not, accept it or not, or like it or not, reality is "as it is."

> Why fret away your life?
> See the willow tree by the river;
> There it is, watching the water flow by.
>
> (Shibayama, 1970, p. 261)

Pay attention to what reality brings you, both Morita's therapy and Yoshimoto's Naikan advise. Check out reality directly. Don't simply accept what I or anyone else tells you about the way things are. See for yourself. Your understanding of psychology must not be founded solely on what you read in some textbooks or hear in lectures. It must be experiential, or it will not be of maximum usefulness to you.

Both elements of constructive living have an action emphasis. It isn't enough to accept feelings, it isn't enough to feel gratitude; it is important to *do* something constructive, something purposeful. We owe the world for our existence. We will never find life satisfaction without making efforts to repay that debt. Being mature and psychologically healthy doesn't mean feeling good all the time. Maturity means acting responsibly and positively, whether we feel good or not, grateful or not.

Finally, both elements of constructive living look pragmatically at what is possible and what is impossible. Morita therapy advises that we cannot change our feelings directly by our wills, that we cannot control other people directly, and that we cannot control completely the outcome of our efforts. We do our best to influence these uncontrollable aspects of our lives, but we must accept what reality actually brings us. Naikan therapy recognizes that we cannot directly change what happened in our past. We can influence our way of looking at the past, our attitude toward the past, and we can work to create a new past by our actions in the present. But as events flow into the past they are fixed forever. We must accept them as reality. Being clear about what is possible and what is impossible in life helps us to avoid wasting attention and energy; we become wiser about the proper directions in which to invest our efforts.

> Not knowing how close the Truth is to them,
> Beings seek for it afar—what a pity!
> It is like those who being in water
> Cry out for water, feeling thirst.
>
> (Shibayama, 1970, p. 93)

References

Fujita, C. (1986). *Morita therapy*. New York: Igaku Shoin.

Ishiyama, F. I. (1983). A case of severe test anxiety treated by Morita therapy. *Canadian Counsellor, 17*(4), 172–174.

Ishiyama, F. I. (1986a). Morita therapy: Its basic features and cognitive intervention for anxiety treatment. *Psychotherapy, 23*(3), 375–381.

Ishiyama, F. I. (1986b). Positive reinterpretation of fear of death: A Japanese (Morita) psychotherapy approach to anxiety treatment. *Psychotherapy, 23*(4), 556–562.

Ishiyama, F. I. (1987). Use of Morita therapy in shyness counseling in the west: Promoting clients' self-acceptance and action taking. *Journal of Counseling and Development, 65,* 547–551.

Iwai, H., & Reynolds, D. K. (1970). Morita therapy: The views from the west. *American Journal of Psychiatry, 126*(7), 1031–1036.

Kondo, A. (1953). Morita therapy: A Japanese therapy for neurosis. *American Journal of Psychoanalysis, 13,* 31–37.

Kora, T. (1965). Morita therapy. *International Journal of Psychiatry, 1*(4), 611–640.

Kora, T., & Ohara, K. (1973). Morita therapy. *Psychology Today, 6*(10), 63–68.

Morita, S. (1983). *Seishin ryoho kogi [Lectures on psychotherapy].* Tokyo: Hakuyosha.

Murase, T. (1974). Naikan therapy. In T. Lebra & W. Lebra (Eds.), *Japanese culture and behavior.* Honolulu: University of Hawaii Press.

Ohara, K., & Reynolds, D. K. (1968). Changing methods in Morita psychotherapy. *International Journal of Social Psychiatry, 14*(4), 305–310.

Reynolds, D. K. (1976). *Morita psychotherapy* (English, Japanese, and Spanish editions). Berkeley: University of California Press.

Reynolds, D. K. (1977). Naikan therapy—An experiential view. *International Journal of Social Psychiatry, 23*(4), 252–264.

Reynolds, D. K. (1980). *The quiet therapies.* Honolulu: University of Hawaii Press.

Reynolds, D. K. (1981a). Morita psychotherapy. In R. Corsini (Ed.), *Handbook of innovative psychotherapies* (pp. 489–501). New York: Wiley.

Reynolds, D. K. (1981b). Naikan therapy. In R. Corsini (Ed.), *Handbook of innovative psychotherapies* (pp. 544–553). New York: Wiley.

Reynolds, D. K. (1983). *Naikan psychotherapy: Meditation for self-development.* Chicago: University of Chicago Press.

Reynolds, D. K. (1984a). *Playing ball on running water.* New York: Morrow.

Reynolds, D. K. (1984b). *Constructive living.* Honolulu: University of Hawaii Press.

Reynolds, D. K. (1986). *Even in summer the ice doesn't melt.* New York: Morrow.

Reynolds, D. K. (1987). *Water bears no scars.* New York: Morrow.

Reynolds, D. K. (in press). *Flowing Bridges, Quiet Waters.*

Reynolds, D. K., & Kiefer, C. W. (1977). Cultural adaptability as an attribute of therapies: The case of Morita psychotherapy. *Culture, Medicine, and Psychiatry, 1,* 395–412.

Reynolds, D. K., & Yamamoto, J. (1972). East meets west: Moritist and Freudian psychotherapies. *Science and Psychoanalysis 1,* 187–193.

Reynolds, D. K. & Yamamoto, J. (1973). Morita psychotherapy in Japan. In J. Masserman (Ed.), *Current psychiatric therapies, 13,* 219–227.

Shibayama, Z. (1970). *A flower does not talk* (Sumiko Kudo, Trans.). Rutland, VT: Tuttle.

Suzuki, T., & Suzuki, R. (1977). Morita therapy. In E. D. Wittkower & H. Warnes (Eds.), *Psychosomatic medicine*. New York: Harper & Row.

Suzuki, T., & Suzuki, R. (1981). The effectiveness of inpatient Morita therapy. *Psychiatric Quarterly, 53*(3), 201–213.

Takeuchi, K. (1965). On Naikan. *Psychologia, 8,* 2–8.

WESTERN PERSPECTIVES

8

The Four Forces of Psychotherapy

ROBERT J. LUEGER
ANEES A. SHEIKH

*"Taken as a whole, (the field) is a patchwork quilt of incompat-
ible designs. In this domain men speak with voices of authority
saying different things in different tongues, and the expectant
student is left to wonder whether one or none are in the right."*

Murray, 1938, p. 103

"Everybody has won and all must have prizes."

Lewis Carroll, *Alice in Wonderland,* quoted in
Smith, Glass, & Miller, 1980

Three models of psychotherapy—behaviorism, psychoanalysis
and humanism—are well known to professional therapists and are recognized by the public. Less familiar is the transpersonal model of psychotherapy, which, according to some sources (e.g., Boorstein, 1980),
constitutes a fourth force in psychology. This chapter presents a discussion of all four forces in American psychotherapy, along with a few
concluding remarks comparing them.

The history of psychotherapy in America during the first half of the 20th century is largely the history of psychoanalysis (the first force). During the 1950s, the monopoly of psychoanalysis was seriously challenged by the emergence of behavioristic approaches to therapy (the second force). These two forces continued to dominate the field well into the 1960s, at which time a group of prominent psychologists launched the movement of humanistic psychology (the third force). These psychologists, including Carl Rogers, Abraham Maslow, Frederick Perls, Rollo May, and Anthony Sutich, were "unwilling to reduce the psyche to a complex of neurological reflexes and interacting forces" (Grof, 1984, p. vii) and were reluctant to base their conclusions about human nature on research with animals and emotionally deranged people. This movement emphasized individual freedom and the ability of human beings to determine their own development. Unlike the psychoanalysts and the behavior therapists, they refused to subscribe to the notion "that the individual is reducible to a series of logical, causative, deterministic propositions" (Belkin, 1987, p. 173).

Although the third force quickly gained popularity, a few influential professionals felt that its emphasis on "growth and self-actualization was still too narrow and limited" and that this new movement had shied away from clear recognition of "spirituality and transcendental needs as intrinsic aspects of human nature" (Grof, 1984, p. vii). These shortcomings gradually led to the birth of the fourth force, the transpersonal approach to psychology and psychotherapy. During the 1980's, this movement has developed rapidly, as evidenced in the emergence of several organizations devoted to this orientation (e.g., the *Journal of Transpersonal Psychology*, the Association of Transpersonal Psychology, the California Institute of Transpersonal Psychology, the International Transpersonal Association, etc.).

THE FIRST FORCE: PSYCHOANALYTIC PSYCHOTHERAPY

Without question, the dominant school of psychotherapy in the 20th century has been the psychoanalytic model. The emerging concepts and ideas of the Viennese physician, Sigmund Freud, received American recognition with the presentation by Freud and his entourage at Clark University in 1908. In the ensuing 80 years, the principles of psychoanalytic thought have not only guided psychotherapy, but they have permeated Western culture through literature, art, religion, and social studies. Although many people with a shallow exposure to the history of the psychoanalytic model are prone to see a unitary model, two distinct traditions—classical psychoanalysis and ego psychoanalytic theory—have emerged as disciples and detractors have sought to clarify or expand original Freudian axioms. Classical psychoanalysis reflects a refinement of Freud's seminal ideas without change in the core mechanisms of psychic functioning. Ego psychoanalytic theories have developed on alternate premises and conclusions.

A comprehensive review of classical psychoanalysis and ego psychoanalytic theories is beyond the scope of this chapter. Instead, the core premises and concepts of each approach will be highlighted, and the implications for therapeutic practice will be discussed. Stages of the therapeutic process will be described, and some effort will be made to identify signs of therapeutic efficacy in each of the psychoanalytic models.

Classical Psychoanalysis

Freud introduced a topography of mental operations that was arranged in a vertical hierarchy of conscious, preconscious, and unconscious. This vertical hierarchy stood in contrast to one proposed by Freud's contemporary, Pierre Janet, which was horizontal in zones of awareness and unawareness (Hilgard, 1977). This vertical rather than horizontal conception of consciousness becomes important in understanding applications of psychoanalytic psychotherapy. In addition to this topography, Freud proposed a tripartite structure of mental operations, which were grouped according to id, ego, and superego functions. Each of these sets of functions includes ideational-affective processes distributed over the topographical layers and developmental influences in the formation of the psyche. Id functions derive out of impulses that drive action; superego functions represent introjections of values primarily expressed as inhibitions of impulses; and ego functions reflect efforts to deal with reality through the energy supplied by the id impulses.

Whereas the topography and structure of mentalistic operations gives the psyche form and substance, it is the dynamic investment of psychic energy that constitutes the processes of these operations. Freud used a closed energy system to model the investment of this energy of the psyche. Psychic energy derives from metabolic processes, which also feed other body systems and, as such, must be replaced once expended. Once generated though, this energy is infused in libido or sexual drives and in aggressive drives. Impulses, and thus energy, have their point of origin in the psychic system in id functions. The arousal of an impulse induces a state of tension, which in turn is reduced when that impulse is gratified. Thus Freud's dynamic model is a tension-reduction model as well. The hypothetical beginning and ending point of any mental operation is a tensionless homeostatic state.

A key feature of the classical psychoanalytic model is the primacy of id functions. Once again, ego functions derive their energy from id processes, and thus represent less direct and less fulfilling means of meeting id-originated needs. The resulting residue of psychic energy complicates subsequent operations. Superego functions derive their energy in much the same way, although they lack the executive quality of ego functions and are juxtaposed to id drives. From this perspective, the development of ego and superego functions necessarily involves a neurotic process of inefficiently invested psychic energy.

Freud postulated stages of psychosexual development that parallel biological maturation of a cephalocaudal (head to tail) nature, from mouth to sphincters to genital zones and puberty. The corresponding stages—oral, anal, phallic, and genital—represent successive, qualitatively distinct organizations of ideations, affects, and actions. An arrest of development within any one of these stages is called a *fixation*. Fixations are important to understanding character neuroses and regressions under conditions of duress. Fixations will limit the organization of cognitive, affective, and action parameters, and render the fixated individual vulnerable along one or more of the cognitive, affective, or action domains.

Fixations are comprised of constellations of ideation-affective energy that have been inefficiently invested. These constellations are energy complexes that draw any subsequent energy; they interfere with gratification of impulses and threaten loss of control. The term *"fuero"* has been applied to these energy complexes (Cameron & Rychlak, 1985); it has its origin in the Spanish feudal era and roughly translates to "a debt or favor" owed by virtue of the issuance of a prior favor. For example, a feudal lord might have provided food or livestock to his subjects, whereupon he might request those subjects to bear arms for him in order to thwart invasion or to pursue a conquest. In psychotherapy, these action-cognition-affection complexes must be unbound so that the associated energy can be more efficiently invested in the dual business of the psyche—namely, satisfying id impulses while responding adaptively to environmental demands.

Two processes are important in the investment and distribution of psychic energy. *Cathexis* is the investment of instinctual energy in a need-gratifying object. The energy of an id impulse is cathected in both primary (id) and secondary (ego, superego) objects. The process of investing energy in secondary and less-satisfying (albeit, more environmentally adaptive) objects is called *displacement*. The other process of importance is that of catharsis. *Catharsis* involves the release of energy bound by *fueros*, unacceptable impulses, defensive maneuvers, and fixations. This release of energy, this catharsis, is fostered by a relationship in which defenses can be relaxed, and it is central to the Freudian therapeutic process of free association.

In free association, the individual in therapy says whatever comes to mind no matter how trivial the thought or association might seem. The goal of psychoanalytic psychotherapy, whether classical or ego function oriented, is to make the unconscious conscious. Thus psychoanalytic therapy is an insight therapy. Symptoms are signs of inefficiently invested energy and failure to develop and adapt, but also they are distortions of the true nature of unacceptable impulses. Through free association, one learns the nature of blocked, unacceptable impulses and invests the freed energy in more efficient and realistic processes.

Resistance dulls the kinetic effort to resolve blocked impulses and gain insight. As such, resistance is a symptom of conflicted impulses in that the central investigative process is inhibited in cognitive, affective, and conative domains. Once again, the presence and nature of resistance must come into awareness before resolution can be achieved on unconscious conflicts. Letting go of symptoms and resolving resistance gives partial release to bound energy and enables control of impulses to be established.

Ego Psychoanalytic Theory

An alternate approach within the psychoanalytic model emphasizes the role of ego functions using the structure and dynamic processes of classical psychoanalysis. Heinz Hartmann is often credited with proposing the autonomous ego (Hall, Lindzey, Loehlin, & Manosevitz, 1985), which does not require displacement of energy from id impulses in biological maturation, but which has its own source of psychic energy. The ego psychoanalytic model proposes that the autonomous ego develops functions comprised of perceptual and cognitive processes that have a basis in brain activity. The role of ego functions is not only to adapt to the demands of the external world, but also to gain mastery of those elements in a proactive manner. Thus ego functions are driven by a mastery or effectance motive (White, 1959) independent of id processes.

If the functions of the ego are both to defend and to master, then the processes of the ego are both defensive and actively adaptive. Defense mechanisms, introduced and advocated by Freud as a form of displacement, were embellished in the work of Anna Freud who sought to remain loyal to the classical psychoanalytic model. Defense mechanisms operate effectively outside awareness and are distortions of reality in the face of working through unacceptable impulses. As such, they were considered to be maladaptive in any long-term developmental sense. Repression and denial are among the most basic and widely employed defense mechanisms, but projection, reaction formation, and identification are closely identified in various character neuroses. Defense mechanisms are evident to the observer when affect does not fit the demands of the situation, when affect and cognition are inconsistent, and when actions are taken without awareness of propelling affect. From the ego psychoanalytic perspective, defense mechanisms are a pervasive but more primitive control of unacceptable id impulses. As such, they are palliative measures of need-reality regulation to be engaged when more advanced, efficient efforts to gain mastery fail. Moreover, under conditions of great duress when no other adaptive course is available (e.g., under torture, in concentration camps, or in the face of environmental catastrophes), defense mechanisms serve an adaptive function of removing the individual psychologically.

Built-in coping mechanisms, such as talking it out, crying, and ritualistic reenactment, offer cathartic relief of bound energy (Menninger, 1963). These built-in mechanisms usually are employed with little awareness but are considered less palliative than defense mechanisms. Cognitive controls (Klein, 1954; Santostefano, 1978), such as leveling-sharpening, are a perceptual defense that limits or expands the amount of information demanding assimilation from the environment. Cognitive controls are in an intermediate category between the built-in and the most effective mastery efforts. Finally, problem-solving efforts represent the highest level of ego adaptation but require the greatest focus and the highest developmental processes (Bellak & Goldsmith, 1984; Loevinger, 1966).

More recent developments in ego psychology have emphasized the balance of ego resources and the demands of the environment in assessing adaptation (Bellak & Goldsmith, 1984). From this perspective, lifestyle adaptation involves the incorporation of defense mechanisms in vocational and family life (Vaillant, 1977), as well as resiliency through alternative resources (Block & Block, 1987). Therapies based on this ego psychoanalytic model involve identification of coping styles, mastery components (e.g., skills and abilities), and characterological defense mechanisms, and involve the uncovering of unacceptable impulses and superego inhibitions.

Current Practice

Many therapists who practice within the frame of the psychoanalytic model probably use an amalgamation of classical and ego psychoanalytic theories. The original drive-reduction motivational model is often supplanted not only by effectance motivation, but also by self-actualization motives (Kohut, 1971). The classical emphasis on childhood traumatic neuroses and the myth of bad parents is found less frequently than an emphasis on the character of the individual and on the internalized interpersonal (e.g., object relations) patterns, which are a product of the psychosocial, psychosexual developmental processes. Thus pattern and structure, interpersonal and intrapsychic, and present and developmental aspects of problems and issues are the objects of focus.

The mode of therapeutic delivery has changed as well. The authoritarian stance of the therapist vis-à-vis the patient, copied from the medical model, has evolved into a more egalitarian model that emphasizes collaboration and sharing between the therapist and the patient. Erikson (1950) was one of the first psychoanalytic therapists to emphasize mutuality or equality between the patient and therapist, "in which the observer who has learned to observe himself (sic) teaches the observed to become self-observing" (p. 15). Bibliotherapy may be used with patients in psychotherapy who may not have prior exposure to psychoanalytic concepts. In short, the aim of the patient in psychoanalytic psychotherapy is to learn to accept his or her past and to more fully experience the present (Prochaska, 1979).

Generally, psychoanalytic psychotherapy remains an approach most effectively applied with verbal, insight-motivated individuals who are capable of "adaptive regression in service of the ego" (Bellak & Goldsmith, 1984) and who maintain a resilient core of intact reality awareness. Greenson (1967), who perhaps has written most authoritatively on the essence of psychoanalytic psychotherapy, says, "People who do not dare regress from reality and those who cannot return readily to reality are poor risks for psychoanalysis" (p. 34). Thus borderline, schizotypal, schizoidal, personality disordered, and schizophrenic or manic-depressive individuals are poor candidates for the psychoanalytic enterprise.

Components of Psychoanalytic Psychotherapy

Whereas classical psychoanalysis uses free association as the method of exchange, current practice involves a more directive effort from the therapist. The initial task is to form a *therapeutic alliance* with the part of the patient's ego that seeks relief from discomfort and is rational enough to reason that the analyst's contributions can produce healing. The scope of this therapeutic alliance is dependent on the capacity of the ego to integrate other functions of the psyche to address the challenge at hand. Thus the alliance formed with the dominant ego state of a person with multiple personality will differ from the id-aligned functions of a histrionic personality and the superego-driven ego integrates of the obsessive-compulsive person. Expansion of the therapeutic alliance can, but not always will, reflect therapeutic growth.

Resistance can appear at any point in therapy, from the initial session to termination. Signs of resistance include missed appointments, coming late to sessions, dramatic recoveries, desire to terminate therapy abruptly, repressed dreams, and an inability to regress within the scope of therapeutic permission. Most patients, although they acknowledge the theoretical possibility of resistance, do not believe that resistance exists in their actions, feelings, or thoughts. Therefore, what patients often must understand is that resistance is an inescapable facet of being human. Accepting this premise and the interpretation of the therapist affects a temporary neurosis that has the potential to be therapeutically positive.

Creating such a neurosis disrupts the egosyntonic state of the individual and poses a challenge to the processes of the ego. An axiom of psychoanalytic psychotherapy is that all that is egosyntonic must become ego-alien to make the therapeutic process possible (Goldman & Milman, 1978). This is easy to say, but hard to accomplish. Tampering with the egosyntonic self, activates defense mechanisms (e.g., rationalization, projection, denial, or isolation); patients justify, excuse, find convenient targets for their self-hatred, refuse to accept adverse evidence, or acknowledge all as true without an affective component.

The therapist's warmth and humanness allow the therapeutic alliance to develop in spite of the patient's resistance. As part of this development, the patient experiences feelings for the therapist in a process called *transference.* The experienced feelings often reflect displacement of feelings from significant others in the patient's life to the therapist. This shift of introjects from significant others in the patient's past to the therapist might take the form of embarrassment over something said, fears of being reproached by the therapist, a submissiveness or compliance with an authority figure, a sense of buddyship, or anger at being held accountable. Object relations theories (Klein, 1954) hold that transference originates in the earliest interpersonal relationships of infancy and represents the narcissistic result of failed separation-individuation. It is valuable to identify the presence of transference in the therapeutic relationship, for it teaches the patient about the nature of his or her interpersonal dynamics and defensive strategies. The therapist might begin by explaining that the therapy does not create the transference, but merely brings transference processes to be activated and developed within the therapeutic relationship. The therapist can facilitate the manifestation of transference dispositions by being passive or opaque, by focusing on aspects of life other than on the present, by concentrating on dreams and fantasies, by scheduling multiple visits within a week, by repeatedly interpreting resistances, by showing compassion and unconditional acceptance, or by acting a role that has been assumed by a significant other in the patient's life.

The therapist uses *analytic confrontation* to ensure that the patient is focusing on and is aware of the specific feelings, actions, cognitions, or experiences that are being analyzed. Greenson (1967) offers several examples of analytic confrontation: "You seem to be angry towards me. You seem to have sexual feelings for me" (p. 304). These specific experiences are further elaborated and clarified by the therapist after the confrontation has been made. Again Greenson offers an example: "He would like to beat me to a pulp, literally grind me up and mush me into a jelly-like mass of bloody, shiny goo. Then he'd eat me in one big 'slurp' like the goddamned oatmeal his mother made him eat as a kid" (p. 304). This process of elaboration bears the technical name of *analytic clarification.*

With the affective, cognitive, and conative dimensions of an experience elaborated, the therapist uses *interpretation* to make conscious the unconscious meaning, the source, and the developmental history of a specific psychic event. The patient is quite vulnerable at this point, and the interpretation of the therapist goes beyond the organized experience of the patient, so that a transference neurosis is activated. Of course, therapists are not always accurate in their interpretation of psychic events. Those interpretations that are accurate tend, gradually, to result in growth and change for the better.

The insights obtained from interpretations of resistance and transference must be accommodated in a process called *working through.* For Freud, working through involved the process of continually reviewing the observed events of a session in an effort to obtain new understandings and perspectives both for therapist and client. This compulsive effort required great patience from the therapist and deep commitment from the patient. Freud coined the term "repetition compulsion" to describe the patient's tendency to repeatedly enact past experience without memory of that experience. In the therapeutic process, therapist and patient use repetition compulsion to gain insight.

Many psychoanalytic therapists consider *dream interpretation* to be an indispensable component of psychoanalytic psychotherapy. Dreams convey current concerns of patients as experiences are self-interpreted. Dreams contain memories of long-forgotten events, repressed thoughts and feelings about parents and siblings, and current attitudes reflecting different aspects of the self (real versus ideal) as well as attitudes toward the therapist. Various psychoanalytic theorists have interpreted the role of dreaming differently. Freud distinguished between the manifest content of dreams and the latent content, which reveals the wish fulfillment of drives or impulses. The transformation of latent content into manifest content was labeled "dream work." This transformation includes the condensation or compression of a number of ideas into a single image, the displacement of objects so that one person or a part of one person might stand for another person, and the symbolization that an object represents of a set of ideas. These components of the dream—manifest content, latent content, dream work, condensation, displacement, and symbolization—require interpretation from the therapist.

Jung (1961) rejected the notion of wish fulfillment in dreams; he focused on the manifest content of the dream as the true source of understanding about the psyche. Rather than a distorted symbolization of drives, dreams are a part of nature and express as best they can, a personal experience in the context of a collective history and a current environment. For Adler (See Hall, Lindzey, Loehlin, & Manosevitz, 1985), dreams are a reflection of the life style of the individual and provide insight into his or her social interest and competitive strivings for superiority. Sullivan (1953) examined dreams for insights into the patient's current source of anxiety, and Horney (See Hall, Lindzey, Loehlin, & Manosevitz, 1985) analyzed the potential of the dream for developing the patient's awareness of the real self. The interpretation of dreams by each theorist and the focus of each theory highlight the unique role of dreams in the spectrum of psychoanalytic personality theories.

Whether experiences of the patient are confronted, clarified, or interpreted is somewhat influenced by the *countertransference* that exists between therapist and patient. Conflicts within the therapist can contaminate the therapeutic value of a transference neurosis. Such conflicts include the need to be accepted as a therapist, the need to be liked by patients, the need to keep money flowing into the practice, difficulties related to the expression of hostility, reactions to guilt inductions, perfectionistic strivings, narcissistic needs for admiration, and difficulties related to sex and intimacy. Social and situational pressures in the therapist's life can influence his or her unconscious response to a patient in therapy. Unresolved developmental experiences of the therapist, such as sibling rivalry or envy, can be resurrected by the therapeutic process.

Focused emotional statements directed to the therapist influence the therapist's state of being. Cohen (1952) has identified some of the signs of countertransference in the following events:

> The therapist has an unreasonable dislike for the patient.
> The therapist feels little or no emotional response toward the patient.
> The therapist likes the patient excessively.
> The therapist dreads upcoming sessions with the patient.
> The therapist feels unusually vulnerable to the patient's criticism (p. 64).

> The therapist is angrily sympathetic with the patient regarding mistreatment by an authority figure.
> The therapist feels impelled to do something active in respect to the patient.
> The patient appears in the therapist's dreams.

Stages in Psychoanalytic Psychotherapy

Many investigators of psychoanalytic psychotherapy have identified three stages in the therapy process—the initial phase, the middle phase, and termination. In the initial phase, three goals must be achieved: (1) the patient must come to see the therapist as trustworthy, competent, and capable of helping—in sum, a positive transference must be established; (2) the patient must switch from a defensive stance (i.e., of attributing the source of his or her concerns to external events) to a growth-oriented, risk-taking ownership for his or her feelings, thoughts, and actions; and (3) a working alliance must be established in which both therapist and patient are commonly committed to changing at least some aspect of the patient's experience. The exact number of sessions needed to fulfill these three conditions will vary according to the qualities of the patient, the parameters of the meetings, and the actions and qualities of the therapist; however, 8 to 12 sessions are commonly required.

The second or middle phase is often considered the heart of the psychoanalytic therapeutic process. Typically it is the longest period of the three states for it contains the bulk of the self-exploration, interpretation, working through, and resolution of presenting symptoms and characterological problems and issues. Although Freud was quite clear in specifying what should happen in the initial and termination phases of psychotherapy, he left the middle phase rather unorganized in deference to the complexity, idiosyncrasy, and variability in characterological issues.

The final or third stage of psychoanalytic psychotherapy is termination. A rule-of-thumb heuristic popular with many analytic therapists is that the length of termination will be determined by the length, intensity, and depth of the middle phase. Sullivan (1953) identified two criteria for termination: (1) the patient must know himself or herself as much the same person as he or she is known by others and (2) the patient must acquire an awareness of the illusions ("parataxic distortions" to Sullivan) that govern interpersonal relationships. Implicit in these two criteria is a greater level of self-insight, a more objective reality awareness, and a sense of personal control to alter selective events of one's life experience. Underlying all these gains is a closer harmony between the unconscious and conscious aspects of experience. The process of termination involves separation and coming to terms with loss. The patient mourns for the unfortunate character patterns of the neurotic self and for the real relationship with the therapist. These losses involve an element of sadness, but they are also liberating. As the patient works through these feelings, he or she often is led to take another (or initial) look at concerns about loss and death, especially as he or she has come to know loss through personal experience. Much of this effort involves making a distinction between leave-taking and fear of death or loss through death. During the termination phase, it is not uncommon for patients to regress temporarily to old mood states and old interpersonal problems. The adage, "Things get worse before they get better," appears to be operative in the termination phase.

Efficacy of Psychoanalytic Psychotherapy

Early efforts to assess the efficacy of psychotherapy focused on challenges to the efficacy of psychotherapy in general (Eysenck, 1952) and on the relative contributions of psychoanalytic and behavioral approaches to therapy (Eysenck, 1960). This dichotomy between psychoanalytic and behavioral therapy was made more complex by the consideration of client-centered and Gestalt approaches in the 1960s and by the introduction of cognitive-behavioral techniques in the 1970s. The effect was to garner support for an eclectic approach to psychotherapy in which techniques chosen from therapies of a particular persuasion are used to address various aspects of the patient's presenting issues. The application of meta-analysis as a research tool has failed to support such an eclectic approach (Shapiro & Shapiro, 1982; Smith, Glass, & Miller, 1980). Instead, the cumulative evidence to date from meta-analysis seems to support a pluralistic approach to psychotherapy in which therapists operating within a particular frame of reference are equally effective in reducing the discomfort of a patient's presenting complaints and in producing life-style change. Meta-analysis indicates that psychoanalytic psychotherapy is as effective as any other theoretical type of psychotherapy. Although this conclusion is likely to sound bland to dogmatic psychoanalytic psychotherapists who have accumulated a wealth of procedural evidence (intuitive) to support their therapeutic efforts, it may be as strong a statement as the method of meta-analysis allows, given the existing sources of validating evidence.

Other efforts to document the efficacy of psychoanalytic psychotherapy, notably the Menninger Psychotherapy Research Project (Wallerstein, 1986) and the Vanderbilt psychotherapy studies (Strupp, 1980), have found support for psychoanalytic psychotherapy. Reports from successfully treated patients usually indicate a deeper grasp of the meaning of their presenting symptoms, of the role that the symptoms play, and of the hidden gains in maintaining a neurotic character style. Patients also report greater insight into the ways in which the environment affects them and in which they, in turn, affect the environment. Out of this perspective, comes a more realistic acknowledgment of the role of internal factors in responses to the environment. Patients generally report more positive feelings about themselves and about others, and they are less defensive and more aware of evidence of defensiveness. Evidence for significant character change is less consistent; patients often persist in their ongoing character style, albeit with greater awareness if the dimensions of their feelings, thoughts, and actions.

Outcome studies of the processes of psychoanalytic psychotherapy reveal many similarities to other insight therapies. Therapists usually begin the therapy with an assessment and diagnosis to determine whether therapy should support the ego, uncover impulses, or change the external conditions of life. Therapists strive to develop a safe and trusting relationship, are more active and directive, and are likely to control the transference process. Free association and the couch are not frequent components of psychoanalytic psychotherapy in the current practice.

THE SECOND FORCE: BEHAVIOR THERAPY

The second great school of psychotherapy to emerge in the 20th century came from the learning and conditioning theories and is collectively known as behavior therapy. Although this school frequently is perceived by the public as a single approach to changing behavior, in fact it reflects a heterogeneous heritage of learning theories and thus is quite diverse. Major differences in the philosophy of human nature, in the nature of evidence, in metaphysical issues (e.g., efficient and final cause) and in the meaning of behaviors, distinguish behavior therapy from the psychoanalytic therapies. In practice, however, similarities are evident; despite the flying fur of scuffling dogmatists, behavior therapy and psychoanalytic therapy have common elements.

The Basis of Behavior Therapy in Various Learning Theories

Behavior therapy owes much of its philosophical basis to the British empiricists, notably Locke and Hume. The mechanistic view of phenomena places the "organism" in relationship to an external environment, which is the source of action and behavior. Aristotle's elucidation of efficient cause as involving a temporal relationship of antecedent event and consequence and his explication of the nature of evidence serve as cornerstones of most learning theories.

Thorndike (1905) capitalized on both of these philosophical sources in proposing an association theory of learning. Each element of learning involves a chain of events: stimulus (antecedent event), response (behavior), and consequence (reward). "Learning" is applied to the association between stimulus and response. The reward serves to strengthen this association and thus ensure the reappearance of the response under similar circumstances. Although subsequent learning theories have shifted the point at which learning occurs, the three basic elements of antecedent, behavior, and consequence have characterized behavior therapy. Thorndike's theory and similar theories of learning can be identified as stimulus-response (S-R) theories.

Ivan Pavlov's conditioning experiments identified the important elements of the stimulus-stimulus learning theories, which are more popularly identified under the heading of classical conditioning. In classical conditioning, a naturally occurring stimulus that produces a physiological-behavioral response is paired with another stimulus that would not ordinarily produce that response. This conditioned stimulus produces a conditioned response similar to the response elicited by the natural stimulus. The "learning" occurs in the pairing of the two stimuli rather than in the stimulus-response relationship.

In the United States, John Watson (1900) championed the principles of classical conditioning as well as the dogmas of empirical behaviorism. Others applied these principles to the treatment of clinical problems, such as children's fears (Jones, 1924), enuresis (Mowrer & Mowrer, 1938), tics and stuttering (Dunlap, 1932), and alcoholism (Ichok, 1934). Many, if not most, of these efforts were made by academicians who had embraced the behavioral theories because of their scientific rigor and empirical verifiability.

In South Africa and later in the United States, Joseph Wolpe (1958) formulated the principles of "reciprocal inhibition," which along with Mowrer's theory of avoidance learning ushered in an alternative approach to anxiety disorders. Using a combination of classical conditioning and stimulus-response principles, Wolpe reduced many clinical problems to phobic anxieties. Wolpe identified the following 14 counterconditioning techniques to treat phobias: assertive responses, sexual responses, relaxation responses, systematic desensitization, conditioned avoidance responses, anxiety relief responses, aversion therapy, feeding responses, respiratory responses, interview-induced emotional responses, abreaction, correcting misconceptions, thought stopping, and drugs. Lazarus (1958) used the term "behavior therapy" to describe Wolpe's therapy procedures, and Eysenck (1959) further explained behavior therapy as the application of "modern learning theory" to emotional disorders. Flush with enthusiasm for the prospects of behavior therapy, emboldened with empirical evidence of their efficacy, and perhaps buoyed with zeal for the behavioral doctrine, Eysenck (1959) declared, "Get rid of the symptom and you have eliminated the neurosis" (p. 163). Behavior therapists rallied to Eysenck's clarion call and began to accumulate evidence that eventually established the efficacy of Wolpe's and Mowrer's systematic desensitization with phobias.

Other learning theories were revealed by Hull (1943) and Tolman (1932) and Spence (1956). The role of incentives, cues, and drive states were defined in ways that linked motivation with external rewards. Distinctions were established between learning and performance, between drive states and incentives, and between cues and reinforced behaviors. Although it is grossly unfair to summarize this rich lore of research so briefly, the fruits of learning research enabled behavior therapists to speak with greater clarity about the elements of learned behaviors, to sharpen the specificity of the learning process, and to qualify the conditions under which learned behaviors can be eliminated. The focus on cue-based learning opened the door to later considerations of "internal" cognitive processes replete in cognitive-behavioral therapies.

Radical behaviorism was introduced by B. F. Skinner (1953) with the zeal of John Watson and the confidence of Eysenck. Skinner's reworking of Thorndike's S-R theory placed greater emphasis on the response-reinforcement relationship and thus has been labeled a R-Rf learning theory. According to radical behaviorism, emitted responses that are followed by a reinforcer are repeated. Schedules of reinforcement differ along two dimensions, fixed/variable and ratio/interval and will influence the acquisition and retention of an emitted response. Emitted behaviors that operate on the environment and are reinforced are referred to as *operant behaviors*. The critical variable in the control of operant learning is the nature of the consequences or contingencies that sustain it. Behaviors can be shaped, generalized, discriminated, and extinguished through control of consequences.

The widest application of operant learning principles occurred in token economy treatments. Systematic reward systems were developed, often for chronic mentally ill, mentally retarded or alcoholic patients, that would govern nearly all aspects of the treated individual's awake time. Elaborate point systems, tokens redeemable for tangible rewards or actions, and penalties for undesirable behaviors (response-cost) were established. Although complete token economies usually have been reserved for residents of stable, long-term treatment centers, partial reward systems have been developed for adolescent, medical, and elderly living environments.

Although Skinner did not deny the existence of thoughts (the proverbial "black box"), he did attempt to reduce the emphasis placed on thoughts by intrapsychically oriented theorists. Skinner (1953) considered thoughts to often be a fiction to account for poorly defined behaviors and to be an irrelevant aspect of human experience. After all, he reasoned, history is filled with the deeds of men and women with little or no evidence of what those people were thinking. Speeches and written communications may have survived, but they are behaviors rather than thoughts. The net effect of this position was to emphasize behaviors and their consequences in therapy to the exclusion of the accompanying thoughts.

The radical behaviorist's dogmatic insistence on observable events, on scrutiny of target behaviors, and on use of time to mark the occurrence of behaviors resulted in a reduction of molar behaviors to micro actions within a well-defined context over a measured time period. Carefully charted behaviors related to the problem behaviors or symptoms became the focus. Thus the frame of operant conditioning was in the present rather than in historical events of development. Finally, the use of prescribed interventions with consequences over marked periods or intervals and subsequent removal of the conditions of learning tested the hypotheses of the behavior therapists. These baseline-treatment-baseline designs (A-B-A) have provided observable evidence of changes in defined target behaviors.

Behavior therapy expanded at an exponential rate through the 1960s so that new journals were established and societies formed. By 1970, behavior therapy was officially recognized by the American Psychiatric Association for its potential contributions to the successful treatment of certain disorders. Behavior therapy also began to gradually lose its "clean lines" as other aspects of experience received greater attention. Lazarus (1971) introduced multimodal therapy, which separated clinical problems into behavior, affect, sensation, imagery, cognition, interpersonal exchanges, and drug ingestion. Lazarus's multimodal therapy can be understood as an extension of Wolpe's therapy techniques, but it has been seized by many current therapists as an eclectic method for integrating environmentally oriented learning theories with internally oriented therapies.

Cognitive Behavior Therapies

The cognitive learning theories that emerged in the span of time from 1930 to 1975 more often took a back seat to the drive reduction theories of Hull and Spence, the radical behaviorism of Skinner, and the reciprocal determinism of Wolpe. Beginning with Tolman's (1932) cue-based learning and continuing with Dollard and Miller's (1950) imitation learning and Bandura and Walters's (1963) observational learning, cognitive theories were attempts to account for unobservable learning reflecting the processing of information. Common to these theories were efforts to define thinking in terms of explicitly observable behaviors and learned responses relating to environmental events. Thus an experimentally controlled target person's behavior might be reproduced by an attentive observer whose own subsequent behavior can be consensually validated as changing due to the exposure. Although the cognitive behavior theories share many features of the response-reinforcement theories, radical behaviorists have been most vocal in challenging the need for a thinking construct to account for the mediating events in question. Also Skinnerians are more apt to emphasize the affective effects of reinforcement, whereas, cognitive behavioral learning theories have emphasized the power of thoughts to elicit affect. As such, cognitive behavior learning theories can be interposed on an associationistic learning paradigm. Antecendent events (stimuli) in the social and physical environment elicit responses (thoughts), which in turn have consequences (reinforcement value) that strengthen or weaken the stimulus-thought relationship. This antecedent-behavior-consequences (A-B-C) paradigm has been adopted by Ellis (1970) in rational emotive therapy; it also is the basis of Meichenbaum's (1977) *Cognitive Behavior Modification.*

Components of Behavior Therapy

Shapiro (1951) introduced two of the basic components of behavior therapy: the *single case design* and the *functional analysis of behavior.* Most behavior therapy, like psychoanalytic or humanistic therapies, begins with an interview attending to the presenting problems or issues. In this interview, the therapist seeks greater clarity and focus for the client's responses, be they overt or covert; greater specification of antecedent or stimulus events preceding the responses (i.e., clarification of the situational stimuli); and an enumeration of consequences that accrue to the individual for the responses made. The therapist might make use of overt behavior, self-report, or imaginary experiences to analyze the antecedent-behavior-consequence chains. With an array of possibilities for each of these three components in mind, the therapist then begins to systematically test for the problematic chain by controlling the conditions under which each of the elements can vary. Ideally this functional analysis of behavior is conducted through repeated observations of a single client in ways that all other explanations for the persistence of the problem behavior can be eliminated as alternative explanations for the behavior in question. Likewise, the addition of behaviors formerly absent is evaluated by removing the conditions (antecedent events or consequences) that effect the desirable behavior. The end product of this process is *situation and response specificity*. Implicit in this approach is the axiom that behavior will be consistent across situations only to the extent that the parameters of the situation/consequence chain are similar.

Behavior therapists focus on *behavioral deficits*, such as the absence of assertive behavior or failure to engage others (social withdrawal), and on *behavioral excesses*, such as explosions of anger, tics, compulsions, binge eating, and impulsiveness. The frequency and duration of these behavioral deficits and behavioral excesses are observed through event sampling and time sampling techniques, respectively.

Whereas the goal of the A-B-A design of the single case method is to demonstrate that the executed interventions are indeed the active ingredients of the observed change, the behavioral analysis is continually modified and refined as more information is gained. The behavior therapist is interested in areas of adequate and optimal functioning in addition to the presenting complaints. A hallmark of behavior therapy is the attempt, whenever possible, to quantify behavioral descriptions in terms of frequencies of behaviors. Thus the therapist assesses how many aggressive, avoidance, or self-punitive responses are made or how many delusional statements are verbalized. The client may be enlisted to observe his or her own behavior through self-monitoring schemes. This self-focus often has the positive therapeutic effect of altering the client's existing personal constructs so that greater specificity of behavior chains is achieved and presenting complaints are expressed concretely as frequencies or durations of specific response. A classic case of behavior analysis in which a woman inpatient "compulsively" hoarded towels serves to illustrate this metamorphosis: instead of labeling her hoarding as "compulsive," a behavior therapist would say that she folded and piled 98 towels in a 45-minute period. The behavior therapist avoids the implicit "why" question by addressing "when," "where," "who," "what," and "how" the behavior occurs.

Shapiro's functional analysis of behavior was applied to covert rather than overt responses in the efforts of Kanfer (Kanfer & Karoly, 1972) to increase self-control. Meichenbaum (1977) incorporated functional analysis of behavior as an organizing framework for teaching clients how to use *self-talk* (thoughts) to mediate stimulus-action (behavior) sequences. The self-talk component subsequently was incorporated in efforts to control the impulsive responding of children and to control pain, among other applications.

Meichenbaum's procedures for training self-talk include a six-stage sequence: (1) the therapist first says aloud what he or she is thinking as he or she performs the desired response; (2) the therapist repeats the desired response while saying softly what his or her guiding thoughts are; (3) the therapist performs the desired response silently but obviously "thinking" as conveyed by facial changes and gestures; (4) the client is encouraged to perform the desired response while saying aloud what the therapist has modeled; (5) the client is instructed to say softly the self-talk he or she has been learning; and (6) the client is encouraged to perform the desired response while thinking to himself or herself. Social and physical reinforcers are used under varying schedules of reinforcement. Whereas the client is taught to use the self-talk, say-aloud technique as a universal problem-solving procedure, situations are considered largely unique so that the procedure must be tailored to the stimulus demands as each new situation is encountered.

Techniques of Behavior Therapy

At the risk of achieving parsimony through reductionism, the techniques associated with the various theories of learning—association learning, classical conditioning, radical behaviorism, and cognitive learning—are here considered collectively and are organized according to whether they are largely antecedent, response, or consequences oriented. Other cataloguing efforts have offered a more in-depth description of the various techniques (Cautela, 1977; Lueger, 1986; Mahoney & Arnkoff, 1978). Representative techniques within each of the three categories will be highlighted as examples of the category.

Antecedent Techniques. *Stimulus control, flooding,* and *aversion therapy* are three behavior therapy techniques that primarily focus on the stimulus or antecedent conditions to change behavior. A simple example of stimulus control occurs when the newly committed dieter cleans all of the junk food out of the cabinets. The absence of a ready stimulus will not elicit the undesired behavior of "binging" on high-calorie sweets. Flooding therapy involves using prolonged, high-intensity exposure to a feared stimulus to reduce the fear-eliciting value of the stimulus. A simple example of flooding is the socially shy new teacher who overcomes a fear of public speaking by lecturing frequently. A more perverse account has been offered by G. Gordon Liddy in his autobiography; he captured, held, and "ate" rats that formerly elicited terror for him. Although flooding can be effectively practiced covertly through imagined scenes, in vivo practice of flooding has been shown to be generally superior to covert application of flooding.

Response Techniques. The bulk of behavior therapy techniques are largely response focused. Wolpe's (1958) *systematic desensitization* involves an attempt to reduce the fear evoked by a threatening situation by teaching incompatible antianxiety responses such as deep muscle relaxation, measured breathing, and pleasant imagery. Once these incompatible relaxation responses have been learned and practiced, the fearful individual is progressively exposed to a graded hierarchy of anxiety-generating situations. Successful mastery of each fear-producing situation (through practice of incompatible relaxation responses and therapist support and encouragement) reduces the frequency and duration as well as the intensity of the avoidance response. Systematic desensitization is effective with covert exposure, although actual exposure generally is more effective.

Behavioral rehearsal and cognitive restructuring are two other general classes of response-focused behavior therapy techniques. *Behavioral rehearsal* is a procedure that is used to replace deficient or inadequate social responses. Such skills often are practiced in role play encounters in which the therapist both models and plays the part of a significant other in the client's life. A specific application of behavioral rehearsal is assertion training.

Cognitive restructuring is used to introduce more adaptive self-verbalizations where maladaptive thoughts are at issue. The therapist assumes a didactic role in instructing the client about the efficacy of self-statements. Among these cognitive restructuring techniques are: rational emotive therapy, which operates on the premise that irrational thoughts play an important role in the client's subjective distress;

self-instructional training, which seeks to introduce an effective private monologue that enables the individual to successfully perform a designated task (e.g., driving a car or computing the square root of a number); and cognitive therapy, which, like rational emotive therapy, holds that irrational thoughts and fantasies cause distress. Beck (1963) has championed the use of cognitive therapy to highlight undue attention to failures, magnification of negative outcomes, minimization of positive outcomes, and arbitrary inferences about personal responsibility that individuals with anxiety disorders and depression make.

Coping-skills techniques are generally oriented toward improving performance under stressful conditions. A mixture of relaxation training, rehearsal, self-instruction, distraction, and stimulus control can be used to facilitate the development of coping skills. *Covert modeling* involves the mental rehearsal of a task, such as visualizing the flight of a basketball in a perfectly executed freethrow. The individual might visualize a perfect performance (*mastery modeling*) or imagine being confronted with obstacles and eventually overcoming those obstacles (coping modeling). *Problem-solving techniques* are another form of coping skills in which the specific target response has not been defined before encountering the situation; instead, problem-solving training attempts to teach a learning set that will enable the individual to select the most effective target responses for further enhancement through coping-skills training or cognitive restructuring.

Consequences Techniques. Self-reward, whether overt or covert, and self-punishment are behavior therapy techniques that primarily use consequences to alter behavior. The token economy efforts discussed earlier are the most systematic approaches. A variant of negative reinforcement and token economy is the response-cost technique, which has been used successfully with impulsive children. More often though, consequences are mixed with antecedent or response techniques in an effort to alter behavior along desired lines.

The Current Practice and Efficacy of Behavior Therapy

The combination of situational specificity, scientific rigor, and zealous adherence to principle has resulted in a therapeutic approach in which the behavior therapist assumes a directive role toward the client. This involves drawing attention to behaviors, educating the client about alternatives, modeling new skills, and indoctrinating the client to change principles. Interventions generally are more limited in time and focused on presenting complaints. Behavior therapists generally have disdained, at least in principle, the use of constructs to explain behavior. Likewise, they have tried to eschew internal explanations of the status of an individual.

In reality, however, behavior therapists may be functioning more like therapists of other theoretical persuasions (Nelson & Hayes, 1986). Namely, many behavior therapists have found the demands of current client problems too pressing for lengthy studies of frequency and duration; they have found that clients push for a "bigger picture" that ties together past, present, and future; and they have resorted to the use of internal constructs, if not purposefully, at least as a convenience of communication. In short, behavior therapy has become, at least in a significant number of therapists' offices, less of a dogma and more of a repertoire of techniques that can be adapted to the specific behaviors.

The issues of therapeutic efficacy raised in Eysenck's (1953) polemic against internal construct psychotherapy, the exuberant claims of success with phobias (82% success rate, by many standards), and the technique-problem matching fervor that has come with reasoned, empirically derived procedures produced a confidence among many behavior therapists by the late 1970s that behavior therapy was the most effective therapy for certain presenting problems.

The results of meta-analyses of therapy outcome studies in which a behavioral technique was contrasted at least against a comparison group (Smith, Glass & Miller, 1980) have not been kind to these assertions of therapeutic superiority. A more focused meta-analytic study (Shapiro & Shapiro, 1982) also failed to support the superiority of behavior therapy over techniques derived from other schools of thought. Nevertheless, behavior therapy has been shown to be as effective as any other systematic school of therapy. Moreover, controversies about the utility of meta-analytic approaches to study refined behaviors leave open the possibility that more specific and powerful analyses will still endorse the use of specific skills with specific problems.

THE THIRD FORCE: HUMANISTIC PSYCHOTHERAPY

The humanistic approach to psychotherapy focuses on the inherent tendency of humans to develop all their capacities in ways that serve to maintain or enhance the whole of the person. Central to this approach is an emphasis on the self as an organizing principle of development and an emphasis on insight into the phenomenology of experience. Humanistic therapists attempt to facilitate a greater congruence between the self and experience through a process of reintegration.

The humanistic approach encompasses existential, client-centered, Gestalt, and experiential psychotherapies. Kurt Goldstein (1940) had an influence on many of the psychotherapy systematizers in the humanistic approach, including Maslow, Rogers, Perls, and Gardner Murphy, and was himself influenced by Andreas Angyal, Max Wertheimer, and John Hughlings Jackson. Goldstein emphasized the unity, organization, and coherence of the human personality. Four basic precepts of the humanistic approach to psychotherapy are credited to Goldstein:

1. Human beings function as organized wholes. In Goldstein's formula, the whole person is equal to the sum of the parts of that person plus an emergent quality.

2. Human beings have one basic motive—self-actualization. Self-actualization is the drive by which the person is moved; normal persons have a tendency toward activity and progress, whereas the tendency to release tension is a phenomenon of pathological life.

3. The normal individual seeks to equalize organismic tension. There is a tendency toward order and "centeredness," that enables the individual to seek growth experiences while tension is equilibrated rather than discharged. A balance of needs and drives (to be translated as "pressure") rather than a reduction of tension guides the person forward.

4. The person must cope with stressful environments. A developing person must "come to terms" with the limits and demands of the environment. In contrast to the behaviorists, Goldstein says that forced responsiveness to stimuli or bondage to environmental stimuli is, again, a condition of nongrowth, if not psychopathology. Anxiety is the subjective experience that danger to one's existence is immanent. The ordered or centered individual is more immune to catastrophic experiences than is the disordered individual.

Existential Therapy

Existential theories of personality also emphasize the emergent, becoming qualities of the individual. Existence, or "being in the world," encompasses the person and his or her environment as a unity. "Being" and "world" are inseparable because they are both a creation of the individual; the phenomenological world reflects the meaning the individual ascribes to the environment as well as the meanings adopted from significant others. Existence is a constant flow from nonbeing into being and back again. Too much awareness of meaninglessness leads to conditions of dread known as *existential anxiety*. Disregarding reality (lying) is a way of not allowing existential anxiety into being, but this leads to neurotic anxiety and inauthenticity. The presenting complaints of clients thus reflect a decision that they must act on their neurotic anxiety. An honest examination of existence is the formula for ridding the self of symptoms. Thus the goal of existential therapy is authenticity, or the aspects of self and world that have been closed off by lying.

Medard Boss and Ludwig Binswanger (See Hall, Lindzey, Loehlin, & Manosevitz, 1985) used the philosophies of Kirkegaard, Heidegger, Camus, and Tillich in developing the elementary principles of the existential-therapy approach. The methods they used, however, probably owed more to the psychoanalytic training each received. Through free experiencing the client is encouraged to express himself/herself more freely and honestly with regard to the present moment, and by emphasizing choice the client is confronted with the risk of changing a fundamental aspect of his or her existence and abandoning the security of symptoms and inauthenticity.

Victor Frankl's (1965) concept of *logotherapy* is a more developed system of existential psychotherapy and will serve, for purposes of illustration, to highlight the elements of existential therapy. The logotherapist interprets, confronts, persuades, and reasons with the client in an effort to raise consciousness and to convince the client to take a more responsible look at the existential vacuum that his or her life has become. The technique of gaining psychological distance from oneself in order to gain perspective is found throughout logotherapy. Frankl's (1965) categorical imperative, "So live as if you were living already for the second time and as if you had acted the first time as wrongly as you are about to act now" (p. 216) illustrates the distancing directive and the paradoxical nature of therapists' statements to clients. Humor, or laughing at oneself, is encouraged as a means of putting things in perspective. *Paradoxical intention* is a therapeutic distancing technique in which the therapist encourages the client to do the very thing that he or she is dreading. *Dereflection* is another technique in which the therapist ignores that with which the client is obsessed and instead directs attention to the "right activities" or more positive aspects of life.

Gestalt Therapy

Fritz Perls (1969), who began his work at the South African Institute for Psychoanalysis and continued in California, has championed uniqueness, honesty, and spontaneity in his Gestalt therapy. Gestalts are perceptual organizations of sensory experiences that maintain the integrity of the person and reflect a continual process of bringing completeness to an individual's needs. Thinking, particularly future-oriented thinking, has the effect of distancing one from the true experience that is more authentically found in the senses. Thus Gestalt therapy seeks to increase sensory awareness in the present. By losing more and more of one's "mind," one can experience with all of the senses the reality of oneself. This process is called *satori*, or waking up. In waking from an intellectual trance, one can see all that one is. Thus one begins to shed the *maya* (alienated, phony self) in favor of awareness of being in one's environment.

Gestalt therapists are directive but must remain spontaneous to be effective. The simple goal of a therapist is to keep the client in the present and to avoid client maneuvers that seek to maintain the phony self. Therapists engage in role playing, use therapist self-disclosure, act to frustrate the client's efforts to manipulate the therapy into a more maternal or paternal relationship, and demand through confrontation on the "hot seat" that the client be more honest and open with himself or herself. The latter effort can involve purposive stripping of the client's dignity to protect a phony existence. Dreams are analyzed because they are held to be spontaneous aspects of personality. The therapist educates the client in the use of the pronoun "I" rather than the more impersonal "it." Humor, comic relief, and high drama all are used to reduce tension, release joy, and generally focus on deeds rather than words. Thinking is considered a means of avoiding the present. Anxiety also reflects a preoccupation with the future rather than with the present and must be transformed into excitement rather than ruminative dread. Finally, the therapist practices anything but unconditional positive regard toward the client in an effort to head off the pursuit of security through sameness, which robs one of the richness of possibilities.

Maslow's (1968) major contribution to humanistic psychotherapy is his explanation of existence and being (becoming) needs in a hierarchy. Again, self-actualization is the highest level of motivating need and is the primary motivator of the developing person. Safety, love, belongingness, self-esteem, and physiological needs must be satisfied before one is developmentally engaged by self-actualization needs. An irreversible process characterizes progression through these needs. Higher-order needs become more important whether frustrated or satisfied. Although Maslow endorsed the unity of being and existence and the importance of becoming, he took issue with other aspects of the existential approach. In particular he seems to have rejected the alienating qualities of the world in favor of a more sanguine view of how the world facilitates the actualization of self.

Client-Centered Therapy

Carl Rogers's (1951) self-theory emerged from his therapeutic experience with clients. Unconditional positive regard is the key attitude of therapist toward client, in order to affect growth and realization of emergent capabilities. Incongruence between self and experience and between ideal self and realized self is the source of the presenting complaints that brings an individual to see a therapist. An inherent need for positive regard exists in each individual. Rogers says that we learn to need love. Self-esteem is established normatively under conditions of worth—that is, positive regard from important other(s) is withheld, conditioned, or withdrawn contingent on the actions of the individual. Experience, unintegrated under these conditions of worth, is "subceived," or not fully articulated in awareness. Defensive reactions lend a cognitive rigidity to efforts to understand and integrate experience so that events are interpreted in absolute terms, are overgeneralized, or are channeled according to limited information-processing strategies.

In his theory of personality, Rogers defines the self as an organizing, conceptual gestalt of "I" and "me" characteristics, of perceptions of "I" or "me" relations to others and to the physical environment, and of values that inform those relationships. Self, thus defined, is fluid, changing, available to awareness, but not necessarily *in* awareness. Rogers's conception of self borrows heavily from William James's (1890/1950, 1902/1961) "self-as-object" and "self-as-process."

Congruence and incongruence can exist on three levels: (1) between self as perceived and the actual experiences of the individual; (2) between the phenomenological field and reality as it truly is; and (3) between self as one is and self as one would like to be. Thus the triple efforts of the therapist are to raise consciousness, expand awareness, and integrate valuation with experience.

In Rogerian humanistic psychotherapy, the client directs the flow of therapy so that the role of the therapist is to be nondirective. Instead, the therapist uses reflection, accurate empathy, and unconditional positive regard to facilitate the self-discovery by the client. Elementary to Rogerian therapy is Wittgenstein's (See Prochaska, 1979) axiom that expression and experiencing are a unity. Experiences are created by expression, and the richer the expression of the client, the fuller the life experience of the person.

Like psychoanalytic therapy, Rogerian client-centered therapy is an insight psychotherapy. The nondirective therapist of client-centered therapy, however, enables the client to discover and own aspects of experience rather than providing synthetic recathexis of bound instinctual energy. Through paraphrasing and accurate empathic reflection, the therapist identifies and articulates feelings with experiences. Therapist statements such as "You feel . . . because . . ." help the client release, express, and own his or her most powerful feelings. This cathartic effect enables the client to own his or her emotions and brings the focus to feelings of the moment. The transformation can be seen from initial stages of therapy in which the client talks about emotional experiences outside himself or herself (e.g., "These new tax forms are really driving me crazy") to later phases of therapy in which the same experience is owned (e.g., "I am despairing of ever finishing these tax forms on time").

Greater immediacy is a positive outcome in client-centered therapy. Awareness of feelings as well as thoughts and action tendencies enables the client to experience life with greater richness and minimizes denial, distortion through projection, and rationalization. Anxiety, the product of incongruent aspects of self, is reduced in successful therapy but gains acceptance as a natural sign of a need for more immediacy.

Current Status and Applications of Client-Centered Therapy

The union of client-centered techniques with behavioral (Truax & Carkhuff, 1967) and with cognitive behavioral (Egan, 1987) principles has led to training programs that accent the basic listening skills of the Rogerian approach to therapy. The addition of problem-solving strategies (Egan, 1987) to these basic listening skills has addressed the criticisms that (1) client-centered therapy, carried to its extreme, results in a narcissistic preoccupation with experiencing, and (2) the positive products of psychotherapy cannot be enumerated and measured.

Basic listening skills begin with physical attending, as summarized by the mnemonic, *SOLER*. The therapist should (1) face the client *S*quarely, (2) maintain an *O*pen posture toward the client, (3) *L*ean toward the client, (4) maintain comfortable and appropriate *E*ye contact, and (5) (paradox of paradoxes!) *R*elax. Along with physical attending, the therapist should use the basic paraphrasing formula, "You feel . . . because . . . ," in which the appropriate client affect is paired with the relevant life experience as related by the client. A nonformula version might less conspicuously integrate feeling and experience as follows: "He failed to arrive at the expected time and you became progressively more worried that something might have happened to him."

Accurate empathy not only requires identification of the right family of emotion, but also discernment of the appropriate intensity and concreteness of expression. *Advanced accurate empathy* involves a greater level of insight and perhaps some degree of *challenging* to bring the client to a new level of awareness of his or her experience and emotion: "You worry about him when he's late, but I sense that it's more than that; you have a hard time letting him go his own way." *Immediacy* is a form of advanced accurate empathy and challenging that keeps the focus of the client on the present. *Helper self-disclosure* is a sparingly used technique in which the therapist uses personal experience in an attempt to give information of value to the client.

The identification of therapist-client behaviors through the Truax and Carkhuff and the Egan methods has enabled psychotherapy evaluators to assess changes related to process variables in Rogerian therapy. In addition, the training of counselors and psychotherapists has been greatly facilited. One positive effect is that client-centered techniques have gained new respect as rigorous and demanding therapeutic techniques. Another positive effect is that a selection and quality control factor has been added to the development of therapists/counselors— that is, personal qualities that enable a therapist to use the client-centered model (e.g., attentive listening, patience, labeling of affect, warm relating to clients, focusing of issues, teaching skills, etc.) can be assessed in the training phase of therapy development.

Effect sizes, which are standardized units of change on outcome variables, drawn from meta-analytic studies (Smith, Glass, & Miller, 1980) of psychotherapy indicate that client-centered therapy is as effective as other schools of therapy. Insufficient data on Gestalt therapy do not permit similar comparisons, but studies of group therapies (Bednar & Kaul, 1978) indicate that Gestalt techniques can be effective relative to some other group psychotherapies. Eclectic approaches to psychotherapy would seem to use the basic listening skills of the client-centered method, but supplement those skills with problem-solving techniques of other theoretical approaches (e.g., systematic desensitization, dream analysis).

THE FOURTH FORCE: TRANSPERSONAL PSYCHOTHERAPY

The term "transpersonal" literally means "beyond the personal" or "beyond personality." Those who subscribe to transpersonal psychology feel that when human beings identify only with the body, the ego, or the personality, they have an extremely limited view of themselves.

Consequently, transpersonal psychology has expanded the domain of investigation to encompass the spiritual dimension of human beings (Vaughan, 1984). Each issue of the *Journal of Transpersonal Psychology* contains a list of the categories of interests, experiences, and events that come under the term "transpersonal." This list includes:

> Meta-needs, transpersonal process, values and states, unitive conscious-ness, peak experiences, ecstasy, mystical experience, being, essence, bliss, awe, wonder, transience of self, spirit, sacralization of everyday life, one-ness, cosmic awareness, cosmic play, individual and species-wide synergy, the theories and practices of meditation, spiritual paths, compassion, transpersonal cooperation, transpersonal realization and actualization and related concepts, experiences, and activities.

Anyone who practices psychotherapy within the foregoing broad con-text is termed a transpersonal psychotherapist.

> Transpersonal psychotherapy includes the full range of behavioral, emo-tional and intellectual disorders as in traditional psychotherapies as well as uncovering and supporting strivings for full self-actualization. The end result of psychotherapy is not seen as successful adjustments to the pre-vailing culture, but rather the daily experience of that state called libera-tion, enlightenment, individuation, certainty or gnosis according to various traditions. (Fadiman, 1980, p. 36).

As Boorstein (1980) points out, this approach to therapy is different from the traditional systems more in orientation and scope than in meth-ods or techniques. It transcends the traditional constricting views of our potential and extends the field of inquiry into areas that are largely ignored by the other three forces in psychotherapy (Tart, 1969, 1975; Walsh & Vaughan, 1980).

The Development of the Transpersonal Perspective

D. E. Harding (1972) shares the following experience:

> A peculiar quiet, an odd kind of alert limpness or numbness came over me. Reason and imagination and all mental chatter died down. For once words really failed me. Past and future dropped away. I forgot who and what I was. . . . It was as if I had been born that instant, brand new, mindless, innocent of all memories. There existed only the Now. . . . I had lost a head and gained a world. . . . Here it was, this superb scene . . . utterly free of me. . . . Its total presence was my total absence . . . it felt like a sudden waking from the sleep of ordinary life. . . . It was self-luminous

reality for once swept clean of all obscuring mind. It was the revelation at long last, of the perfectly obvious . . . there arose no questions, no reference beyond the experience itself, but only peace and a quiet joy, and the sensation of having dropped an intolerable burden. (pp. 23–24)

Over the years, an increasing number of individuals have experienced a variety of "nonhabitual states of consciousness" such as the above, which go beyond the usual confines of space and time (Fadiman, 1980; Grof, 1984; Walsh & Vaughan, 1983). For many, such events have been extremely powerful and have had important implications for their relationships, life styles, motivations, identities, and philosophies (Walsh & Vaughan, 1983; White, 1973). These emotionally important but unusual experiences led to a search in the literature for accounts that could explain them satisfactorily (Fadiman, 1980).

As Fadiman (1980) points out, the search within mainstream Western psychology turned out to be largely fruitless. Convincing discussions of transcendent experiences, or what Sutich (1968, 1980) calls the "ultimate states," were found to be conspicuously missing from the literature. There were a few exceptions, however. These included William James's (1950, 1961) explorations into higher consciousness, Jung's (1961, 1968) investigation of the individuation process, Assagioli's (1965) incorporation of spiritual practices into psychotherapy, and Maslow's (1968, 1971) inquiries into self-actualization and peak experiences. Since all of these theorists had been influenced to varying degrees by Eastern spiritual and psychological disciplines, the search naturally was directed to an exploration of these systems; the relevance of these disciplines to emerging Western needs was readily noticed (Fadiman, 1980).

One of the most salient results of this search was the recognition of the transcendent unity that exists between almost all ancient traditions; for example, Hinduism, Buddhism, and Sufism maintain that the ego (the lesser self) or the *phenomenal self* must be transcended in order to connect with the real self or *cosmic self* and to establish a genuine sense of unity with nature (Fadiman, 1980; Grof, 1984; Gurdjieff, 1968; Shah, 1970, 1972; Yogananda, 1972). As A. R. Arasteh (1980), in his book on Sufism says, the cosmic self "is not what environment and culture develop in us, but is basically the product of the universe in evolution." The cosmic self or transpersonal self embraces all our being; whereas "the phenomenal self designates only a part of our existence. The phenomenal self has separated us from our origin, that of union with *all of life*" (p. ix). The transpersonal self is that "part of us which has access to the perennial wisdom" (Vaughan, 1984, p. 25).

As Walsh and Vaughan (1983) state, it seems that "in the utmost depths of the human psyche, when all dualism and exclusivity have been dropped, awareness finds no limits to identity and directly experiences itself as beyond both time and space: that which humanity has traditionally called God" (p. 404). Walsh and Vaughan (1980) draw our attention to the convergence of the world's great religions: "The Kingdom of heaven is within you" (Christianity); "Look within, thou art the Buddha" (Buddhism); "By understanding the Self all this universe is known" (Hinduism); "He who knows himself, knows his Lord" (Islam).

From the transpersonal perspective, Eastern and Western approaches to health and growth are seen as complementary, and the confluence of the two streams is deemed desirable. The integration of ancient wisdom and modern knowledge permeates the writings of a number of prominent Western thinkers, such as Tart (1969), Grof (1975, 1980), Wilber (1977, 1980), Walsh (see Walsh & Shapiro, 1983), Fadiman (1980), and Vaughan (1984). Their efforts have made it "scientifically respectable to assert alternates, views of reality that are as substantial, consistent, and functional as the ones that are accepted within traditional Western psychology" (Fadiman, 1980, p. 37).

Grof (1975, 1984) and Wilber (1977) perhaps have been most influential in the integration of Eastern and Western approaches and in giving direction to the transpersonal perspective.

Grof (1980), who explored therapy under the influence of LSD, observed the following four major types or levels of experience: (1) abstract or aesthetic experience dealing with impressive perceptual changes in the environment; (2) psychodynamic experience pertaining to significant memories, affective issues, or unresolved conflicts from the past; (3) perinatal experiences or experiences dealing with birth, aging, pain, agony, disease, or death; and (4) experience of a transcendent, transpersonal, archetypal, or mystical nature.

The image of human beings and the model of personality that emerge from Grof's research appear much closer to Eastern philosophy than to Freudian or behavioristic concepts (Grof, 1980). Also it seems, as Grof suggests, that different systems of therapy and healing deal with different layers of the experience.

Ken Wilber (1977) presents an impressive overview of the entire spectrum of consciousness. He considers consciousness to be a continuum with unity at one pole and complete dualism at the other. Wilber observes that most psychological or spiritual systems deal with only one segment of this continuum. Yet the ultimate aim of psychotherapy should be to lead the client farther down the road toward unity rather than to allow him or her to remain fixed at any point along the way (Fadiman, 1980).

A Transpersonal Model

Walsh and Vaughan (1980) identified four major dimensions of the transpersonal model of the person. These include *consciousness, conditioning, personality,* and *identification.* They view consciousness as the essence of being human. Ordinary consciousness is seen as "a defensively contracted state" (p. 15) of diminished awareness. In order to grow one must let go of this defensive condition and remove obstacles in the way of the recognition of our limitless potential. An extensive body of literature from a variety of cultural traditions maintains that these higher states are attainable.

According to the transpersonal model, most of us are more tightly trapped in conditioning than we realize, but it is possible to free ourselves (Walsh & Vaughan, 1980). The goal of transpersonal psychotherapy is basically to release our consciousness from this "conditioned tyranny" (Ram Dass, 1977). Attachment is considered to be one important form of conditioning and to play a pivotal role in the causation of suffering.

Unlike most other psychological systems, the transpersonal model states that there is more to us than our personality. It is considered to be only one facet of our being. "Health is seen as primarily involving a disidentification from personality rather than modification of it" (Walsh & Vaughan, 1980, p. 16). One of the goals of transpersonal psychotherapy is to nurture those aspects that permit a person to disidentify from the restrictions of the personality and to recognize his or her identity with the total self (Fadiman, 1980; Speeth & Fadiman, 1979).

Like a variety of Eastern disciplines, transpersonal psychology recognizes identification not only with external objects, but also with internal phenomena (Walsh & Vaughan, 1980). In fact, the latter is considered even more important than the former. Identification with mental content is considered to interfere seriously with our experience of expanded states of consciousness. Transcending all identification is believed to lead to the experience of a "variety of states of consciousness in which perception is described as nondualistic; the individual feels himself or herself to be connected with, one with, or actually to *be* the whole universe" (Walsh & Vaughan, 1980, p. 18).

THE FOUR FORCES COMPARED

Wilber's (1977) continuum of consciousness is a useful reference for comparing the four forces of psychotherapy. Again, consciousness is a continuum with complete unity at one pole and complete dualism at the other. The concept of unity means that no two things in the universe can be completely separated or differentiated from each other. Dualism infers that all things in the universe are separate and independent. Psychoanalytic, behavioral, and humanistic therapies address only one segment of this continuum, whereas, transpersonal psychotherapy is directed toward the achievement of greater unity. We now will examine the extent to which each of the four psychotherapies leads the client down the continuum toward unity.

The goal of psychoanalytic psychotherapy is the release of bound energy through the resolution of unconscious conflicts. Release occurs when that which is unconscious is made conscious. Affect is unified with awareness (cognition), and the individual shifts toward a higher level of developmental integration with the benefit of the freed energy. Although greater unity is effected, additional conflict is endemic to human maturation. Increasing civilization is accompanied by more neurosis, because freed energy can never be fully invested in the existing organization of development. The goals of a tension reduction model are inertia or entropy, neither of which is a viable, sustained state of human living. Thus the individual is continually in conflict, and the dualistic unconscious and conscious elements of experience prevail.

Behavior therapy is directed toward reducing behavioral excesses or rectifying behavioral deficits. Clearly defined target behaviors become the focus of the therapy, but other aspects of experience are rendered temporarily irrelevant. Although the target behaviors might change in the continuing therapy process, the focus changes successively and sequentially rather than expansively. Awareness, meaning, and existence are pertinent to behavior therapy only as responses to antecedent conditions in a specific situation. Any sense of unity is bound to the stimulus parameters; "cosmic" can be understood only from the changes witnessed among the individual's behavioral repertoire.

Humanistic psychotherapy has emphasized the phenomenal self as an organizing principle of growth and change. Whether the phenomenal self is understood as a defensive alignment (the "not me"), as an awareness of competencies (the "good me"), or as a goal (self-actualization), it designates only part of existence. Rogerian therapy moves toward unity through increasing realization of the client's potential. Insight produces this realization in a process similar to that found in psychoanalytic psychotherapy. Unconscious aspects of experience are more fully appreciated by verbal labeling of affect as feelings and by attaching meaning to the now enriched experience. As unintegrated experience becomes integrated, the phenomenal self is correspondingly transformed. Despite its greater articulation and complexity, the enriched phenomenal self continues to separate existence by holding gains against conditions of worth.

Existential psychotherapy more closely resembles transpersonal therapy in its pursuit of unity than any other force of therapy. Maslow's peak experiences and Boss and Binswanger's *Dasein* come closest to the transpersonal cosmic unity and to Wilber's end point of complete unity of consciousness. Perhaps unfortunately, existential psychotherapy also has pursued self-actualization and peak experiences as therapeutic goals. Although self-actualization serves as a useful beacon for the therapeutic process, the striving-to-become separates the client from the process of being. As Frankl (1965) noted, self-actualization is a by-product of living (being), not a goal to be pursued. In pursuing self-actualization, the client invariably fails to achieve the highest level of unity.

In addition to the continuum of consciousness, the four forces of psychotherapy can be compared on the basis of richness of constructs, empirical verifiability, or intuitive verifiability. The four forces have different ages of existence and different levels of exposure among practicing psychotherapists. The "older" therapies, psychoanalytic and behavioristic, are superior on all these dimensions relative to the "newer" humanistic and transpersonal therapies. Nevertheless, the *utility* of any psychotherapeutic model is directly related to the degree of its differentiation and the boundedness of its constructs. A comprehensive theory can account for a wide range of human experience, even if it is inherently dualistic.

Let us return to Wilber's continuum of consciousness. The four forces of psychotherapy also might be compared according to how much of the spectrum of dualism/unity they account for, rather than whether unity is addressed. Most critics of personality theories have regarded psychoanalytic psychotherapy to be a comprehensive theory of personality in that it accounts for a large amount of human experience. Also, psychoanalytic theory has provided succinct definitions of important therapeutic constructs, such as transference and therapeutic alliance, that are important to the practice of psychotherapy in all four forces. Humanistic psychotherapy is potentially useful for addressing an extensive amount of human experience. However, humanistic psychotherapy has provided fewer useful constructs for the conduct of psychotherapy than has psychoanalytic therapy. Behavior therapy has provided many useful techniques of psychotherapy but is based on a small number of essential constructs of learning. Techniques involve learned responses that must be matched to antecedent events. Although the underlying essentials of theory are nearly universal, the techniques must be refashioned to fit the specifics of the situation under consideration. Despite its narrow treatment focus, behavior therapy has the potential of addressing much of human experience.

How does the transpersonal model of psychotherapy compare with the other three forces in the number of useful constructs of therapeutic change? Walsh and Vaughan (1980) have treated the transpersonal force as an inclusive model with four dimensions—consciousness, conditioning, personality, and identification. That is, the transpersonal model incorporates the therapeutic elements of the other three forces but goes beyond to the cosmic unity. The behavioristic approach explains and controls phenomena related to conditioning; the humanistic and psychoanalytic approaches handle issues of personality; and the transpersonal model efficaciously explains phenomena of consciousness. The significant contribution of the transpersonal model is the added emphasis on experience beyond the usual into the spiritual.

In practice, the dilemma is whether a therapist should practice as an ideological partisan or as an eclectic. The partisan (e.g., the psychoanalyst, the radical behaviorist, the reflective Rogerian) stays with the principles and techniques of a particular mode of therapy, whereas the eclectic uses techniques as they fit regardless of theoretical purity. Lazarus (1971) was an early proponent of eclectic practice. Accused of theoretical sloppiness, if not contradiction, the eclectic therapist is likely to take satisfaction and confidence from the precision of the technique-to-problem fit. Meta-analyses of psychotherapy outcomes have failed, however, to support any school of practice over the others in treating specific problems. Contrary to common sense and conventional wisdom, different therapies are not more effective with different problems. Despite such negative outcome research findings, the intuitive validity of practicing eclectically probably is sufficient to ensure its continued existence. The role of transpersonal therapy in eclectic practice is addressing the spiritual domain of experience.

An important issue for the transpersonal model (and for the existential model as it was espoused early on) is the dilemma of how to mark change in a way that satisfies the tenets of science. With knowledge, the scientific psychotherapist strives to predict and control human behavior. Proper evidence allows the therapist to be something other than a shaman or priest. The therapist should be able to recognize (however belatedly) that something is happening, what it is, what might be bringing that event about, and what the next most likely sequels are. In marking change it might not be necessary to measure it. Family therapists, particularly those with a systems perspective, often assume that change is an ongoing process that is better marked by qualitative rather than quantitative guides. Such an approach to the measurement of psy-chotherapy outcomes is acceptable to many psychoanalytic therapists but is not well received by those with a more traditional empirical per-spective. The transpersonal model will have to ingeniously address the change measurement issue to acquire the respect of the scientific, medi-cal, and insurance communities.

Finally, the lessons of history learned by the first three forces of psychotherapy can be valuable to the fourth force. Psychoanalytic ther-apy has been expanded to account for competency motives. Behavior therapy has admitted covert behaviors (thoughts) to be treated on a par with overt behaviors. Client-centered humanistic therapy has become more directive, and existential therapy has converted *being* into goals to be pursued. The transpersonal force must continue to derive its essence from the spiritual domain, while it expands and accommodates itself to a broad range of human experience.

References

Arasteh, A. R. (1980). *Growth to selfhood.* Boston: Routledge & Kegan Paul.

Assagioli, R. (1965). *Psychosynthesis.* New York: Viking Press.

Assagioli, R. (1973). *The act of will.* New York: Viking Press.

Bandura, A., & Walters, R. (1963). *Social learning and personality development.* New York: Holt.

Beck, A. T. (1963). Thinking and depression, I. Idiosyncratic content and cogni-tive distortions. *Archives of General Psychiatry, 9,* 324–333.

Bednar, R. L., & Kaul, T. J. (1978). Experiential group research: Current perspec-tives. In S. L. Garfield & A. E. Bergin (Eds.), *Handbook of psychotherapy and behavior change: An empirical analysis* (2nd ed.) (p. 725–768). New York: Wiley.

Belkin, G. S. (1987). *Contemporary psychotherapies.* Chicago: Rand McNally.

Bellak, L., & Goldsmith, L. A. (1984). *The broad scope of ego function assessment.* New York: Wiley.

Block, J. H., & Block, J. (1987). The role of ego-control and ego-resiliency in the organization of behavior. In P. Karoly & J. J. Steffen (Eds.), *Advances in child behavioral analysis and therapy* (Vol. 3). Lexington, MA: Lexington Books.

Boorstein, S. (1980). *Transpersonal psychotherapy.* Palo Alto, CA: Science and Behavior Books.

Cameron, N., & Rychlak, J. F. (1985). *Personality development and psychopathol-ogy, a dynamic approach* (2nd ed.). Boston: Houghton Mifflin.

Cautela, J. R. (1977). Covert conditioning: Assumptions and procedures. *Journal of Mental Imagery, 1,* 53–64.

Cohen, M. B. (1952). Countertransference and anxiety. *Psychiatry, 15,* 231–243.

Dollard, J., & Miller, N. (1950). *Personality and psychotherapy.* New York: McGraw-Hill.

Dunlap, K. (1932). *Habits: Their making and unmaking.* New York: Liveright.

Egan, G. (1987). *The skilled helper* (3rd ed.). Belmont, CA: Brooks/Cole.

Ellis, A. (1970). *The essence of rational psychotherapy: A comprehensive approach to treatment.* New York: Institute for Rational Living.

Erikson, E. H. (1950). *Childhood and society.* New York: Norton.

Eysenck, H. J. (1952). The effects of psychotherapy: An evaluation. *Journal of Consulting Psychology, 16,* 319–324.

Eysenck, H. J. (1953b). *Uses and abuses of psychology.* Baltimore: Penguin.

Eysenck, H. J. (1959). Learning theory and behavior therapy. *Journal of Mental Sciences, 105,* 61–75.

Eysenck, H. J. (1960). *Behavior therapy and the neuroses.* New York: Pergamon Press.

Fadiman, J. (1980). The transpersonal stance. In M. J. Mahoney (Ed.), *Psychotherapy process: Current issues and future directions.* New York: Plenum Press.

Frankl, V. E. (1965). *The doctor and the soul: From psychotherapy to logotherapy.* New York: Knopf.

Goldman, G. D., & Milman, D. S. (Eds.). (1978). *Psychoanalytic psychotherapy.* Reading, MA: Addison-Wesley.

Goldstein, K. (1940). *Human nature in the light of psychopathology.* Cambridge, MA: Harvard University Press.

Greenson, R. R. (1967). *The technique and practice of psychoanalysis* (Vol. 1). New York: International Universities Press.

Grof, S. (1975). *Realms of the human unconscious.* New York: Viking Press.

Grof, S. (1980). Theoretical and empirical basis of transpersonal psychotherapy. In S. Boorstein (Ed.), *Transpersonal psychotherapy.* Palo Alto, CA: Science and Behavior Books.

Grof, S. (Ed.). (1984). *Ancient wisdom and modern science.* Albany, NY: State University of New York Press.

Gurdjieff, G. I. (1968). *Meetings with remarkable men.* New York: Dutton.

Hall, C. S., Lindzey, G., Loehlin, J. C., & Manosevitz, M. (1985). *Introduction to theories of personality.* New York: Wiley.

Harding, D. E. (1972). *On having no head.* New York: Harper & Row.

Hilgard, E. R. (1977). *Divided consciousness: Multiple controls in human thought and action.* New York: Wiley.

Hull, C. L. (1943). *Principles of behavior: An introduction to behavior theory.* New York: Appleton-Century-Crofts.

Ichok, G. (1934). Les reflexes conditonnel et le traitement de l'alcoolique. *The conditioned reflexes and the treatment of alcoholism. Progress in Medicine, 2,* 1742–1745.

James, W. (1950). *Principles of psychology*. Dover, NY: Henry Holt. (Original work published 1890)

James W. (1961). *The varieties of religious experience*. New York: Collier Books. (Original work published 1902)

Jones, M. C. (1924). The elimination of children's fears. *Journal of Experimental Psychology, 1*, 382–390.

Jung, C. G. (1961). *Memories, dreams, and reflections*. New York: Random House.

Jung, C. G. (1968). *The archetypes and the collective unconscious*. Princeton, NJ: Princeton University Press.

Kanfer, F. H., & Karoly, P. (1972). Self-control: A behavioristic excursion into the lion's den. *Behavior Therapy, 3*, 398–416.

Klein, G. S. (1954). Need and regulation. In M. R. Jones (Ed.), *Nebraska symposium on motivation* (Vol. 2) (pp. 224–274). Lincoln: University of Nebraska Press.

Kohut, H. (1971). *The analysis of the self*. New York: International Universities Press.

Lazarus, A. A. (1958). New methods in psychotherapy: A case study. *South African Medical Journal, 32*, 660–664.

Lazarus, A. A. (1971). *Behavior therapy and beyond*. New York: McGraw-Hill.

Loevinger, J. (1966). The meaning and measurement of ego development. *American Psychologist, 21*, 195–206.

Lueger, R. J. (1986). Imagery techniques in cognitive-behavioral therapy. In A. A. Sheikh (Ed.), *Anthology of imagery techniques* (pp. 61–83). Milwaukee: American Imagery Institute.

Mahoney, J. M., & Arnkoff, D. (1978). Cognitive and self-control therapies. In S. L. Garfield & A. E. Bergin (Eds.), *Handbook of psychotherapy and behavior change* (pp. 689–722). New York: Wiley.

Maslow, A. H. (1968). *Toward a psychology of being*. New York: Van Nostrand.

Maslow, A. H. (1971). *The farther reaches of human nature*. New York: Viking Press.

Meichenbaum, D. (1977). *Cognitive behavior modification*. New York: Plenum Press.

Menninger, K. (1963). *The vital balance*. New York: Viking Press.

Mowrer, O. H., & Mowrer, W. A. (1938). Enuresis: A method for its study and treatment. *American Journal of Orthopsychiatry, 8*, 436–447.

Murray, H. L. (1938). *Explorations in personality*. New York: Oxford University Press.

Nelson, R. O., & Hayes, S. C. (1986). The nature of behavioral assessment. In R. O. Nelson & S. C. Hayes (Eds.), *Conceptual foundations of behavioral assessment* (pp. 3–41). New York: Guilford Press.

Perls, F. (1969). *Gestalt therapy verbatim*. Lafayette, CA: Real People Press.

Prochaska, J. O. (1979). *Systems of psychotherapy: A transtheoretical analysis*. Homewood, IL: Dorsey Press.

Ram Dass, B. (1977). *Grist for the mill*. Santa Cruz, CA: Unity Press.

Rogers, C. (1951). *Client-centered therapy*. Boston: Houghton-Mifflin.

Santostefano, S. (1978). *A biodevelopmental approach to clinical child psychology: Cognitive controls and cognitive-control therapy.* New York: Wiley.

Shah, I. (1970). *The way of the Sufi.* New York: Dutton.

Shah, I. (1972). *Thinkers of the East.* Baltimore: Penquin.

Shapiro, D. A. & Shapiro, D. (1982). Meta-analysis of comparataive therapy outcome studies: A replication and refinement. *Psychological Bulletin, 92,* 581–604.

Shapiro, M. B. (1951). An experimental approach to diagnostic psychological testing. *Journal of Mental Science, 97,* 748–764.

Skinner, B. F. (1953). *Science and human behavior.* New York: Macmillan.

Smith, M. L., Glass, G. V., & Miller, J. I. (1980). *The benefits of psychotherapy.* Baltimore: John Hopkins.

Speeth, K., & Fadiman, J. (1979). Transpersonal psychotherapy. In R. Henrik (Ed.), *Psychotherapy handbook.* New York: New American Library.

Spence, K. W. (1956). *Behavior theory and conditioning.* New Haven, CN: Yale University Press.

Strupp, H. H. (1980). Success and failure in time-limited psychotherapy: Further evidence (Comparison 4). *Archives of General Psychiatry, 37,* 947–954.

Sullivan, H. S. (1953). *The interpersonal theory of psychiatry.* New York: Norton.

Sutich, A. J. (1968). Transpersonal psychology: An emerging force. *Journal of Humanistic Psychology, 8,* 77–79.

Sutich, A. J. (1980). Transpersonal psychotherapy: History and definition. In S. Boorstein (Ed.), *Transpersonal psychotherapy.* Palo Alto, CA: Science and Behavior Books.

Tart, C. (Ed.). (1969). *Altered states of consciousness.* New York: Wiley.

Tart, C. (Ed.). (1975). *Transpersonal psychologies.* New York: Harper & Row.

Thorndike, E. L. (1905). *The elements of psychology.* New York: Seiler.

Tolman, E. C. (1932). *Purposive behavior in animals and men.* New York: Century Book Company.

Truax, C., & Carkhuff, R. (1967). *Toward effective counseling and psychotherapy: Training and practice.* Chicago: Aldine.

Vaillant, G. (1977). *Adaptation to life.* New York: Brown.

Vaughan, F. (1984). The transpersonal perspective. In S. Grof (Ed.), *Ancient wisdom and modern science.* Albany, NY: State University of New York Press.

Wallerstein, R. S. (1986). *Forty-two lives in treatment: A study of psychoanalysis and psychotherapy.* New York: Guilford Press.

Walsh, R., & Shapiro, D. H. (1983). *Beyond health and normality: Explorations of exceptional psychological well-being.* New York: Van Nostrand Reinhold.

Walsh, R. N., & Vaughan, F. E. (1980). Comparative models of the person and psychotherapy. In S. Boorstein (Ed.), *Transpersonal psychotherapy.* Palo Alto, CA: Science and Behavior Books.

Walsh, R., & Vaughan, F. (1983). Towards an integrative psychology of well-being. In R. Walsh & D. H. Shapiro (Eds.), *Beyond health and normality: Explorations of exceptional psychological well-being.* New York: Van Nostrand Reinhold.

Watson, J. (1919). *Psychology from the standpoint of a behaviorist.* Philadelphia: Lippincott.

White, J. (Ed.). (1973). *The highest state of consciousness.* New York: Doubleday.

White, R. W. (1959). Motivation reconsidered: The concept of competence. *Psychological Review, 66,* 297–333.

Wilber, K. (1977). *The spectrum of consciousness.* Wheaton, IL: Quest.

Wilber, K. (1980). *The Atman project.* Wheaton , IL: Quest.

Wolpe, J. (1958). *Psychotherapy by reciprocal inhibition.* Palo Alto, CA: Stanford University Press.

Yogananda, P. (1972). *The autobiography of a yogi.* Los Angeles: Self-Realization Fellowship.

9

Hypnosis: Historical and Social Psychological Aspects

LORNE D. BERTRAND
NICHOLAS P. SPANOS

"The Commission has unanimously come to the conclusion that there is nothing to show that the fluid of animal magnetism exists and that, consequently, this non-existent fluid can serve no useful purpose."

Report of the French Commission of Inquiry
on Mesmerism, 1784

The notion of hypnosis is associated with a constellation of unusual experiences and behaviors that are viewed as being discontinuous

Preparation of this chapter was supported by a Social Sciences and Humanities Research Council of Canada Doctoral Fellowship and a Natural Sciences and Engineering Research Council of Canada Postdoctoral Fellowship awarded to the first author, and a grant from the Medical Research Council of Canada held by the second author.

We thank Betty Bayer, Margaret de Groh, and Carol Scott for critically reading earlier versions of this paper.

237

from everyday social actions. These phenomena include heightened responsiveness to suggestion, a purported loss of conscious control over behavior, and alterations in subjective experiences that are supposedly specific to hypnosis (for reviews see Spanos, 1982, 1986b). Historically, the apparent discrepancy between "normal" behavior and hypnotic phenomena has led a number of theorists to explain hypnotic behavior by positing various esoteric and unusual psychological and physiological mechanisms (Ellenberger, 1970; Sarbin, 1962). As a result, the idea of hypnosis has, in a sense, taken on a "life of its own"; hypnosis has come to be viewed as an identifiable and distinct mental entity or state rather than an explanatory metaphor used to describe a particular form of social behavior. Within this "altered state" framework, the role of social psychological factors in accounting for hypnotic phenomena is deemphasized. Altered state hypotheses are premised on the notion that hypnotic phenomena are highly unusual and, therefore, require the positing of unusual explanatory mechanisms.

When people engage in behavior that does not conform to normative expectations, observers tend to attribute the behavior to unusual internal causes rather than to situational or contextual variables (Bromley & Shupe, 1981; Garfinkel, 1967; Leifer, 1969; Szasz, 1961). Along with the emphasis that traditional and contemporary "special process" theorists have placed on esoteric explanations of hypnotic phenomena has gone a deemphasizing of the social and historical climates in which these phenomena occurred. Throughout this chapter, we shall argue that hypnotic phenomena can be understood in terms of the normative processes that guide and maintain more mundane forms of social interaction. Our position holds that an analysis of hypnosis in these terms precludes the necessity of positing the existence of special states of consciousness as explanatory concepts.

We shall begin with an overview of the current status of the "state/ nonstate" controversy in hypnosis and proceed to a discussion of how behaviors currently associated with hypnosis evolved out of earlier religious and philosophical ideas. Altered state theorists sometimes use hypnosis as an explanation for various historical phenomena. For instance, it is sometimes claimed that hypnosis was employed unwittingly by ancient and medieval priests, temple healers, and exorcists to produce both religious prophecy and "miraculous" healing. We shall argue that this use of current notions of hypnosis to explain historical events is misleading and that a more parsimonious understanding of these events can be gained by eschewing modern altered state notions and analyzing the events in their historical context.

STATUS OF THE STATE/NONSTATE CONTROVERSY

Traditional accounts have portrayed hypnosis as an altered state of consciousness that is fundamentally different from waking. These accounts emphasize the subjective reports of involuntary behavior frequently elicited from highly susceptible hypnotic subjects as well as the increased responsiveness to suggestion and the purported distortions in sensory functioning, perception, and memory that often accompany hypnotic procedures (Bowers, 1976; Hilgard, 1977a, 1977b; Kihlstrom, 1985; Kihlstrom, Evans, Orne, & Orne, 1980; Orne, 1959).

However, this view of hypnosis has not gone unchallenged. For instance, Barber (1969) and Barber, Spanos, and Chaves (1974) discussed the results of a large number of studies indicating that brief instructions designed to enhance subjects' motivation and involvement in the experimental situation are as effective as hypnotic techniques in producing heightened responsiveness to suggestions. This point deserves emphasis. Many psychologists as well as lay people continue to hold the misleading assumption that hypnotic procedures are uniquely potent in enhancing responsiveness to suggestions for pain reduction, amnesia, age regression, hallucination, and other seemingly unusual behaviors. In fact, it is probably this implicitly held assumption more than any other that lends popular support to altered state formulations. Nevertheless, this assumption is simply incorrect. Nonhypnotic procedures of various types have been shown time and again to be just as effective as, and sometimes even more effective than, hypnotic procedures at facilitating response to suggestions for pain reduction (Barber & Hahn, 1962; Evans & Paul, 1970; Spanos, Radtke-Bodorik, Ferguson, & Jones, 1979), hallucination (Barber & Calverley, 1964; Graham, 1970; Spanos, Bridgeman, Stam, Gwynn, & Saad, 1983; Spanos, de Groot, Tiller, Weekes, & Bertrand, 1985), age regression (Barber & Calverley, 1965; Spanos, de Groot, Tiller, Weekes, & Bertrand, 1985), and many other traditional hypnotic phenomena. In addition, despite the attempts of numerous investigators to uncover stable psychological and physiological correlates of the supposed "hypnotic state," consistent findings have not been forthcoming (Barber, 1970; Sarbin & Slagle, 1979; Sheehan, 1979; Wagstaff, 1981). Such results have lent support to the view that hypnosis is not a separate entity or state, but rather is a social response that is explicable in terms of the same concepts as those used to explain other social interactions. This perspective does not resort to special psychological or physiological processes to account for hypnotic behavior, but instead describes such behavior as a goal-directed or strategic role enactment that is guided by the context in which it takes place (Sarbin, 1967; Sarbin & Coe, 1972; Spanos, 1982, 1986a; Wagstaff, 1981).

It is important to note that descriptions of hypnotic behaviors (as well as other social behaviors) in terms of role enactments does not imply faked behavior and corresponding confabulated reports of subjective experiences (Coe, 1983; Goffman, 1961; Sarbin & Allen, 1966). Instead, this perspective regards hypnotic responding as a role enactment in which contextual factors guide actors to interpret their goal-directed actions as involuntary happenings (Sarbin, 1983; Spanos, 1986b). The hypnotic situation implicitly conveys to subjects the expectation that their behavior should occur automatically and without their conscious control (Spanos, in press). For example, the instructions given in most situations ask people to *do* something (e.g., "Please take the cup to the sink"). Such instructions implicitly define the subject as the instigator of the action requested. In contrast, hypnotic suggestions are worded passively to imply to subjects that something will happen to them. Unlike standard requests or instructions, hypnotic suggestions do not ask subjects explicitly to enact overt behaviors, rather they inform subjects that a particular behavioral event will occur, while inviting them to engage in imaginings that are consistent with the occurrence of the behavior (Spanos, 1982). For instance, "imagine a force attracting your hands toward each other. . . . As you think of this force pulling your hands together, they will move together" (Weitzenhoffer & Hilgard, 1959, pp. 21–22). This suggestion can be interpreted as including two components: (1) subjects are tacitly requested to enact a specific behavior, and (2) they are instructed to disclaim responsibility for this behavior. Consistent with this notion, subjects are more likely to rate their responses as involuntary happenings when they are administered suggestions as opposed to direct instructions that imply voluntary behavior (Spanos & Barber, 1972; Spanos & de Groh, 1983; Spanos & Gorassini, 1984; Weitzenhoffer, 1974).

The elicitation of suggested behavior that is rated as feeling nonvolitional can be understood in terms of modern causal attribution models (Bem, 1967, 1972). From this perspective, subjects regard their behavior as involuntary because the context in which it occurs cues them to believe that the behavior should occur involuntarily. The cultural myths surrounding the notion of hypnosis, coupled with the information conveyed by suggestions, certainly foster a view of hypnotic behavior as an involuntary happening rather than a self-generated action. Given these considerations, many subjects engage in the required behavior and then disavow responsibility for this behavior by focusing on the elements of the context that legitimize attributions of nonvolition. Thus, these subjects may come to interpret their behavior as an automatic occurrence when, in fact, it was a strategic and purposeful response to the demands of the situation (Spanos, Rivers, & Ross, 1977).

This formulation has been supported by the results of two recent experiments on hypnotic amnesia (Bertrand & Spanos, 1985; Spanos & de Groh, 1984). In both of these studies, hypnotically amnesic subjects frequently reported engaging in some form of cognitive distraction strategy that led to failures in the recall of previously learned material. However, most of these subjects also reported that their amnesia had been an involuntary occurrence. Thus, although subjects were cognizant of the strategies they utilized during the hypnotic tasks, they frequently downplayed or ignored the importance of these strategies in bringing about their responses and instead viewed these responses as involuntary happenings.

The goal-directed nature of hypnotic responding also has been demonstrated by recent studies that focused on the countering of suggested responses. For example, Spanos, Cobb, and Gorassini (1985) gave excellent hypnotic subjects several suggestions calling for simple motor responses (e.g., arm lowering). Subjects in several groups were instructed to counter (i.e., resist) the suggested responses (e.g., "Try to prevent your arm from lowering"). Some subjects were informed that deeply hypnotized subjects are unable to resist suggestions while others were informed that the ability to resist is a sign of very deep hypnosis. When the inability to resist was presented as a sign of deep hypnosis, most subjects failed to counter the suggestion and indicated afterwards that they were unable to do so despite serious efforts. On the other hand, when the ability to resist was defined as a sign of deep hypnosis, almost all subjects successfully countered each suggestion and defined their responses as voluntary rather than as involuntary. Spanos, Radtke, and Bertrand (1984) obtained related findings for hypnotic amnesia. In this case, the same excellent hypnotic subjects first indicated that they were unable to recall the words covered by the amnesia suggestion. Later, however, when they were led to believe that successful recall would define them as being deeply hypnotized, all of these "amnesic" subjects recalled all of the supposedly forgotten test words. In short, even excellent hypnotic subjects retain voluntary control over their suggested responses. Frequently, however, the wording of suggestions and other contextual variables lead them to self-present as having lost such control. Somewhat paradoxically, subjects are able to convey the impression convincingly of having lost control over their responses only by retaining such control and employing it judiciously to meet the changing demands of the hypnotic test situation (Spanos, 1982).

Given that little experimental evidence has accrued in support of hypnosis as involving special or unique psychological processes, the puzzling question of why such views continue to be held by many investigators remains. Coe (1983) has provided an interesting partial answer to this query. He argues that special rewards are provided to clinical practitioners and researchers who adhere to special process views of hypnosis. For instance, within the domain of clinical hypnosis, presenting hypnosis as a special state maintains hypnotic intervention procedures as therapeutic tools that are different from other clinical techniques and thus are somehow "special." This leads to a view of hypnotherapists as possessing an exclusive and powerful tool that is not available to other practitioners. Consequently, a special demand is placed upon the services of these therapists, leading to a steady stream of clients and referrals from other practitioners. The view of hypnotherapy as a special technique is also legitimized by the professional hypnosis societies, which publish specific guidelines for the education and training of hypnosis practitioners and which, like other guilds, attempt to limit competition by restricting the use of hypnosis to those whom they certify as possessing the "special training" required to use this powerful and mysterious tool. With respect to experimental researchers, Coe (1983) emphasized the special recognition accorded to altered state theorists by the professional hypnosis associations. This recognition is conferred through such avenues as membership on the editorial boards of the professional journals and the awarding of special prizes and distinctions to prominent state theorists.

Coe (1983) does not suggest that such considerations are the sole reason for the maintenance of beliefs in hypnosis as an altered state. However, his perspective certainly indicates that special rewards are set aside for proponents of this position. Such social rewards for adhering to a particular point of view undoubtedly play a role in the perseverance of such beliefs in the face of contrary evidence (Berger & Luckmann, 1966; Schein, Schneier, & Barker, 1961).

In summary, misconceptions about the nature of hypnosis remain prevalent, and these misconceptions reinforce the view that hypnosis represents a distinct psychological entity. This view has obscured not only our understanding of phenomena traditionally associated with hypnosis, but also the manner in which numerous authors have discussed historical events that bear resemblance to current hypnotic phenomena. These historians have attempted to trace the entity "hypnosis" through the ages in the same way that medical historians have attempted to trace the occurrence of diseases like tuberculosis or syphilis down through the ages. As a result, historians of hypnosis have tended to emphasize selectively certain similarities between various historical phenomena and some of the phenomena currently associated with hypnosis. However, because of their bias toward viewing hypnosis as an internal entity, the social climates in which these historical phenomena occurred typically are downplayed or even ignored (Spanos & Gottlieb, 1979).

In the subsequent sections of this chapter, we shall focus on several phenomena that have been regarded as illustrative of the operation of hypnosis in historical times. We shall attempt to show how these phenomena can be conceptualized in terms of contextual factors operating in these historical situations, without the necessity of postulating "hypnotic" states of consciousness. In the final section, an example of how a social psychological analysis may be applied to the clinical disorder of multiple personality will be presented.

HYPNOSIS IN HISTORICAL PERSPECTIVE

Hypnosis in Antiquity

The notion that hypnosis is a distinct entity has led to the hypotheses that hypnotic processes operated, but either went undetected or were misunderstood, long before the terms "mesmerism" or "hypnosis" came upon the historical scene. For example, various authors have suggested that historical phenomena such as Biblical exorcisms, Egyptian temple healings, and Asclepian dream healings in ancient Greece can be explained in terms of hypnotic processes (Edmonston, 1986). Such interpretations make the implicit assumption that current notions concerning the operation of hypnosis as an altered state are correct and can be used to explain historical events that share certain similarities with present-day happenings (Spanos, 1978; Stam & Spanos, 1982; Stocking, 1965). A basic difficulty in these formulations is that the complex social contexts in which these happenings occurred are deemphasized for the sake of comparison with current ideas. When the historical context of such events is taken into account, there is little need to propose esoteric explanatory concepts, and when such explanations are used, they are merely redundant and obscure an accurate depiction of these events (Spanos, 1983a). To illustrate our point, we shall discuss one historical phenomenon that a number of authors have explained using hypnosis, the Asclepian dream healings in ancient Greece. Our analysis is based on that provided by Stam and Spanos (1982).

The cult of Asclepius was a religious healing sect in ancient Greece from the fourth century B.C. onward. Modern historians have focused on the so-called dream healings, or incubations, practiced by this cult.

During these dream healings, the patient slept in the temple and was supposedly visited by the god Asclepius in a dream. During this dream, the god either cured the patient outright or offered a prescription for a cure (Edelstein & Edelstein, 1945).

Numerous 19th-century authors proposed animal magnetism and somnambulism as explanations for the dream healings (Edelstein & Edelstein, 1945). More recently, authors have proposed hypnosis (Kroger & Fezler, 1976; Ludwig, 1964; MacHovec, 1975, 1979; Pulos, 1980). These hypotheses suggest that hypnosis was used (probably unwittingly) during the night to guide the patients' experiences while they awaited the appearance of the god in a dream.

Much of the evidence concerning a role for hypnosis in the dream healings consists of selective citations from sources of questionable credibility. For instance, much of the information regarding the events of the incubations was derived from Aristophanes's (448–380 B.C.) play *Plutus*. Arsitophanes, however, was a comic poet, and his writings regarding the healings must be placed within this context (Edelstein & Edelstein, 1945; Phillips, 1973). Nevertheless, a number of modern authors have selectively chosen passages from this play in support of their views of the healings. For example, in one scene from the play, a clandestine witness to the proceedings is described. The witness sees the god accompanied by two enormous snakes cure the blindness of a sleeping friend. Some authors have interpreted this passage to mean that during the incubation period priests disguised as gods and accompanied by trained snakes entered the temple and cured the sick via hypnotic suggestion (MacHovec, 1979). However, as discussed by Stam and Spanos (1982), this interpretation is questionable. It is dubious at best to accept the writings of a comic poet at face value "without making allowance for poetic fantasy and comic license" (Edelstein & Edelstein, 1945, p. 146). In addition, there is no evidence to suggest that the temple priests attempted to heal the sick by tricking them into believing that the priests were gods. Even in the play, it was the god and not a disguised priest who affected the cure. In fact, the god was never seen by anyone awake. The visions of the god reported by the sick were dream visions (Edelstein & Edelstein, 1945; Kerényi, 1947–1960).

In sum, reconstructions of Asclepian dream healings in terms of hypnotic suggestions are based primarily on selective citation from secondary sources of dubious validity and on the implicit assumption that hypnosis is an identifiable state or entity that can be induced without the knowledge of either the subject or the hypnotist. Certainly, it is not unreasonable to hypothesize that expectations of a cure were engendered by various temple practices or that these heightened expectations may have produced beneficial effects in some patients (Stam & Spanos, 1982). The efficacy of positive attitudes and expectations in almost any treatment procedure is recognized widely (Barber, 1981, 1984; Frank, 1973). However, acceptance of this fact is very different from assuming that temple priests unwittingly made use of hypnosis to bring about cures.

Emergence of the Mesmeric Role

Modern notions of hypnosis grew out of Mesmer's (1781–1980) work on animal magnetism. As is well known, Mesmer believed that a "subtle fluid" permeated the universe, including the human body. Disease resulted from an imbalance of this fluid within the body, and cure of disease was accomplished by redistributing the flow of fluid. Redistribution of fluid in the sick could be brought about by the transmission of magnetic fluid from certain healthy individuals (magnetizers) to the sick. The roots of Mesmer's theorizing can be traced to the scientific *zeitgeist* of his era. A predominant notion in the 18th century was that of the "ether," which was believed to be a pervasive fluid that filled all matter (Darnton, 1970; Ellenberger, 1970; Sarbin, 1962). Mesmer built on the popular notion of this fluid and proposed that its imbalance in the human body was responsible for illness.

By the early 19th century, the constellation of behaviors that came to characterize Mesmerism were well delineated. Mesmerism consisted of a set of rather unusual behaviors that occurred within the delimited social context of the mesmeric relationship. The behaviors included convulsions in response to the "passes" of the mesmerist, amnesia for the events of the mesmeric session, demonstrations of increased intelligence and clairvoyance, and the perception of these behaviors occurring outside of the patient's voluntary control (Spanos & Gottlieb, 1979).

As the role of the magnetized patient became more clearly defined, so too did the role of the mesmerist. The magnetizer's personal characteristics, faith in the procedure, and the "moral purity" of his undertaking quickly came to be viewed as crucial to treatment. The personal characteristics of the magnetizer were perceived as more virtuous and desirable than those of the patient, thereby helping to legitimize the status differential between magnetizer and patient. The mesmerist-patient relationship came to be regarded as a confrontation between good and evil, with the mesmerist representing the moral good of health and the patient representing the moral evil of disease (Spanos & Gottlieb, 1979).

The unusual behaviors associated with mesmerism were viewed as the automatic result of underlying physiological change. However, the behaviors associated with mesmerism depended upon the particular school of animal magnetism with which a particular mesmerist identified (Dingwall, 1968). In addition, two French commissions created in 1784 to investigate Mesmer's claims found that certain behaviors such as convulsions, catalepsy, and paralysis only occurred if the subjects knew they were being magnetized (Ellenberger, 1970). Such evidence, of course, underscores the importance of contextually generated expectations and beliefs in the elicitation and maintenance of mesmeric behavior. Nevertheless, an important question remains: Why did the particular constellation of unusual behaviors associated with magnetism come to coalesce into a coherent social role? Spanos and Gottlieb (1979) suggested that the mesmerist-patient relationship grew out of the secularization of earlier exorcist-demoniac roles. These authors pointed out that cases of demonic possession were fairly frequent during the 18th and early 19th centuries, coincident with the popular rise of Mesmer's animal magnetism. Both the exorcist and mesmerist roles were characterized by "laying on of hands," or mesmeric "passes," (Owen, 1971; Rose, 1971). The role of the exorcist, like that of the mesmerist, involved the development of an appropriate attitude toward himself and his procedures. Despite the fact that the exorcist's power was seen as deriving from God, his personality and attitude were conceptualized as being crucial in effecting a cure. The exorcist, like the mesmerist, construed his activity as a moral confrontation between good and evil. The notions of authority and submission were prevalent in the context of exorcism as well as mesmerism. The exorcist was viewed as constantly in control, and the domoniac remained submissive to him (Oesterreich, 1966; Spanos, 1983a).

Spanos and Gottlieb (1979) also pointed to a number of similarities between the roles of the demoniac and the magnetized patient. For instance, convulsions were an almost invariable accompaniment of possession and also were exhibited frequently by magnetized patients. Similarly, heightened intellectual functioning and clairvoyance followed by spontaneous amnesia for the events occurring during possession were frequent occurrences (Oesterreich, 1966). These behaviors, of course, also were observed among magnetized patients. Possession was experienced as involuntary by the demoniac and was defined as such by society at large (Spanos, 1983a). Thus the possessed saw themselves and were viewed by others in much the same way as magnetized subjects were seen—as automatons submissively responding to the wishes of some agency external to the self.

These similarities in the roles of exorcist/demoniac and mesmerist/patient are not the only evidence that the mesmeric role was modeled on earlier demoniac enactments. Spanos and Gottlieb (1979) also pointed out that clerics and mesmerists were well aware of the similarities in the effects they each produced and often reinterpreted each other's practices in their own terms. Mesmerism came to be identified by many clergy and laypeople as a special case of demonic possession, and this identification continued to be maintained throughout the 19th century. Within this framework, the magnetized subject was viewed as the innocent victim of diabolical influence, and the magnetizer was seen as the evil witch or sorcerer who controlled the demon's activities.*

The converse of this identification of mesmerism with possession also was apparent, and a number of mesmerists interpreted exorcisms as the result of magnetic influence. For example, Mesmer (1781–1980) himself reinterpreted the exorcisms of John Joseph Gassner, a Catholic priest, as examples of mesmerism. These reinterpretations typically indicated that exorcism had been effective because the priests who employed it unknowingly made use of mesmeric techniques (Spanos & Gottlieb, 1979).

From Demonology to Neurology

By the mid-19th century, the medical community frequently interpreted both possession and magnetism in terms of hysteria (Drinka, 1984; Ellenberger, 1970). Explanations of physiological functioning or of behavior in terms of universal fluids or ethers fell into disfavor with increasing scientific knowledge. Scientific and medical thinking during this period were influenced by a rise in both the popularity and status of neurology. This change in the scientific *zeitgeist* produced two important changes in theorizing about possession and mesmerism. First, it replaced previous supernatural and "fluidist" hypotheses of these phenomena with naturalistic accounts that were more in keeping with 19th-century scientific thinking. Second, the neurological position placed these phenomena securely under the rubric of disease.

This point of view was perhaps most strongly supported by Charcot, who contended that hysteria was a disease and that only hysterics could manifest the signs of *grand hypnotisme*. Charcot frequently drew attention to similarities between symptoms of hysterics and the behavior of the demonically possessed of previous centuries as evidence that the

---

*As an aside to this observation, we have found that some subjects visiting our laboratories who are members of certain charismatic Christian sects refuse to undergo hypnotic testing because they believe that hypnosis will leave them unprotected against possession by demons.

possessed had, in reality, been suffering from the disease hysteria (Charcot & Marie, 1892; Charcot & Richet, 1887–1972). Charcot's identification of hypnosis with nervous disease was undoubtedly facilitated by the fact that many of the central' "symptoms" of magnetism (when divorced from the social context in which they occurred) lent themselves easily to neurological interpretation (e.g., convulsions). Relatedly, many of the odd behaviors that have remained a part of the modern hypnotic role probably received initial legitimation in 19th-century medical circles because their superficial resemblance to the symptoms of neurological disease encouraged their conceptualization as medical symptoms (Wagstaff, 1981). These behaviors continue to be conceptualized as "symptoms" of hypnosis and have become enshrined as such on modern hypnotic susceptibility scales. The misleading medical names still applied to these behaviors clearly reflect their historical origins (e.g., "amnesia" as opposed to attempted forgetting; "analgesia" as opposed to redirecting thoughts away from pain; "hallucination" as opposed to imagining; "catalepsy" as opposed to stiffening and failing to bend a limb). The 19th-century medical accounts of these behaviors, like earlier accounts in terms of demonic possession, reinforced the notion that these behaviors occurred involuntarily and, like the symptoms of other diseases, were not under the patient's control (Drinka, 1984; Spanos & Gottlieb, 1979).

Using the notion of hysterical disease as an explanation for possession and mesmerism did little to promote an understanding of the behaviors associated with these phenomena. Despite the point of view proffered by some psychiatric writers and historians that hysteria represents a disease entity that can be traced throughout the centuries (Veith, 1965; Zilboorg & Henry, 1941), there is no universally accepted definition of the term. On the contrary, the term is highly ambiguous and historically has referred to a wide conglomeration of relatively unusual and dramatic, but often unrelated, behaviors (Chodoff, 1974; Chodoff & Lyons, 1958; Janet, 1925; Szasz, 1961; Ullmann & Krasner, 1969; Ziegler & Imboden, 1962). This array of behaviors included spontaneous amnesia, fugue states, convulsions, sensory and motor disturbances in the absence of demonstrable organic pathology, heightened suggestibility, hallucinations, anorexia, a host of sexual disturbances, and a personality configuration variously described as vain, coquettish, frigid, and so on (Spanos & Gottlieb, 1979). There is no evidence to support the contention that this compilation of behaviors subsumed by the term "hysteria" reflects a unitary disease process or has a common etiology (Slater, 1965). Furthermore, there is little evidence to suggest that the behavioral referents for the term hysteria in ancient times were similar to the constellation of behaviors labeled as hysteria in the 19th and 20th centuries.

The popularity of the diagnosis "hysteria" in the 19th century should be understood in terms of the concurrent rise in the status of psychiatry as a medical discipline. The emphasis in medical theorizing was on the compilation of various symptoms into delineated syndromes. Hysteria may be viewed as an example of this medicalization process. Even though hysteria was often employed as a catch-all diagnosis that covered a wide variety of behaviors, many of which were unrelated, the medicalization of these behaviors served to reify hysteria as an internal disease entity (Szasz, 1961). It should be kept in mind that 19th-century practitioners of psychiatry were also the discipline's first historians and were intent on legitimizing the notion that certain behavioral deviancies were really diseases. The reification of hysteria as a disease entity was facilitated by demonstrating that this disorder had an ancient history. The symptoms of this "disease" now could be traced from Asclepian temples through 16th-century possessed nuns and Mesmer's magnetized patients to 19th-century hysterics. In short, psychiatric histories legitimized the medical mythologies that provided the underpinning for the emergence of psychiatry as a medical discipline (Drinka, 1984; Spanos, in press).

An important result of the acceptance of a disease model of hysteria was that the primary causes of the disorder were viewed as internal. Thus interpersonal factors that might have reinforced or maintained the behaviors were relegated to positions of secondary importance or even ignored (Spanos & Gottlieb, 1979). A number of authors have taken issue with this disease model and have proposed that so-called hysterical behaviors reflected learned, interpersonal strategies designed to communicate dissatisfactions and/or to obtain various types of social reinforcement (Smith-Rosenberg, 1972; Spanos, 1983a; Spanos & Gottlieb, 1979; Ullmann & Krasner, 1969). Given that hysteria was viewed as a legitimate illness, adopting that role led to attention and rewards that otherwise were unavailable to the patient (Spanos & Gottlieb, 1979).

As posited by Spanos and Gottlieb (1979), a social role conceptualization applied to the history of possession, hysteria, and mesmerism acknowledges that disease theorists have been correct in pointing to behavioral similarities associated with these notions. Where the disease perspective lacks theoretical viability is in its acceptance of the behavioral commonalities as deriving from a unitary disease process. A social role theory suggests that the manifestations of possessed behavior were maintained for centuries as a coherent social role because the status of the demoniac became associated with a number of important social functions. For example, "when coupled with exorcism procedures, the role provided a means of reintegrating deviants into the social community, served as a proselytizing device, and in various ways supported the religious and moral values of the community" (Spanos & Gottlieb, 1979, p. 541).

Coincident with the gradual shift from possession to hysteria from the 16th through the 19th centuries were changes in the behaviors associated with patients' performance. As behavioral deviance came to be defined increasingly in medical terms, those behaviors that were not amenable to explanations based upon organic pathology gradually became less frequent (e.g., vomiting pins, speaking in a demonic voice, defining oneself as possessed). Conversely, behaviors that could easily be subsumed under a medical rubric remained apparent (e.g., convulsions, sensory-motor disturbances, vague physical complaints) (Spanos & Gottlieb, 1979).

In the late 18th and 19th centuries many patients treated with magnetism and hypnotism, both in and outside of hospitals, were defined as hysteric (Drinka, 1984; Ellenberger, 1970). In other words, they were individuals who were already adept at enacting many of the behaviors that, with the guidance of the mesmerist, quickly coalesced into the role of the magnetized subject. For example, a number of investigators have described how the lower-level staff and students working with Charcot were afraid of displeasing or contradicting him. Therefore, with varying degrees of subtlety, they shaped patients to display the constellation of behaviors they believed their supervisor wanted to see. The patients, often anxious to please and desirous of being at the center of attention, guided their role enactments of *grand hypnotisme* on the basis of cues provided by the staff (Drinka, 1984; Ellenberger, 1970; Spanos & Gottlieb, 1979).

The Dissociation Perspective

Despite the doubts cast upon Charcot's propositions concerning hypnosis, notions of a relationship between hypnosis and hysteria persisted well into the 20th century. For example, in attempting to develop a theory for both hypnotic phenomena and hysteria, Janet (1925) perpetuated Charcot's characterization of hypnosis as psychopathological in nature. Janet's explanation of hypnotic phenomena revolved around the concept of *dissociation*. Briefly stated, dissociation theory relied upon the notion that behavior was governed by constellations of ideas that normally functioned simultaneously or in sequence. In certain individuals, a weakness in the nervous system resulted in a splitting or dissociation of these constellations of ideas from one another. Within these dissociated constellations, various behaviors that normally occurred with the patient's awareness and voluntary control became functionally isolated from the constellation of ideas that constituted the "conscious self" and from conscious control.

Janet's propositions were attractive initially because they appeared to account for not only hypnotic behaviors, but also other types of so-called splitting phenomena such as multiple personality and fugue states. However, a major difficulty in this position was the failure of one of its central propositions to gain experimental support. As Ellenberger (1970) pointed out, one important prediction of dissociation theory as applied to hypnosis was that the events occurring while the patient was hypnotized would not be remembered after the patient was awakened. In fact, however, spontaneous posthypnotic amnesia was seen rarely, and when posthypnotic amnesia was suggested explicitly during hypnosis, recall could be reinstated easily after awakening by the simple verbal instruction "Now you can remember." In addition, as Pattie (1956) noted, systems that purportedly were isolated from, and inaccessible to, consciousness continued to influence conscious behavior. For example, in studies of retroactive interference, results have indicated that information for which subjects supposedly are amnesic continued to affect the recall of material that was not covered by the amnesia suggestion (Graham & Patton, 1968; Mitchell, 1932; Stevenson, Stoyva, & Beach, 1962). These observations placed serious doubts upon Janet's theory, and subsequent investigators rejected his position outright (Hull, 1933; White & Shevach, 1942).

Because of the allure of the dissociation position in explaining the apparent automaticity of hypnotic responding, the notion was given new life by Hilgard (1974, 1977a, 1977b) in his theory of neodissociation. This formulation held that dissociated experiences typically remain outside of the hypnotic subject's awareness. Nevertheless, these dissociated subsystems can be "contacted" by the experimenter and thereby can report on the experiences that supposedly occur at an unconscious level. This proposition was tested initially in studies of hypnotic analgesia (see Hilgard, 1979 for a review). According to Hilgard (1979), only the "hypnotized part" of hypnotically analgesic subjects experiences a reduction in consciously perceived pain (i.e., "overt pain"). However, a "hidden part" of the subjects (i.e., a "hidden observer") continues to experience the painful stimulation at its full intensity at an unconscious level (i.e., "hidden pain"). The hypnotized part and the hidden part are separated by an "amnesic barrier," and thus hypnotized subjects typically are not aware of high levels of pain experienced by their hidden part.

In a series of studies, Hilgard and his associates explicitly informed hypnotically analgesic subjects that they possessed a hidden part that remained aware of everything that occurred during hypnosis despite suggestions to the contrary. Afterwards, subjects' hidden parts were contacted and requested to make pain estimates. Subjects' hidden pain ratings tended to be higher than their overt pain ratings.

Spanos and Hewitt (1980) argued that hidden observer responding is not a reflection of a preexisting dissociated subsystem, but rather is an experimental creation resulting from a strategic enactment carried out by subjects in response to the instructions contained in Hilgard's experimental procedure. The instructions used in these studies explicitly informed subjects that they possessed a hidden part that remained aware of everything that happened around them during hypnosis. Spanos and Hewitt (1980) reasoned that subjects' responses to a hidden observer manipulation would vary depending upon the information given to them regarding the characteristics of their hidden part. They gave one group of subjects Hilgard's instructions implying that their hidden part was more aware than their hypnotized part. However, a second group was told that their hidden part was even *less* aware of their surroundings than their hypnotized part. Subjects given Hilgard's "more aware" instructions reported more hidden than overt pain, while subjects administered the "less aware" instructions reported even less hidden than overt pain.

These results were not consistent with Hilgard's notion of dissociated subsystems that remain more aware of pain than the hypnotized subsystem. Instead, they suggest that the hidden observer is an experimental creation that reflects subjects' strategic attempts to fulfill task demands (Spanos, 1983b). Adding support to this conclusion, Spanos, Gwynn, and Stam (1983) found that the *same* subjects could be induced to report successively both more *and* less hidden pain when first one response and then the other was defined as indicative of deep hypnosis.

In summary, the experimental data do not support the contention that hypnosis involves a dissociation of various cognitive subsystems from conscious awareness. Behaviors that, on the surface, may appear to reflect dissociation are more profitably viewed as strategic enactments carried out by subjects in response to task demands. Despite the lack of empirical support for the dissociation position, this notion is still a popular and frequently employed explanatory concept in clinical practice. In the following section, we shall discuss one well-known clinical phenomenon associated with the notion of dissociation, that of multiple personality.

A CLINICAL EXAMPLE: MULTIPLE PERSONALITY

The resurgence of the concept of dissociation can be seen not only in current theorizing about hypnosis, but also in various clinical realms, most notably in discussions of multiple personality syndrome. In this section, we shall discuss the notion of multiple personality and indicate how this phenomenon may be understood without recourse to special psychological processes. From our social psychological perspective, multiple personality is explicable as a role enactment in which contextual factors guide and maintain the symptomatic behaviors (Spanos, 1986b, in press).

There are a number of similarities among the behaviors that characterize hypnosis and those considered indicative of multiple personality. These commonalities can be grouped into three categories: (1) actors temporarily appear to lose control over their behavior, and experience it as an involuntary happening; (2) control for this behavior is transferred from the self to "hidden" mental parts, selves, or agencies; and, (3) actors frequently are amnesic for the information that is accessible to their "hidden selves" (Spanos, in press). These similarities suggest that theoretical accounts appropriate for hypnotic phenomena also may be useful in elucidating the phenomenon of multiple personality.

Traditional accounts of multiple personality have employed psychodynamic formulations, and emphasize early developmental traumas as antecedents to the disorder. From this perspective, multiple personality patients (i.e., multiples) are viewed as the victims of unconscious processes that temporarily displace the "normal self" and become manifest as new identities (Allison & Schwarz, 1980).

Reported cases of multiple personality were relatively common around the turn of the present century (Sutcliffe & Jones, 1962; Taylor & Martin, 1944); however, until the early 1970s, the number of cases reported was few. Since the mid-1970s there has been a dramatic upsurge in the number of reported cases (Boor, 1982; Greaves, 1980; Rosenbaum, 1980). Relatedly, some psychotherapists are much more likely than others to diagnose multiple personality. According to Gruenewald (1971), most therapists do not see even one case of multiple personality throughout their entire careers. Nevertheless, several modern psychotherapists each have dealt with over 50 such cases (Allison & Schwarz, 1980; Bliss, 1980, 1984a; Kluft, 1982).

The disproportionate number of cases diagnosed by a few therapists may reflect the expertise gained by these clinicians in recognizing the symptoms of multiple personality and, in turn, correctly diagnosing the disorder (Allison & Schwarz, 1980; Rosenbaum, 1980; Watkins & Johnson, 1982). On the other hand, an alternative hypothesis arising from a social role perspective suggests that these therapists have become experts not in diagnosing a previously existing condition, but in producing a situation and providing the cues that will foster and maintain enactments of multiple personality (Spanos, in press).

This social role perspective maintains that multiples are involved actively in using available information to create a social impression that is congruent with their perceptions of the situational demands and with the interpersonal goals they are attempting to achieve (Spanos, Weekes, & Bertrand, 1985; Sutcliffe & Jones, 1962). According to this formulation, psychotherapists often play an important function in the generation and maintenance of this role enactment. Therapists sometimes encourage patients to adopt the role of being a multiple, provide them with information about how to enact the role convincingly, and provide "official" legitimation for the different identities their patients enact (Orne, Dinges, & Orne, 1984; Spanos, Weekes, & Bertrand, 1985; Sutcliffe & Jones, 1962). Thus the different frequencies with which some investigators diagnose multiple personality may not reflect differences in diagnostic expertise so much as the use of diagnostic and therapeutic practices that unwittingly encourage patients to adopt and maintain the multiple personality role.

The limited case report data support the social role hypothesis that therapists sometimes subtly encourage and then validate multiple personality enactments. For example, Prince (1930) actually provided names for the secondary personalities that emerged during therapy for his famous patient, Eve. In a more recent case, a woman had difficulty remembering a sexual incident with her husband. At this point, her therapist "instructed Linda to close her eyes and asked to speak to the one who had carried out the act" (Smith, Buffington, & McCard, 1982, p. 21). It was only after this instruction that a secondary personality emerged.

A number of therapists make use of hypnotic procedures to discover and communicate with secondary personalities. From a social role perspective, hypnotic procedures do not have intrinsic properties that facilitate the discovery of hidden personalities (Spanos, Weekes, & Bertrand, 1985). However, such procedures frequently are presented to the patient as a means of contacting "hidden parts" and as an aid to recalling events that may be inaccessible or "repressed." In fact, some therapists recommend that hypnotic procedures be used explicitly to "call forth" and identify secondary personalities (Allison & Schwarz, 1980; Bliss, 1980, 1984b; Brandsma & Ludwig, 1974). For example, in the well-known case of Kenneth Bianchi (the "Hillside Strangler"), who was implicated in the rape-murders of several California women, the clinician prefaced the use of hypnosis by describing it to Bianchi as a tool for uncovering hidden aspects of personality (Schwarz, 1981). It was during this hypnotic interview that Bianchi first manifested a secondary personality.

Once a secondary personality has become manifest in the clinical situation, the procedures used by the therapist may serve to validate and sustain this behavior. For example, Allison and Schwarz (1980) state that patients are frequently reluctant to accept that they are multiples; in such cases, the therapist should actively persuade them to accept this diagnosis. In addition, therapists typically converse at length with each "personality," giving each a unique name and obtaining from each detailed information about their origins, functions, and habits, as well as information about what "they" know and don't know about each other (Spanos, in press). Once patients are defined as multiples, they obtain validation for their enactments in a broader social context. Kohlenberg (1973), for example, reported that the staff of a ward housing a multiple typically conversed and interacted with each of his three "personalities" in a different manner. These considerations suggest that enactments of multiple personality may be understood in terms of the role-validating context that guides and maintains these enactments.

A recent experiment conducted in our laboratory provided research evidence to support this position (Spanos, Weekes, & Bertrand, 1985). Our subjects were university students asked to role play an accused murderer undergoing a psychiatric evaluation. One group was exposed to a "hypnotic" interview that was modeled closely after a hypnotic interview conducted with Kenneth Bianchi (see Schwarz, 1981 for a description of this case). As in the Bianchi interview, our subjects were "hypnotized" and told that there might be another part of them and that the "psychiatrist" (actually an experimenter who was role playing also) would like to communicate with that other part. The "psychiatrist" then attempted to contact the subjects' hidden parts. A control group underwent the same psychiatric interview without any mention of hypnosis.

Results of this study indicated that, although no mention of multiple personality was made to subjects in either group, more than 80% of subjects given the Bianchi interview exhibited characteristics of a multiple personality. For example, these subjects adopted a different name and referred to their primary identity in the third person. None of the control subjects enacted another personality or adopted a different name during the initial interview.

During a second session, subjects were reminded to continue role playing, and those in the experimental group were again "hypnotized." Subjects who had reported a different identity during the first session were given a cue to reinstate their "hidden part." While the "psychiatrist" was in communication with this "part," subjects completed two psychological tests (a sentence completion test and a semantic differential inventory). After finishing these tests, subjects were "awakened" and their "primary personality" (i.e., the character they were role playing) completed the same tests. Control subjects simply completed the two tests twice in succession. The results of this testing were straightforward. Subjects who had displayed another "part" gave responses on the two testings that were markedly and consistently different. A similar pattern is frequently obtained with clinical cases of multiple personality. In such cases, the identities of multiples are frequently extreme opposites in terms of preferences, emotionality, and behavior (Ludwig, Brandsma, Wilbur, Benfeldt, & Jameson, 1972; Smith et al., 1982; Thigpen & Cleckley, 1957; Watkins & Johnson, 1982).

In a replication and extension of the Spanos, Weekes, and Bertrand (1985) study, Spanos, Weekes, Menary, and Bertrand (1986) pretested experimental and control subjects on the psychometric tests in a session prior to the one in which they received the treatment manipulation. In addition, subjects completed the schizophrenia and psychopathic deviate subscales of the Minnesota Multiphasic Personality Inventory (MMPI) as well as the semantic differential and sentence completion inventories. Results of this study replicated the original findings. Over half of the subjects interviewed using the Bianchi technique manifested a secondary personality, whereas none of the control subjects exhibited this response. In addition, subjects who were classified as multiples gave significantly different responses on all of the psychometric tests when each personality was assessed. Control subjects did not differ on their responses from pre- to post-test.

The findings of our role playing studies suggest that cues for the enactment of a multiple personality role are present in some therapy situations and that subjects can identify and utilize these cues to produce enactments of this syndrome. It is important to remember that our experimental instructions were based on the protocol used in an actual clinical setting. If subjects participating in a one-hour experimental session can produce convincing enactments of multiple personality, it seems reasonable to assume that such information given in a therapy situation can produce similar results.

CONCLUDING REMARKS

As we have discussed throughout this chapter, behaviors that appear to be unusual often are assumed to result from special or unusual processes that operate outside the actor's sphere of volitional control. The history of hypnotic phenomena has provided an example of this process. Because the behaviors associated with hypnosis differ from those encountered in everyday social life, investigators have posited esoteric mental states or processes as explanations for these behaviors. This practice has led to a discounting of the social and contextual factors that guide and validate the enactments that are carried out in these situations.

We have argued throughout that "unusual" phenomena such as hypnosis, hysteria, demonic possession, and multiple personality are interpersonal activities, and an analysis of their interpersonal nature renders "special process" explanations unnecessary. In the case of each phenomenon, the associated behaviors are profitably viewed as strategic role enactments that are guided and legitimized by high-status professionals, whether they are hypnotists, physicians, priests, or therapists. A perspective that examines the contextual factors that guide and validate these enactments offers more explanatory power then the invocation of ill-defined "special process" theories.

References

Allison, R. B., & Schwarz, T. (1980). *Minds in many pieces: The making of a very special doctor.* New York: Rawson, Wade.

Barber, T. X. (1969). *Hypnosis: A scientific approach.* New York: Van Nostrand.

Barber, T. X. (1970). *LSD, marijuana, yoga, and hypnosis.* Chicago: Aldine.

Barber, T. X. (1981). Medicine, suggestive therapy, and healing. In R. J. Kastenbaum, T. X. Barber, S. C. Wilson, B. L. Ryder, & L. B. Hathaway (Eds.), *Old, sick, and helpless: Where therapy begins.* Cambridge, MA: Ballinger.

Barber, T. X. (1984). Changing "unchangeable" bodily processes by (hypnotic) suggestions: A new look at hypnosis, cognitions, imagining, and the mind-body problem. In A. A. Sheikh (Ed.), *Imagination and healing.* Farmingdale, NY: Baywood.

Barber, T. X., & Calverley, D. S. (1964). An experimental study of "hypnotic" (auditory and visual) hallucinations. *Journal of Abnormal and Social Psychology, 63,* 13–20.

Barber, T. X., & Calverley, D. S. (1965). Toward a theory of "hypnotic" behavior: Effects on suggestibility of five variables typically induced in hypnotic induction procedures. *Journal of Consulting Psychology, 29,* 98–107.

Barber, T. X., & Hahn, K. W. Jr. (1962). Physiological and subjective responses to pain producing stimulation under hypnotically-suggested and waking-imagined "analgesia." *Journal of Abnormal and Social Psychology, 65,* 411–418.

Barber, T. X., Spanos, N. P., & Chaves, J. F. (1974). *Hypnosis, imagination and human potentialities,* New York: Pergamon.

Bem, D. R. (1967). Self-perception: An alternative interpretation of cognitive dissonance phenomena. *Psychological Review, 74,* 183–200.

Bem, D. R. (1972). Self-perception theory. In L. Berkowitz (Ed.), *Advances in experimental social psychology* (Vol. 6). New York: Academic Press.

Berger, P. L., & Luckmann, T. (1966). *The social construction of reality.* New York: Doubleday.

Bertrand, L. D., & Spanos, N. P. (1985). The organization of recall following hypnotic suggestions for complete and selective amnesia. *Imagination, Cognition, and Personality, 4,* 249–261.

Bliss, E. L. (1980). Multiple personalities: A report of 14 cases with implications for schizophrenia and hysteria. *Archives of General Psychiatry, 37,* 1388–1397.

Bliss, E. L. (1984a). A symptom profile of patients with multiple personalities, including MMPI results. *Journal of Nervous and Mental Disease, 171,* 197–202.

Bliss, E. L. (1984b). Hysteria and hypnosis. *Journal of Nervous and Mental Disease, 172,* 203–206.

Boor, M. (1982). The multiple personality epidemic: Additional cases and inferences regarding diagnosis, etiology, dynamics, and treatment. *Journal of Nervous and Mental Disease, 170,* 302–304.

Bowers, K. S. (1976). *Hypnosis of the seriously curious.* Monterey, CA: Brooks/Cole.

Brandsma, J. M., & Ludwig, A. M. (1974). A case of multiple personality: Diagnosis and treatment. *International Journal of Clinical and Experimental Hypnosis, 22,* 216–233.

Bromley, D. G., & Shupe, A. D. (1981). *Strange gods: The great American cult scare.* Boston, MA: Beacon Press.

Charcot, J. M., & Marie, P. (1892). Hysteria. In D. Hack Tuke (Ed.), *Dictionary of psychological medicine.* London: Churchill.

Charcot, J. M., & Richet, P. (1972). *Les demoniaques dans l'art.* Amsterdam: B.M. Israel. (Original work published 1887)

Chodoff, P. (1974). The diagnosis of hysteria: An overview. *American Journal of Psychiatry, 131,* 1073–1078.

Chodoff, P., & Lyons, H. (1958). Hysteria, the hysterical personality, and "hysterical" conversion. *American Journal of Psychiatry, 114,* 734–740.

Coe, W. C. (1983). *Trance: A problematic metaphor for hypnosis.* Paper presented at the 91st annual meeting of the American Psychological Association, Anaheim, CA.

Darnton, R. (1970). *Mesmerism.* New York: Schocken Press.

Dingwall, E. J. (1968). *Abnormal hypnotic phenomena* (Vol. 1). New York: Barnes & Noble.

Drinka, G. F. (1984). *The birth of neurosis.* New York: Simon and Schuster.

Edelstein, E. J., & Edelstein, L. (1945). *Asclepius: A collection and interpretation of the testimonies* (2 vols.). Baltimore, MD: Johns Hopkins University Press.

Edmonston,, W. E. Jr. (1986). *The induction of hypnosis.* New York: Wiley.

Ellenberger, H. F. (1970). *The discovery of the unconscious.* New York: Basic Books.

Evans, M. B., & Paul, G. L. (1970). Effects of hypnotically suggested analgesia on physiological and subjective response to cold stress. *Journal of Consulting and Clinical Psychology, 35,* 362–371.

Frank, J. D. (1973). *Persuasion and healing: A comparative study of psychotherapy.* Baltimore, MD: Johns Hopkins University Press.

Garfinkel, H. (1967). *Studies in ethnomethodology.* Englewood Cliffs, NJ: Prentice-Hall.

Goffman, E. (1961). *Encounters: Two studies in the sociology of interaction.* Indianapolis, IN: Bobbs-Merrill.

Graham, K. R. (1970). Optokinetic nystagmus as a criterion of visual imagery. *Journal of Nervous and Mental Disease, 151,* 411–414.

Graham, K. R., & Patton, A. (1968). Retroactive inhibition, hypnosis, and hypnotic amnesia. *International Journal of Clinical and Experimental Hypnosis, 16,* 68–74.

Greaves, G. R. (1980). Multiple personality 165 years after Mary Reynolds. *Journal of Nervous and Mental Disease, 168,* 577–595.

Gruenewald, D. (1971). Hypnotic techniques without hypnosis in the treatment of a dual personality. *Journal of Nervous and Mental Disease, 168,* 577–595.

Hilgard, E. R. (1974). Toward a neodissociation theory: Multiple cognitive controls in human functioning. *Perspectives in Biology and Medicine, 17,* 301–316.

Hilgard, E. R. (1977a). *Divided consciousness.* New York: Wiley.

Hilgard, E. R. (1977b). The problem of divided consciousness: A neodissociation perspective. *Annals of the New York Academy of Sciences, 296,* 48–99.

Hilgard, E. R. (1979). Divided consciousness in hypnosis: The implications of the hidden observer. In E. Fromm & R. E. Shor (Eds.), *Hypnosis: Developments in research and new perspectives (2nd ed.).* Chicago: Aldine.

Hull, C. L. (1933). *Hypnosis and suggestibility.* New York: Appleton.

Janet, P. (1925). *Psychological healing* (2 vols.). New York: Macmillan.

Kerényi, C. (1960). *Asklepios: Archetypal image of the physician's existence* (R. Manheim, Trans.). London: Thames & Hudson. (Original work published 1947)

Kihlstrom, J. F. (1985). Hypnosis. *Annual Review of Psychology, 36,* 385–418.

Kihlstrom, J. F., Evans, F. J., Orne, M. T., & Orne, E. C. (1980). Attempting to breach posthypnotic amnesia. *Journal of Abnormal Psychology, 89,* 603–616.

Kluft, R. P. (1982). Varieties of hypnotic interventions in the treatment of multiple personality. *American Journal of Clinical Hypnosis, 24,* 230–240.

Kohlenberg, R. J. (1973). Behavioristic approach to multiple personality: A case study. *Behavior Therapy, 4,* 137–140.

Kroger, W. S., & Fezler, W. D. (1976). *Hypnosis and behavior modification: Imagery conditioning.* Philadelphia: Lippincott.

Leifer, R. (1969). *In the name of mental health: The social functions of psychiatry.* New York: Science House.

Ludwig, A. M. (1964). An historical survey of the early roots of mesmerism. *International Journal of Clinical and Experimental Hypnosis, 12,* 205–217.

Ludwig, A. M., Brandsma, J. M., Wilbur, C. B., Benfeldt, F., & Jameson, D. H. (1972). The objective study of a multiple personality: Or, are four heads better than one? *Archives of General Psychiatry, 26,* 298–310.

MacHovec, F. J. (1975). Hypnosis before Mesmer. *American Journal of Clinical Hypnosis, 17,* 215–220.

MacHovec, F. J. (1979). The cult of Asklipios. *American Journal of Clinical Hypnosis, 22,* 85–90.

Mesmer, F. A. (1980). *Mesmerism* (G. J. Bloch, Ed. and Trans.). Los Altos, CA: Kaufmann. (Original work published 1781)

Mitchell, M. B. (1932). Retroactive inhibition and hypnosis. *Journal of General Psychology, 7,* 343–358.

Oesterreich, T. K. (1966). *Possession: Demoniacal and other.* Secaucus, NJ: Citadel Press.

Orne, M. T. (1959). The nature of hypnosis: Artifact and essence. *Journal of Abnormal and Social Psychology, 58,* 277–299.

Orne, M. T., Dinges, D. F., & Orne, E. C. (1984). On the differential diagnosis of multiple personality in the forensic context. *International Journal of Clinical and Experimental Hypnosis, 32,* 118–169.

Owen, A. R. G. (1971). *Hysteria, hypnosis, and healing.* London: Dobson.

Pattie, F. A. (1956). Theories of hypnosis. In R. M. Dorcus (Ed.), *Hypnosis and its therapeutic applications.* New York: McGraw-Hill.

Phillips, E. D. (1973). *Greek medicine.* London: Thames & Hudson.

Prince, M. (1930). *The dissociation of personality.* London: Longmans, Green.

Pulos, L. (1980). Mesmerism revisited: The effectiveness of Esdaile's techniques in the production of deep hypnosis and total body hypnoanaesthesia. *American Journal of Clinical Hypnosis, 22,* 206–211.

Rose, L. (1971). *Faith healing.* Middlesex: Penguin.

Rosenbaum, M. (1980). The role of the term schizophrenia in the decline of diagnoses of multiple personality. *Archives of General Psychiatry, 37,* 1383–1385.

Sarbin, T. R. (1962). Attempts to understand hypnotic phenomena. In L. Postman (Ed.), *Psychology in the making.* New York: Knopf.

Sarbin, T. R. (1967). The concept of hallucination. *Journal of Personality, 35,* 359–380.

Sarbin, T. R. (1983). *A contextual analysis of nonvolition in hypnosis.* Paper presented at the 91st annual convention of the American Psychological Association, Anaheim, CA.

Sarbin, T. R., & Allen, V. C. (1966). Role therapy. In G. Lindzey & E. Aronson (Eds.), *The handbook of social psychology* (Vol. 1). Reading, MA: Addison-Wesley.

Sarbin, T. R., & Coe, W. C. (1972). *Hypnotic behavior: The psychology of influence communication.* New York: Holt.

Sarbin, T. R., & Slagle, R. W. (1979). Hypnosis and psychophysiological outcomes. In E. Fromm & R. E. Shor (Eds.), *Hypnosis: Developments in research and new perspectives.* (2nd ed.). Chicago: Aldine.

Schein, E. H., Schneier, I., & Barker, C. H. (1961). *Coercive persuasion: A sociopsychological analysis of the "brainwashing" of American civilian prisoners by the Chinese communists.* New York: Norton.

Schwarz, J. R. (1981). *The Hillside strangler: A murderer's mind.* New York: New American Library.

Sheehan, P. W. (1979). Hypnosis and the process of imagination. In E. Fromm & R. E. Shor (Eds.), *Hypnosis: Developments in research and new perspectives* (2nd ed.). Chicago: Aldine.

Slater, E. (1965). Diagnosis of "hysteria." *British Medical Journal, 29,* 1395–1399.

Smith, R. D., Buffington, P. W., & McCard, R. H. (1982). *Multiple personality: Theory, diagnosis, and treatment.* New York: Irvington.

Smith-Rosenberg, C. (1972). The hysterical woman: Some reflections on sex roles and role conflict in 19th century America. *Social Research, 39,* 652–678.

Spanos, N. P. (1978). Witchcraft in histories of psychiatry: A critical analysis and an alternative conceptualization. *Psychological Bulletin, 85,* 417–439.

Spanos, N. P. (1982). A social psychological approach to hypnotic behavior. In G. Weary & H. L. Mirels (Eds.), *Integrations of clinical and social psychology.* New York: Oxford.

Spanos, N. P. (1983a). Demonic possession: A social psychological analysis. In M. Rosenbaum (Ed.), *Compliant behavior.* New York: Human Sciences Press.

Spanos, N. P. (1983b). The hidden observer as an experimental creation. *Journal of Personality and Social Psychology, 44,* 170–176.

Spanos, N. P. (1986a). Hypnotic behavior: A social-psychological interpretation of amnesia, analgesia, and "trance logic." *Behavioral and Brain Sciences, 9,* 449–467.

Spanos, N. P. (1986b). Hypnosis, nonvolitional responding, and multiple personality: A social psychological perspective. In B. Maher & W. Maher (Eds.), *Progress in experimental personality research* (Vol. 14). New York: Academic Press.

Spanos, N. P. (in press). Hypnosis, demonic possession, and multiple personality: Strategic enactments and disavowals of responsibility for actions. In C. Ward (Ed.), *Altered states of consciousness and mental health: A cross-cultural perspective.* New York: Sage.

Spanos, N. P., & Barber, T. X. (1972). Cognitive activity during hypnotic suggestion: Goal-directed fantasy and the experience of nonvolition. *Journal of Personality, 40,* 510–524.

Spanos, N. P., Bridgeman, M., Stam, H. J., Gwynn, M., & Saad, C. L. (1983). When seeing is not believing: The effects of contextual variables on the reports of hypnotic simulators. *Imagination, Cognition, and Personality, 2,* 195–209.

Spanos, N. P., Cobb, P. N., & Gorassini, D. R. (1985). Failing to resist hypnotic test suggestions: A strategy for self-presenting as deeply hypnotized. *Psychiatry, 48,* 282–292.

Spanos, N. P., & de Groh, M. M. (1983). Structure of communication and reports of involuntariness by hypnotic and nonhypnotic subjects. *Perceptual and Motor Skills, 57,* 1179–1186.

Spanos, N. P., & de Groh, M. M. (1984). *Effects of active and passive wording on response to hypnotic and nonhypnotic instructions for complete and selective forgetting.* Unpublished manuscript, Carleton University, Ottawa, Canada.

Spanos, N. P., de Groot, H. P., Tiller, D. K., Weekes, J. R., & Bertrand, L. D. (1985). "Trance logic" duality and hidden observer responding in hypnotic, imagination control, and simulating subjects: A social psychological analysis. *Journal of Abnormal Psychology, 94,* 611–623.

Spanos, N. P., & Gorassini, D. R. (1984). Structure of hypnotic test suggestions and attributions of responding involuntarily. *Journal of Personality and Social Psychology, 46,* 688–696.

Spanos, N. P., & Gottlieb, J. (1979). Demonic possession, mesmerism, and hysteria: A social psychological perspective on their historical interrelations. *Journal of Abnormal Psychology, 88,* 527–546.

Spanos, N. P., Gwynn, M. I., & Stam, H. J. (1983). Instructional demands and ratings of overt and hidden pain during hypnotic analgesia. *Journal of Abnormal Psychology, 92,* 479–488.

Spanos, N. P., & Hewitt, E. C. (1980). The hidden observer in hypnotic analgesia: Discovery or experimental creation? *Journal of Personality and Social Psychology, 39,* 1201–1214.

Spanos, N. P., Radtke, H. L., & Bertrand, L. D. (1984). Hypnotic amnesia as a strategic enactment: Breaching amnesia in highly susceptible subjects. *Journal of Personality and Social Psychology, 47,* 1155–1169.

Spanos, N. P., Radtke-Bodorik, H. L., Ferguson, J. D., & Jones, B. (1979). The effects of hypnotic susceptibility, suggestions for analgesia, and the utilization of cognitive strategies on the reduction of pain. *Journal of Abnormal Psychology, 88,* 282–292.

Spanos, N. P., Rivers, S. M., & Ross, S. (1977). Experienced involuntariness and response to hypnotic suggestions. *Annals of the New York Academy of Science, 296,* 208–221.

Spanos, N. P., Weekes, J. R., & Bertrand, L. D. (1985). Multiple personality: A social psychological perspective. *Journal of Abnormal Psychology, 94,* 362–376.

Spanos, N. P., Weekes, J. R., Menary, E., & Bertrand, L. D. (1986). Hypnotic interview and age regression procedures in the elicitation of multiple personality symptoms: A simulation study. *Psychiatry, 49,* 298–311.

Stam, H. J., & Spanos, N. P. (1982). The Asclepian dream healings and hypnosis: A critique. *International Journal of Clinical and Experimental Hypnosis, 30,* 9–22.

Stevenson, D. R., Stoyva, J., & Beach, H. D. (1962). Retroactive inhibition and hypnosis. *Bulletin of the Maritime Psychological Association, 11,* 11–15.

Stocking, G. W. (1965). On the limits of "presentism" and "historicism" in the historiography of the behavioral sciences. *Journal of the History of the Behavioral Sciences, 1,* 211–218.

Sutcliffe, J. P., & Jones, J. (1962). Personal identity, multiple personality, and hypnosis. *International Journal of Clinical and Experimental Hypnosis, 10,* 231–269.

Szasz, T. S. (1961). *The myth of mental illness.* New York: Hoeber-Harper.

Taylor, W. S., & Martin, M. F. (1944). Multiple personality. *Journal of Abnormal and Social Psychology, 39,* 281–300.

Thigpen, C. H., & Cleckley, H. (1957). *The three faces of Eve.* New York: Fawcett.

Ullmann, L. P., & Krasner, L. (1969). *A psychological approach to abnormal behavior.* Englewood Cliffs, NJ: Prentice-Hall.

Veith, I. (1965). *Hysteria.* Chicago: University of Chicago Press.

Wagstaff, G. F. (1981). *Hypnosis, compliance, and belief.* New York: St. Martin's Press.

Watkins, J. G., & Johnson, R. J. (1982). *We, the divided self.* New York: Irvington.

Weitzenhoffer, A. M. (1974). When is an "instruction" an "instruction"? *International Journal of Clinical and Experimental Hypnosis, 22,* 258–269.

Weitzenhoffer, A. M., & Hilgard, E. R. (1959). *Stanford hypnotic susceptibility scale, forms A and B.* Palo Alto, CA: Consulting Psychologists Press.

White, R. W., & Shevach, B. J. (1942). Hypnosis and the concept of dissociation. *Journal of Abnormal and Social Psychology, 37,* 309–328.

Ziegler, F. J., & Imboden, J. B. (1962). Contemporary conversion reactions: II. Conceptual model. *Archives of General Psychiatry, 66,* 279–287.

Zilboorg, G., & Henry, G. W. (1941). *A history of medical psychology.* New York: Norton.

10

Current Conceptual Trends in Biofeedback and Self-Regulation

PATRICIA NORRIS

The spirit is the master, imagination the tool, and the body the plastic material. . . . The power of the imagination is a great factor in medicine. It may produce diseases in man and in animals, and it may cure them. . . . Ills of the body may be cured by physical remedies or by the power of the spirit acting through the soul.

Paracelsus, Father of Modern Medicine

The field of biofeedback, formally, is about 20 years old; the term "biofeedback" was coined at the first meeting of the Biofeedback Society of America (then named the Biofeedback Research Society) in 1969. However, the first psychophysiology experiment using biological feedback to the subject was probably that conducted by J. H. Bair at the turn of the century (Bair, 1901). He undertook a study to teach subjects to activate the muscles used to wiggle their ears. Using mechanical levers that transmitted a tiny pressure change to a steel pen that scratched paper on a revolving drum, he provided the subjects with immediate feedback of their efforts. Soon they were able to learn to twitch their ears. He also recorded careful introspections of the accompanying mental states. Bair conducted the study because of his interest in volition and his desire to explore the nature of the will.

For most of this century there was little interest in volition, awareness, and introspection. A resurgence of these interests in the early sixties led to the exploration of self-regulation using feedback. Presently biofeedback work, especially in research, is conducted under two separate and distinct conceptual paradigms—(1) the drug and operant conditioning model and (2) the self-regulation model. The drug model and the operant conditioning model of research assumes that "specific effects" of biofeedback can and should be studied independently of subject variables such as expectations, instructions and strategies, and relaxation (Shellenberger & Green, 1986). This dualistic approach, which tries to separate any mental and psychological events from the biological changes being monitored, is in contrast to the self-regulation model, which is based on the principles that psyche and physiology are inseparable, that any perturbation of one results in comparable and complementary change in the other, and that this fact must be taken into account in any research or clinical therapy with biofeedback.

Clinical work, too, has been provided under both these models, but it seems clear that as clinicians continue the use of biofeedback in therapy, they move more and more into the area of self-regulation. With the advent of a capacity to provide moment-by-moment biological feedback, certain distinctions existing previously in modern, Western scientific paradigms—distinctions between conscious and unconscious processes, between cortical and subcortical processes, between the voluntary and involuntary nervous systems—are being eroded. Control of the autonomic nervous system is no longer conceptualized as being only unconscious and involuntary. Self-regulation and voluntary control have a history that goes back thousands of years and has roots in both the East and the West. In the last decade, advances in physical and biological sciences have begun to elucidate the mechanisms necessary to transform these long-standing empirical sciences into modern technological science. In this chapter, some of these conceptual trends, connected with the self and with volition, will be explored and the importance and usefulness of this approach will be discussed.

Emotion, Cognition, and Volition

In the past decade there has been an explosion of new research and new knowledge in the areas of brain biochemistry and neurobiology highlighted by the discovery of the endorphins and a myriad of neuropeptides. The role of the limbic system and the hypothalamic-pituitary axis in human emotions, as well as the biochemical basis of these emotions, and their integration with higher cognitive functions is beginning to be understood. It is the limbic-hypothalamic-pituitary axis that has been conceptualized as the biologic basis, the rationale, for the mediation of biofeedback-assisted self-regulation (Green, Green, & Walters, 1970). See Figure 10.1, page 269.

It is commonly accepted that emotional states have a role in health and disease and in immune functioning. It is now becoming evident that the neuropeptides provide a physiologic basis for emotions. Very recent discoveries have shown that the neuropeptides are "immunopeptides" as well—that is, the cells of the immune system not only have receptors for the various neuropeptides, but they also make these neuropeptides themselves (Pert, Ruff, Weber, & Herkenham, 1985).

A new field of self-regulation, variously termed "psychoneuroimmunology," "neuroimmunomodulation," or, more simply, "behavioral immunology"—mind and immunity—sheds new light on the old mind-body problem. Self-regulation, learned with biofeedback and visualization, demonstrates that what we think and feel and visualize have biological consequences that can promote healing. Biofeedback provides the modern, technological objectification and verification of the effects of emotions, cognitions, and visualizations on physiological processes, which in turn mediate visceral behavior and immune system behavior.

To a certain degree, concepts of biofeedback and self-regulation training combine Eastern and Western approaches to healing. The present trends in biofeedback therapy are both a reflection of and a contribution to current trends in self-regulation therapies. This is especially true of the psychologies related to healing and psychophysiological psychotherapy. The renewed interest in psychosomatic medicine and the emerging and rapidly expanding field of psychoneuroimmunology attest to the fact that the psyche is reemerging in psychology.

It has been said that in an attempt to separate itself from religion and to emulate physics and hard science, in the old Newtonian model, psychology first lost its soul, then lost its mind, and finally lost consciousness! But now, it seems, psychology has regained consciousness and is awake and moving again.

Consciousness has reentered the theoretical framework of behaviorism in cognitive-behavioral therapy. The cognitive therapy movement has its basis in the view that beliefs interact with situational factors to result in feelings and behaviors (Emery & Tracy, 1987). For Beck and Emery (1985), cognitive-behavioral therapy consists of a series of strategies to correct distorted and maladaptive thinking, to restore health and healthy homeostatic functioning. The therapy is based on a theory of psychopathology that recognizes the reciprocal relationship between the cognitive, emotional, somatic, and behavioral systems. This is similar, in the mind-body connection, to the psycho-physiological principle stated by Green and Green (1977) as part of the rationale for psychophysiological self-regulation (PSR):

> Every change in the physiological state is accompanied by an appropriate change in the mental-emotional state, conscious or unconscious; and conversely, every change in the mental-emotional state, conscious or unconscious, is accompanied by an appropriate change in the physiological state. . . . This [closed] principle, when coupled with volition, allows a natural process—*psychosomatic self-regulation*—to unfold. (pp. 33–34)

Self-regulation has been a part of the lexicon of biofeedback training and therapy since the term "biofeedback" was first chosen in 1969 to describe the investigations into voluntary control of various internal processes (Basmajian, 1963; Brener & Hothersall, 1966; Brown, 1970; Budzynski, Stoyva, & Adler, 1970; Green, Green, & Walters, 1969; Hnatiow & Lang, 1965; Kamiya, 1962, 1968; Mulholland & Runnals, 1962; Peper & Mulholland, 1970; Stern & Lewis, 1968). Much of the early work was collected in the *Aldine Annuals* (1970–1978) under the title "Biofeedback and Self-Control." The Biofeedback Society of America titled its journal *Biofeedback and Self-Regulation.* In an editorial in the journal's first issue, Johann Stoyva (1976) defined self-regulation as "the endeavor to modify voluntarily one's own physiological activity, behavior, or process of consciousness" (p. 2).

The Idea of a Volitional Self

It has not been obvious to everyone working in the area of biofeedback what has always been implicit in the idea of feed*back*—namely, that feedback is feed-back to a *self* and that voluntary control over usually unconscious autonomic processes, autonomic self-regulation, by definition means *conscious* self-regulation. If it is not conscious, it is not intentional, and if it is not intentional, it is not voluntary control.

The study of consciousness and volition is playing an increasingly important role in the behavioral sciences. Although controversies are not all resolved, concepts of a volitional self permeate the paradigms of all the behavioral sciences. In psychodynamic psychotherapy, a psychology of the self is articulated by Heinz Kohut (1977). In *The Restoration of the SELF,* Kohut and his followers place the self at the center of personality development and examine the role of the self in health and disease. Concepts of consciousness, belief, meaning, and volition in theories of behaviorism and cognitive behavior therapy are compared and contrasted by top practitioners in these fields (Michelson & Ascher, 1987). For comprehensive examinations of the importance of self, consciousness, and volition in biofeedback training and psychophysiological therapy, see Green (1979), Green and Green (1977), Green, Green, & Walters (1969, 1970), Lacroix (1986), Norris (1986), and Shellenberger and Green (1986).

Biofeedback and Self-Regulation

Biofeedback training is the continuous monitoring and amplifying of an ongoing biological process of a person, and the feeding back or displaying of this information to that person's cortex, to their conscious awareness. This allows the individual to intentionally self-regulate the physiological activity being monitored by observing the effects of each self-regulation strategy. Many physiological processes have been thus monitored and fed back, and regulated or influenced by the observing self. These include heart rate and other cardiac behavior, vascular changes, hydrochloric acid production, gastrointestinal motility, striate muscle activity, brain rhythms, evoked potentials, and even blood glucose and insulin levels.

Learning to modify or regulate a physiological process—that is, training the whole body—actually means training the central nervous system. For example, training for vascular changes in the hands, or in any other part of the body, is really training the part of the hypothalamus that regulates blood flow to that part of the body to respond to visualization and the intention to make the change. We are not directly aware of our central nervous system, of course, but only of contents of consciousness.

It is becoming apparent, and acceptable, that consciousness and volition are the most essential factors in developing self-regulation skills in the central nervous system, regardless of which neurologic and biochemical mechanisms of the body and brain are employed. This is equally true of striate and neuromuscular skills and of smooth muscle and autonomic skills. Memory in the body is not really in the tissues, for either type of activity, but is stored in appropriate brain centers. Whether we are learning to walk, serve a tennis ball, decrease gastrointestinal motility, or regulate heart rate, we are not really training our body, we are training our brain. We are gaining cortical control over subcortical processes. We are learning to exert conscious control over the unconscious.

Figure 10.1 is a cybernetic model of the underlying neurological and psychological principles (Green & Green, 1977). The caption explains in

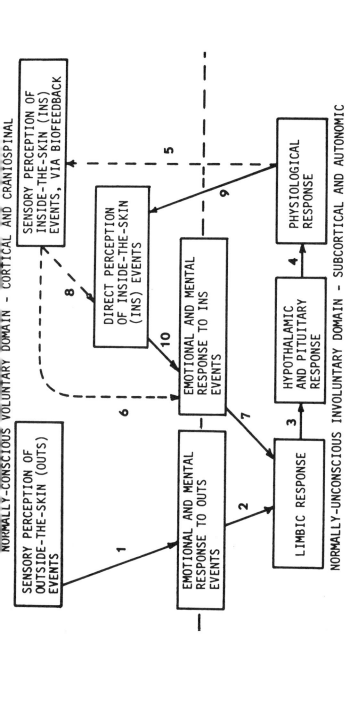

FIGURE 10.1. Simplified operational diagram of self-regulation of psychophysiologic processes. Sensory perception of external event leads to a physiologic response along arrows 1 to 4. When the physiologic response is monitored and displayed (arrow 5) to a person, the emotional and mental response to the feedback (arrow 6) results in a new limbic response. This in turn effects the neural-humoral pathways (arrows 3 and 4) modifying the physiologic response, completing the feedback loop and facilitating voluntary control. Biofeedback practice increases a person's sensitivity to internal events, and arrow 8 develops, followed by arrows 9 and 10. External feedback becomes unnecessary as direct perception of inside-the-skin events becomes sufficient for maintaining self-regulation skills. Reprinted with permission from Green & Green (1977).

condensed form how the system works. The central nervous system is represented, as well as the emotional and mental parts of ourselves of which we are most aware. This is a highly simplified diagram of processes that occur simultaneously in the voluntary and involuntary neurological domain and in the conscious and unconscious psychological domain. The upper half of the diagram represents the normal domain of conscious processes—processes that take place in awareness or have ready accesses to awareness. The boxes labeled "emotional and mental response" have been placed on the midline of the diagram, divided by the horizontal center line into conscious and unconscious parts in order to show that they are partly conscious and partly unconscious.

The lower half of the diagram represents processes of which we are normally unaware. The basic neurological and neurohumoral information associated with the diagram was known several decades ago (MacLean, 1949; Masserman, 1941; Papez, 1937; Penfield & Rasmussen, 1950). Both Masserman and MacLean published their articles in *Psychosomatic Medicine*. Masserman showed that the hypothalamus was not the "seat of the emotions," as had been thought, and MacLean identified the limbic system as the "visceral brain," the emotional brain, implicated in psychosomatic disease. However, even though the physiological and psychological processes may be as intimately related as the two halves of a zipper, it is increasingly being recognized that the mind-body system is open, not closed, and can be directed or programmed by volition.

The most significant implication of Figure 10.1 is that self-regulation training is first of all *awareness training* (direct perception of internal processes, see arrow 9); second, it is a potent tool in *visualization training*, as intentionality is brought to bear, via visualization, to create physiological change (see arrows 10, 7, 3, 4, and 9).

Yoga and Self-Regulation

For the last 5,000 years, the self-regulation experts of India have taught their students to consciously self-regulate their psychological and psychophysiological processes. Many other people around the world have used various aspects of self-regulation in their rituals, particularly in healing rituals, for centuries.

When Elmer and Alyce Green established the Voluntary Controls Program at the Menninger Foundation and began speaking and writing about voluntary control of internal states, many people mistakenly equated self-regulation of biological processes with paranormal capacities. The news that migraine patients were self-regulating an autonomic process (vascular behavior) to ameliorate headaches led to opportunities to examine individuals who had accomplished self-regulation. Daniel Ferguson, chief of psychosomatic services at the Veterans Administration Hospital in St. Paul, Minnesota, and a graduate of the Menninger School of Psychiatry, brought a yogi, Swami Rama, to the Voluntary Controls Program in 1970. Ferguson and two other physicians had observed the Swami obliterate his pulse and make other striking physiological changes during a cardiovascular examination. Ferguson thought that since yoga and biofeedback are both methods of teaching self-regulation, they might have something in common, and perhaps a study in Elmer Green's lab at the Menninger Foundation could find out what was actually happening. Eventually, Swami Rama came to the Menninger Foundation for a 5-week period, during which a series of experiments were conducted.

In one experiment, the Swami stopped his heart from pumping blood by deliberately putting it into atrial flutter for 17 seconds. During this time, his heart rate averaged 360 beats per minute. The EKG record of this experiment (Figure 10.2) was shown to a cardiologist at the Kansas University Medical Center, who identified it as atrial flutter. The chambers of the heart do not fill properly, the valves do not work properly, the pulse vanishes, and blood pressure drops precipitously. This state is often followed by full cardiac arrest. In this case, however, the Swami drew in his solar plexus, took a breath, and restored his heart beat to normal. His wires were removed, and he gave a lecture on how it was done.

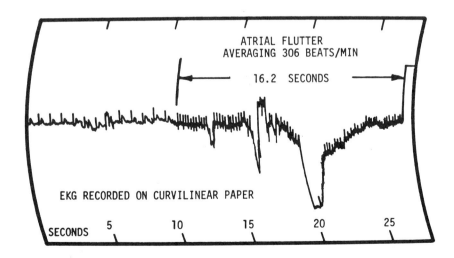

FIGURE 10.2   Voluntary atrial flutter demonstration by Swami Rama, The Menninger Foundation, 1970. Reprinted with permission from Green & Green (1977).

In another experiment, the Swami controlled vascular behavior in his hand so that two areas of his right palm, 2 inches apart, were made to differ by 10° Fahrenheit. He said that he would cause the left side of his right hand to increase in temperature and the right side to decrease. Thermistors were attached to the two sides of his palm (see Figure 10.3), and his hands were placed palm up on a plywood platform in front of him. During the experiment, which lasted about 20 minutes, he did not move his hands. They remained in an open, palms-up, relaxed position.

Swami Rama said that this particular feat was one of the hardest psychophysiological controls he had learned, even more difficult than "heart stopping." Therefore, it is of significance for biofeedback that a college graduate student, upon learning of this demonstration, taught himself to accomplish the same voluntary control of blood flow to the two sides of his hands in 1 week. He was able to do this because he had the assistance of two thermal biofeedback machines to give him a second-by-second display of his efforts to control differential palm temperatures. For the Swami, it was necessary to focus upon the most subtle sensory and attentional cues, and a change probably had to be significant before he could detect it. For the student, a change as slight as

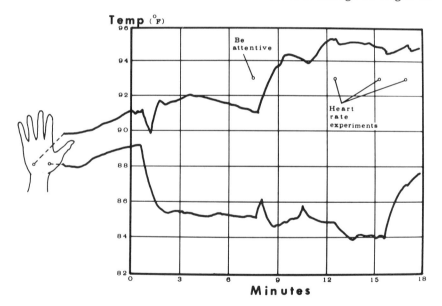

FIGURE 10.3 Simultaneous warming and cooling of the hand. Swami Rama's demonstration of voluntary control of blood flow in the right hand caused the left side to become pink and the right side gray. Reprinted with permission from Green & Green (1977).

$1/100°$ F was instantly made visible via the biofeedback instruments. By constantly monitoring the effects of his visualizations, he easily gained similar control of the vascular behavior of his hands. Swami Rama immediately saw that biofeedback instruments were useful and wanted to take some with him back to India. He thought biofeedback could be useful for speeding up certain aspects of yogic training, and furthermore, he thought biofeedback monitoring of internal processes could help "separate the fakers from the fakirs" (Green & Green, 1977).

Self-regulation is greatly facilitated and enhanced by the use of biofeedback. Biofeedback serves as a human sensory extension, in the same way that a telescope or a microscope serves as a sensory extension. Thermal biofeedback with a meter or digital display allows one to see directly the increase or decrease of circulation in the area of the body where the thermistor is placed. Heart rate biofeedback allows one to see directly beat-by-beat changes in heart rate and thus to detect changes that accompany any intentional strategies to increase or decrease heart rate.

Later another expert of self-regulation, Jack Schwarz, demonstrated control of pain and bleeding in the lab by thrusting a 7-inch sailmaker's needle through his biceps, while simultaneously maintaining autonomic calm, demonstrated by warm hands, a calm pulse, and predominately alpha brain rhythms. Eventually, Alyce, Elmer, and Judith Green and Elda Hartley took a portable psychophysiological laboratory to India and examined a number of individuals with superior voluntary control. They then produced a film called *Biofeedback: The Yoga of the West* (Hartley, 1974).

The important point of dramatic instances of self-control, from cardiovascular self-regulation and pain control to fire walking, is that they represent aspects of hidden human potential, a part of our heritage as conscious, volitional human beings. These demonstrations and research findings have powerful implications for self-regulation and self-healing.

HIERARCHY OF SELF-REGULATION

The scientific study of self-regulation in western European societies began around the middle of the 19th century, when medical and biological scientists turned their attention to hypnosis, self-suggestion, and the scientific study of learning. Although I. P. Pavlov is best known for his work in classical conditioning, according to A. S. Romen, a Russian psychiatrist, his investigations were particularly significant in structuring a scientific approach to psychophysiological self-regulation. He proposed and supported a materialistic basis for the study of hypnotic suggestion and self-suggestion. He addressed the problem of sleep and the physiological understanding of hysteria (Pavlov, 1951; Romen, 1981). Clinical hypnotists such as Janet, Charcot, and Mesmer laid an early foundation for psychophysiological change resulting from hypnotic suggestion, and during the first half of this century scientific study of self-regulation through voluntary control of internal states got underway (Jacobson, 1938; Luthe, 1965; Schultze & Luthe, 1959). Hypnosis as a therapeutic tool is again gaining prominence and is frequently used in combination with biofeedback and other psychophysiological therapy techniques (Brown & Fromm, 1987; Wickramasekera, 1976).

Healing that takes place with biofeedback-assisted self-regulation is sometimes dismissed as a suggestion effect or as a placebo effect. This, however, does not really constitute a dismissal. Neither the power of suggestion nor the placebo effect is a fake. The *power* of suggestion lies in the physiological changes that take place as a result of it; and the *effect* of the placebo is the physiological effect that occurs as a result of what the recipient believes the placebo to be. Any internal physiological response to hypnotic suggestion, to a placebo, to self-hypnosis and self-suggestion, and to an image or visualization, is a self-regulation response. What differentiates them is the degree of conscious volition or intentionality employed. We can think of these in terms of a hierarchy of self-regulation, with the position on the hierarchy determined by the degree of awareness and volition; at the top of the hierarchy lies voluntary control.

Placebo Effect as Self-Regulation

Placebos are, by definition, inactive. But the placebo effect is both active and specific. The same inactive ingredient—a "sugar pill"—can cause nausea and vomiting when posing as an emetic, pain relief when posing as an analgesic, sleepiness when posing as a hypnotic, and wakefulness when posing as an amphetamine. The reaction, of course, is caused by the "name"—the meaning—given to the placebo and by the ensuing visualization and expectation of the named change occurring, not by the contents of the pill.

In one well-known experiment, a group of women with continuous, severe morning sickness were given either an antiemetic or a placebo. A number of the women responded to the placebo with cessation of the nausea and vomiting. In the next phase of the experiment, these women were given ipecac, a powerful emetic, still under the guise of an *anti*emetic, with no return of their nausea. Their self-regulation, brought about by visualizing the cessation of nausea, had more powerful effects than the emetic.

Effects on Physiology of Suggestion

Suggestion can have a powerful effect on physiology if it is accompanied by belief. A person may start sneezing on seeing a bowl of artificial flowers of a type to which they are allergic, because they believe them to be real. Upon learning that they are artificial, the sneezing stops. In the first instance, the person visualized an allergic reaction, and the lower brain centers, which control that reaction, responded with the same neurohumoral sequelae that accompany exposure to an actual antigen. In the same way, healing suggestions can have remarkable effects. In the introduction to *The Healing Heart* (Cousins, 1983), Bernard Lown describes a patient who was critically ill with irreparably damaged cardiac muscle following a massive heart attack. With congested lungs, uncontrollably rapid heart rate, chaotic arrhythmia, and labored breathing, he required both oxygen and an intravenous drip of cardiac stimulant to keep him alive. On rounds at his bedside Dr. Lown told his attending staff that the patient's heart had a "wholesome, very loud third sound gallop," which denotes that the heart is straining to the point of failure. Following this, the patient unexpectedly improved and was discharged from the hospital. Later Dr. Lown asked him about his "miraculous" recovery, and he responded that he not only knew what had happened but even the exact moment when it happened.

> I was sure the end was near and you and your staff had given up hope. However, Thursday morning when you entered with your troops, something happened that changed everything. You listened to my heart; you seemed pleased by the findings and announced to all those standing about my bed that I had a wholesome gallop. I knew that the doctors, in talking to me, might try to soften things. But I knew they wouldn't kid each other. So when I heard you tell your colleagues I had a wholesome gallop, I figured I still had a lot of "kick" to my heart and could not be dying. My spirits were for the first time lifted, and I knew I would recover.

The perceived suggestion changed his belief, his visualization, and his heart behavior.

Barber (1984) made a thorough review of 30 years of research using suggestion to alter physiology, culminating with the unambiguous conclusion that words *can* direct specific autonomic physiological events. It seems clear that autonomic physiological control by suggestion is mediated in the same way that physiological control is mediated under any other circumstances, by the same limbic-hypothalamic-pituitary mechanisms that always mediate the autonomic process. As Green (1979) has pointed out, these lower brain centers behave in the same way (except perhaps in degree) whether the brain sees danger, thinks it sees danger, or imagines it sees danger. In other words, perception of an object and the image of that object are neurologically similar events in the cortex, and the lower brain centers cannot tell the difference.

Hypnotic Self-Regulation

In a hypnotherapy workshop conducted by Erika Fromm and Daniel Brown, I saw a wonderful film of a Cesarean section conducted with hypnosis, with no local or general anesthetic. The obstetrician performed both the surgery and the hypnosis, telling his patient just what he was doing as he was doing it and maintaining conversation with her. At the point when he was ready to open the uterus and lift out the baby, he informed her that he was ready to do so and would be very busy for the next few minutes but did not want to lose communication contact. He asked her if she could sing a song to welcome her baby into the world, which she proceeded to do, without a quiver in her voice.

Dentists have frequently used hypnosis to help patients experience pain-free extractions and fillings. During World War II, when narcotics were not always available, this was commonly practiced among military dentists. It was then a simple matter to add the instruction that there would be little bleeding and rapid healing, and indeed these patients did bleed less and did heal more rapidly than those receiving traditional anesthesia. At the Third International Congress on Ericksonian Approaches to Hypnosis and Psychotherapy, Kay Thompson, a Philadelphia dentist, reported that people with hemophilia, whose blood normally did not clot, could prevent themselves from bleeding during surgery and extractions, using self-hypnosis. Since it has been shown that with the aid of biofeedback both increase and decrease of blood flow to an area can be learned, such training could prove useful to individuals with hemophilia.

Theoretically, any process that can be controlled by hypnosis also can be controlled voluntarily without hypnosis. Obviously, the obstetrician had no internal control of the patient's body; the patient herself was controlling the internal events (relaxation, absence of pain) by self-regulation. In practice, however, it would be most difficult and beyond the capacity of most of us without training to undergo major surgery without either anesthesia or hypnosis. On the other hand, many people have learned to control the pain of minor surgery, dental procedures, and so on. When Jack Schwarz gave a demonstration of control of pain and bleeding at the Veterans Administration Hospital in Topeka, thrusting the large sailmaker's needle through his biceps, the feat was duplicated by a psychiatrist with only a slight prompting from Schwarz in the middle of the experiment, when the psychiatrist momentarily lost concentration and confidence.

Wadden and Anderton (1982) found in their review of the clinical uses of hypnosis that suggestion is largely ineffective for controlling behavior involving the skeletal muscle systems, such as eating behavior and smoking; in contrast, hypnotic suggestion does affect physiological responses involving the smooth muscle systems of the autonomic nervous system. For such physiological processes as gastric motility and secretions, cerebral blood flow, bronchial airway activity, and wart remission—all presumably outside an individual's control—verbal suggestions can produce greater physiological change. This general finding was reached by a large number of independent investigators who often noted the greater strength of the positive relationship between suggestion and the change in so-called involuntary processes. Biofeedback clinicians are finding the same thing to be true of visualization and intentionality; visualizations in the form of intentional formulas act with immediacy and directness on autonomic nervous system processes.

Voluntary Control of Internal States

Voluntary control speaks of volition and choice. With biofeedback, the effects of the suggestion, the belief, and the visualization on the internal process being monitored can be seen objectively. An important component of true self-regulation is *knowing* that we know. This is one of the ways in which awareness is essential to the operation of voluntary control. The ability of conscious intentions to influence the internal process being monitored are instantly available to consciousness. Eventually the person learning self-regulation knows just what to do and how to do it and can bring about the desired physiological change under essentially any circumstances. Psychophysiological self-regulation is really under *voluntary* control when one can exert this control "in the crunch," when one can warm hands and feet on a ski lift 50 feet above the ground in a cold wind or reduce autonomic arousal on an airplane that has gone into full emergency procedure because of engine trouble. For patients who need to reverse a severe symptom when it suddenly arises, such as extreme tachycardia, a rheumatoid arthritis flare up, or colonic spasm, this degree of voluntary control is essential. The importance of this is clearly illustrated by the following case.

Mary D. is a 35-year-old married professional woman with one child. She has Marfan's syndrome, characterized by tall stature, joint hyperextensability, scoliosis, and ocular and cardiovascular abnormalities. Despite these conditions, she was in good health until she suddenly suffered an "aortic dissection" that occurred while she was driving her car. She managed to stop her car and, realizing no one would stop, rolled out on the highway before she lost consciousness. Shortly after being taken to the hospital, she had open-heart surgery. She received an aortic valve replacement and bypass grafts of her aorta and pulmonary vein. She has a double-barreled aorta resulting from the dissecting aneurysm, which reaches down nearly to the juncture of the femoral arteries. She was referred for psychophysiological therapy by one of her physicians for the amelioration of resulting symptoms (e.g., shortness of breath, loss of stamina, and anxiety). She was initially heavily stressed, fearing that death was imminent. With the aid of biofeedback training, she learned to deepen her breathing, increase circulation to any desired area of her body, and to slow her heart rate. She is now able to control stress reactions and prevent the vasoconstriction that normally accompanies stress and arousal. She has learned to avoid additional strain on her heart and on the aorta, without having to avoid the vicissitudes of life.

At the beginning of therapy, when stress of any sort caused her heart rate to increase noticeably, she could hear her heart rate increase, which would cause fear and panic. The sound made by her artificial aortic valve is clearly heard by anyone sitting next to her and sounds quite loud internally. Hearing this increase would cause her heart to beat faster still, and a vicious circle of anxiety and accelerating heart rate would ensue. At these times, she would feel quite out of control and at the mercy of her body. During self-regulation training, as she gained confidence in her ability to control autonomic symptoms of stress, the situation changed. Now when she hears her aortic valve speeding up from stress or anxiety from any source, she almost always can reverse it by using self-regulation strategies she has learned (e.g., deep diaphragmatic breathing, peripheral vasodilation, and visualizing a calm and steady heart beat). For the most part, she feels in charge of her body's responses.

This degree of voluntary control is useful, and often necessary, to achieve. We have the potential to achieve this level of control over many autonomic processes, and thereby we can develop a much heightened sense of our own autonomy, healing ability, and self-mastery, psychologically as well as physiologically.

VOLUNTARY CONTROL AND HEALING

In the present decade, self-regulation strategies have found their way into virtually every clinical area, including both medical and psychological treatment. In fact, it is as mistaken to say that an illness is strictly physical or strictly psychological as it is to separate the mind from the body in a dualistic manner. The psychophysiological principle previously stated affirms that even a broken leg or any other physical malady resulting from an accident will generate mental and emotional changes that will affect healing. Likewise, every psychological illness is reflected in the body in a myriad of ways.

It has become fashionable to say that biofeedback is disappointing, not living up to its promise, by those ignoring the self-awareness–volition link. Meanwhile as biofeedback training has become more and more identified with self-regulation training and the acquisition of internal skills, a proliferation of biofeedback-assisted self-regulation techniques has occurred in many diverse areas of human health and performance. It would be impossible to cover all of them in this chapter; therefore, only a few areas representative of the changes taking place will be focused upon.

Everyone familiar with the biofeedback literature is familiar with the general postulate that any biological process that can be continuously monitored and fed back to an individual can be brought under some degree of conscious control. So far, I believe, this has been shown to be true. This concept can be expanded and made more specific with the statement that any internal process that can be triggered or controlled by suggestion, perception, experience of stress, or any psychological process *without* volition also potentially can be brought under *voluntary* control. It is a cortical-subcortical connection that we can learn to make voluntarily. This concept was expressed by Elmer Green (in Hartley, 1974): "If there is such a thing as psychosomatic illness, then obviously there is such a thing as psychosomatic health. . . . If we can make ourselves sick [involuntarily], then perhaps we can learn to [voluntarily] make ourselves well."

We have long known that the muscles of the heart, stomach, and intestines have responded to images and emotions; thinking of something frightful leads to fear, which leads to vascular and intestinal responses. Biofeedback is showing that these same "involuntary" muscles also respond to volition and visualization. Biofeedback is making this knowledge and these abilities accessible to everyone, and biofeedback is making our potential for conscious control of the unconscious scientific, measurable, and verifiable (Norris, 1986).

The *Diagnostic and Statistical Manual of Mental Disorders*, DSM-III-R (American Psychiatric Association, 1987), describes a major diagnostic category on Axis I as "Psychological Factors Affecting Physical Condition," stating that the category can be used to describe disorders that have been called "psychosomatic" or "psychophysiological." Common examples given include tension and migraine headache, angina pectoris, painful menstruation, sacroiliac pain, neurodermatitis, rheumatoid arthritis, asthma, tachycardia, arrhythmia, gastric ulcer, duodenal ulcer, cardiospasm, pylorospasm, nausea and vomiting, regional enteritis, ulcerative colitis, and frequency of micturition. These are all among the conditions that have been successfully treated with psychophysiological therapy, using biofeedback to objectify and verify self-regulation. These are examples of the psychophysiological disorders that are routinely treated in biofeedback and behavioral medicine clinics. Disorders of the circulatory system that can be controlled or eliminated with self-regulation include Raynaud's disease, Burger's disease, intermittent claudication and other peripheral vascular disorders, and circulatory complications accompanying diabetes and other illnesses. Respiratory disorders treated successfully for increased comfort and function include asthma, and chronic obstructive pulmonary diseases; gastrointestinal disorders include esophageal spasm, ulcers, irritable bowel syndrome, and inflammatory bowel disease; cardiovascular diseases include hypertension, tachycardia, preventricular contractions, and mitral valve prolapse. These are some of the major psychophysiological disorders especially amenable to improvement by self-regulation.

Anxiety disorders, including panic disorders and phobias of all sorts ranging from simple phobias (e.g., fear of snakes or writing checks) to complex disorders (e.g., agoraphobia), are treated effectively with biofeedback-assisted self-regulation training. Performance anxiety and test anxiety are situational problems that virtually disappear when psychophysiological self-regulation is learned to the point where it can be applied in a situation that otherwise would have triggered the anxiety attack.

The physiological concomitants—in fact, the diagnostic criteria—of anxiety disorders include: motor tension, which commonly takes the form of trembling, twitching, muscle tension and aches or soreness, restlessness, and easy fatigability (APA, 1987). If an individual learns neuromuscular control of various muscle groups and can quiet the muscles at any time, then, ipso facto, these symptoms do not appear. The diagnostic criteria of anxiety disorders also include *autonomic hyperactivity:* shortness of breath, tachycardia, sweating or cold, clammy hands, dry mouth, dizziness or lightheadedness, nausea, diarrhea, or other abdominal distress, hot or cold spells, frequent urination, and trouble swallowing. Since an individual can gain control of autonomic arousal, lower the autonomic tone to very relaxed levels, learn slow and deep diaphragmatic breathing, and learn to slow the heart rate voluntarily, then panic attacks can be aborted.

Following the discovery that humans could recognize and influence the production of and abundance of alpha brainwave rhythms (Kamiya, 1962, 1968), a number of interesting clinical uses of brainwave biofeedback emerged. It is noteworthy that one of these is in an area that might have seemed a very unlikely candidate for voluntary control—namely, the reduction and suppression of seizures in epilepsy (Finley, Smith, & Etherton, 1975; Lubar, 1975; Lubar & Bahler, 1976; Sterman, 1973). Barry Sterman's work with voluntary suppression of seizures began after he observed that some of the cats he had trained to produce sensory motor rhythm sleep spindles in some sleep studies were, at a later occasion, producing them to avoid seizures upon exposure to a convulsant in an unrelated experiment (Sterman, 1972). He observed this because each previously trained cat assumed a posture and stance associated with their earlier rewarded sleep spindle behavior. Cats not previously trained and exposed to the convulsant had seizures, and the trained cats had sleep spindles instead. Fortunately, Sterman immediately realized the possible significance of this and decided to try to same sensorimotor techniques with human subjects. Both research and clinical treatment protocols have grown continuously under Sterman's guidance since that time.

This work has evolved in a number of ways. Self-regulation of brain rhythms is being used by a growing number of clinicians in the treatment of epilepsy, and it also has been found useful in the treatment of various other conditions, including attention deficit disorders, pain, anxiety, obsessive-compulsive disorders, alcoholism, and insomnia.

The etiology of psychophysiological disorders is often complex and may include some genetic predisposition, as well as learned habitual response patterns to stress. Factors such as nutrition and exercise, psychodynamic and environmental stress, and target-organ vulnerability often play a role in the development of psychophysiological disorders. Psychophysiological therapy is multimodal and may include cognitive-behavioral strategies, counseling, suggestions for nutritional changes and for exercise. The major tools include biofeedback-assisted relaxation training, biofeedback-assisted systematic desensitization, deep diaphragmatic breathing, visualization, and exploration of preexisting conscious and unconscious imagery for discovering underlying meanings. Images of the psychophysiological process help in the construction of intentional, healthy visualizations.

PSYCHOPHYSIOLOGICAL HEALING AND CONSCIOUSNESS

Very frequently, when a person experiencing a psychophysiological disorder becomes deeply relaxed, underlying psychodynamic material related to their condition becomes available to consciousness. For this reason, psychotherapy is often greatly facilitated, on the one hand, and the psychogenic causes of the condition are uncovered and worked through, on the other. In such cases, it does not make sense to try to separate the psyche from the physiology in therapy.

Conscious-Unconscious Coordination

The following cases, with similar diagnoses (polycythemia and thrombocythemia, both myeloproliferative diseases) and similar consistent psychodynamic correlates, clearly illustrate this relationship between physical and psychological factors.

Some years ago, a colleague referred to us another professional therapist, a 40-year-old male psychologist in training analysis, who had a myeloproliferative disease expressing itself in severe thrombocytosis. His platelet counts were approximately four times normal, and chemotherapy to reduce his platelets was being contemplated by his hematologist. The colleague and the patient, Mark, lived in another state, and it was proposed that Mark come for a week or more of intensive therapy, a treatment paradigm already being used for cancer patients and others. Although I was unfamiliar with this condition, my colleague was convinced that the type of treatment program I use with cancer patients would be effective for this patient as well. Mark and I had several telephone conversations during which we decided that, if nothing else, the stress management aspects of the therapy would be worthwhile, especially since his thrombocytosis always worsened under stress. His thrombocytosis had been diagnosed following a routine blood test; he was asymptomatic. His platelet count was 1,265,000 (normal range is 200,000 to 400,000), and subsequent blood tests found his platelet count fluctuating in the 1,200,000 to 1,300,000 range.

Mark said he was fearful of the consequences of this disorder, including the danger of stroke due to arterial blocking, the possibility of internal bleeding (he said his platelets "in general" might not be much good), the possibility of myelofibrosis, and a risk of the illness going into leukemia. Certainly there was risk of leukemia, if not treated, and an even greater likelihood of eventually contracting leukemia if treated with chemotherapy.

Patient history revealed that his parents were last-moment escapees from the Holocaust. During the process, his mother suffered a miscarriage. A couple of years later, his parents were settled safely in a large city in the United States, and Mark was born. His infancy was fairly normal and happy, until at age 5, he contracted Reyes Syndrome. During its course, he experienced almost total loss of motor control, including the ability to walk, talk, feed himself, and control his bladder and bowel sphincters; he became like a helpless baby in diapers once again. He said this irreparably changed his relationship with his mother and created many psychological issues of protection, overcompensation, and overprotection.

Psychophysiological therapy consisted of training in self-regulation of autonomic nervous system responses, primarily by means of thermal training and breathing exercises; of neuromuscular relaxation to the point of muscle quietness; and of visualization and imagery techniques. Imagery was used to explore and bring to the surface unconscious images Mark held of his disease and also to explore associated emotional issues. Visualizations were employed as intentional formulas, to guide the body into more healthy ways of reacting and into a generally more favorable physiological state.

Initially Mark was extremely labile autonomically, and he was fascinated by identifying many of the thoughts and feelings that in him were associated with rapid increase of sympathetic arousal. We experimented with how contents of consciousness affected his sympathetic nervous system, reflected in electro-dermal response (EDR) and hand temperature responses. He practiced many hours a day and made voluminous notes and observations.

Prior to his arrival at the Menninger Biofeedback and Psychophysiology Center, Mark and I had discussed visualization procedures on the telephone, and he had formed some mental constructs of his bone marrow as being wildly proliferative, with the megakaryocytes (the developmental precursors of platelets) popping out platelets like steam out of a steam kettle. However, in the initial guided imagery tour of his body, all his images of bone marrow and the process of platelet formation were of barren and decimated areas; he found these images very surprising in view of his intellectual understanding of myeloproliferative processes. When he visualized his bones and bone marrow, he saw them as very empty with almost no platelets; but when he imagined his blood stream, it seemed stuffed with nothing but platelets.

Toward the middle of his stay, Mark became aware of feelings of anxiety and depression, particularly about the usefulness of visualization. As autonomic relaxation and exploratory imagery deepened, he began to have dreams and images of special meaning. A series of images reminded him of how hard it was for him to play as a child. He had images and memories of the beloved physician from his childhood who was like a father figure to the whole family, and whom he remembered not only as a mentor but also as being exceedingly protective. He also had informative images of his running; he had been running up to 30 miles a week, engaging in this activity in a serious, even harsh and punitive way. He began to understand his resistance to visualization, both in terms of a reluctance to play and also as a reluctance to assume *self*-regulation at the possible expense of giving up *external* protection. He then found it possible to come closer to his internal body images and to interact with them more, to feel emotionally and kinesthetically more connected to his body. He felt that he had passed the desire to see his blood as being good, but "keeping its distance," not wanting it to get too intimate, too "huggy-kissy" as he called it. Following this, the visualization process proceeded with ease.

By the time he was ready to return home, after a week of training, Mark was comfortable with two effective visualizations, (1) the quieting of the sympathetic activation of his bone marrow and (2) the production of platelets as normal and sufficient. He had also established an excellent degree of autonomic self-regulation.

In follow-up examinations, his platelet count has been going down for the last 4 years, although it still is not quite down to the normal range. About 6 months following his therapy, he had one platelet count over 1,000,000, which he was able to bring back down in less than a month, at the next test. This was the last time he had platelet counts that high. During the first year, counts were generally between 800,000 and 900,000. Two years later the counts were between 600,000 and 800,000, and he was planning to be married. Perhaps most importantly, he reports that "things changed enormously" in his life, in his attitude toward himself, his work, and his illness. He said that his training analyst told him that he was far less "doomsday" than he had been, and it started with his trip to Kansas. He said that he was making many changes in his ways of relating and, most significantly, *something* inside him felt very different. At present, 5 years later, he reports that he has had a continuous decrease of platelet counts (one count was close to the 400,000 range) and that he retains the other gains he has made.

Very shortly thereafter, the next patient with a myeloproliferative disorder was referred by his physician. George, a 43-year-old unemployed man from our local area, came once a week for self-regulation training. He had been diagnosed 4 1/2 years earlier with polycythemia vera, in which there is hyperplasia of all bone marrow elements (erythrocytes, megakaryocytes, granulocytes, and fibroblasts). His spleen was enlarged, he had headaches several times a week, and every 2 weeks he required a phlebotomy to withdraw a pint of blood. He also had experienced a loss of mental function, particularly memory function, including the ability to recognize common words, presumably as a result of brain ischemia due to blockage of microarterioles caused by the excessive production of blood platelets. In addition, he had gout. This could usually be controlled with Indocin, but the problem had been with him for 3 weeks without ceasing at the time he first was seen.

Treatment consisted of both thermal and muscle biofeedback. The goals were a daily period of deep relaxation of both autonomic and neuromuscular systems, defined by physiological parameters, and the ability to relax quickly when he experienced the onset of a stressor. Initially George exhibited considerable muscle tension as well as autonomic tension. As he learned to achieve deep autonomic relaxation, he began to talk about feelings of depression. He reported that both his siblings were handicapped (one was retarded and the other had had polio). His parents, and he himself, had relied upon him to be the healthy one and held high expectations for him, but they never recognized or praised his accomplishments. He frequently found himself feeling that he was not doing enough, not working hard enough, or giving up too easily. Remarkably, he also was a long-distance runner who would push himself hard, even to the point of crawling to finish the distance he had set out to attain.

By the 5th week of training, he reported that his hematocrit was 53, down from the previous reading of 61; he appeared less depressed and said that he had "decided to live," to see his kids grow up. He noted that, whereas his running had been punishment before, he was now taking a different attitude: for instance, he now took time off if he was tired instead of pushing and berating himself. He began to recognize that he always had been on guard against threats from outside, and he began to visualize that he was safe and secure, that nothing was attacking him.

Four months later, George had gone 4 months without a phlebotomy. He began a part-time job at a sheltered workshop for the mentally retarded and was feeling satisfaction at the contributions he was making. His relationships with his children and others were improving. He was playing more and controlling his temper better. At the end of treatment, after 7 months, he was much less depressed, had worked through issues of guilt and low self-esteem, and was much improved physically. This improvement has been sustained over the last 4 years.

The third patient was a 67-year-old woman, Martha, living with her husband in semiretirement. Initially she was referred by her physician for headaches that were a result of her diagnosed condition of essential thrombocytosis. Her physician was interested (if somewhat skeptical initially) to hear of the results of psychophysiological therapy on the blood disorders of the other two patients and looked forward to collaboration.

At first, the central dynamics for this patient did not seem similar to those of Mark and George. She was happily married, and her children were grown. As she began to acquire the ability to relax deeply, she began to experience recurrent old memories and sorrows regarding emotional hardships and pain experienced by her children when they were small. Then followed a series of images of her own childhood and of her mother during a period in which they experienced a great hardship. Her father left the family with no support, and her mother had to take in laundry. Martha became responsible for herself and her younger siblings, and for helping her mother eke out a meager subsistence.

Now she was becoming conscious of experiencing many threats to the well-being of her children, not only in the memory of their early years but also in the present.

When Martha began treatment, her platelet counts averaged 1,019,000. Her symptoms included frequent, intense headaches and chronic tiredness. She was motivated to improve her condition and eager to avoid imminent medical treatment. In a short time she mastered deep autonomic and neuromuscular relaxation, and she replaced rapid, shallow thoracic breathing with deep, relaxed diaphragmatic breathing. As we explored contributing events in her life she became aware of many times when she felt that a great deal of responsibility fell upon her shoulders, when she had to do well, push hard, and maintain strengths. Major events included the death of her oldest brother from a mastoid infection after a long illness just before he graduated from high school and the death of her second oldest brother in the war in 1943. She took care of her mother, who "had a very hard time of it," and they had to scrimp a good deal. Her father, who had returned home, often took the last penny for drinking and finally left the family permanently when Martha was a senior in high school. He never sent money for family support.

As Martha became increasingly able to master the physiological accompaniments of her worries, she became increasingly aware of her tendency to worry and feel anxious about life problems that her children were facing in their young adulthood. She became able to relate these fears to her own childhood, and she resolved a number of deeper fears and feelings of inadequacy to meet threats. During this time her platelet counts were decreasing slowly but steadily; quarterly tests showed platelet counts of 893,000, 853,000, 830,000, 735,000, and 726,000. She is headache free, has more energy, and feels the practice has added an important dimension to her life, quite apart from its effects on platelet counts. Chemotherapy to decrease platelets proliferation was avoided, and recently her physician told her that she needed to have blood tests only once a year.

These three cases illustrate something significant that investigators and clinicians are beginning to understand. It appears that the images we hold, consciously or unconsciously, tend to be implemented in the body. In the case of the polycythemia and thrombocythemia patients, the unconscious imagery seems to be, *no matter how much defense there is, it is not enough.* Throughout the ages some healers have maintained that consciousness and volition are the most crucial factors in health, and modern neurochemistry is beginning to unravel the mechanisms whereby this takes place. Consciousness, visualizations, and volition are triggers of neuropeptide action.

Neuroscientists have agreed for a long time that emotions are mediated by the limbic system of the brain. Also, it is becoming increasingly clear that the limbic system, the seat of emotions in the brain, is also the focal point of receptors for neuropeptides (Pert et al., 1985). According to Candace Pert, chief of brain biochemistry, neuroscience branch of the National Institutes of Mental Health, neuropeptide behavior is associated with specific states of consciousness and with alterations in those states. Can it be that the constant apprehension of possible threat on the part of these three patients generated neuropeptide signals to the bone marrow to strengthen the defensive system way beyond what was needed? Pert states further than when we document the key role that emotions, expressed through neuropeptide molecules, play in affecting the body, it will become clear how emotions can be a key to the understanding of disease.

Psychoneuroimmunology

The rapidly growing field of psychoneuroimmunology is also being furthered by advances in the study of neuropeptides and their receptors. Pert and her colleague Michael Ruff have found receptor sites on human monocytes for every neuropeptide they have studied. The emotion-affecting peptides actually appear to control the routing and migration of monocytes, which are so pivotal in immune system response. Pert points out that cells of the immune system not only have receptors for various neuropeptides, but also make the neuropeptides themselves; they can make the same chemicals that control mood in the brain. These findings are beginning to demonstrate the mechanisms for clinical psychoneuroimmunology. It is not just a question of "how the mind controls the body," but also of how the brain and the immune system influence and control each other. Thus thoughts, images, and visualizations appear to influence and control brain cells directly and immune cells indirectly.

Biofeedback has a crucial role to play in clinical psychoneuroimmunology. The role of stress in immune suppression is well established, and now studies are beginning to show that decreasing stress alone can produce immune enhancement. Barbara Peavey (1982) collected a group of 16 individuals with high stress and low immunity, measured by white cell count and by phagocytic capacity of neutrophils. She divided them into two groups and taught one group self-regulation and relaxation, using both EMG (for muscle relaxation) and temperature (for sympathetic nervous system relaxation) training, to criterion levels showing good relaxation; the other group served as controls. When the highly stressed biofeedback group learned to relax to criteria, there was a direct effect on immunity; their neutrophils were functioning significantly better than at their own pretreatment levels and also significantly better than the untreated controls.

However, the reason I teach voluntary control of as many physiological processes as possible to cancer patients and patients with other life-threatening illnesses is not primarily to manage stress, although managing stress is also of great value to these patients. Of primary importance is the gained *certainty*, experientially and existentially, that they *can* control these processes that are capable of being fed back. This builds confidence that they can equally influence processes that we do not at present have the capacity to monitor and feed back on a moment-by-moment basis, like increasing natural killer cell activity at a tumor site. The role of experience in changing one's belief system and one's world view cannot be overestimated (Norris, 1986).

The combination of biofeedback and imagery has proven to be an outstanding strategy for working with cancer patients. With biofeedback, patients learn to warm their hands, then their feet, and then any part of their body that they turn their attention to. Increasing circulation to an injured or hurting part of the body can reduce pain and promote healing, giving objective evidence of "doing some good" with visualizing. The patients also learn increased muscle control, heart rate control, and electrodermal control. Biofeedback provides convincing experiential proof to their cortex and to their unconscious that control is indeed taking place. It is not hard for patients to believe that with this degree of control they also can direct immune system activity with their visualizations.

I have worked with more than 100 cancer patients, and in our group we have seen a good many more, in adjunctive cancer therapy. Many types of cancer are represented, and patients have ranged in age from

5 years old to the elderly. In the absence of control groups and statistical analysis, these cases comprise a collection of well over 100 anecdotes. They are anecdotes, however, that are well documented and carefully followed. Most of these patients continue to outlive medical expectations for their survival. For all of them, the quality of life is greatly improved, with increased physical and psychological comfort. In our program we teach people to mobilize all the healing resources of their body, particularly their immune system, to help make them stronger than the cancer.

Our protocol is designed to help patients restore and/or maintain the greatest possible level of health, with the rationale that cancer will have less chance of taking over a healthy, optimally functioning body. Nutrition and exercise play the same role recognized as important in prevention, helping their healthy parts be more resistant to the spread of cancer and also minimizing adverse side effects of medical treatment. Biofeedback-acquired self-regulation skills promote deep relaxation, stress and pain management, and experiential knowledge of conscious participation in body regulation and healing. Exploration and transformation of beliefs, attitudes, and expectations relevant to healing are undertaken, with a recognition that every expectation, every belief, every conscious and unconscious image, is a visualization that tends to become actualized in the body.

Most importantly, patients are guided to an accurate understanding of their present condition and of the images they hold; to a clear, objective and subjective sense of their own internal processes; to an understanding of the desired results and efficaciousness of their medical treatment; to a visualization of the chemotherapy or radiation as a powerful ally to their own healing resources; and to a visualization of their immune system overcoming the cancer, with the knowledge that the cancer cells are weak, confused, and disorganized, whereas the immune system is potent, competent, and in tune with nature.

Consciousness, visualization, and volition, which we all accept as existential and experiential facts, are generators of neuropeptide and neurotransmitter behavior, and initiate immune system responses. Refined experiments are showing that very specific activities of the immune system can be elicited by voluntary control. Jeanne Achterberg (Achterberg & Lawlis, 1988) reported at a recent medical conference that neutrophiles and T cells can be modified differentially by visualization, by focusing attention specifically on one or the other of these immune-system components with information about its development and function. Students from Southern Methodist University were divided into two groups. One group was taught the morphology, location, and function of T cells, and the other group learned the morphology, location, and function of neutrophils. This study is showing definite trends. There are statistically significant differentials in T-cell counts for those visualizing functioning T cells, without changes in neutrophils or other immune components; conversely, those visualizing neutrophils have statistically significant differentials in neutrophil counts, without other immune cellular changes.

Most biofeedback therapists utilize visualization and imagery constantly when teaching psychophysiological self-regulation, regardless of their degree of awareness of this process and its correlates. Biofeedback "signals"—changes in the feedback indicating physiological change—in the absence of external physical stimuli (e.g., receiving a shock or a drug) are the direct result of image and visualization constructs. External stimuli in the form of suggestion and instruction operate by evoking or creating images and visualizations in the cortex.

Multiple Personality and States of Consciousness

With every change in consciousness, there is always a corresponding change in the body. This is illustrated most dramatically in the case of multiple personalities. Since the minds and bodies of persons with multiple personalities go through profound and measurable changes, they offer exciting new proof of the human capacity for instantaneous psychophysiological reorganization. Different personalities within one person have different brain wave patterns, different handedness, and different allergies. Cases have been reported in which one personality of a multiple needed a different eyeglass prescription, in which one but not others was color blind, and even one in which one of the personalities was diabetic.

Therapists have recognized that multiple personalities are not the sole province of persons identified with multiple personality disorder. John Beahrs, like many therapists who have worked with multiple personalities, believes we are all composed of a number of subpersonalities, a division of labor in the psyche to face a variety of life situations (Beahrs, 1983). William James dealt with the concept of subpersonalities, which he called "our various selves." Identifying and integrating subpersonalities is a central therapeutic strategy of psychosynthesis. Roberto Assagioli defined subpersonalities as all the traits, beliefs, and functions organized around the different roles we play in life, such as child and parent, boss or subordinate, and those in different social groups; very different and often antagonistic traits are often displayed in different roles. "Ordinary people shift from one to the other without clear awareness, and only a thin thread of memory connects them; but for all practical purposes they are different beings—they act differently, they show different traits" (Assagioli, 1965, p. 75).

Both Assagioli and Beahrs have found that becoming conscious of and then orchestrating the various subpersonality roles is a healthy strategy that we all can learn to use more effectively. Beahrs, who worked with the famed hypnotists Milton Erikson and Ernest Hilgard, has the hypnotherapist's perspective on the unconscious; rather than a seething cauldron calling for suppression, he sees it as the source of life and growth. It is perhaps most accurate to think in terms of each person's total consciousness, including the levels of consciousness—the conscious, the entire preconscious, and the unconscious. Paradoxical as it may sound, what we ordinarily think of as consciousness has many interruptions and becomes unconscious in sleep or anesthesia, for instance; the "unconscious," on the other hand, is *always* conscious, monitoring and recording the external world as well as the internal environment. Although continuity of consciousness is illusive, unconscious experience can be brought to consciousness by various means.

The literature on multiple personalities is replete with indications of rapid healing capacity (Braun, 1986; Putnam, 1984; Wilbur, 1984). Bennet Braun, a Chicago psychiatrist who has studied a large number of persons with multiple personalities, notes that these changes in physiology are similar to those that can be brought about by hypnosis. Theoretically, there are no changes brought about by hypnosis that cannot be brought about by voluntary control. After all, the hypnotist holds no strings within the body of the subject. The person is controlling all the changes in physiology, whether consciously or unconsciously. Biofeedback and visualization therapies are showing that conscious control of the unconscious can be learned, perhaps of any organic system over time—including the healing system (O'Regan, 1987)—and surely of any system that can be affected by personality shifts or by hypnosis.

An interesting potential is suggested by a multiple personality I have been working with, using visualization and imagery. Rosa has four identified adult personalities and several child personalities of various ages. We began biofeedback therapy to alleviate pain and muscle tension associated with temporomandibular joint dysfunction and to develop ways to ameliorate anxiety and decrease physiological stress responses. Techniques for reducing sympathetic nervous system overresponding were utilized by a teen personality to abort destructive tantrums. Gradually, all the alternate personalities were being taught biofeedback strategies. This appears to have an important secondary effect of helping the various personalities integrate in awareness and communication with *each other,* simultaneously with the increased conscious/unconscious integration within *one* personality that self-regulation demands.

CONCLUDING REMARKS

Biofeedback plays a central role in self-regulation therapies because it provides the experiential and the objective proof that change is happening, a necessary ingredient of learned skills. This chapter only touches on a few of the biofeedback/self-regulation areas of application. In psychiatry, medicine, education, athletics, the performing arts, and even astronaut training, biofeedback and self-regulation are enhancing human potential to be well, to excel, to survive. With the aid of electronics, biofeedback is showing how internal states respond to volition and imagery. Biofeedback makes this knowledge and these abilities accessible to everybody; it makes conscious control of the unconscious scientific, measurable, and verifiable.

According to Roger Sperry, in the 1981 Nobel Prize in Medicine lecture, cognitive introspective psychology and related cognitive science can no longer be ignored experimentally, or written off as "a science of epiphenomena" or as something that must in principle reduce eventually to neurophysiology. The events of inner experience, as emergent properties of brain processes, become themselves explanatory causal constructs in their own right, interacting at their own level with their own laws and dynamics. The whole world of inner experience (the world of the humanities), long rejected by 20th-century scientific materialism, thus becomes reorganized and included within the domain of science.

The growing interest in teaching self-regulation skills with biofeedback and visualization in our schools (as well as in sports, the performing arts, and any area where peak performance is desired) represents an exciting opportunity to expand our innate abilities in a powerful way, with ever-increasing benefits to society and the well-being of our world. The process of learning biofeedback and visualization techniques evokes both enthusiasm and capacity for greater self-responsibility in our healing processes. By becoming experientially aware of the possibilities of healing and transformation; we can respond in new ways and gain an understanding of our inner ability to heal ourselves.

References

Achterberg, J., & Lawlis, F. (1988, January). *Psychoneuroimmunology: Implications for cancer therapy*. Paper presented at the 21st Annual Medical Symposium of the A.R.E. Clinic, Phoenix, AZ.

Aldine Annuals, 1970–1978. Biofeedback and self-control: An Aldine Annual on the regulation of bodily processes and consciousness. Chicago: Aldine.

American Psychiatric Association. (1987). *Diagnostic and Statistical Manual of Mental Disorders* (3rd ed.). Washington, DC: Author.

Assagioli, Roberto. (1965). *Psychosynthesis: A manual of principles and techniques.* New York: Hobbs, Dorman.

Bair, J. H. (1901). Development of voluntary control. *Psychological Review, 8,* 474–510.

Barber, T. X. (1984). Changing "unchangeable" bodily processes by (hypnotic) suggestions: A new look at hypnosis, cognitions, imaging, and the mind-body problem. In A. A. Sheikh (Ed.), *Imagination and Healing.* Farmingdale, NY: Baywood.

Basmajian, J. V. (1963). Control and training of individual motor units. *Science, 141,* 440–441.

Beahrs, J. (1983). *Unity and multiplicity: Multilevel consciousness of self in hypnosis, psychiatric disorder and mental health.* New York: Brunner/Mazel.

Beck, A. T., & Emery, G. (1985). *Anxiety disorders and phobias: A cognitive perspective.* Philadelphia: Center for Cognitive Therapy.

Braun, B. G. (Ed.). (1986). *Treatment of multiple personality disorder.* Washington, DC: American Psychiatric Press.

Brener, J., & Hothersall, D. (1966). Heart rate under conditions of augmented sensory feedback. *Psychophysiology, 3,* 23–28.

Brown, B. B. (1970). Recognition of aspects of consciousness through association with EEG activity represented by a light signal. *Psychophysiology, 6,* 442–452.

Brown, D. P., & Fromm, E. (1987). *Hypnosis and behavioral medicine.* Hillsdale, NJ: Erlbaum.

Budzynski, T. H., Stoyva, J. M., & Adler, C. S. (1970). Feedback-induced muscle relaxation: Applications to tension headache. *Journal of Behavior Therapy and Experimental Psychiatry, 1,* 205–211.

Cousins, N. (1983). *The healing heart.* New York: Norton.

Emery, G., & Tracy, N. L. (1987). Theoretical issues in the cognitive-behavioral treatment of anxiety disorders. In L. Michelson & L. M. Ascher (Eds.), *Anxiety and stress disorders.* New York: Guilford.

Finley, W. W., Smith, H. A., & Etherton, M. D. (1975). Reduction of seizures and normalization of the EEG in a severe epileptic following sensorimotor biofeedback training: Preliminary study. *Biological Psychology, 2,* 189–203.

Green, E. E. (1979). Psychophysiologic correlates of expectancy. Presidential address, Biofeedback Society of America, San Diego.

Green, E. E., & Green, A. M. (1977). *Beyond biofeedback.* New York: Delacorte.

Green, E. E., Green, A. M., & Walters, E. D. (1969). Feedback technique for deep relaxation. *Psychophysiology, 6,* 371–377.

Green, E. E., Green, A. M., & Walters, E. D. (1970). Self regulation of internal states. In J. Rose (Ed.), *Progress of cybernetics: Proceedings of the International Congress of Cybernetics.* London: Gordon and Breach.

Hartley, E. (1974). *Biofeedback: The yoga of the west* [Film]. Cos Cob, Ct: Hartley Productions.

Hnatiow, M., & Lang, P. J. (1965). Learned stabilization of heart rate. *Psychophysiology, 1*, 330–336.

Jacobson, E. (1938). *Progressive relaxation.* Chicago: University of Chicago Press.

Kamiya, J. (1962). Conditioned discrimination of the EEG alpha rhythm in humans. Lecture to the Western Psychological Association, San Francisco.

Kamiya, J. (1968). Conscious control of brain waves. *Psychology Today, 1*, 57–60.

Kohut, H. (1977). *The restoration of the self.* New York: International Universities Press.

Lacroix, J. M. (1986). Mechanisms of biofeedback control: On the importance of verbal (conscious) processing. In R. J. Davidson, G. E. Schwartz, & D. Shapiro (Eds.), *Consciousness and self-regulation* (Vol. 4). New York: Plenum Press.

Lubar, J. F. (1975). Behavioral management of epilepsy through sensorimotor rhythm EEG biofeedback conditioning. *National Spokesman, 8*, 6–7.

Lubar, J. F., & Bahler, W. W. (1976). Behavioral management of epileptic seizures following EEG biofeedback training of the sensorimotor rhythm. *Biofeedback and Self-Regulation, 1*, 77–104.

Luthe, W. (1965). *Autogenic training.* New York: Grune & Stratton.

MacLean, P. D. (1949). Psychosomatic disease and the "visceral brain." *Psychosomatic Medicine, 2*, 338–353.

Masserman, J. H. (1941). Is the hypothalamus a center of emotion? *Psychosomatic Medicine, 2*, 3–25.

Michelson, L., & Ascher, L. M. (1987). *Anxiety and stress disorders.* New York: Guilford.

Mulholland, T., & Runnals, S. (1962). Evaluation of attention and alertness with a stimulus-brain feedback loop. *Electroencephalography and Clinical Neurophysiology, 4*, 847–852.

Norris, P. A. (1986). Biofeedback, voluntary control and human potential. *Biofeedback and Self-regulation, 11*(1), 1–29.

Norris, P. A., & Porter, G. (1987). *I choose life: The dynamics of visualization and biofeedback.* Walpole, NH: Stillpoint Publishing.

O'Regan, B. (1987). Inner mechanisms of the healing response program. *Noetic Sciences Review, 5*, 6–8.

Papez, J. W. (1937). A proposed mechanism of emotion. *Archives of Neurology and Psychiatry, 38*, 725–743.

Pavlov, I. P. (1951). *Collected works* (Vol. 3, Book 2). Moscow-Leningrad:

Peavey, B. S. (1982). *Biofeedback assisted self-regulation: Effects on phagocytic immune system.* Unpublished doctoral dissertation, North Texas State University, Denton, TX.

Penfield, W., & Rasmussen, R. (1950). *The cerebral cortex of man: A clinical study of localization of function.* New York: Macmillan.

Peper, E., & Mulholland, T. B. (1970). Methodological and theoretical problems in the voluntary control of electroencephalographic occipital alpha by the subject. *Kybernetik, 7,* 10–13.

Pert, C. B., Ruff, M. R., Weber, R. J., & Herkenham, M. (1985). Neuropeptides and their receptors: A psychosomatic network. *Journal of Immunology, 135*(2), 820s–826s.

Putnam, F. (1984). The study of multiple personality disorder: General strategies and practical considerations. *Psychiatric Annals, 14,* 58–61.

Romen, A. S. (1981). *Self-Suggestion and its influence on the human organism.* Armonk, NY: M. E. Sharpe.

Schultz, J., & Luthe, W. (1959). *Autogenic training: A psychophysiologic approach in psychotherapy.* New York: Grune & Stratton.

Shellenberger, R., & Green, J. A. (1986). *From the ghost in the box to successful biofeedback training.* Greeley, CO: Health Psychology Publications.

Sperry, R. (1982). Some effects of disconnecting the cerebral hemispheres. Nobel lecture, 8 December 1981. *Bioscience Reports, 2,* 265–276.

Sterman, M. B. (1972). *Studies of EEG biofeedback training in man and cat.* Highlights of the 17th Annual Conference, VA Cooperative Studies in Mental Health and Behavioral Sciences, pp. 55–60.

Sterman, M. B. (1973). Neurophysiologic and clinical studies of sensorimotor EEG feedback training: Some effects on epilepsy. *Seminars in Psychiatry, 5,* 507–524.

Sterman, M. B. (1977). Clinical implications of EEG biofeedback training: A critical appraisal. In G. E. Schwartz & J. Beatty (Eds.), *Biofeedback: Theory and research.* New York: Academic Press.

Stern, R. M., & Lewis, N. L. (1968). Ability of actors to control their GSR's and express emotions. *Psychophysiology, 4,* 294–299.

Stoyva, J. (1976). Self-regulation: A context for biofeedback (Editorial). *Biofeedback and Self-Regulation, 1,* 1–6.

Wadden, T. A., & Anderton, C. H. (1982). The clinical uses of hypnosis. *Psychological Bulletin, 91*(2), 215–243.

Wickramasekera, I. (Ed.) (1976). *Biofeedback, behavior therapy and hypnosis: Potentiating the verbal control of behavior for clinicians.* Chicago: Nelson Hall.

Wilbur, C. (1984). Multiple personality and child abuse. In B. G. Braun (Ed.), *Symposium on Multiple Personality, Psychiatric Clinics of North America, 7,* 3–8.

11

Psychosomatic Illness: A New Look

CAROL E. MCMAHON
ANEES A. SHEIKH

If there be nothing new, but that which is hath been before,
how are our brains beguiled which, laboring for invention, bear
amiss the second burden of a former child.

William Shakespeare, *Sonnet 59*

INTRODUCTION

The year 1989 marks the 50th anniversary of a scientific enlightenment. With the publication in 1939 of the first issue of *Psychosomatic Medicine* came formal sanction of scientific pursuit of psychosomatics in medical theory and research. Time was apparently overripe for this development, for within two decades the psychosomatic movement became evident on an international scale. Entering the 1960s, a dozen journals representing England, France, Italy, Switzerland, West Germany, Argentina, the United States, and Japan had joined the pursuit. Expansion of membership in professional societies for psychosomatic research has been logarithmic (McMahon & Koppes, 1976), and vigor of growth seems not to have abated.

296

Though perennially current in the East, the reality of psychosomatic phenomena was a revolutionary realization for the West. Moved by the facts of emotion-related illness and justified by psychoanalytic theory with its hypothesis of psychogenesis, advocates of psychosomatics over- came forceful intellectual resistance to concepts of mental influence. Insisting that mind *caused* bodily changes, they urged that all illness be conceived in a psychosomatic framework. The pioneers were confident in the expectation that "psychosomatic" would in due course become the type of all medicine.

Thus it is appropriate at this half-century point to assess the degree to which the initial promise has been fulfilled. This chapter traces the modern history of the psychosomatic movement focusing principally on unresolved issues of causation of psychosomatic illness. It is argued that lack of fundamental explanation of the mind-body relationship has pro- hibited the thorough going revolution in medicine anticipated by the pioneers. An alternate model of causation based upon a three-dimen- sional model of human nature is introduced.

THE STATUS OF THE REVOLUTION

Assessing the movement's current status, its strength in numbers might well satisfy the founders' expectations. So also perhaps might its diversi- fication of interests and expansion to include specialized subareas such as psychoneuroimmunology and psychoneuroendocrinology. The tally of disorders classified as psychosomatic has grown steadily as diseases formerly conceived in exclusively physical terms have joined the ranks. Psychophysiological relationships scarcely envisioned by the pioneers (including a proposed association of mental imagery, immune function, and cancer) are discussed with heretofore uncommon openness.

Alternate therapies have appeared on the scene, met the test of re- search, and been credited with clinical effectiveness. Furthermore (as in the case of biofeedback), these innovative healing strategies have re- sisted restrictive medical classification as useful solely in "psychiatric" applications.

Scientists are newly aware of anomaly, having acknowledged the fail- ure of the medical model to explain various events. Placebo effects, yogic feats, hypnosis wart cures, and "spontaneous" remission are among the phenomena now conspicuous as requiring explanation in terms of holis- tic functioning.

The term "holism," despite its ambiguity and lack of formal definition, has entered lay and professional vocabularies signifying an innovative and presumably superior mode of conceiving and treating illness. The literature on mind-body relationships has grown to vast proportions in half a century, consisting by and large of correlations determined through empirical studies, though epidemiological and case studies have likewise contributed to a formidable body of psychophysiological knowledge.

By these indications an impression may be created that the expectations of the pioneers have been satisfied. Yet several unanswered questions counteract this impression and create a sobering influence. For instance, is it problematic that no consensus has been reached on the fundamental question of the mind-body relationship? Is it satisfactory for progress that "physical" processes continue to be conceived as both necessary and sufficient conditions for psychosomatic illness? Need we be troubled by the largely atheoretical character of the science, or need we be dismayed by the recent deletion of the diagnostic classification "psychosomatic disorder" from the *Diagnostic and Statistical Manual of Mental Disorders* (DSM III)? More troublesome still, have we squarely confronted the fact that voluntary self-regulation of autonomic mechanisms, and holistic events themselves, are both logically and biologically impossible given our underlying dualistic definition of human nature?

These are indeed problematic concerns, all of which point to a difficulty that empirical research, however inspired, is powerless to resolve. This difficulty lies at the deepest level of explanation in a metaphysical hard core of assumptions regarding human nature. The dualism of René Descartes forms the philosophical basis of medical science, specifying that mind and body are permanently estranged, mutually exclusive entities. The prohibitive implications of this philosophy of isolationism are clearly evident in medical history, and we must search here in the underlying determinants of medical theory and practice for an explanation as to why the psychosomatic revolution has not completed its cycle.

PSYCHOSOMATIC ILLNESS IN HISTORICAL PERSPECTIVE

In the Victorian era of the mid-1800s, orthodox physicians experienced particular difficulty curing so-called neuropaths or functional nervous cases. The mission of medicine in the 19th century was to identify the physical basis of pathology, but this form of illness resisted such analysis.

Neuropaths were sufferers from disorders known today as psychosomatic, whose complaints of headache, backache, chronic fatigue, dyspepsia, and so forth constituted a thorn in the side of early modern medicine, both clinically and theoretically. In cases of functional nervous disorders, the pathology could not "be brought under the observation of even the best aided senses. What the microscope can see we call structural—what the microscope cannot see we call functional" (Beard, 1881, p. 114).

In the 1800s mechanistic physiopathology held exclusive sway. The body was considered a machine governed by mechanistic laws, and the mind an "immaterial substance." The notion of psychological causation of somatic events was beyond consideration, as it was understood to imply a logical and therefore a biological impossibility. The "contents of the mind," among which emotions were included, were incapable of affecting matter in any way (McMahon, 1975a, 1976a).

But although no organic derangement could be found in cases of functional nervous disorders, these conditions often had tangible physiological manifestations. Thus, while such disorders stubbornly refused to disclose structural alterations, medicine was as stubbornly convinced of the existence of structural change. A medical author wrote in 1896:

> Not that physical changes do not presumably exist in the intimate elements of structure to which our senses have not yet gained access. We believe confidently . . . that those that come after us will not fail to discover the physical causes of derangements we are now constrained to call functional. (Maudsley, 1896, p. 14)

As a consequence of pervasive mechanistic physiopathology, "functional" became synonymous with "organic disease of undetermined cause," and medicine began a vigorous program of research aimed at identifying the physical causes of functional disorders. "Insanity" was known to be accompanied oftentimes by various forms of observable neuropathology. Even the ancients had recognized this, some citing the relationship in support of the postulate of localization of the mental function in the brain. The case seemed hopeful for isolating the physical causes of insanity, but not so for other functional disorders where no evidence of organic derangement could be found.

Psychological factors, however, seemed reliably to correlate with nervous disorders implying some involvement of mind. Given the metaphysical underpinning of theory, however, a psychological variable could in no way influence a physiological process. Thus it came to be assumed that somatic complaints that were attributed to "nervousness" existed largely in the minds of patients, and nervous disorders were frequently classified as "imaginary ailments" (McMahon, 1975a, p. 127).

In the late 19th century nervous patients were labeled malingerers who either exaggerated symptoms or engaged in outright deception.

William McDougall, a leader in early physiological psychology, traced this historical development:

> While the secrets of the psychoses were indefatigably besieged with the microscope, and with wonderful methods of staining nervous tissue, the nervous disorders were neglected and despised; for they were regarded as merely functional; and that meant that they had no structural basis which the microscope might reveal; and therefore, according to the prevailing mode, they were unreal; they were merely fanciful or imaginary; they were products of the patient's imagination, and therefore to be treated by scolding, derision, or other disciplinary measures. (McDougall, 1926, p. 33)

The lack of benevolence may well have related to the fact that conventional medical methods invariably failed to remedy nervous disorders. Surgeons of the day were accused of "cutting, cauterising and sacrificing numberless hypochondriacal neuropaths" and it was agreed that "nothing is harder to cure than a neuropath" (Janet, 1925, Vol. II, p. 1030).

The nervous disorder was understood as neither mental nor organic illness and therefore was determined not to be a genuine form of pathology. As evidence of this conviction, when such conditions appeared to be the causes of death, they were "not noted as such in the tables of mortality" (Beard, 1881, p. 22). A physical change without a physical cause was a logical impossibility, and an "imaginary" disease could not kill. The fact that nervous disorders seldom did result in death confirmed belief in their imaginary basis.

"Physical hysteria" (the contemporary conversion reaction) was a functional nervous disorder defined in the 1800s as "a malady of the imagination." Its symptoms were "deceptive appearances displayed in bodily functions." In these cases, "the whole energies of the patient's mind are bent on deception" (Jones, 1864, p. 517). Such diseases were understood as "merely the fanciful productions of idle women of inferior constitution" (McDougall, 1926, p. 34). Physicians were advised not to treat these cases unless therapy consisted of measures such as those used in handling "malingering soldiers" (Jones, 1864, p. 520). It was assumed that hysterical patients feigned symptoms of disease because they desired to be ill. Psychosomatic phenomena were thus dismissed or explained away, their existence forbidden by conceptions of the mind and body underlying medical theory.

The Freudian Influence and "Psychogenesis"

As Professor Szasz has demonstrated (1961, p. 42), Freud did not "discover" conversion hysteria, rather he advocated that so-called hysterics be considered ill. Owing to the influence of Freudian theory with its explanation of psychogenetic or mental causation, the condition known as "physical hysteria" became prototypical of newly conceived "functional" illness. As an instance of psychogenesis, the conversion reaction had a cause residing beneath the level of consciousness and identifiable by psychoanalysis. The formerly prohibited concept of causation of physical by mental events was justified by Freud's argument: "a disturbance that can be set right by means of psychic influences can itself have been nothing else than psychical" (in Ferenczi, Abraham, Simmel, & Jones, 1921, p. 11), and each instance of successful outcome of psychotherapy reinforced the belief in psychological origin of this type of disorder. The situation in the 1920s was characterized thus:

> By degrees a marked silence fell over the mechanistic school, and attempts were frequently made to explain their former utterances psycho-genetically. The quarrel from now onwards lay entirely between supporters of the various psychological theories. (Ferenczi et al., 1921, p. 11)

Thus mind had a moment of glory as psychogenesis swept the field of causation. The new look was given a new name; "psychosomatic" replaced "nervous" disease, and "holism" was admitted to the vocabulary. At this historical juncture the organic-functional distinction grew obscure as zealous proponents of holism moved toward an iconoclastic position. Many argued for the psychogenesis of organic disease, thereby conceiving *all* illness as psychosomatic.

By the 1940s the functional nervous disorder had been eclipsed by new defining terms:

> It is misleading, and even erroneous, to regard illness of this nature as "nervous disease" . . . . A more appropriate term for disorders of this nature—whether they be "cases of functional disease" or "cases of organic disease"—is "psychosomatic illness." This term is cumbersome but useful. It connotes both an aetiology and a mechanism. As regards aetiology, it indicates that the external agents which provoked the reaction of illness were of a special kind, being neither physical nor chemical nor micro-organic, but psychological. (Halliday, 1938, p. 13)

Having achieved scientific explanation, the nervous disorder became a legitimate object of medical inquiry. Functional nervous disorders were construed initially in exactly the same manner as conversion hysteria: "both conditions are psychogenic, that is to say, they are caused ultimately by a chronic repressed or at least unrelieved tension" (Alexander, 1948, p. 9).

The Pioneers of Holism

Freud's therapeutic argument (i.e., that a condition curable by psychological influences can be none other than psychological in origin) had a profound effect on medicine though victories for the new perspective were hard won. Psychoanalytic theory was itself unacceptable to conservative institutions, and extension of its postulates to various branches of scientific medicine required Herculean efforts. Opponents of psychoanalysis were legion in the early years, and those who accomplished its integration with physical medicine were heroic figures indeed.

With Freud's personal sanction, Smith Ely Jelliffe (1866–1945) championed the cause and argued persuasively that psychic processes initiate and maintain derangements in nervous and physico-chemical metabolic functions. Organic pathology, according to Jelliffe, could be precipitated by conflicts of unconscious origin, and physical symptoms were symbolic of psychic factors motivating them.

From 1902 through the remainder of his life, Jelliffe edited the *Journal of Nervous and Mental Diseases* and with increasing frequency made it a vehicle for disseminating the new concepts. The journal's memorial tribute written by another pioneer, A. A. Brill, stated: "Jelliffe is the father of psychosomatic medicine, and it is pleasing to know that Freud always gave him due credit for it" (1947, in Alexander, Eisenstein, & Grotjahn, 1966, p. 232).

A prestigious figure in internal medicine, Felix Deutsch (1844-1964) protested against the traditional restriction to organic causation, prompting the Neurologic Society in which he held membership to challenge him to claim allegiance to one or the other of these incompatible viewpoints: was he an "internist" or an "analyst"? Yet Deutsch continued to approach pathology in the psychoanalytic mode, and at professional meetings presented the first reports of psychogenic colitis, angina pectoris, and asthma. In *Psychoanalysis and Internal Medicine* Deutsch (1927) (a journal article) used the term "psychosomatic" to describe etiology of various cardiovascular and metabolic disturbances. He insisted upon a perspective of determinism and causality involving a "fusion and interaction" of psychic and somatic events.

By self-definition a conservative anarchist, Franz Alexander (1891–1964) furthered the cause, devoting an impressive career to associating specific organic diseases with particular psychological causes. He demonstrated the applicability of Cannon's physiological model to psychosomatic disorders of the autonomic nervous system, and in 1939 with several colleagues, founded the flagship journal *Psychosomatic Medicine*.

In 1943, Alexander introduced a distinction between conversion hysteria and the "vegetative organ neurosis." This established a separate classification for the latter as "psychophysiological or psychosomatic." The former category had less visible organic pathology and continued to be construed as a "mental" disorder per se; thus "psychosomatic" disorders and "conversion reactions" came to occupy separate classifications in diagnostic manuals of "mental disorders." The distinction between conversion hysteria and the vegetative organ neurosis, however, was an anatomical distinction not a theoretical one. Causation in both instances was presumed "mental."

In the early decades of its existence a popular ridicule placed psychosomatic medicine in the "pre-Osler stage." The tables turned, however, and in its 14th edition medicine's standard textbook, William Osler's *Principles and Practice of Medicine . . . ,* 1942, replaced its first chapter on typhoid fever with one titled "Psychosomatic Medicine." By the 1940s the new perspective appeared to have triumphed.

Misgivings About Mind

The impact of psychoanalytic pioneers was potent enough to combat successfully historic resistance to concepts of causation of physical by mental events. The hypothesis of psychogenesis was instrumental in launching psychosomatic medicine as a formal discipline and in giving initial impetus to the holistic approach. Belief that mental events were causally related to physiological changes awakened broad interest in autonomic functions and in theories of emotion. A link was forged connecting interests of sociologists, neurologists, psychologists, psychiatrists, and other medical specialties, and by the 1950s the movement's force was self-perpetuating. It did not collapse with the passing medical vogue of psychoanalytic theory, and it continued despite the inevitable realization that "psychogenesis" was itself untenable. In the final analysis, the mechanism of causation had not been explained.

The pioneers had themselves expressed occasional misgivings when discussing the precise association of psychic energy and pathophysiology. Jelliffe was by no means content with the final picture and seemed even to concur with critics who accused him of "telling only half the truth." He felt his success may have been greater if he had a "more detailed knowledge of general somatic pathology" (in Alexander et al., 1966).

Carl Gustav Jung (1875–1961) was among those openly critical of the Freudian conception of causality. Jung responded to a presentation by Jelliffe with an explicit statement of the problem. As Jelliffe wrote afterward, Jung had accused him of

mixing physiology and psychology, mind and matter, body and mind . . . .
The things we have come to think of in terms of complements, he insists on
regarding as separate—especially physiology and psychology, which he
seems to think have nothing to do with each other. The idea of the symbol as
an energy container Jung . . . will not follow. (1926, in Alexander et al.
1966, p. 231)

Jung was not alone in recognizing the incompatibility of mental and
mechanistic concepts. Characteristic of his genius, Freud had himself
seen the fundamental problem of explanation. In reference to hysteria
Freud noted that conditions that "involve the leap from a mental process
to a somatic innervation . . . can never be fully comprehensible to us"
(1909/1968, p. 17). In his own writings Freud confined hysterical manifestations of psychic disturbances to voluntary functions—those of the
anatomical "path of the will" as opposed to the historic "path of the
reflexes." Though fundamentally "incomprehensible," evidence confirmed the reality of conversion reactions. But Freud himself saw no
possibility of extension of his model to causation of visceral disturbances. Psychic control of "involuntary" somatic functions violated not
only logic but traditional rules of anatomy and neurophysiology. Proponents of self-regulation carry the same burden today.

The Freudian postulate of psychic determinism succeeded in bringing
causality to all aspects of mental life, but "psychic energy," libidinal impulses, and so forth were not physical constructs, nor had they physical
analogues. So despite the determinism that presumed the mind was as
rigidly ruled by cause and effect as any event in the physical universe, the
interaction dilemma proved no less menacing after Freud than before.

To further challenge psychoanalytic explanation, it was recognized as
early as 1935 that the therapeutic argument justifying psychogenesis
stood on uncertain ground. For instance, Dunbar (1935/1954) discussed
cases of "psychogenic" vomiting, cured by psychotherapy, later recognized as caused by brain tumors. The causation enigma was destined to
alter the course of the holistic movement and to dictate a more conservative approach to theory and research.

Correlations to the Rescue

While explicit use of the concept of psychogenesis grew less frequent
over time, a methodology developed that was designed to evade the
issue of causation. The scientifically sanctioned hypothesis, as expressed
in volume 1 of The Principles of Psychophysiology (Troland, 1932), was
based on "the familiar postulate that consciousness is correlated with,
but distinct from, the cerebral factor in physiological operations" (p. 14).

Marston (1928) looked with dismay upon a growing trend to "abandon all theories, and all previous results and undertake statistical correlations of how all people react under all possible circumstances" (p. 53). Yet Marston praised the "psycho-physiologists" for having "refrained from dogmatic assertion as to the type of causal conception, if any, existing between their two sets of data" (p. 18).

The trend was toward abandoning deeper questions so as to prevent the mind-body problem from posing conceptual difficulties, and in this science achieved resounding success. Mind-body dualism became understood as a "philosophical or semantic" problem rather than a scientific problem. Nemiah (1985, p. 304) described the modern penchant for "avoiding the understanding of the genesis of symptoms," and Lader (1972, p. 300) reminded scientists of the necessity of evading the "mind-body conundrum." Lader recognized that historical resistance to psychosomatics was caused by

> the non-scientific approach and excessive claims made by some enthusiastic advocates of the psychosomatic approach. This approach still seeks chimaeric connections between psyche and soma and believes that emotions "cause" bodily changes. (p. 309)

The philosophical assumption of psycho-physical parallelism furnished the basis for correlation research and, with strict restrictions on semantic usage, a means of evading the mind-body problem. A demarcation of psychological and physical domains was adhered to with rigor, and two sets of theory—separate but equal—allowed conceptual handling of dual subject matters.

With the lost hope for psychogenesis, the search for specific mind-body causal associations was gradually abandoned. Some supporters of psychosomatic medicine explicitly disavowed concepts of mental causation. Sandor Lorand (1973) challenged the American Psychiatric Association's official stance: "In my opinion a number of disease processes have in common physiologic and psychologic factors which, although not causing each other, interact and influence each other, sharing equally in the disease process" (p. 265).

Behaviorism to the Rescue

Psychology's condemnation of mentalism and its subsequent exaltation to scientific repute, inspired similar trends in modern psychophysiology and psychosomatic medicine. To frame concepts in terms of "behaviors" brought a sense of liberation from the causally impotent mind, and the mechanistic, reflexive stimulus-response model helped further to evade an appearance of mentalism. The integration of Cannon's physiology with the stimulus-response model seemed for a time to furnish a scientifically clean picture of pathogenesis wherein by a process of "somatization," energies generated at the psychological level of experience could "translate" into disturbances of somatic function. Rational science seemed finally to have grasped the essence of functional disorders. "Emotional behavior" was credited with the causal potency the immaterial mind lacked:

> An autonomic response, which has been invoked in the interest of homeostatic balance or as an expression of emotional behavior, may become excessive, giving rise to symptoms which have as sound a scientific basis as any produced by organic disease. The term "functional" which we apply quite appropriately to such illness has acquired an unfortunate connotation in ordinary medical practice. There is all too often some implication that the symptoms are "imaginary." (Sheehan, 1943, p. 415)

Symptoms have been considered *real* in inverse proportion to their degree of causation by mind. As the behavioral perspective grew in popularity, focus shifted from psychic or inner events as causal variables to observables. Since "behaviors" were not psychic entities, having more to do with muscles than mentation scientists seemed on safer ground positing relationships between habits or overt actions and illnesses. Life circumstances provided a convenient framework for explanation. "Death of a spouse" and "bereavement" better suited the popular taste than tribulation, misery, and despair. Social and psychological "stressors" became stimuli for autonomic responses. "Type A behaviors" were identified, and the conditioning paradigms of psychology became models for "behavioral medicine." The science of psychophysiology evolved as the field studying what some have termed the "biology of behavior," despite David Graham's (1971) forthright statement that the "behavioral" variable is often used in place of the "equivalent" term—"psychological" variable (p. 22).

As causation by mind waned, mechanism held its ground and research programs diversified. Noting an evolution toward increased scientific discipline Lipowski (1976, p. 17) presented an overview of modern research models. Three types of methodology were identified: (1) epidemiological studies seeking correlations between life events and frequency and severity of morbidity, (2) psychophysiological laboratory investigations correlating various stimuli with electrophysiological response measures, and (3) clinical studies establishing correlations between existing disorders and psychological or social variables. Little tolerance, Lipowski observed, is currently given to poorly defined and difficult to quantify mental variables. Thoroughly purged of the 19th century's "mentalistic hobgoblins," the new correlation methodology brought an energizing feel of "hard science" to the subject matter; the movement's expansion continued, bolstered by the facts of psychosomatics, despite the lack of theory to explain underlying causation.

The Facts of Mental Influence: Imagery Research

In the present decade mounting evidence is again swaying opinion in the direction of potency of conscious processes, and nowhere is causal influence of mental processes on somatic events more evident than in research on the psychophysiology of imagery (Kunzendorf & Sheikh, in press). Conscious control by means of imagery has been explored in various contexts including autonomic self-regulation; influences on chemical composition of bodily fluids; activation of sense organ responses (e.g., in the eye); and, in the burgeoning field of imagination and healing, in treatment and prevention of specific forms of pathology (Sheikh, 1984). Other research encompasses imagery and affect, imagery and motivation, and individual differences where evidence suggests specific attributes of imagery in the psychosomatic patient (Sheikh, Richardson, & Moleski, 1979).

Reviewed in detail, the imagery evidence is brought specifically to bear on the question of conscious control, revealing inadequacies in the dualistic-based models of epiphenomenalism and behaviorism (Sheikh & Kunzendorf, 1984). Specific outcomes of scores of imagery studies violate the predictions of these isolationist models. A full reconciliation of facts with theory will be contingent upon accessing a model that describes the whole, permitting causal interaction in place of isolation of the parts.

CARTESIAN ISOLATIONISM AS A MODEL OF HUMAN NATURE: PROHIBITIVE IMPLICATIONS FOR PSYCHOSOMATIC MEDICINE

A Promise Unfulfilled

Though psychosomatic medicine became a respected scientific enterprise, its present status does not conform to the expectations of its pioneers. To early proponents of the burgeoning movement, its auspicious beginnings signified an impending revolution in medicine. It was their desire and their confident expectation that the psychosomatic approach become the type of all medicine. Indeed, they looked hopefully toward the day when the approach would become so universal as to allow discontinuation of the term "psychosomatic." They found the word less than adequate since it seemed stubbornly to draw attention to duality rather than unity.

According to Dunbar, the encyclopedist of early holism, "Psychosomatic medicine has not to be regarded as a speciality but as an approach to medicine" (1935/1954, p. 35). When the American Psychosomatic Society was organized, its officials stated under "Scope and Philosophy" of the Society: "the concept of psychosomatic medicine as a field, or specialty, of medicine is not inclusive enough . . . the Society is dedicated to the development of sound theoretical and therapeutic principles . . . and their widespread application in clinical practice and medical education" (Weiner, 1971, p. 607). The Academy of Psychosomatic Medicine specified as a major objective "to facilitate total and comprehensive care in the everyday practice of the healing arts" (Howard, 1973, p. 3). Yujiro Ikemi (1974), founder of the Japanese Psychosomatic Society, advocated the psychosomatic approach in "comprehensive management for diseases in various fields of clinical medicine" (p. 156).

It is evident today that the goal of making psychosomatics the favored approach in general medicine has not been fulfilled. In place of enlightening the medical world that all illness must be understood holistically, the "psychosomatic disorder" came to be viewed as a special case of pathology. Some proponents of psychosomatic medicine militated against this eventuality on logical grounds. Graham's (1972) chapter on "Psychosomatic Medicine" in the comprehensive *Handbook of Psychophysiology* correctly noted an arbitrary factor in choice of diseases discussed therein: those included were limited to disorders well researched in terms of psychological correlates. Presumably any disorder might constitute a suitable subject for psychosomatic inquiry. Nevertheless, terminology throughout the chapter points to a separate diagnostic category, and Graham's summary states: "we have considered . . . knowledge and opinion in a number of those illnesses which may be called 'psychosomatic'" (p. 915).

A few critics from within the field have explicitly rejected the concept of a psychosomatic disorder as "a misleading and scientifically sterile one" (Lipowski, 1976, p. 1; see also Weiss, 1974). But the very evident association of psychological factors with the once "nervous" now "stress-related" conditions did, for a time, furnish medicine with a new diagnostic classification.

The "Psychosomatic" Diagnosis

The evolution of "psychosomatic" (or "psychophysiologic") as a diagnostic classification has been traced through standard reference sources and diagnostic manuals (McMahon, 1986) but warrants further discussion. The *Merck Manual,* the most widely used medical text in the world, appeared in its 1st edition in 1899. Its 14th edition was published in 1982.

As dictated by historical constraints, editions prior to the 1950s are devoid of terms implying holistic states or psychological causes of bodily disturbances. The 9th edition of 1956, however, contained a forceful statement of the existence of a special class of disorders called "Psychophysiologic Autonomic and Visceral Disorders." The *Manual* states: "this longer but more exact term is used in preference to 'psychosomatic' disorders" (p. 1296). Conditions listed under this heading match closely with the 19th century's "nervous" disorders and include ulcers, headaches, backache, and so forth.

In the *Manual's* 11th edition of 1966, the discourse on psychosomatic disorders stands as yet unrevised and states: "Today's concept is that psychological upset may sometimes antedate and cause functional impairment and disorders thus produced are instances of Psychogenic Origin" (p. 114). Diagnostic manuals do not reflect frontiers of changing opinion. The movement in the 1960s appears still armed with psychogenesis and confident in its theoretical basis: "In two thirds of his patients, the physician must take into account and *rectify the mechanism* [italics added] whereby psychic tension finds bodily expression" (*Merck Manual,* 1966, p. 115).

The revelation of Freudian theory—that is, that the psychological meaning of the symptom was causally related to its appearance—was irreconcilable with the mechanistic model, and in subsequent editions of the *Manual* the obscurity of the causal "mechanism" took its toll on "psychosomatic disorders," much as it defeated the "nervous" diagnosis of the last century. Subsequent editions of the *Manual* show dwindling use of the concept of psychogenic causation. The 12th edition (1972) shows a major transition involving both loss of ground on claims of causation and a change of direction for the holistic movement:

The focus of psychosomatic medicine has increasingly turned from mechanisms of interaction between physic and somatic processes to the clinical study of individuals' adaptation to illness and disease. Adaptation studies have focused on . . . coping with illness and have attempted to discern those processes that were beneficial and those that were maladaptive. (p. 1366)

In the 1972 edition the familiar tally of disorders remains listed as "psychophysiologic reactions," but terminology describing causation has been substantially diluted. "Psychogenesis" is no longer mentioned. In its place is found the statement: "emotional factors often play a causative or contributory role, though physical symptoms dominate the clinical picture" (p. 1369).

The concept of psychological causation is so thoroughly diluted in the 14th edition (1982) that critical readers might be led to dismiss the concept entirely. This 1982 edition states that the word "psychosomatic" can be used

to refer to conditions in which psychologic factors have some etiologic importance. Even in these disorders, however, the etiology is always complex and multifactorial, and psychologic factors are *not* the only contributors to illness. (p. 1404)

The 1982 volume further states that in a great variety of disorders "psychologic and social stress are entwined . . . however, cause and effect are difficult to disentangle in investigating such associations" (p. 1405). It is allowed that "psychosocial stress" producing conflict may appear "disguised in somatic form with what appear to be symptoms of organic disease." However, "the mechanisms responsible for such symptoms are unclear although they are generally ascribed to tension" (p. 1405). Since cause and effect are indeed difficult to disentangle in the framework of isolationism, causation by mind was ultimately foresaken.

The Psychosomatic Diagnosis Abandoned

The modern evolution of concepts observed in the *Merck Manuals* is paralleled in diagnostic manuals published by the American Psychiatric Association. The 1968 edition of the *Diagnostic and Statistical Manual of Mental Disorders* (DSM-II) confirmed the existence of "Psychophysiologic Disorders" with a specific classification:

This group of disorders is characterized by physical symptoms that are *caused by* [italics added] emotional factors and involve a single organ system, usually under autonomic nervous system innervation. (American Psychiatric Association, 1968, p. 46)

In the 1980 version of this manual (DSM-III) this classification was deleted. In its index the reader seeking "psychosomatic" or "psychophysiologic disorders" is referred to: "Psychological factors affecting physical condition" (p. 492). The mind-body dichotomy lends a dual set of defining properties to this new category. The "physical condition" is defined simply as "a physical disorder." As to "psychological factors": "This manual accepts the tradition of referring to certain factors as 'psychological,' although it is by no means easy to define what this phrase means (p. 303)." The 1987 edition, DSM-III-R, contains no index entry for either "psychosomatic" or "psychophysiologic" disorder.

Thus the causal link forged by psychogenesis after two centuries of denial of a role for mind appears to have been broken. Psychosomatic disorders have been restored to the status of "physical disorders." Still more disquieting for the holistic movement, the establishment of a specific category of "physical conditions affected by psychological factors" seems to imply that physical conditions are not universally thus affected.

Disillusionment Within

These modern developments constitute major deviations from the course charted by the field's founders. In place of becoming the "type of all illness," psychosomatic disorders became a special case of pathology. Rather than achieving the status of the favored approach in general medicine, psychosomatics evolved as a specialty. Wittkower (1960) uncovered evidence of the progressive narrowing trend that established psychosomatic medicine as a separate discipline. From 1939 to 1944, nearly 25% of articles published in *Psychosomatic Medicine* were contributed by neurologists and other medical specialists apart from psychiatry and psychology. From 1955 to 1960 this figure had declined to 9%.

The revolutionary goals of early advocates of holism have not been attained, and despite the breadth and precision of modern research and the extraordinary number of zealous proponents, an increasing feeling of dissatisfaction is apparent in the literature of the past two decades.

We trace a thread of discontent in presidential addresses to the American Psychosomatic Society. In 1970 John Mason stated: "we must face the fact that the psychosomatic approach has not yet had the sweeping, revolutionary impact on medicine of which it appears capable" (in Langley & Brand, 1972, p. 176). Marvin Stein's 1985 address voiced the same concern: "In spite of a considerable amount of clinical and investigative endeavor, the general field of psychosomatic medicine has not made the

progress expected of it" (1986, p. 13). Jenkins' address in the previous year isolated for critical attention a failure to "expand horizons."
Criticisms from without the field might be attributed to traditional historical prejudice against mind, but misgivings voiced by the field's principal advocates are telling indicators of pressing difficulties. Roy Grinker who helped pioneer the field, began his *Psychosomatic Concepts* (1973) with the prefatory statement: "There has been little progress in the field of psychosomatic medicine in the last few decades" (p. ix). Lader (1972) noted that the area of psychosomatic medicine had "lost its pristine promise" (p. 297). Lipowski (1968) commented upon a "spreading sense of disenchantment with the whole concept of psychosomatic medicine" (p. 396). Less reserved in his criticism, Szasz (1961) wrote: "the 'psychosomatic approach' has led neither to better therapies for patients nor to clearer theoretical insights for investigators" (p. 104).

Impediments to Progress

A closer scrutiny of the literature makes possible isolation of specific barriers to progress, and these are clearly products of the legacy of Cartesianism—mind-body isolationism. In Stein's presidential address, our attention is directed to the "tremendous leap from emotions to pathophysiology." He warns that "there may be major theoretical and methodologic flaws which have impeded substantial and fundamental advances in the field of psychosomatic medicine" (1986, p. 13). A case in point concerned the tradition of evasion of the question of the "how" of symptom formation in bronchial asthma: "In the specific psychodynamic causation formulations of bronchial asthma, little or no attention has been paid to the transition from an abstract psychodynamic concept to the specific pathophysiologic change found in asthma, i.e., bronchiolar obstruction" (p. 10).

Bernard Engel's address (1986) focused directly on the logical difficulties that dualism poses for psychosomatic medicine. He described the paradoxical nature of psychoanalytic formulations that "talk about mechanisms" and then "resort to mentalism" when trying to relate mechanistic processes to one another. He further enlightens his audience to the effect that disguising mentalism in behavioristic terminology does not resolve conceptual difficulties:

> The strategy that seems to have become the accepted formulation for dealing with dualism is a complete failure: The dualism explicit in the word, psychosomatic, has been replaced by the dualism implicit in the oxymoron, biobehaviorism. Instead of psychic causes of somatic disorders, we are told

that disease is the result of an interaction between biological (qua, organic) factors and behavioral (qua, mental) factors . . . biobehaviorism is simply a synonym for mind-body dualism. (1986, p. 470)

In an insightful analysis, Dr. Engel demonstrates how neither mind nor mechanism, either separately or combined, furnishes a basis for explanation; he proposes a behavioral approach that avoids "resorting to mind-body interaction" (1986, p. 477).

Previous writers, however, have been oblivious for the most part to the difficulties Dr. Engel brings to light, preferring to cope with rather than to confront the dilemma of isolationism. For this reason we observe another barrier to progress in scientists' justified hesitancy to violate convention when that violation involves assertions that fly in the face of formal logic. Nor will a distinguished scientific career tilt the balance in favor of the community's acceptance of such assertions. Perilous consequences have long been associated with claims of causation of physical by mental events. Though, for a time, science has entertained these hypotheses, they remain continuously at risk of being discarded when increasing knowledge advances the potential of causal explanation in physico-chemical terms. Donald (1972) related such an instance and advised hesitancy in asserting causal relationships:

> An example of how wrong one can be is that for many years shrewd clinicians described two groups among people with acute or chronic respiratory failure, usually chronic bronchitis who were actually ill with pneumonia. They spoke from their experience of "fighters" who were manifestly breathing with great difficulty but battling to remain alive and "nonfighters" who floated gently away and died without apparent dyspnoea or distress. In the last fifteen years it has been shown that the fighters had, in fact, fairly normal PCO_2 levels, their ventilatory response remained normal and they continued to ventilate even though they were suffering from severe dyspnoea. The "nonfighters" have now been shown to be people who had been given oxygen at high PCO_2 levels. They were, in fact, narcotized by carbon dioxide, they were underventilating and died quietly, often on high oxygen. What was an obvious division of a random population into "fighters" and "nonfighters" in fact was describing two different physiological situations. All one can conclude from this is that we must beware of filling in the gaps in our knowledge with this type of false interpretation. (pp. 318–319)

Thus conservatism has been judicious. As Lipowski (1986) observed, the prudent course evades condemnation: The decline and fall of psychogenic theories has led to a sort of backlash, one manifested by the current avoidance of sweeping explanatory formulations linking psycho-social factors and the occurrence of physical illness" (p. 10).

Our conceptual model of the organism permits the existence of *no bodily event* for which complete explanation in physical terms will not be forthcoming. When a physically based explanation does emerge it will be construed as scientific "fact" and perhaps also as an anticipated "breakthrough." Since it conforms to our underlying definition of the real world, the physical explanation will become a more or less stable entry into the body of knowledge. Psychological explanations, however, are perpetually relegated to the realm of speculation. In the wisdom of scientific conservatism, certainty is preferred over attempting to cross the great divide in our vessel with a hole.

A more tangible and distressing barrier to progress is posed by the fact that psychosomatic and psychophysiologic research results do not adapt readily to clinical application. The correlation data do not furnish the battery of "causes and cures" that form clinical medicine's stock in trade. An instance of this difficulty is offered by Ostfeld (1973), who directed critical attention to hypertension research published in *Psychosomatic Medicine* over a 30-year period. Ostfeld presumed that investigators had the following expectations of their work: "pathogenesis of the disease will become illuminated and treatment of it will be improved" (p. 1). According to Ostfeld neither goal has been fulfilled and none of the recent advances in medicine regarding pathogenesis or treatment of hypertension relate to the findings of psychosomatic research.

Yet much recent work has a specifically clinical focus, and from laboratory investigations concerning voluntary control of autonomic functions have come repeated confirmations of "self-regulation" capacities. Events long forbidden by anatomical and theoretical models of organismic functions have now been amply documented. Dramatic psychological outcomes in the direction of restoration of homeostasis and modification of brain wave patterns have been found in association with meditative techniques, "standard relaxation exercises," "autogenic phrases," imagery techniques, and so on (Sheikh, 1984).

Causal potency, however, apparently resides in the mental realm; thus outcomes remain fundamentally inexplicable. Clinical researchers are for this reason forced to maintain a conservative stance. They hesitate to proclaim "victory" over illness and without exception refrain from employing terms implying scientific "breakthroughs."

Psychosomatic research proceeds in the vein of "normal science." A model directing research, as Kuhn (1962) described it, is "like an accepted judicial decision in the common law . . . . an object for further articulation and specification (p. 23). The possibilities for future research along established lines are limitless. The knowledge base is like a vast, free-floating body of empirical findings, largely ungrounded in a unifying theoretical framework. Lacking an accommodating model of the organism, the discipline's "discoveries" are less than "revolutionary"; its clinical innovations fall short of "breakthroughs"; its treatment strategies, no matter how effective, are never "cures"; and the would-be self-regulator, the client trained in voluntary control of autonomic functions, is inwardly convinced before the fact of inherent inability to succeed.

CAUSATION AND A THREE-DIMENSIONAL MODEL OF HUMAN NATURE

The basis of all of these difficulties is our lack of theoretical understanding of holistic functioning. The term "holism" has been employed in recent years to encourage perception of unitary functioning of the organism. Holism, it is argued, is prerequisite for understanding the disease process and for instituting effective therapy. As previously noted, several authors have disparaged use of the term "psychosomatic," as it implies duality of psyche and soma (Dunbar, 1935/1954; Henry, 1972). The literature abounds with recommendations that we achieve an understanding of the "relationship" between mind and body—the relationship upon which holism is presumably based.

It must become our priority to give "the whole" meaning at the deepest level of explanation, and in so doing, to remove constraints on causality that deny the role of mental events. Isolationism has evaded critical scrutiny largely because scientists have failed to entertain the possibility of alternative models of human nature.

As Professor Kuhn (1962) has demonstrated, the philosophical underpinnings of science are accepted as unwritten law or as articles of faith. The mechanistic model led to dramatic advances in physical science and continues to prove its worth in several areas of clinical medicine. In the area of psychosomatics, however, the model has been less accommodating, and a substantial body of logically irreconcilable facts now demands a framework for causal explanation (Sheikh & Panagiotou, 1975).

In light of the dominance both historically (in premodern medicine) and currently (in the East) of nondualistic models of human nature, the holistic objective seems less elusive. In these alternate models we discover a framework for explanation wherein self-regulation is the norm and causation of illness is holistically conceived. What the Cartesian model lacks and what these alternate models share is a third dimension of reality—a vital dimension in addition to mind and matter.

Returning for a moment to our Cartesian roots, we observe the philosopher's introduction of mechanism. Here Descartes (1664/1967) dismisses the biologic soul—the premodern, vital substrate of animal existence—as unnecessary for interpretation of biological events:

> The final summary is as follows: I desire you should consider that these functions in this machine proceed from the mere arrangement of its organs, neither more, nor less than do the movements of a clock, or other automaton . . . It is unnecessary to conceive in it any soul . . . or any other principle of motion, or of life, than its blood . . . agitated by the heat of the fire which burns continually in the heart, and which is in no wise essentially different in nature from all the fires which are met with in inanimate bodies. (vol. 2 p. 276)

If the model appears foreign it is only because intervening centuries have rectified anatomical and physiological errors. In place of the heart as control center and heat as the energy source, science has substituted brain and nervous system as locus of control, and electrochemical impulse has replaced "fire" as the operating principle. Thus, in agreement with a vast accumulation of mechanistic knowledge of the body, the philosophy that captivated the scientific mind in the 1700s has not loosened its tenacious hold.

The mechanical model, however, permits but a linear chain of causal events into which mind or "self," however defined, cannot enter. As history has proven in the case of "nervous" disorders, the model does not permit the existence of psychosomatic illness.

Alternative models that affirm psychosomatic events define the organism differently. In addition to mind and matter, they acknowledge reality of a vital causal substrate. This third phase of reality is designated by many names. For the Chinese, *chi* is the essence of vitality. Vital energy interacts continuously with material events and explains the existence of emotion-related illness. In Indian tradition *kundalini* represents vital energy as a "universal life principle" manifest in all nature's living forms.

The Golden Age affirmed the existence of a vital spirit or biological soul. This soul *was the self* or "I"; it both performed and controlled vital functions. Thought, reason, and will were among the higher faculties of the soul; digestion, respiration, sensation, and movement were among the lower. Though the "animal spirit" proved impossible to dissect or to measure, its existence was an inference from facts. Necessary for successful explanation, the biological soul, with its several faculties, governed and performed all vital functions (McMahon, 1975b, 1986).

Assuming that mind and matter lay equal claim to being real, our problem in the modern age consists entirely of the isolationism that forbids their interaction. A solution may be achieved by adopting a third dimension of reality—one that accounts for and gives equal claim to reality to life itself.

The time-honored dualistic metaphysic made no provision for vitality, thus the question "What is life?" became a Gordian knot modern intellects could never sever. Vast strides in accumulation of knowledge of matter, however, have now pointed our way to a solution. Increasing realization of what matter *is* has, at the same time, demonstrated what vital matter *is not.* It has been determined that a third dimension of reality exists, though it is unaccounted for in the traditional scientific world view.

The Necessity of a Third Dimension

Nobel Prize–winning physicist Erwin Schrödinger (1945) addressed this question: *What Is Life?* His inquiry identified two deficiencies in our view of the world. First, the laws of physics cannot explain the phenomena of living matter; and second, mind is excluded from this view of nature because it is logically inadmissible.

Schrödinger began his inquiry stating that thanks to the

ingenious work of biologists . . . mainly of geneticists . . . enough is known about the actual material structure of organisms and about their functioning to state that, and to tell precisely why, present-day physics and chemistry could not possibly account for what happens in space and time within a living organism. . . . the structure of the vital parts of living organisms differs entirely from that of any piece of matter that we physicists and chemists have ever handled physically in our laboratories or mentally at our writing desks. (p. 2)

Schrödinger explained the persistence of the scientific misconception that vital matter was of a piece with inanimate substance. It had been confidently assumed that statistical physics applied to events within the cell because such events were presumed to involve enormous numbers of single atoms and single atomic processes. If this were the case, "all the relevant laws of physics and physical chemistry would be safeguard even under the very exacting demands of physics in respect to 'large numbers.'" Today it is known that "incredibly small groups of atoms, much too small to display exact statistical laws, *do* play a dominating role in the very orderly and lawful events within a living organism" (p. 17).

For the reader who remains unreconciled to the unsettling notion that the laws of physics cannot explain vital matter, a brief account of Schrödinger's evidence is presented. First, living cells evade the decay of matter to equilibrium. Were the substance of living things governed by the laws of physics, that substance would tend toward a state of thermodynamic equilibrium or "maximum entropy," but instead, as Schrödinger observes, it "keeps going" (p. 69). A body temperature of 98 degrees would create a disordering tendency referred to as "heat motion," sufficient to perturb the genes, but it does not. Were cells subject to the laws of physics, the hereditary code would be promptly destroyed by well-known physical influences such as paramagnetism and diffusion.

Schrödinger was not alone in arriving at this conclusion. Several leading physicists have come by his and by other routes to the conclusion that our world picture requires a third dimension. An entirely new set of principles is necessary to accommodate the phenomena of life.

A second objection to the reigning view of reality is associated with the first. As Schrödinger put it, it has long been assumed that "the physiological processes in the brain of a human thinker . . . would be deciphered and drawn up in terms of the ultimate constituents of matter" (p. 98). This assumption "cut out mind" from the real world. According to Schrödinger, "we do not belong to this material world that science constructs for us. We are not in it, we are outside" (p. 107). Scientists have not noticed the omission because the human body belongs to the world picture. The problem enters "when I feel that I am the author of these bodily goings on . . . then comes the impasse, the very embarrassing discovery of science, that I am not needed as an author" (p. 107). The human body's movements are its own.

The mistake of science, he continues, has been to allow us "to imagine the total display as that of a mechanical clockworks, which . . . could go on just the same for all science knows, without the existence of consciousness." Science has remained "completely ignorant" in this regard (p. 108). Schrödinger quotes famed neuroscientist Sherrington who pointed explicitly to this problem: "physical science . . . faces us with the impasse . . . the blank of 'how' of mind's leverage on matter" (p. 215). As Schrödinger saw it, the paradox posed by the dichotomy is "so painful that it is always meeting with the violent resistance of those who hope to solve it by denying it. In the mind-matter problem," science has never "been able to adumbrate the causal linkage satisfactorily even to its most ardent disciples" (p. 94).

The mind-matter problem becomes unproblematic, however, if matter causally associated with mind is reconceived and endowed with different properties. Several leading physicists have taken what they consider a necessary logical step and have adopted a "biotonic phase" of existence—a third dimension of reality. By appropriating this innovative concept we acquire the means of resolving the interaction dilemma. Achieving a conceptual model of the whole, we derive the possibility of interacting parts.

IMPLICATIONS OF THE NEW PERSPECTIVE

The three-dimensional model and its implications for causation are discussed elsewhere (Weimer, 1976; Weimer & Palermo, 1982). A few points are suggested here, though obviously a beginning and not an end is signified in these concluding paragraphs.

1. *"There is no such thing as a non-physical illness."* This statement by David Graham (1971, p. 121), is harmonious with a three-dimensional interaction model. Assuming that no part exists in isolation, the statement might be differently phrased: all illness is psychosomatic. Current estimates link "stress" to as much as 70 to 90% of illness. If this is indeed the case, 70 to 90% of illness is inadequately explained in exclusively physical terms and requires a holistic framework furnished by a model of causation involving reciprocal influences.

2. *Causation processes as reciprocal influences.* As Weimer (1976) has demonstrated, the linear or "billiard ball" model of causation is not equal to the task of explanation of psychophysiological phenomena. Relationships between phases suggest instead dynamic, reciprocal processes. A continuous loop better represents ongoing processes than a linear chain.

3. *Autonomic events are behaviors.* As Engel has argued (1986, p. 472), autonomic nervous system (ANS) events are as much "behavior" as any mediated by the somatic nervous system. In a holistic model where the concept of self expands to mean more than isolated mind or ego, autonomic processes become acts performed (whether knowingly or unknowingly) by the self-regulator.

4. *Self-regulation is the norm, and personal responsibility is inescapable.* The mechanistic model, which assumed functional autonomy of bodily events, rendered us "victims" of physical illness. The causally impotent mind was necessarily passive witness to autonomous mechanism. Though perhaps an intimidating notion, the interaction model makes us instead "perpetrators" of psychosomatic illness. Therefore, self-regulation methods assume greater

importance as potential means of restoring and maintaining autonomic equilibrium.

5. *"Meaning" acquires significance.* Symptoms of functional illness have long been recognized as embodying meaning. Psychoanalytic theory identified symbolic significance. Other models emphasize defensive utility, secondary gain, and so forth. Meaning, however, being irreconcilable with mechanism, could not be integrated into the causal framework and remained peripheral to medical concerns.

Meaning now comes to the fore as an aspect characteristically human in human disease. Meaning may warrant status on a par with mechanism in diagnosis, treatment, and prevention. If the sufferer is indeed implicated as unwilling perpetrator, comprehension of meaning of symptoms assumes utility as an aspect of effective self-regulation.

6. *Anomalous events must be understood as such.* Events unexplainable in terms of isolationism require explanation in holistic terms. "Spontaneous" remission, placebo effects, and hypnotically induced physiological changes are among many events whose potential significance has not been appreciated for lack of scientific explanation. In each of these anomalies we may eventually find models of normal functioning.

CONCLUDING REMARKS

A model transcending isolationism will empower us to act upon the recommendations of historical proponents of psychosomatics whose entreaties have echoed through the reign of dualism. Over 100 years ago French physician Hippolyte Bernheim, observing the impact of hypnotic suggestions on physiological processes, wrote: "Mind is not a negligible quantity. There is such a thing as psychobiology. There is also such a thing as psychotherapy. This is a powerful lever, and one which the human intelligence and medical therapeutics must turn to full account" (in Janet, 1925, Vol. 1, p. 11). Fifty years of advancement in physical medicine ensued, after which the psychoanalytic pioneers restated Bernheim's position as if the concepts expressed were innovations.

A quarter century subsequent to the Freudian era, Jerome Frank (1975), observing the power of mind in placebo effects, biofeedback, and meditative exercises, urged again that psychotherapeutic methods may assist. He said, "If psychotherapists can persuade physicians of their usefulness, they can make diagnostic, preventive and therapeutic contributions" (p. 200).

The scientific enlightenment that gave psychosomatic medicine its initial impetus was the reality of a unique phenomenon—the causation of bodily events by mental events. Thus, after 50 years of formal existence of psychosomatic medicine, it is manifest that the revolution requires reinforcement. Its culmination will require the logical foundation furnished by an alternative to isolationism. In a three-dimensional interaction model of human nature we find this rational justification, a basis for theory, and an uncompromised means of pursuing the noble objectives of the field's pioneers.

References

Alexander, F. (1948). Fundamental concepts in psychosomatic research: Psychogenesis, conversion, specificity. In F. Alexander & T. M. French, *Studies in psychosomatic medicine.* New York: Ronald Press.

Alexander, F., Eisenstein, S., & Grotjahn, M. (Eds.). (1966). *Psychoanalytic pioneers.* New York: Basic Books.

American Psychiatric Association. (1968). *Diagnostic and statistical manual of mental disorders* (2nd ed.). Washington, DC: Author.

American Psychiatric Association. (1980). *Diagnostic and statistical manual of mental disorders* (3rd ed.). Washington, DC: Author.

American Psychiatric Association. (1987). *Diagnostic and statistical manual of mental disorders* (rev. ed.). Washington, DC: Author.

Beard, G. M. (1880). *Practical treatise on nervous exhaustion* (2nd ed.). New York: William Wood.

Beard, G. M. (1881). *American nervousness.* New York: Arno Press.

Descartes, R. (1967). *Traité del'homme. The philosophical works of Descartes* (Vols. 1 & 2) (E. Haldone & G. Ross, Trans.). Cambridge: Cambridge University Press. (Original work published 1664)

Deutsch, F. (1927). Psychoanalysis and internal medicine. In F. Alexander, S. Eisenstein, and M. Grotjahn, (Eds.). (1966). *Psychoanalytic pioneers.* New York: Basic Books.

Donald, K. W. (1972). In Ciba Foundation Symposium 8. *Physiology, emotion and psychosomatic illness* (pp. 318–319). Amsterdam: North Holland.

Dunbar, H. F. (1954). *Emotions and bodily changes* (4th ed.). New York: Columbia University Press.

Engel, B. (1986). Psychosomatic medicine, behavioral medicine, just plain medicine. *Psychosomatic Medicine, 48*(7), 466–479.

Ferenczi, S., Abraham, K., Simmel, E., & Jones, E. (1921). *Psycho-analysis and the war neurosis.* London: The International Psycho-Analytic Press.

Frank, J. (1975). Psychotherapy of bodily disease. *Psychotherapy and Psychosomatics, 26,* 192–202.

Freud, S. (1968). Notes upon a case of obsessional neurosis. In S. Freud, *Three case histories.* New York: Collier Books. (Original work published 1909)

Graham, D. T. (1971). Psychophysiology in medicine. *Psychophysiology, 8,* 121–131.

Graham, D. T. (1972). Psychosomatic medicine. In N. Greenfield & R. Stanbach (Eds.), *Handbook of psychophysiology* (pp. 839–917). New York: Holt, Rinehart and Winston.

Grinker, R. (1973). *Psychosomatic concepts,* New York: Jason Aronson.

Halliday, J. L. (1938). The rising incidence of psychosomatic illness. *The British Medical Journal, 2,* 11–14.

Henry, J. P. (1972). In Ciba Foundation Symposium 8. *Physiology, emotion and psychosomatic illness* (p. 317). Amsterdam: North Holland.

Howard, J. C. (1973). *Academy of psychosomatic medicine membership directory.* Schering Laboratories.

Ikemi, Y. (1974). Psychosomatic medicine in Japan. *Psychosomatics, 15,* 155–156.

Janet, P. (1925). *Psychological healing* (Vols. 1 & 2), (E. Paul & C. Paul, Trans.). New York: Macmillan.

Jenkins, C. D. (1985). New horizons for psychosomatic medicine. *Psychosomatic Medicine, 47*(1), 3–25.

Jones, C. H. (1864). *Clinical observations on functional nervous disorders.* London: John Churchill.

Kennedy, F. (1918). The nature of nervousness in soldiers. *Journal of the American Medical Association, 71,* 17–21.

Kuhn, T. S. (1962). *The structure of scientific revolutions.* Chicago: University of Chicago Press.

Kunzendorf, R., & Sheikh, A. (Eds.). (in press). *The psychophysiology of mental imagery: Theory, research and application.* Farmingdale, NY: Baywood.

Lader, M. (1972). Psychophysiological research and psychosomatic medicine. In Ciba Foundation Symposium 8. *Physiology, emotion and psychosomatic illness* (pp. 279–320). Amsterdam: North Holland.

Langley, L. L., & Brand, J. L. (1972). The mind-body issue in early twentieth-century American medicine. *Bulletin of the History of Medicine, 46,* 171–179.

Lipowski, Z. J. (1968). Review of consultation psychiatry and psychosomatic medicine III. Theoretical issues. *Psychosomatic Medicine, 30,* 395–422.

Lipowski, Z. J. (1976). Psychosomatic medicine: An overview. In O. W. Hill (Ed.), *Modern trends in psychosomatic medicine.* London: Butterworths.

Lipowski, Z. J. (1986). Psychosomatic medicine, past and present, Pt. II. Current state. *Canadian Journal of Psychology, 31,* 8–13.

Lorand, S. (1973). Correlation between psychiatry and medicine: Historical evaluation of psychosomatic medicine, *New York State Journal of Medicine, 73,* 2665–2669.

Marston, W. M. (1928). *Emotions of normal people.* New York: Harcourt, Brace.

Mason, J. (1972). Presidential address to the American Psychosomatic Society (1970). In L. Langley and J. Brand (Eds.), The mind-body issue in early twentieth century American medicine. *Bulletin of the History of Medicine, 46,* 171–179.

Maudsley, H. (1896). *Responsibility in mental disease.* New York: Appleton.

McDougall, W. (1926). *Outline of abnormal psychology.* New York: Scribner's.

McMahon, C. E. (1975a). The wind of the cannon ball: An informative anecdote from medical history. *Psychotherapy and Psychosomatics, 26,* 125–131.

McMahon, C. E. (1975b). Harvey on the soul: A unique episode in the history of psychophysiological thought. *Journal of the History of Behavioral Science, 11,* 276–283.

McMahon, C. E. (1986) *Where medicine fails.* New York: Trado-Medic Books.

McMahon, C. E. (1976a). Psychosomatic disease and the problem of causation. *Medical Hypothesis, 2,* 112–115.

McMahon, C. E. (1976b). The psychosomatic approach to heart disease: A study in pre-modern medicine. *Chest, 69,* 531–537.

McMahon, C. E., & Koppes, S. (1976). The development of psychosomatic medicine: An analysis of growth of professional societies. *Psychosomatics, 17,* 185–187.

The Merck manual of diagnosis and therapy. (1899). Rahway, NJ: Merck, Sharp and Dohme.

Nemiah, J. C. (1985). Hysteria. *Psychosomatic Medicine, 47*(3), 303–305.

Osler, W. (1942). *Principles and Practice of Medicine Designed for the Use of Practitioners and Students of Medicine* (Fourteenth Edition) New York: Appleton Century.

Ostfeld, A. (1973). What's the payoff of hypertension research? *Psychosomatic Medicine, 35,* 1–3.

Schrödinger, E. (1945). *What Is Life?* Cambridge: Cambridge University Press.

Shakespeare, W. (1977). *Shakespeare's Sonnets* (S. Booth, Ed.) London: Yale University Press.

Sheehan, D. (1943). Physiological principles underlying psychosomatic disorders. *Journal of Nervous Diseases, 98,* 414–416.

Sheikh, A. A. (Ed.). (1984). *Imagination and healing.* Farmingdale, NY: Baywood.

Sheikh, A. A., & Kunzendorf, R. G. (1984). Imagery, physiology and psychosomatic illness. *International Review of Mental Imagery, 1,* 95–138.

Sheikh, A. A., & Panagiotou, N. C. (1975). Use of mental imagery in psychotherapy: A critical review. *Perceptual and Motor Skills, 41,* 555–585.

Sheikh, A. A., Richardson, P., & Moleski, L. M. (1979). Psychosomatics and mental imagery: A brief review. In A. A. Sheikh & J. T. Shaffer (Eds.), *The potential of fantasy and imagination.* New York: Brandon House.

Stein, M. (1986). A reconsideration of specificity in psychosomatic medicine. *Psychosomatic Medicine, 48,* 13–22.

Szasz, T. S. (1961). *The myth of mental illness.* New York: Hoeber.

Troland, L. T. (1932). *The principles of psychophysiology* (Vols. 1–3). New York: Van Nostrand.

Weimer, W. B. (1976). Manifestations of mind: Some conceptual and empirical issues. In G. Globus, G. Maxwell, & I. Savodnik (Eds.), *Consciousness and the brain,* New York: Plenum.

Weimer, W. B., & Palermo, D. (Eds.). (1982). *Cognition and the symbolic processes* (Vols. 1 & 2). Hillsdale, NJ: Erlbaum.

Weiner, H. (1971). *American Psychosomatic Society brochure.* American Psychosomatic Society, Inc.

Weiss, J. H. (1974). The current state of the concept of a psychosomatic disorder. *International Journal of Psychiatric Medicine, 5,* 473.

Wittkower, E. D. (1960). Twenty years of North American psychosomatic medicine. *Psychosomatic Medicine, 22,* 308.

12

Cerebral Laterality: Implications for Eastern and Western Therapies

ROBERT G. LEY
MAURA SMYLIE

Something I owe to the soil that grew,
More to the life that fed,
But most to Allah
Who gave me two separate sides of my head.

I would go without shirts or shoes,
Friends, tobacco, or bread,
Sooner than for an instant
Lose either side of my head.

Rudyard Kipling, in his poem *Kim*

The fact that the human brain is divided into two "halves," or hemispheres, is perhaps the best known aspect of brain anatomy. The impetus for such widespread awareness can be attributed in large part to Robert Ornstein's (1972) seminal book, *The Psychology of Consciousness.* In this book Ornstein described and ultimately popularized the initial scientific findings from Roger Sperry's studies of "split-brain" patients (Sperry, 1966). As a by-product of attempting to control epileptic seizures by severing the corpus callosum and the anterior commissure (a bundle of nerve fibers that joins the two halves of the brain), Sperry and his coworkers vividly illustrated the different cognitive functions, or "experiences," of the left and right cerebral hemispheres. As a result of the initial "split-brain" studies, a firm association between the left hemisphere and verbal/linguistic processes was established and differentiated from the linkage between the right hemisphere and nonverbal, visual-spatial cognitive processes.

In addition to describing the cognitive properties of each hemisphere, Ornstein (1972) further asserted that different modes of consciousness could be construed as evolving from the left and right hemispheres' cognitive styles—analytic versus holistic, respectively. Using cerebral laterality as a metaphor for *personal* cognitive styles, Ornstein implied that a strong tendency existed for individuals to use preponderantly one hemisphere or the other to experience the world and to cognize the information in it. Thus people could be classified according to their "hemisphericity." The notion of individual hemisphericity was extrapolated to groups of individuals: it was suggested that different cultures were more prone to rely on either a left- or right-hemisphere mode of information processing. In short, Ornstein differentiated Eastern and Western modes of experience and related these to hemispheric differences in cognitive style.

Ornstein's creative formulation of "esoteric psychologies," such as Buddhism, Yoga, and Sufism, in terms of the mode of consciousness embodied in their practices and the differential hemispheric functions that may support them was reminiscent of an earlier genre of interest in things that were Eastern. This tradition was best represented by Alan Watts (1961) in his classic book, *Psychotherapy East and West.* Watts argued persuasively that Eastern "ways of life" such as Buddhism, Taoism, Vedanta, and Yoga are neither organized religions or philosophies of life. Rather, they should be considered to resemble psychotherapies, principally because Eastern ways of life and Western psychotherapies are oriented toward changing individuals' consciousness, their experience of themselves, and their relationship to society. Currently, a renaissance of interest in Eastern psychotherapies and other traditions is occurring (as evidenced by the publication of this volume). In part, this renewed interest is due to Western recognition of the therapeutic efficacy of certain constituents of Eastern therapies (e.g., meditation, isolation, or relaxation) as well as a more general cultural and scientific interest in mind and body relationships.

This chapter reexamines Ornstein's thesis in light of the knowledge of hemispheric functions that has accumulated in the last two decades. Furthermore, the ways in which cerebral asymmetries may interact with Eastern psychotherapies will be considered.

THE POPULARIZATION OF THE LATERALITY CONCEPT

As a backdrop to this reappraisal, it is important to be fully acquainted with the truly dramatic dispersion of information about cerebral laterality. Quite simply, the scientific study of brain laterality became a psychological *zeitgeist:* a tenfold increase in research articles in this domain was documented from 1970 to 1980 (Ley & Kaushansky, 1985). Goleman (1977) characterized scientific interest in the differential functioning of the cerebral hemispheres as psychology's most recent "fad." Others labeled an overenthusiastic tendency to pick a pair of polar opposites and assign each to the left and right hemisphere as "dichotomania."

In nonscientific domains, the frequency with which laterality themes appeared in news articles, advertisements, and cartoons in the popular press during the 1970s and 1980s was astounding and testified to the widespread currency of the brain laterality concept. For example, cerebral hemispheric differences have provided the humorous motif in cartoons such as "Peanuts," "Herman," and "Cathy" as well as numerous times in *New Yorker* magazine. Even in Ann Landers's column a letter was published explaining that "Everyone has two brains in his head, a 'yes' brain and a 'no' brain." These "brains" were further associated with the left and right hemispheres. The letter writer concluded that the side of one's head that one slept upon was responsible for producing depressed or happy moods upon awakening in the morning. Judging from these examplars in the popular press, it is clear that laypersons are well aware that the left and right hemispheres "do different things."

Hemispheric differences in function have been used to suggest explanations for behaviors as wide ranging as tennis playing, wine tasting, movie preferences, and conflicts between "cowboys and Indians"—the latter hostilities being due to the belief that Indians are "right-hemisphere types," whereas cowboys think mostly with the left side of their brains. Advertisers have also attempted to capitalize on the appeal to consumers of left- and right-hemisphere functions. For example, Saab, the Swedish automaker, has run a two-page ad that features technical specifications and "hard facts" on the left side of the page and an exotic, visually stimulating photograph of a speeding Saab on the right side of the page.

Apart from the human species, hemispheric dominance and functional cerebral differences have been investigated in animals, ranging from chickens to dolphins. In short, a thorough review of the laterality concept in scientific articles and the popular press indicates that most cognitive functions and bodily parts, ranging from taste preferences to the nasal cycle, have been formulated in terms of the different properties of the left and right hemispheres. However, the greatest impetus for the popularization of the laterality concept came not from the popular press, but rather from educators.

THE RIGHT-BRAIN MOVEMENT

In 1977, the *Brain/Mind Bulletin* anointed the year as "the year of the right brain." Such an appellation reflected a changing trend, particularly in humanistic circles and progressive educational settings, wherein an emphasis on logical, analytic thinking and verbal skills had been developed within the school system at the expense of more intuitive, creative, nonlinear, holistic approaches to thinking and education. It was believed that the former emphasis reflected the dominance of the left hemisphere in Western culture. Progressive educators rued the historical, implicit disparagement of right-brain properties, such as imagery and creativity. A value judgment underlying the changing educational emphasis was that right-brain functions were more precious, unique, and valued, and thus in need of nurturing. Additionally, specific educational programs were necessary to foster right-brain thinking. However, right-brainedness came to be replaced by "whole-brainedness" as a more desired cognitive state and pedagogical goal (Ley & Kaushansky, 1985).

Within educational circles, the transition from a supposed left-hemisphere-dominant school system to a right-brained and then ultimately to a whole-brained classroom capitalized on a number of myths about brain laterality. The most fundamental myth governing the right-brain educational movement was the misguided notion that people are either left-brained or right-brained individuals. This notion is founded on another fallacious assumption, namely, that only one hemisphere or one half of the brain is used at any given time or for any cognitive activity and that cerebral activity alternates or otherwise flips back and forth between the two hemispheres. Although unquestionably there are individual differences in emotionality, linguistic skills, imaging, and spatial abilities, it is simply not the case that a particular hemisphere has sole responsibility for a particular cognitive task. Rather, the differences are relative rather than absolute ones, even for well-lateralized cognitive functions. It is almost certainly the case that educational programs that are oriented toward training the right hemisphere simply foster greater individual use of nonverbal problem-solving strategies: They do not change the balance or use of each hemisphere (Ley & Kaushansky, 1985).

THE BASICS OF CEREBRAL LATERALITY

Despite widespread awareness of the fact that the brain is divided and specialized for different cognitive functions, it should be apparent from the formulations of right-brain educators, that many misconceptions about hemispheric functioning exist (Ley & Kaushansky, 1985). One of the most basic principles of brain and behavior relationships is that each hemisphere controls movements in the opposite half or side of the body. This means that sounds coming to the left ear, objects in the left visual field, and sensations in the left hand will be almost exclusively projected to the right hemisphere. Conversely, stimuli in the right side of space or on the right half of the body are projected to the left hemisphere (Bryden, 1982). An example of this cross-wiring is the occurrence of a left-side paralysis of the arm, leg, or facial musculature following a right-hemisphere brain injury.

Various clinical and research strategies have confirmed that the two cerebral hemispheres are specialized for different cognitive functions. Commencing in the mid–19th century, the work of European neurologists showed that damage to certain portions of the left hemisphere resulted in language disturbances called "aphasias." Aphasias were rarely observed to follow instances of right-hemisphere damage; consequently, it was inferred that the left hemisphere was specialized for most language and verbal processes. The strong association between language skills and the left hemisphere combined with the importance of language as a communication medium created the opinion that the left hemisphere was the "dominant" one.

Subsequent research has shown that the left hemisphere is responsible for processing the phonological, syntactic, and semantic aspects of language (Segalowitz, 1983). A left-hemisphere advantage for linguistic functions has been demonstrated in auditory and visual domains as well as for motor tasks involving the left and right hands. Despite the left hemisphere's greater involvement in the reception and production of language, it is not the case that the right hemisphere is idle or impotent during linguistic processes. Some recent clinical evidence derived from split-brain patients has shown a rudimentary language capacity in the right hemisphere. Also, it is well known that right-hemisphere information processing capacity is involved with highly emotional or imageable words (Bryden & Ley, 1983). Furthermore, although gender, handedness, cognitive style, and experimental task difficulty can weaken or otherwise modify the strength of the association between the left hemisphere and language functions, the association nonetheless remains the most robustly established hemispheric function (Bryden, 1982).

In contrast to the left hemisphere, the right hemisphere dominates for a variety of nonlinguistic visual-spatial functions (Ornstein, Herron, Johnstone, & Swencionis, 1979). Experimentation demonstrated that the right hemisphere was relatively superior for recognizing and processing environmental sounds and many musical functions, including tone recognition; in fact, it is the right hemisphere that regulates the intonation in ordinary speech (Segalowitz, 1983). Also, the right hemisphere plays a predominant role in the recognition of faces and emotions (Ley & Bryden, 1983). Finally, the right hemisphere is more involved in mental imaging (Ley, 1983).

Despite research findings linking specific functions to each hemisphere, it is important to be aware that such differences relate more to the "style" of information processing rather than the information that is being processed. In other words, it is not so much the case that each hemisphere is uniquely specialized to work with different "things," (e.g., the left hemisphere with phonemes and the right hemisphere with musical tones), rather, it is that each hemisphere is organized structurally to provide a different cognitive style. Each style is more or less well adapted to processing different types of information. As mentioned previously, as a result of the explosion of laterality research in the 1970s the left hemisphere came to be characterized as a logical, analytic, and sequential processor, whereas the right hemisphere was described as a holistic, Gestalt, and diffuse processor.

Given such characterizations, it is easy to see why the left hemisphere predominates for processing language and the right hemisphere is relatively superior for face recognition. However, recent research has challenged the appropriateness of characterizing the left and right hemispheres as analytic and holistic processors, respectively (Sergent, 1982). Sergent has suggested that the left hemisphere is best suited for "detailed" processing, that which can be most aptly considered "high-resolution" or "high-frequency" information. In contrast, the right hemisphere is a better processor of larger, nondetailed, "low-frequency" information. Somewhat radically, Sergent has asserted that both hemispheres analyze and both perceive wholes, but that it is the rate or the "fineness" of detail that determines hemispheric advantages for particular stimuli.

Similar to Sergent's reformulation of hemispheric processing styles, rapidly accumulating laterality research continues to modify past, well-established axioms, such as the linkage between the right hemisphere and emotional processes. Three possible explanations for lateralization of emotional processes now exist: first, that emotions are better recognized by the right hemisphere; second, that control of emotional expression is regulated principally by the right hemisphere; and third, that the right hemisphere is specialized for negative emotions, whereas the left hemisphere is specialized for positive emotions (Ley & Strauss, 1986).

These competing formulations are modified further when one considers the possibility that lateral asymmetries for different emotions may vary, and when one distinguishes emotional *perception* from emotional *expression*. Also, each hemisphere may have different rates of arousal (Heilman & Van Den Abell, 1979); it may be that the left hemisphere dominates approach behaviors (in regard to emotion), whereas the right hemisphere governs avoidance behaviors (Davidson & Fox, 1983). Furthermore, personality and individual defense mechanisms further attenuate the once supposedly strong association between the right hemisphere and emotion. Finally, some research is suggesting that the *within* hemispheric differences, with respect to structural organization, may ultimately prove to be more influential than the *between* hemispheric differences (Levy, 1983). This is especially the case in regard to gender differences in recognition ability. All of these considerations or modifications provide abundant substantiation for Kosslyn's (1987) view that the neuropsychological literature on lateralization is typified by "ubiquitous variability."

EASTERN THERAPIES

Prior to examining possible interactions between Eastern psychotherapies and brain laterality, a brief review of Eastern therapies is in order. Rather than focus on the range and diversity of Eastern approaches (which are described throughout this volume), Japanese psychotherapies have been selected, largely because each one represents a well-articulated set of therapeutic techniques, which then allows for a more direct comparison to Western approaches and the elucidation of potential underlying hemispheric mechanisms.

Reynolds (1980) has written extensively on the "quiet therapies," including Morita psychotherapy, Naikan, Shadan, Seiza, and Zen. Reynolds has deemed these Japanese psychotherapies "quiet ones" inasmuch as each one involves considerable personal isolation and introspection. In fact, these attributes are suggested in the name of each Japanese therapy. For example, Naikan is derived from the Japanese words for "inner" (*nei*) and "observation" (*kan*). When these words are combined, they mean "introspection." Similarly, *seiza* is derived from *sei* (meaning "quiet") and *za* (meaning "sitting"), which denotes the principal therapeutic task in the treatment method. *Shadan* is the Japanese word for "isolation." Zen has evolved from the Japanese pronunciation of the Chinese word *ch'an*, which was derived from the Sanskrit *dhyana*, which means "meditation."

Although there is a discernible North American tendency to construe Eastern philosophies, and by extension Eastern therapies, as mystical (and therefore perhaps unscientific), the foregoing Japanese psychotherapies offer much pragmatic advice and invoke techniques for resolving life's basic problems. Before considering the extent to which cerebral lateralities might influence the style and tasks of Eastern therapies, it is useful to summarize their nature.

Morita and Naikan Therapies

Morita and Naikan therapies are the most widely practiced of the Japanese psychotherapies. Inasmuch as Reynolds has expertly described the development and nature of these therapies in Chapter 7, there is no reason to reiterate that information. However, to allow for contrast with other Japanese therapies, such as Seiza, Shadan, and Zen, Morita and Naikan will be summarized briefly here.

Morita psychotherapy is a rather directive therapy in which the patient progresses from isolated bed rest and enforced inactivity to light manual tasks (e.g., cleaning) to heavy work, (e.g., farming or gardening). The most important phase of Morita therapy is the "life training" period in which patients continue to work but gradually increase their social interactions, often through recreational activities, until they reenter the community. Morita therapy is oriented toward the treatment of Shinkeishitsu neuroses, which center on social anxieties, unassertiveness, and inferiority. A principal goal of Morita therapy is to facilitate the patient's interactions with others, through work and play, despite anxiety about such involvement.

In contrast to Morita therapy, Naikan therapy is based upon meditation. Clients are assigned topics upon which to meditate. Meditative exercises frequently focus upon the client's relationship to significant others. The "Sensie," who functions as a therapist, sits with the client and listens to his or her confessions. As in Morita therapy, during the initial phase of Naikan therapy the client is isolated from all others except the Sensie.

Naikan therapy emphasizes a client's responsibility for the trouble he or she has caused significant others. It aims to develop the personal awareness of that which one has received from others relative to what one has given to others. Contemporary social relationships come to be understood in light of the client's relationship to his or her parents, particularly the mother. Naikan therapy promotes strong emotions as the client reappraises himself or herself and restructures the past.

Shadan

Shadan therapy is also known as Ansei or "rest" therapy, and resting is the principal component of this treatment. The Shadan therapist believes that maladaptive thoughts or feelings are similar to any physical illness, and that prolonged bed rest and isolation are curative. Quite simply, the neurotic or unhealthy mind needs to rest so that restorative psychic energy can accumulate.

Similar to the initial phase of Morita therapy, Shadan procedures involve the patient being isolated and in bed. Initially, the patient is required to rest in bed, eat three meals daily, and only undertake natural body processes. Gradually, over a number of days, the patient is introduced to and required to complete simple tasks, such as computation or letter writing. Eventually, the daily mental work assignments are graduated to readings about nature and then to readings about human beings. Such mental work is not in the service of a diversion, but rather for elucidation.

Seiza Therapy

Seiza, or "quiet sitting" therapy, like Shadan therapy, is based upon natural healing properties that are associated with rest, isolation, and relaxation. In Seiza therapy, the patient is trained to breathe properly and sit quietly. The therapy involves two 30-minute sessions daily, one in the morning and another in the evening.

With respect to the sitting position for Seiza therapy, the client sits with a straight back. The legs are bent backwards and tucked under the buttocks, which rest on the insteps of the feet. The feet are crossed and hands are gently clasped or folded on one's lap. The body position and posture are quite exact, yet comfortable. In addition to the proper seating posture, appropriate breathing is the second necessary aspect of Seiza. The prescribed body posture facilitates correct breathing, and the focal point for such breathing is the body's center of gravity, or *"tanden,"* which is a few inches below the navel. In Seiza, the exhalation phase of breathing is emphasized and is approximately four times greater in duration than that which is required for the inhalation phase. During exhalation, air is gradually released through the nose. Once the sitting posture is perfected and the breathing technique mastered, the client's mind is to focus on the *tanden,* and a deep, meditative state is achieved. Quite simply, the goal of Seiza is to sit quietly.

Zen

In Reynolds's (1980) authoritative book on Eastern psychotherapies, he includes Zen among the techniques that he reviews, despite its status as a religion. Zen adherents construe the practice of Zen as a form of self-discipline that can improve emotional and psychological well-being.

Zen meditative techniques remain something of a novelty in the Western world, despite the popularization of transcendental meditation (TM) in the mid-1960s. The original ground swell of interest associated with TM can be attributed in large part to the Beatles being devotees of Maharishi Mahesh Yogi. In the last 20 years, interest has increased further due to people's interest in Eastern cultures and religious philosophies such as Buddhism, Sufism, and Zen.

Zen involves numerous techniques that aim to guide the practitioner to a state of *satori*. *Satori* represents a major shift in one's experience of oneself and is considered a step toward enlightenment. Zen sitting is an important method for facilitating the experience of *satori*.

The first type of Zen sitting is called Bompu Zen and involves sitting in a lotus position and breathing deeply, which promotes good physical health, relaxation, and improved sleep and work habits. In Bompu Zen, one learns to concentrate, minimize outside distractions, and control one's mind. Initially, in Bompu, the person counts each breath, which promotes mental concentration. Four other forms of Zen are described by Reynolds (1980), although their practice is intended to assist the person in developing supernormal powers, self-awareness, and enlightenment.

Reynolds reports that Zen sitting is often an adjunct to Morita therapy; indeed, the various Japanese therapies briefly reviewed here share many common features, including an emphasis on experience rather than theory and on personal development rather than symptom relief. Each therapy stresses self-discipline, and the therapist functions as a directive guide. Isolation, meditation, and relaxation are cornerstones and common elements to each therapy.

Similarly, each of the Japanese therapies seeks to alter individual, egocentric consciousness; in this regard, the Japanese techniques can be compared to other Eastern methods, such as Buddhism, Taoism, Vedanta, and Islamic Sufism, in which meditation is a common practice as well.

WESTERN BRAIN RESEARCH ON ASPECTS OF EASTERN THERAPIES

Freud regarded meditation as a regressive, infantile, and maladaptive attempt to fuse with a mother (Watts, 1961) or as a means to reexperience intrauterine life (the so-called *Nirvana* principle). Since Freud, Western psychotherapists and researchers have not been charitable toward or frankly that interested in Eastern therapies. However, in the mid-1970s American studies of the specific and nonspecific components in a variety of psychotherapies and the examination of common therapeutic change mechanisms (Frank, 1974) may have served to divert some attention to non-Western techniques or, at least, Eastern aspects of Western psychotherapies (e.g., meditation).

Over the last two decades, Western psychological researchers have devoted some effort to investigating the processes that occur in Eastern therapies. It is beyond the purview of this chapter to comprehensively review this research, although much of it focuses on the therapeutic effects associated with isolation or sensory deprivation (Suedfeld, 1975). More general attempts have been made to establish the psychophysiological correlates of meditation, and by now it is well-established that meditation, similar to hypnosis and progressive relaxation, results in decreased autonomic arousal, including lower blood pressure, respiration, heart rate, and muscle tension (Goleman, 1977).

Initial interest in the electrical activity of the brain (EEG) during meditation naturally led to a consideration of hemispheric differences during meditative states. In general, the EEG studies of meditators have produced contradictory results. For example, researchers have found both increases and decreases in, as well as a lack of alpha activity, during meditation (Shapiro, 1982). Unfortunately, much of the research methodology is lacking with respect to meeting standard psychometric criteria (e.g., adequate control groups, baseline or pretreatment measures, and appropriate sample sizes). Furthermore, an operational or consensual definition of meditation has been difficult to achieve. For instance, it is a gross oversimplification to assume that all types of meditation involve an attempt to eradicate verbal thinking from the mind, as many believe. This misconception was consequently linked to another misguided notion that any meditative practice (perhaps by virtue of its Eastern trappings) exclusively prompted or was linked isomorphically to right-hemisphere mentation. As mentioned above, such linkage was taken as a given during the 1970s when all things creative, mystical, transcendental, or "off-beat" were considered the province of the right hemisphere.

Most certainly, meditation takes many forms, ranging from concentrated attention on a meditative object (e.g., a vase or *mantra*) to an active internal dialectic replete with vigorous verbal thinking. However, at the broadest level of analysis, all meditative techniques involve attending and concentrating as well as turning attention from the external to the internal.

Quite clearly, much research on meditation was undertaken during the 1970s right-brain movement and the accompanying over-valuing of all right-hemisphere processes or characteristics. As mentioned earlier, the original conception guiding this research was that meditation would facilitate cognitive processing in the right hemisphere and decrease or occlude left-hemisphere activity. A study representative of this approach is that undertaken by Warrenburg and Pagano (1982). These researchers compared the performances of novice and experienced transcendental meditators (as well as nonmeditators) on a battery of verbal, musical, and spatial cognitive tasks. The results were not definitive, but the researchers concluded that individuals who are predisposed to learning TM are also inclined toward, or more interested in, altering their attentional focus from a left-hemisphere-dominant to a right-hemisphere-dominant mode. This conclusion is a rather gratuitous one, aligned with the school of thought that people characteristically utilize (exclusively) one hemisphere or the other to attend, perceive, and cognize the world.

Somewhat differently, Meissner and Pirot (1983) have shown that transcendental meditation influences the information processing of *each* cerebral hemisphere. Using a reaction time research paradigm in which subjects were to manually respond to an auditory verbal stimulus, it was found that subjects who were experienced meditators did not show the expected right ear (left hemisphere) advantage *after* they had meditated. In contrast, nonmeditator control subjects showed the expected right ear, left-hemisphere response bias. It seemed that after meditation, meditating subjects displayed a suppressed response to auditory stimuli that were delivered to the left hemisphere, whereas their reaction times were facilitated for stimuli arriving at the left ear and transmitted to the right hemisphere. Meissner and Pirot concluded that meditation is an attentional strategy that disrupts the usual hemispheric biases of the brain. A similar finding was earlier demonstrated by Pagano and Frumkin (1972) after meditating TM subjects were tested for their memory of various musical tones. Experienced meditators displayed enhanced right-hemisphere functioning in the aftermath of their meditation.

These findings suggest that meditation may exert something of a priming effect by differentially activating the right hemisphere, subsequently rendering it a more efficient processor of stimuli directed to it. Ley (1984) has found similar right-hemisphere priming effects for highly emotional and imageable words. Thus it may well be that a variety of forms of meditation may engender affective or imageable experiences that are not verbally mediated and that lead to a relative increase in right-hemisphere activation. It should be remembered that this assertion is conjectural and lacks empirical verification.

In the 1980s, Western research on meditation became methodologically sounder. Consequently, a much clearer picture between cerebral dominance and meditation has been shown. For example, although it is accepted generally that meditation leads to decreased electrocortical arousal, there is some evidence that experienced meditators demonstrate more alpha activity than nonmeditators, even when they are not meditating (Delmonte, 1984). It is unclear whether to attribute this rather remarkable difference to the fact that prospective meditators possess the characteristic prior to becoming experienced meditators or whether meditation causes such a difference. Delmonte asserts that meditation may begin with left-hemisphere-type activity, which gives way to more characteristic right-hemisphere functioning as the meditation progresses. However, it appears that during advanced meditation, the so-called no-thought state, overall left- and right-hemisphere activity is diminished and relatively balanced.

WESTERN THERAPIES AND THE LATERALITY CONCEPT

Ley (1979) has written at length on the implications of laterality research for Western psychotherapeutic practice. Using cerebral asymmetries as a metaphor, he has asserted that many therapeutic approaches, ranging from psychoanalytic to behavioral, might be construed as efforts to decode a right-hemisphere repository of nonlinguistic emotions and images. Ley has suggested that right-hemisphere advantages for processing affective and imageable stimuli might further mediate therapist-client communication and interactions. Thus various psychotherapeutic strategies and techniques can be considered attempts to create a therapeutic atmosphere that encourages right-hemisphere mentation. Ley has detailed the ways in which the therapeutic setting, the therapeutic "words," and the therapeutic task conspire to develop a right-hemisphere environment. For a comprehensive description of this thesis refer to Ley (1979).

Given this formulation, it is interesting to speculate on the possibility that the setting for some Eastern therapies is not unlike sensory deprivation conditions, which have a tendency to facilitate right-hemisphere experiences (e.g., vivid images or affects). The meditative, reflective, or isolated setting for Japanese therapies may disproportionally engender right-hemisphere mentation. As well, the client's posture in Japanese therapies likely influences the nature of the thought processes, and it is no surprise that prolonged bed rest or Zen sitting prompts regression and strong emotion. This is particularly important during the first phases of Morita, Shadan, and Seiza therapies, inasmuch as it has been shown that earlier childhood memories are prompted when subjects are reclining (Berdach & Bakan, 1967).

In recent years, some innovative Western psychotherapies have emerged, which have obvious Eastern accouterments. For example, Gallegos (1985) describes a method of using "animal symbolism" and imagery to stimulate the client's expressive imagination. Gallegos claims that this method produces "metaphoric descriptions" that are related to the Indian *shakra* system, and he believes that animal imagery can be used to integrate oneself.

Likewise, "aroma therapy" has appeared in the therapeutic marketplace. Reportedly, it is based on the mood-altering power of scents (e.g., lavender, tangerine, or rose), which are used in conjunction with massage. Scented oils are rubbed onto the body, based on the premise that "When you smell something, it registers on the right side of the brain . . . the side associated with memory, pleasure, and creativity" (Roebuck, 1986, p. 1). Again, as should be evident by now, such reasoning is specious, not supported by laterality research, and appears to be borne of a desire to "shoehorn" a particular "therapy" into a laterality context or an Eastern tradition. Until such radical or innovative therapies achieve an appropriate degree of acceptability, they must be regarded as novelties or therapeutic confections that lack a theoretical foundation and empirical support, despite the originator's effort to graft the techniques onto a laterality model.

Similar to these radical therapies, some educators have advocated the integration of Eastern and Western techniques to improve students' cognitive performance. For example, Yellin (1983) advocates combining biofeedback, Yoga, and the Lozanov method to enhance learning among learning-disabled or retarded students. The Lozanov method combines music, drama, physical exercises, and relaxation techniques for prelearning preparation. The shared heritage with Eastern psychotherapeutic practices is apparent, but empirical validation of the teaching program's efficacy is lacking (Ley & Kaushansky, 1985).

CONCLUDING REMARKS

In general, there is surprisingly little solid, empirical evidence to substantiate the once-prevalent notion that all things Eastern naturally and exclusively engage the right hemisphere. Although the concept of cerebral laterality has had considerable heuristic value as a metaphor for providing novel conceptualizations of individual and cultural experiences, such extrapolations are often very distant from any data base. For example, although Robert Ornstein (1972) provides a cogent argument for viewing Western society as dominated by the left hemisphere, there is scant evidence to support his view or the contrasting position that Eastern ways of life are dominated by the right hemisphere.

In partial support of his thesis, Ornstein (1972) describes one such study that he conducted in which subjects read the Sufi tales of Idris Shah. Shah's Sufi tales are replete with metaphor, imagery, and humor. Ornstein succeeded in demonstrating that such tales (and their stimulus attributes) arouse greater right-hemisphere activity than do factual, technical passages. Even withstanding some methodological shortcomings to Ornstein's study, it is a considerable leap of faith to believe that stable, enduring differences in hemispheric activation typify and distinguish the members of each culture.

The possibility that particular cultures use a specific hemisphere for information processing is easily refuted. First, in order to support this notion one must adhere to a number of beliefs about cerebral laterality that are unfounded neurologically. Second, those who have advocated the Eastern equals right hemisphere and Western equals left hemisphere position have assumed that Eastern and Western brains are organized similarly. Almost certainly this is not the case, especially in light of Levy's (1983) estimation, that even within Western (e.g., North American) society "no more than 15% of the population" demonstrate the classical pattern of association between the left hemisphere and language and the right hemisphere and visual-spatial processes.

The neat transposition of a Western model of laterality into (or onto) an Eastern head is untenable because most probably the Eastern brain is organized and lateralized somewhat differently. Cortical hemispheric differences probably evolve due to historical differences between Eastern and Western linguistic systems. For example, research suggests that the Japanese language uniquely influences Japanese brain development. A speech disorder specialist in Tokyo found that his patients' brains were lateralized for language much differently than that which had been shown in North America. For Japanese subjects, the Japanese vowel sound "ah" activated the left hemisphere, yet it activates the right for Western subjects. Also, traditional Japanese musical tones and environmental sounds prompted left-hemisphere activation among Japanese subjects, whereas such stimuli have repeatedly demonstrated right-hemisphere advantages among North American subjects (e.g., typically, Caucasian undergraduate university students) (Segalowitz, 1983).

Although such findings must be considered provisional, inasmuch as they were summarized from a Japanese book entitled *"The Japanese Brain,"* which has not been translated into English, the findings nonetheless converge with North American findings that written and spoken forms of Oriental languages lead to different localization of language (Segalowitz, 1983). In short, although there is a small body of research support for the notion that meditation leads to a relative activation of the right hemisphere, it must be remembered that these findings are derived almost exclusively from studies of North American Caucasian meditators. Thus there is no reason to assume that similar hemispheres or intrahemispheric mechanisms will support the meditative exercises of the Japanese, Chinese, Indian, or Pakistani.

As Watts (1961) rightly claimed, many Eastern philosophical and religious traditions should be construed as psychotherapies or healing techniques. It may well be that greater linkage between Eastern and Western therapies and their possible hemispheric substrates will be forthcoming from psychoimmunological studies of the relationship between the mind, disease, and healing processes. For example, there is some evidence that asymmetrical differences exist in neurotransmitter distribution within the dopaminergic and cholinergic systems of the left hemisphere in contrast to the noradrenergic and seratonergic systems of the right hemisphere. Thus, even at a neurochemical level, there is a functional asymmetry of brain organization associated with particular physical pathology and associated psychological states.

It would not be surprising if a variety of healing techniques, both Eastern and Western, influence the distribution of neurochemicals. Some support for this conjecture can be drawn inferentially from the clinical and research literature on imagery and healing. Countless imagery techniques exist to assist individuals suffering from a variety of physical maladies and psychological woes (Sheikh, 1983). Given the relationship between imagery and the right hemisphere and evidence of hemispheric shifts in depression, Ley and Freeman (1984) have hypothesized that cerebral lateral differences mediate the relationship between helplessness, despair or depression, and the immunosuppression that constitute many diseases.

In conclusion, just as the right-brain movement in education gave way to the whole-brained classroom, a belief that Eastern therapies exclusively engaged the right hemisphere has been superseded by an empirically based understanding that both hemispheres are engaged in activities such as meditation. However, some slight differences in activation of the left and right hemisphere may occur, although the size and direction of the hemispheric changes (from left to right or vice versa) is perhaps more profoundly influenced by the ethnicity and gender of the practitioner, rather than the practice.

Somewhat ironically, it has perhaps been only the Western devotee of Eastern healing or Eastern therapeutic traditions that has the slightest interest in which half of his or her brain is being activated. Given that meditation and Yoga have been practiced similarly for perhaps 1,000 years, it is a peculiarly North American orientation to either alter or investigate the practice in order to enhance its effectiveness or to try to do it better. Unquestionably, Eastern therapies are whole-brained activities and electrophysiologically, both hemispheres are active. It is the development and integration of both hemisphere's processes, rather than the exclusion or subordination of one or the other (if that was possible), that is most likely to lead to optimal psychological and emotional functioning. Even in a metaphoric sense, it is the integration and complementarity of left- and right-hemisphere cognitive styles that is important. It is clear that people, cultures, and therapeutic practices should not be viewed simply or strictly as left-brained or right-brained.

References

Berdach, E., & Bakan, P. (1967). Body position and free recall of early memories. *Psychotherapy: Theory, Research and Practice, 4,* 101–102

Bryden, M. P. (1982). *Laterality: Functional asymmetry in the intact human brain.* New York: Academic Press.

Bryden, M. P., & Ley, R. G. (1983). Right hemisphere involvement in imagery and affect. In E. Perecman (Ed.), *Cognitive processing in the right hemisphere.* New York: Academic Press.

Davidson, R. J., & Fox, N. A. (1983). Asymmetrical brain activity discriminates between positive and negative affective stimuli in human infants. *Science, 218,* 1235–1237.

Delmonte, M. (1984). Electrocortical activity and related phenomena associated in meditation practice: A literature review. *International Journal of Neuroscience*, 24, 217–231.

Frank, J. D. (1974). *Persuasion and healing*. New York: Schocken.

Gallegos, E. (1985). Animal imagery, the chakra system, and psychotherapy. *Hakomi Forum*, Winter, 19–25.

Goleman, D. (1977). Split-brain psychology: Fad of the year. *Psychology Today*, 11, 89–90.

Heilman, K. M., & Van Den Abell, T. (1979). Right hemispheric dominance for mediating cerebral activation. *Neuropsychologia, 17*, 215–221.

Kosslyn, S. M. (1987). Seeing and imagining in the cerebral hemispheres: A computational approach. *Psychological Review, 94*(2), 143–175

Levy, J. (1983). Cerebral asymmetry and the psychology of man. In M. Wittrock (Ed.), *The brain and psychology*. New York: Academic Press.

Ley, R. G. (1979). Cerebral asymmetries, emotional experience and imagery: Implications for psychotherapy. In A. A. Sheikh & J. J. Shaffer (Eds.), *The potential of fantasy and imagination*. New York: Brandon House.

Ley, R. G. (1983). Cerebral laterality and imagery. In A. A. Sheikh (Ed.), *Imagery: Current theory, research and application*. New York: Wiley.

Ley, R. G. (1984). Right hemispheric processing of emotional and imageable words. In A. A. Sheikh (Ed.), *International Review of Mental Imagery*. New York: Human Sciences Press.

Ley, R. G., & Bryden, M. P. (1983). Right hemispheric involvement in imagery and affect. In E. Perecman (Ed.), *Cognitive processing in the right hemisphere*. New York: Academic Press.

Ley, R. G., & Freeman, R. J. (1984). Imagery, cerebral laterality and the healing process. In A. A. Sheikh (Ed.), *Imagery and healing*. Farmingdale, NY: Baywood.

Ley, R. G., & Kaushansky, M. (1985). The 4Rs: Readin, 'ritin, 'rithmetic, and the right hemisphere. A review of the brain laterality model for education. In A. A. Sheikh (Ed.), *Imagery in education*. Farmingdale, NY: Baywood.

Ley, R. G., & Strauss, E. (1986). Hemispheric asymmetries in the perception of facial expressions by normals. In R. Bruyer (Ed.), *The neuropsychology of face perception and facial expression*. Hillside, NJ: Erlbaum.

Meissner, J., & Pirot, M. (1983). Unbiasing the brain: The effects of meditation upon the cerebral hemispheres. *Social Behaviour and Personality, 11*(1), 65–76.

Ornstein, R. (1972). *The psychology of consciousness*. San Francisco: Freeman.

Ornstein, R., Herron, J., Johnstone, F., & Swencionis, C. (1979). Differential right hemisphere involvement in two reading tasks. *Psychophysiology, 16*, 398–401.

Pagano, R. R., & Frumkin, L. R. (1972). The effect of transcendental meditation on iconic imagery. *Biofeedback and Self-Regulation, 4*, 313–322.

Reynolds, D. K. (1980). *The quiet therapies: Japanese pathways to personal growth*. Honolulu: University Press of Hawaii.

Roebuck, R. (1986, June 15). Aroma therapy. *Toronto Star*, Cl.

Segalowitz, S. J. (1983). *Two sides of the brain*. Englewood Cliffs, NJ: Prentice-Hall.

Sergent, J. (1982). The cerebral balance of power: Confrontation or cooperation. *Journal of Experimental Psychology: Human Perception and Performance, 8*, 253–272.

Shapiro, D. H. (1982). Overview: Clinical and physiological comparison of meditation with other self-control strategies. *American Journal of Psychiatry, 139*, 267–274.

Sheikh, A. A. (1983). *Imagery: Current theory, research and application*. New York: Wiley.

Sperry, R. W. (1966). Hemispheric deconnection and unity in conscious awareness. *American Psychologist, 23*, 723–733.

Suedfeld, P. (1975). The benefits of boredom. *American Scientist, 63*(1), 60–69.

Warrenburg, S., & Pagano, R. (1982). Meditation and hemispheric specialization: Absorbed attention in long term adherence. *Imagination, Cognition and Personality, 2*(3), 211–229.

Watts, A. (1961). *Psychotherapy East and West*. New York: Pantheon Books.

Yellin, D. (1983). Left brain, right brain, super brain: The holistic model. *Reading World, 23*(1), 36–44.

13

Psychoneuroimmunology: Toward a Mind-Body Model[1]

KENNETH R. PELLETIER[2]
DENISE L. HERZING

Every transformation of man . . . has rested on a new picture of the cosmos and the nature of man.

Lewis Mumford

TOWARD A MODEL OF MIND-BODY INTERACTION

This chapter began as an attempt to develop a theoretical model for integrating the data in the rapidly evolving area of psychoneuroimmunology (PNI) and thereby to guide future research. However, during the course of a detailed analysis of the original study methodologies,

---

[1]This chapter is an expanded version of a recently published paper in *Advances* (Pelletier & Herzing, 1988). It is included here with permission from the Institute for the Advancement of Health.
[2]Research supported by grants from the Institute of Human Development.

discussions with key researchers in the area, and a consideration of the linkage between the stress and psychoneuroimmunological data, it became increasingly clear that the database for such a model was inadequate. In order to meet the need of proposing a model wherein seemingly discrepant or incomplete findings may be integrated and understood, an approach that is different from a general critical review of the literature is in order. Given both this need and the increasingly evident limitations of the data, the objective of this critical review is twofold: (1) to develop a tentative model of mind-body-environmental interaction appropriate to the current research in PNI and (2) to identify the specific limitations of the present database by defining the areas where further research would appear to be most promising to generate the iterative interaction between theory and data required to generate a comprehensive model of mind-body interaction. Developing such a model would have profound implications beyond PNI, since it could provide a model for the assessment of other subtle energy systems, including meditation, visualization, relaxation therapies, hypnosis, acupuncture, homeopathy, and electromagnetic influences upon the body. It would also provide a model of the potential for limb and organ regeneration. Although any conclusions must be tentative at present, the rudimentary aspects of a comprehensive model are beginning to emerge.

BACKGROUND—NATURAL AND BIOLOGICAL SCIENCES

Many models have been proposed to elucidate the interaction between body and mind in health and between matter and energy in the natural sciences. Plato (1929) reflected that body and mind are separate but that the health of the body and mind is affected by imbalance from which disease states occur. Descartes's reflections on body and mind and the interpretation of Descartes's statements have been discussed and debated by Jennings (1985). His review of Descartes's original texts points to Descartes's belief in the continuity between energetic and particulate matter in the living organism. However, Descartes's later phenomenological mentations on the nature of mental being were conducted under a very specific state of self-observation. In this specific mental state, Descartes failed to observe other states of consciousness in his own mental being. His methodological error failed to define the continuum of mental experience and led to the incorrect conclusion that mind and body were discrete and separate.

Continuity of the mind-body system is supported by models in the natural sciences, particularly by quantum physics (Zukav, 1979). Albert

Einstein stated that matter and energy are equivalent and interchangeable. He contended that there are no absolute particles but that all matter is fluid and plastic. Bohr developed the complementarity principle, demonstrating the wave-particle nature of subatomic particles depending on experimental conditions (See Pert, 1987). Jumping ahead a bit, the complementarity principle is receiving attention in the receptor site research of the PNI realm. Evidence suggests that all neuropeptides may be made up of one molecule and that changes in the configuration of this molecule result in new information that differentiates neuropeptides from one another (Pert, 1987). This change in configuration is so instantaneous that researchers have speculated that the receptors for the neuropeptides have both a wave-like and a particulate character. Although this modeling is highly speculative, it is indicative of the wealth of insight in the natural sciences paradigm that might lend insight into the increasingly subtle energy models of mind-body interaction. Among the other basic insights from quantum physics that may prove applicable is the uncertainty principle, which has been defined by Heisenberg (see Pelletier & Herzing, 1988) and which describes the effect of the observer on changing the system. This principle was subsequently demonstrated by Einstein, Podolsky, and Rosen who found that two electrons from a single atom spinning away from each other were affected by each other's behavior, suggesting that the parts of the whole cannot be separated from each other (see Pelletier & Herzing, 1988). This observation is also supported by Bohm's (1980) theory of implicate-explicate order, which describes the futility of trying to separate the observer from the observed and the part from the whole. Quantum field theory later described a field for each type of particle and suggested that it is the interaction of these fields that make up reality and create a system of interaction.

Systems theory has also played a major role in the attempt to comprehend the interaction of mind and body. Bertalanffy (1968) stated that a whole is different and more than the sum of its parts. According to his theory, it is the flow of energy across boundaries and the aspects of higher levels of complexity and order emerging from open systems that are expanding and interacting with the environment that defines the whole. More recently, Prigogine and Stengers's (1984) theory of dissipative structures formulates that living things are open systems and thrive above states of equilibrium that demand entropic prediction from the laws of thermodynamics. According to this theory, living systems are able to exchange energy with the environment and therefore are stabilized by change and flow of information, thus avoiding entropy and the collapse of the system. In his theory, there is no hierarchical structure;

instead there is an interweaving of levels of complexity. Another promising area in a systems approach to mind-body interaction is that of Karl Pribram (1987) at Stanford University. After working for years in the area of neurophysiological research, Pribram theorized that the brain works in the same way as a hologram—that is, storing complete information that is available in each of its "parts." According to Pribram, humans have access to all information through attention mechanisms or through neural inhibition, suggesting that there is a higher level of control exerting its influence on the physical systems of the body.

With specific reference to psychoneuroimmunological principles, Pert (1987) and Cunningham (1986) have both formulated systems theories of an informational nature to address the mind-body system. These theories interpret the basic immune and neurological systems in informational terms. Immune system cells are analogous to actors playing out a role of reciprocal communication and exchange of information both between other immune cells and to the nervous system. Since Pert's research is pivotal in this area, it will be discussed more fully later in this chapter. At this point one of Pert's observations is of great importance:

> The word I would stress in regard to this integrated system is network . . . what we have been talking about all along is information. Perhaps, then, mind is the information flowing among all of these bodily parts. Maybe mind is what holds the network together. I think it is possible now to conceive of mind and consciousness as an emanation of emotional information processing, and as such, mind and consciousness would appear to be independent of brain and body. (Pert, 1987)

Basic communication skills such as pattern recognition, message coding and decoding, and transmission abilities are characteristic of these two systems. That these systems interact with higher cognitive levels and that they display similar attributes suggest that there are principles and organizational rules governing these complex interactions. These principles have been labeled as *supercedent properties* and are characteristic of larger systems. Although supercedent properties may not be evident from the mechanisms of the "parts," these properties emerge from the interaction of the "whole."

One such supercedent theory is that of Nobel laureate Roger Sperry (1986). According to Sperry, consciousness is an emergent property of a whole system that cannot be predicted by its parts. He recommends that mental and spiritual forces should be reinstated at the top of the hierarchy of the brain's causal control; and furthermore, they should be accorded primacy in determining what we are and what we do. Furthermore, he states that the more highly evolved "macro" characteristics of all things exert downward influence over the lower "micro" characteristics of the parts. He asserts that this central control power of the belief system of an individual has potential control over social behavior and possible health consequences. This emergent quality of mind has led to speculation and discussions of definitions of mind and criteria for defining mind in other organisms (Gallup, 1985). Sperry infers that the conscious experience of an organism must causally determine the patterns of neural firing without interfering with physical or chemical laws of neural processing. Thus conscious experience, or the emergence of purpose and meaning, is given primacy in determining a person's actions and is thereby able to exert a downward control over the properties at a physiological and physical level. Sperry explains that in simple terms the dispute amounts to whether a newly evolved whole interacts completely through the properties of its parts, or whether whole systems in nature are, in addition, controlled by novel emergent properties of their own and whether the holistic properties in turn have a downward influence over the components.

Increasingly, researchers in the physical and biological sciences are either explicitly or implicitly adopting a systems approach that provides the observer with an interactive role between the self and environment in a subtle energy model. This conscious interaction theory points the way toward a basic PNI model that may focus researchers upon critical hypotheses. Additionally, a systems model of ongoing interaction between the mind and body could provide a means of interpreting the clinical evidence of psychosocial phenomena and their health consequences.

There is an anachronistic and inaccurate division between the concepts of mind and body proposed by Descartes and the overwhelming evidence in the physical sciences for the continuity between matter and energy and the emergent properties of whole systems. For this reason, we will review the clinical and experimental medical literature with a working hypothesis that the mind-body continuum is a critical interacting network that is of major causative and supercedent importance in determining ultimate states of both disease and health. By exploring the current medical literature from this viewpoint, a new framework emerges that incorporates the mind-body system into study designs and analysis and also stimulates further testable hypotheses of this concept.

PSYCHONEUROIMMUNOLOGY

A great deal of data explicating the relationship between the central nervous system (CNS) and the immune system has emerged in the field of PNI (Ader, 1981, 1983). Numerous connections between the central nervous system and the immune system (e.g., nerve endings in the thymus, lymph nodes, spleen, and bone marrow) suggest a complex, communicative, and interactive system between the brain and the immune system. Noradrenergic sympathetic fibers also innervate the tonsils, appendix, and the Peyer's patches of the small intestine. Additionally, cells of the immune system respond to chemical signals from the CNS via neuroendocrines, neuropeptides, neurohormones, and neurotransmitters (including epinephrine, norepinephrine, histamine, and dopamine). To date, the best overview of the immune system is by Myrin Borysenko (1987) of the Tufts University School of Medicine. Given these complex connections and subtle interactions, the influence of psychological and psychosocial factors may well determine the immunological consequences of exposure to a variety of "invading" stressors—psychological as well as physical stressors.

One last critical caveat must be noted. Any state of health or disease is the end result of a complex interaction between such factors as genetics, age, sex, personality, environment, bacteria, viruses, carcinogens, and a host of other factors, some of which are yet to be discovered. There is considerable difficulty in determining direct versus indirect immunological effects of any behavioral state. Questions of a direct effect of a psychological factor upon immunity are complicated by a multiplicity of associated changes in diet, behaviors that are detrimental to one's health (e.g., cigarette smoking, alcohol consumption), environmental changes, and sleep disruption, all of which are also known to influence the immune system. Although the focus here is on PNI, there is no attempt to reduce this complexity to one monolithic theory. Many of these other factors may prove to be equally important or even more important, but consideration of these is clearly beyond the scope of this discussion. Evidence is emerging from numerous studies indicating that such subtle relationships between mind and body may swing the balance between health and illness, life and death.

STRESS AND IMMUNOSUPPRESSION

From the outset it is important to note a somewhat polarized opinion among researchers in the PNI field. One group tends to see the PNI research as an outgrowth of longstanding stress research, while others tend to see it as a new and separate field of inquiry. Our position is clearly the former since there is significant overlap between stress and psychoneuroimmunological research. PNI has begun to provide the biochemical "missing link" between the neurophysiological research of the 1950s through the 1970s and the clinical-experimental data that was not explicable on that basis alone. Most recently, Kiecolt-Glaser and her colleagues (1987) presented an excellent review of this controversy and cited their reservations concerning a simplistic, reductionistic linkage between stress and the PNI data. However, they did conclude that there is significant overlap between the stress and PNI areas, for both basic and epidemiological studies in both areas have found greater morbidity and mortality among specific populations. While the more biologically oriented PNI researchers and clinicians may prefer not to drag the increasingly complex issues of stress and coping into this new field, that stance is neither possible nor desirable. For the purposes of this chapter, *stressor* refers to the stimuli per se, while *stress* refers to the neurophysiological and subjective responses to the stimuli. Issues of coping styles and mediators between the stressor and the stress response will be elaborated later in this chapter.

Immunological effects of stress are not always clear; neither are they only unidirectional. A number of variables, including chronicity, age, duration, and genetic and temporal characteristics of the stressor, may be factors that determine the ultimate health outcome. Such variables and the literature discussing the enhancement of immune system parameters will not be discussed here, although we recognize them as an important area. Most studies link disease with general stressors (Jemmott & Locke, 1984; Palmblad, 1981). Others have linked disease to specific factors, such as depression (Schleifer et al., 1984), loneliness (Kiecolt-Glaser et al., 1984) and hopelessness (Goodkin, Antoni, & Blaney, 1986). Experimental and natural stressors that decrease immunocompetence include sleep deprivation (Palmblad, Petrini, Wasserman, & Akerstedt, 1979), epinephrine administration (Crary, Hauser, et al., 1983; Crary, Borysenko, et al., 1983), norepinephrine administration (Kraus, Locke, & Kutz, 1984), corticosteroids (Frey, Walker, Frey, & de Weck, 1984), and unemployment (Arnetz et al., 1987). A few studies appear to indicate stress-induced enhancement of some aspects of immune function, but this data is too uncertain to evaluate at present. Although the detailed process of direct effects of stressor interaction and immunosuppression is still undocumented, immunological measures made during natural and experimental stressors have begun to elucidate the process.

Several studies have reported the relationship between parameters of immunological functioning and academic exam stress (Dorian, Keystone, Garfinkel, & Brown, 1982; Jemmott et al., 1983; Kiecolt-Glaser et al., 1984). In the study by Dorian et al. (1982), examination stress was correlated with a decrease in lymphocyte proliferation among psychiatry residents as compared with matched control groups. Jemmott et al. (1983) reported a decrease in the rate of secretory immunoglobulin A (S-lgA) during academic stress in first-year dental students as compared to baseline and periods of little academic stress. Kiecolt-Glaser et al. (1984) reported decreased lymphocyte proliferation among medical students on the first day of final exams as compared to preexam and postexam periods. Medical students had diminished natural killer (NK) cells and diminished helper T-cells, and their lymphocytes had a drastically reduced ability to produce interferon—an NK cell mediator—during examinations. These specific immunological measures indicate possible mechanisms for the general links between stressors and subsequent illness or mortality. However, the degree of immunological impairment necessary to increase susceptibility to disease is currently undetermined.

Studies on the stress of bereavement and immune function suggest that bereavement may inhibit lymphocyte proliferation (Bartrop, Lazarus, Luckhurst, Kiloh, & Penny, 1977; Schleifer, Keller, Cammerino, Thornton, & Stein, 1983). Bartrop et al. (1977) found that bereaved spouses had lower lymphocyte proliferation 8 weeks after the spouse's death, but not 2 weeks after the death. The matched control group of this study did not differ from the bereaved group in T– and B–cell counts or serum immunoglobulins. Schleifer et al. (1983) also found diminished lymphocyte proliferation after bereavement in husbands of women who had terminal breast cancer. In addition, no differences in T– and B–cell counts were observed in the individuals before or after the death of the spouse. In a recent critical review, Workman and La Via (1987) reported that total T-lymphocytes, T-suppressor cells, and T-helper cells were consistently unaffected by stressors, while lgA, granulocyte activity, NK cell activity, numbers of monocytes, total lymphocytes, and B-lymphocytes showed inconsistent findings for stress effects. Their review also indicated that both PHA and Con A, responsiveness of both mitogens that activate T-lymphocytes, was consistently depressed with stressors, suggesting that stress affects the cellular activation process. At this time, the epidemiological evidence from the bereavement data indicates that mortality is higher after conjugal bereavement only among older widowers. Data regarding widows are uncertain, and the precise immunological mediators remain undefined.

Animal immunological research, a literature base that is larger than that on humans, is another source of evidence and support for the relationship between psychological and immunological variables in humans. Animal studies indicate similar immune reactivity to stressors. In animals, stress has been found to reduce immunocompetence in humoral immunity (Edwards & Dean, 1977; Edwards, Rahe, Stephens, & Henry,

1980), cell-mediated immunity (Joasoo & McKenzie, 1976; Laudenslager, Reite, & Harbeck, 1982; Reite, Harbeck, & Hoffman, 1981), and enhanced susceptibility to neoplastic disease (Riley, 1981), infectious disease (Mohamed & Hanson, 1980), and autoimmune (Amkraut, Solomon, & Kraemer, 1971) diseases. Stressful events, such as overcrowding (Brayton & Brain, 1975; Davis & Read, 1958), exposure to high intensity sound (Jensen & Rasmussen, 1963), and exposure to a predator (Hamilton, 1974), have also shown a correlation to increased susceptibility to infections. Direct modulation of immunological parameters under stress include antibody levels (Michaut et al., 1981) and lymphocyte cytotoxicity and proliferation (Borysenko & Borysenko, 1982; Monjan, 1981; Russell et al., 1984). Most recently, Shavit and Martin (1987) reviewed the animal data linking stress, opiate mediators, and subsequent immunological status. They concluded that foot-shock stress suppresses immunity and decreases animal resistance to tumors. This suppressed immunity is mediated by opioid peptides and can be experimentally replicated by morphine injections. Additionally, inescapable shock results in immunosuppression, and the CNS together with opioid peptides help mediate this effect. Results of their review lend evidence to the data from both human and animal results indicating that the psychological state of helplessness is immunosuppressing. It seems that animals as well as humans show immunomodulation under stressors, but the psychological factors modulating immunocompetence are still unclear.

Behavioral conditioning of the animal immune system also demonstrates the possibility of altering immune responses through experience and raises questions of the behavioral impact upon immunity (Ader & Cohen, 1981; Bovbjerg, Ader, & Cohen, 1984). That animals can "learn" to suppress their immune response may have implications for the management of immune diseases through behavioral modification techniques and conditioning. Reactions of animals to uncontrollable versus controllable stress (Laudenslager, Ryan, Drugan, Hyson, & Maier, 1983; Seligman, 1975) have demonstrated that rats show a decreased immune function only when they receive uncontrollable shock. This suggests that when animals are "helpless" or "hopeless" under a stressor, their immune systems are affected. When given "control" over the situational stressor, rats (and their immune systems) are able to cope. Clearly, "predictability" and "controllability" of the stressor is a major mediating factor in determining the ultimate stress response. Additionally, Seligman's (1975) work demonstrated that rats receiving inescapable shock rejected implanted tumor cells less effectively than rats given control over the shocks they received. Although generalizations directly from animal studies should be made with caution, Seligman's factor of "control" over the stressor appears to have significant implications for the psychological factor of control for humans who feel helpless or hopeless. At this time, the evidence in the animal research of PNI clearly indicates that experimental stressors do reproducibly modify specific immunological parameters. Also it is clear that immunosuppression is much more frequently reported than immunoenhancement. Whether the latter is more difficult to induce than the former, or whether it is even possible, is an important research issue left unanswered at present.

Studies of animals are particularly valuable because they are usually characterized by greater experimental control than are human studies. The hypothesis that psychological variables influence immunological functioning is made more tenable by animal studies, although important differences in immune systems among mammalian species indicate the need for caution in generalizations from animals to humans. In addition, the possible similarities and differences in social structure and psychological factors between species or between individual animals may make it necessary to control for such factors in experimental situations. Animal models may raise different questions about the measurement of "emotion" and "stress," the least of which is whether we can extrapolate such studies to humans. This caution is particularly true in the often-cited linkage between the animal "learned helplessness" model and human depression, which is clearly much more complex. With a trend of research away from dealing with simplistic and one-dimensional, external stressors, there is a trend toward a more precise definition, in psychological terms, of how people and animals react to and perceive those events as individuals and in a social context.

In addition to this caution regarding linkage between animal and human models, researchers must also be cautioned to conduct their experiments with animals using the same compassionate and minimally · invasive methodologies that are an integral part of review procedures with humans.

AFFECT-INDUCED IMMUNOMODULATION

Explicit, quantifiable influences of affective factors in immune-related illnesses are currently under investigation. General reviews of psychological and emotional factors that can alter resistance to infectious diseases have been written by Kaneko and Takaishi (1963) and Solomon and Amkraut (1981). A variety of illnesses have been weakly linked to affective factors, including allergic diseases (Dirks, Robinson, & Dirks, 1981; Kleiger & Kinsman, 1980), autoimmune disorders (Moos &

Solomon, 1964; Solomon & Moos, 1965), infectious diseases (Canter, 1972; Kasl, Evans, & Niederman, 1979), and neoplastic disease (Riley, 1981; Shekelle et al., 1981). Albeit weak, these links may indicate a consistent mechanism at work under different stressors.

It is suspected that the affect dimension of many illnesses is mediated through immunomodulation. At the National Institutes of Mental Health, Pert (1986, 1987) has reviewed and discussed the connections and communication system between the limbic system, neuropeptides, and the immune system. She believes that these emotion-affecting neuropeptides control the migration of human monocytes in healing and disease. Mood or emotionally modulated areas of the brain, the amygdala and hypothalamus, have 40 times the number of neuropeptide receptors than other areas in the brain, suggesting that these substances function in the biochemical mediation of emotion. The presence of neuropeptide receptors on immune cells, as well as the ability of these cells to learn, recall, and produce neuropeptides themselves, suggest (1) an interactive network of information flow between the brain and immune system and (2) a system in which direct control of emotions may have immunological consequences. Every neuropeptide receptor is evident on human monocytes, which play a pivotal role in the immune system by communicating with B- and T-cells. This evidence from Pert's research underscores the role of brain-mediated neuropeptides to influence immunity through the bidirectional functions of endogenous opiates. Neurophysiological evidence of increased neural firing in the hypothalamus of the rat during immune challenge suggests that the brain receives information about the status and activity of the immune system (Besedovsky, del Rey, & Sorkin, 1983; Besedovsky, Felix, & Haas, 1977). That neuropeptides may be involved in biochemical mediation of emotion and function to communicate between the brain and immune system is not a new observation, but it is one that recently finds increasingly supportive evidence.

If neuropeptides mediate emotion in the limbic system, either through normal pathways or through immune-cell production, then emotional modulation, via cognitive control, may direct the movement of immune cells via the production of neuropeptides by the CNS or the immune cells themselves. This suggests that the brain can communicate through the limbic system to the immune system or that the immune system can communicate to the brain through the limbic system. In this scenario, the limbic system, or emotional perception, would be the site of message translation. In another possible scenario, the brain would have direct access to the immune system via direct CNS links, circumventing the limbic system, and vice versa. If the immune system and the nervous system are so closely linked, it is possible that mental/emotional illness may show concomitant immune system abnormalities (some evidence exists to verify this). That there are emotional as well as cognitive channels that may modulate the immune system also suggests that personality, emotional stability, and cognitive control or awareness of situational variables may have direct immunological consequences on health.

Although these quite convincing findings have been interpreted as some of the best evidence for the direct, causal influence of mind and emotions on immunity, there are alternative explanations that must be considered. There are genetic factors that determine brain development, left-right laterality, personality, and immunity. Immunity markers, such as NK cell activity, may be genetic markers for personality and affective disorders rather than caused by them. Personality or emotional states may be linked to socioeconomic factors that have demonstrable effects on higher disease rates in cancer, infections, and heart disease. Finally, genetic and/or environmental factors may have an impact upon both psychological and immunological parameters resulting in a noncausal linkage. A correlation seems evident, but causation remains an open issue.

IMMUNOENHANCEMENT—EFFECT OR ARTIFACT?

Stress has been generally demonstrated to induce immunosuppression, and this finding has led to the question of whether or not stress management may be related to enhanced immune function. Understanding the factors that modulate the immune system may lead to the application of these factors to enhance immune function. Psychological influences that contribute to immunoenhancement of the cellular immune function include the relaxation technique utilized by Kiecolt-Glaser et al. (1985). In this study, geriatric residents were taught progressive relaxation and guided imagery techniques. When compared with the control group, the experimental group showed a significant increase in NK activity as well as a decrease in antibodies to the herpes simplex virus, showing better control of the virus by the immune system. Humor (Cousins, 1981), positive attitudes and humorous film stimuli (Dillon, Minchoff, & Baker, 1985), and exposure to humanistic films (McClelland & Kirshnit, 1984) have provided evidence of immunoenhancement possibilities. In McClelland and Kirshnit's study, students exposed to a film about Mother Teresa's work caring for the sick and poor showed increased S-lgA levels regardless of whether they outwardly approved of her work or not. It has been argued that salivary lgA production is related to upper respiratory tract infections, but the actual clinical significance of IgA variability is uncertain. Reports by Hall, Longo, and Dixon (1981) indicated that the subconscious suggestion, via hypnosis, of increasing lymphocyte activity and function, showed an actual increase in the number of lymphocytes in some patients, especially those easily hypnotized. Both the McClelland and Kirshnit (1984) and the Hall et al. (1981) studies suggest that information and suggestions may enter our stream of awareness on an unconscious level and may enhance immune function regardless of whether we are outwardly aware of an effect or emotional reaction. These studies also suggest the possibility of increasing our own ability to enhance and control our immune system through conscious or unconscious suggestion or through exposure to positively enhancing stimuli.

Actually the phenomenon of immunoenhancement is controversial, if it exists at all. Results from visualization and improved cancer outcome related to relaxation therapy and hypnotic induction have been reported (Borysenko, 1987; Simonton, Matthews-Simonton, & Creighton, 1978). However, Ornstein and Sobel (1987) indicate that although there have been many claims for the effects of positive attitude and imagery on diseases, there is little convincing scientific support that they alone can cure serious illness. Several options are possible: (1) enhancement may simply be the restoration of normal baseline functions; (2) selective suppression of certain cells in the immune system may produce the illusion that others are enhanced; (3) there may be a "rebound" effect in which a stressor temporarily suppresses an immune marker, which then rebounds to an apparent higher value when the stressor ceases; or (4) it may be possible to actually enhance immunological responses above baseline, but these extremely complex issues are far from resolution. Clinical significance of immunological variability is unknown, and there is no empirical basis to determine the magnitude of immunological impairment necessary to be causally linked to increased disease susceptibility, onset, or intervention.

MEDIATION PATHWAYS

Neuroendocrine pathways were the first to be proposed as mediation pathways between stress and impaired immune function. Cannon's (1926) fight or flight response and Selye's (1950) general adaptation syndrome constitute the classic studies in this area. Considerable evidence for both pathways exists (see Jemmott & Locke, 1984). It is clear that stress results in immune suppression in most basic and clinical-experimental trials. Chronic stress may particularly result in immunosuppression by acting through the hypothalamic-pituitary-adrenal pathway. Under stress, the hypothalamus produces a corticotropin-releasing factor that triggers the secretion of adrenocorticotropic hormone (ACTH) by the pituitary. In turn, ACTH stimulates the adrenals to secrete the corticosteroid hormones, which result in immunosuppression. In addition to the corticosteroids, the stress response also results in the production of brain chemistries (including epinephrine, endorphins, dopamine, and prostaglandins), which also suppress the cellular production of antibodies (Pelletier, 1977). Although the current thinking is that chronic, sustained, Type II stress has a more detrimental effect on health and immunity than acute, short-term, Type I stress (Pelletier, 1977), there is still insufficient data to conclusively evaluate the relative immunological impact of chronic versus acute stressors. This question needs to be clarified in order to link specific stress response patterns to subsequent health status.

Receptors for a variety of hormones and neurotransmitters that are produced during stress have been discovered on lymphocytes (Bishopric, Cohen, & Lefkowitz, 1980; Borysenko & Borysenko, 1982). Considerable evidence exists for immunological reactivity to corticosteroids and catecholamines (Claman, 1972; Fauci, 1978) and for the direct effect of neuropeptides on immunological reactivity (Ahlquist, 1981; Claman, 1972). But many other stress-related hormones may modulate immunity. Receptors for opioid peptides on T-lymphocytes, morphine, and enkephalins were discovered by Wybran, Appelboom, Famaey, and Govaerts (1979), and receptors for beta-endorphins were discovered by Hazum, Chang, and Cuatrecasas (1979). These opioid peptides have been shown to enhance lymphocyte response (Gilman, Schwartz, Milner, Bloom, & Feldman, 1982) and to contribute to tumor growth (Lewis et al., 1983). Understanding this complex interaction between hormones and immunocompetence is still incomplete, but a higher level of interaction is also suggested by current research on direct CNS influence.

Direct anatomical links between the nervous and immune systems have recently been discovered. Autonomic innervations in the thymus and spleen have been reported (Bulloch & Moore, 1981; Fujiwara, Muryobayashi, & Shimamoto, 1966; Williams et al., 1981). Given this direct neuroanatomical evidence of a relationship and possible pathways of communication between the nervous and immune system, it seems plausible that immunomodulation is not entirely dependent on neurohormonal mediation. Other evidence of immunoregulation by the CNS includes a role for sensory neurons as efferent links to the immune system via the release of substance P, a peptide associated with pain sensation (Tecoma & Huey, 1985). When the known pathway of the stress response is considered in light of this more recent research indicating direct autonomic nervous system fibers linked to the thymus, spleen, lymph nodes, and bone marrow, a more complete model of mind-body, bidirectional interaction begins to emerge. How these fibers affect the cells of the immune system is uncertain, but the pathways appear to be bidirectional. If and how the immune system uses these fibers to signal the presence of antigens to the brain is also unknown. Activated lymphocytes do produce neurotransmitters and neuromodulating hormones, so there is a possible mechanism of communication between immune cells and autonomic fibers. Although this model is promising, there are many, many questions left unanswered at this point. However, if the autonomic nervous system is in direct communication with the immune system, and given that the autonomic nervous system can be monitored and regulated by cognitive control, the role of the mind's regulation in determining subsequent immunocompetence should be more seriously researched as a direct, causative agent.

PSYCHOSOCIAL STUDIES: CONSCIOUS AND SUBCONSCIOUS MEDIATION

Conscious Mediation of Psychoneuroimmunology Activity

Considerable evidence exists as to the importance of individual differences in coping mechanisms and how this may determine ultimate immunocompetence. The person's adaptive response to stress is being viewed increasingly as at least equally important as the stressor itself. This relationship has been most succinctly defined by Lazarus and Folkman (1984) in their definitions of stress and subsequent coping behavior. Stress is a "relationship between the person and the environment that is appraised by the person as taxing or exceeding his or her resources and endangering his or her well-being." They define coping as "constantly changing cognitive and behavioral efforts to manage specific external and/or internal demands that exceed the resources of the person." What may be most important in the Lazarus and Folkman research is that it provides a critical missing link between the simplistic earlier models that linked life change scores to disease outcome and the more complex and interrelated PNI data. Individuals with poor coping skills do evidence greater immune disruption in response to stressors, and this finding should prove important in predicting both individual responses and in formulating more precise behavioral interventions. Their innovative research has convincingly demonstrated that the stress-response relationship is a systemic one involving a mind-body-environmental response. Reductionistic approaches to understanding stress, coping, and the subsequent research in PNI is simplistic and inaccurate.

In addition to a systems approach in the stress literature, the role of conscious will in regulating intention has been reviewed by Libet (1985). Our attitudes, perceptions, and personality traits may have direct consequences on whether a stressor is able to manifest itself in the body. Although these stressors may influence immunological function, psychological processes that mediate those influences contribute to the ultimate immunological impact. A variety of host characteristics that mediate the influence have been identified in humans; they include mood (Kiecolt-Glaser et al., 1984; Linn, Linn, & Jensen, 1982), personality characteristics (Jemmott et al., 1983), coping style (Lazarus, 1970; Locke et al., 1984; Schwartz, 1983; Weinberger, Schwartz, & Davidson, 1979), suppressed anger (Jemmott & Locke, 1984; Pettingale, Greer, & Tee, 1977), hopelessness (Pettingale, Morris, & Greer, 1985), psychological vulnerability (Canter, Cluff, & Imboden, 1972), inhibited power motivation (McClelland, Alexander, & Marks, 1982; McClelland, Floor, Davidson, & Saron, 1980; McClelland, Locke, Williams, & Hurst, 1978), affective defensiveness and inattention to distress (Derogatis, Abeloff, & Melisaratos, 1979; Jemmott et al., 1983; Jensen, 1984; McClelland et al., 1980; McClelland & Jemmott, 1980; Polonsky, Knapp, Brown, & Schwartz, 1985; Rogentine et al., 1979; Temoshok & Fox, 1984), and daily hassles (Lazarus, 1970). The same external event may be perceived differently between individuals, and individual responses to stress have been reported (Canter, 1972; Canter et al., 1972; Jemmott et al., 1982; McClelland et al., 1980). Personality factors also have been correlated with specific diseases. For example, cancer has been correlated with nonassertiveness, the inability to express emotion (Kissen, 1967), and hopelessness (Goodkin et al., 1986); rheumatoid arthritis has been correlated with perfectionism, compliance, subservience, nervousness, restlessness, reserve, and anger (Solomon, 1981); and cardiovascular disease has been associated with Type A behavior (Friedman & Rosenman, 1974). With regard to the reputed "cancer-prone" personality, it is important to note that the studies to date do not convincingly demonstrate the existence of such a personality complex. This vast amount of literature points to the importance of assessing individual styles of coping with stress. Specifically, the impaired ability to express emotions, particularly anger, may be a risk factor or marker for the presence of cancer, but definitive conclusions are unwarranted by the data now available.

Ultimately, the area of PNI that is of greatest interest will be attempts to restore, stabilize, or enhance immunocompetence to sustain or enhance optimal states of health. There is so much more known about disease than health; thus, this latter area holds the greatest potential for major discoveries. Data from the major prospective research by Thomas, Krush, Brown, Shaffer, and Duszynski (1982), of the Johns Hopkins University School of Medicine, indicate that healthy individuals appear to have positive relations with their parents during childhood, strong self-esteem, an optimistic outlook, relative lack of depression, and a marked ability to cope with stress. On the negative side, 1,337 medical students who indicated less closeness to parents, less satisfactory personal relationships, and ambivalence or personal avoidance on the Rorschach, had a relative risk of cancer later in life that was three to four times that of the group judged to be of better psychological health. Given these findings, virtually all of the negative aspects of these qualities have been thought to be immunosuppressing in psychoneuroimmunological studies. Will these positive dimensions be found to be equally profound in stabilizing or enhancing human immunity as the basis for optimal health?

Answering this question is ultimately the most challenging, intriguing, and significant issue raised by the PNI research. Can psychotherapeutic or behavioral interventions directly enhance immune function and thereby prevent the onset or alter the course of diseases involving human immunity? To date the behavioral interventions implying, but not proving, such efficacy are clinical biofeedback, meditation, autogenic training, Jacobson's progressive relaxation, hypnosis, general relaxation, behavior modification, and visualization techniques. These constitute mind-body technologies that might be harnessed and applied with increasing specificity. It is critical to note that just as stress and subsequent immunological responses cannot be simplistically reduced to a monolithic theory, it is equally ludicrous to subsume the range, subtlety, and complexity of such behavioral interventions under the monolithic concept of the relaxation response. Future applications of behavioral interventions in the mind-body area will focus on more precise pairing of individual diagnosis with the specific, subtle differences among the systems listed previously to enhance the clinical outcome. PNI is complex, and the behavioral interventions will involve specific mind-body techniques coupled with other behavioral dimensions, such as diet, exercise, social support, and modification of the physical environment.

There are already several lines of inquiry that may prove to be positive in this area. Focusing on how people react to external events in a positive manner, Kobasa (1982) identified and measured a style of coping she names "hardiness," which modified the relationship between stress and illness. Hardiness style includes aspects of commitment, control, and challenge about a stressful event. People low in hardiness were more susceptible to illness than people scoring high in hardiness. For these low scorers of hardiness, lack of social support was associated with increased illness.

Positive and immune-enhancing visualization techniques also have shown specific immunological consequences (Hall et al., 1981). In this study, people under hypnosis visualized their white blood cells as "sharks" attacking the germs in their body. Younger people had a better response to this technique in general; but people who were easily hypnotized showed an increase in the numbers of lymphocytes after hypnotic sessions. Kiecolt-Glaser et al. (1985) found that relaxation and guided-imagery techniques prompted a significant increase in NK activity in a geriatric population. Most recently, Coates and Greenblatt (1986, 1987), of the University of California School of Medicine in San Francisco, conducted a study indicating that such interventions may prevent or at least delay the progression of AIDS in seropositive males.

One of the most significant studies in the PNI area was reported in the *Annals of Internal Medicine* (Smith, McKenzie, Marmer, & Steele, 1985). Researchers at the University of Arkansas College of Medicine worked with a 39-year-old female who was an experienced meditator. After establishing a baseline on immunological measures, the woman was able to voluntarily reduce both the induration of her delayed hypersensitivity skin test reaction and in vitro lymphocyte stimulation to varicella zoster. Subsequently, she was able to allow her reaction to return to baseline. She was given a skin test weekly for 9 weeks. During weeks 1 to 3, she reacted normally; during weeks 3 to 6 she was asked to inhibit her reactions; and during weeks 6 to 9, she was again asked to react normally.

This study is one of the most innovative research models to indicate that a practiced individual can voluntarily regulate a specific immune response through meditation and visualization. Such research designs and findings are highly significant and are consistent with earlier research in biofeedback, in which Pelletier and Peper (1977) provided the first unequivocal evidence that adept meditators could voluntarily control pain, bleeding, and infection from self-inflicted puncture wounds. It is essential to recognize the importance of working with individuals who are practiced in mind-body techniques, rather than relying upon large numbers of inexperienced subjects. If researchers wanted to study concert pianists, it is unlikely that they would learn a great deal from randomly selected novices and their finger exercises. There is evidence that exceptional individuals can voluntarily alter neurophysiological and immunological functions at will. By studying these occurrences, we may be able to determine the capacity and the means for the average person. Most importantly, this voluntary regulation can be used therapeutically to increase or decrease immune response depending upon what is required in a particular disease. Applications of such techniques involving empowerment, self-efficacy, and autonomic regulation range from primary prevention to adjunctive interventions to the possibility of developing noninvasive, nontoxic, tertiary interventions.

Presently, a study is being developed to determine whether or not a small number of healthy meditators using specific meditation and visualization practices in the Nyingma tradition of Tibetan Buddhism can bidirectionally exert a systematic influence upon immunity. If such a direct, causal, replicable effect can be demonstrated between mind and immunity, the second phase will be to determine if normal, untrained, but motivated volunteers can learn such techniques. If that is accomplished, then such mind-body strategies will be used for a population with immune or autoimmune diseases to determine if progression and/or outcome can be altered in a positive direction. A potentially significant clinical application would be with autoimmune diseases, since psychosocial factors have been associated with the onset and/or progression of a range of such disorders, including systemic lupus, Crohn's, ulcerative colitis, rheumatoid arthritis, diabetes, and myasthenia gravis. There appears to be no empirical basis for such factors in multiple sclerosis, although that disease is commonly misrepresented in this category of disorders. These are relatively recent and small studies, but they may point the way for new possibilities for increasing our ability to control our own immune systems not by the avoidance of negative stressors but instead by the use of positive emotional strategies.

It is clear that studies of the effect of stress on humans need to take a broader approach, and since we can access a human's inner psychological experience, studies should incorporate the individual's coping style and personality characteristics into research design. Since reductionistic designs are only able to isolate individual stressors and not the perception and coping skills that the individual applies to handling stress, a cognitive approach may be in order. Although the task of assessing an individual's relationship and pattern of dealing with the world is far from easy, it is possible that we will miss the richness of such a complex modulation system and its subsequent health benefits unless we give primacy to the cognitive translation by the individual mind.

Human research literature of these coping abilities and variation in individual subjects is supported by studies with animals. Research on animals has indicated that psychosocial factors, such as restraint, crowding, rotation, and predation pressures, can affect immune function (Borysenko & Borysenko, 1982; Monjan, 1981; Rogers, Dubey, & Reich, 1979). Host characteristics of animals that contribute to final immunological outcome have been measured. They include: perceived control (Laudenslager et al., 1983; Sklar & Anisman, 1980), type of coping response (Sklar & Anisman, 1980), historical experience with the stressor (Solomon, Levine, & Kraft, 1968), and operant conditioning (Ader & Cohen, 1975; Gorczpynski, Macrae, & Kennedy, 1982). We have no direct way of knowing what an animal's inner psychological experience is. The range of animal behavior that has evolved to alleviate anxiety or stress is unknown and may possibly be a variable in experimental animal studies as well as in human studies.

Subconscious Mediation of Psychoneuroimmunology Activity

Much of the information we receive from our environment enters out of awareness through the subconscious. Hypnotic procedures are among the most effective interventions that allow access to this dimension of mind. Hypnosis has been suggested as a model for studying the cognitive and psychological factors that influence biochemical factors of physical disease, and suggestions that hypnosis and visualization may enhance immune function have been put forth. Recent attention has been directed toward the psychological and cognitive factors involved in hypnosis that influence the recovery from diseases. Hypnotic induction may be capable of directly influencing immunological systems. General reviews have been written by Bowers and Kelly (1979), Hall (1983), and Jemmott and Locke (1984). High hypnotizability may be an important factor in the production of alterations in the immune system (Bowers & Kelly, 1979). Among the immunological parameters influenced by hypnosis are: alterations in hypersensitivity of skin response (Black, 1963; Black, Humphrey, & Niven, 1963), contact dermatitis (Ikemi & Nakagawa, 1962), alleviation of chronic uriticaria (Kaneko & Takaishi, 1963), viral warts (Surman, Gottlieb, Hackett, & Silverberg, 1973), direct shifts in immunomodulation with mental imagery (Hall et al., 1981), inhibition of allergic skin reaction (Clarkson, 1937), inhibition of asthma and hayfever allergic symptoms (Mason & Black, 1958), inhibition of dog allergy (Perloff & Spiegelman, 1973), alleviation of ichthyosiform erythrodermia (Mason, 1952), decreases in plasma 17-hydroxycorticosteroid concentrations and cortisol levels (Sachar, Cobb, & Shor, 1966; Sachar, Fishman, & Mason, 1965), and inhibition of the Mantoux reaction (Black et al., 1963). It is interesting to note that in the Mantoux histological samples there were no differences; only in the reactive swelling aspect was there a hypnotic effect. That is, hypnosis inhibited the swelling component of the Mantoux reaction but not the cellular component. Although the relaxation aspect of hypnosis can account for decreases in adrenal corticoid hormones, enhancement of immune responses cannot. A neural rather than a humoral mechanism has been suggested for alterations in immune responses during hypnosis, since the vascular component of the Mantoux response was affected and since adrenergic nerve endings have been found in the spleen and thymus (Mason, 1961; Rogers et al., 1979). Based on the hypnosis data, the autonomic nervous system is clearly sensitive to conscious and subconscious mediation, which affects aspects of immune function.

When addressing the complex and varied interactions of the conscious and subconscious between individuals, it is essential to consider the psychological and social attributes that modify perception. Virtually all the psychological adaptation that individuals go through has been labeled as stress. But just as the immune system and nervous system react to incoming information, people react to the meaning of information from their environment (Lazarus & Folkman, 1984). Even though the function of a specific bit of information may be objectively measured, its interpretation and meaning to the individual may vary according to the total context of that individual's self and social perception. The possibility that the immune system may be modulated by conscious psychological coping responses to minimize the impact of natural and experimental stressors would suggest that before a response occurs on a physical level, the total immunocompetence takes place on the higher and more complex level of human consciousness.

PSYCHOSOCIAL INFLUENCES ON PSYCHONEUROIMMUNOLOGY

Evidence is accumulating that positive social support is necessary for a person's health. Supportive interactions among people and cultures may affect our ability to resist illness. The sense of belonging and affiliation has been reported to be a basic human need (Maslow, 1943; Murray, 1939). General reviews on social support and its health consequences are provided by Dohrenwend and Dohrenwend (1974), Mechanic (1977), Pelletier (1977, 1979), and Pilisuk and Parks (1986). As Pilisuk and Parks point out, there is now abundant evidence to show that such support may be one of the critical elements distinguishing those who remain healthy from those who do not. Social support presumably works to prevent illness by maintaining homeostasis or by enhancing the immune system. But how can external environmental stressors, on the negative side, or psychosocial support systems, on the positive side, get "into" the psychoneuroimmunological network? Given the links between psychological, neurological, and immune responses, the clinical-experimental observations, that both positive and negative aspects of social support can have a profound influence on health, become more comprehensible.

Both the positive and the negative influences of social support have been documented. Positive and supportive associations, such as community support and close associations, have been linked to better health and lower absenteeism (Cassel & Tyroler, 1961), lower incidence of cancer and heart disease (Phillips, 1975), and reduced hospital stays (Mumford, Schlesinger, & Glass, 1982). Human companionship has been linked to better health in married persons versus singles (Bloom, Asher, & White, 1978; Kraus & Lilienfeld, 1959). The importance of community and support groups is evident in Japanese culture (Syme, 1982). Japan has the highest life expectancy in the world, and their intimate community bonds seem to be the protecting factor. Social support and interaction seem to enhance the healing abilities of our bodies. Likewise, the negative influence of the lack of social stability and social connectedness, often termed "social marginality," has been linked to a variety of behavioral, physical, and psychological illnesses, including: arthritis (Cobb, Kasl, French, & Norstebo, 1969), tuberculosis (Chen & Cobb, 1960), hypertension (Harburg, Erfurt, & Chape, 1973), schizophrenia and depression (Brown, Bhrolchaim, & Harris, 1975; Brown, Davidson, & Harris, 1977; Brown & Harris, 1978; Hammer, 1963; Mishler & Scotch, 1963), coronary disease (Froland, Brodsky, Olson, & Stewart, 1979), and general mortality rates (Berkman & Syme, 1978). The negative effect of the loss of close ties is further elaborated in a study by Parkes, Benjamin, & Fitzgerald (1969) of the link between bereavement and high coronary mortality. In this study, the rate of coronary mortality was substantially higher for newly bereaved spouses, especially men. Social support as a modifier of bereavement has been reported by Raphael (1977) and Lowenthal and Haven (1968). Direct immune dysfunctioning has been linked with marital quality and disruption (Kiecolt-Glaser et al., 1987). It seems that our place in the community and our interaction in a larger social structure may play an instrumental role in keeping us healthy. At this point in time, three large, prospective, community-based studies, as well as the vast majority of clinical-experimental trials, indicate that an intact social support system reduces both morbidity and mortality. It is likely that we need substantial longitudinal studies linking social support, stress and coping measures, immunological parameters, subsequent health indicators, and control groups to clarify what appears to be an increasingly important mind-body mediator.

General psychosocial factors such as emotional stability, personality, and life stress also have been linked to immune disorders such as cancer (Fox, 1981), to autoimmune diseases (Solomon, 1981), and to infectious diseases (Blank & Brody, 1950; Cohen-Cole et al., 1981; Holmes, Hawkins, Bowerman, Clarke, & Joffe, 1957; Ishigami, 1919; Jackson et al., 1960; Katcher, Brightman, Luborsky, & Ship, 1973; Roark, 1971; Totman & Kiff, 1979). Specific psychosocial factors, including life events and family routines (Boyce et al., 1977), ego strength (Greenfield, Roessler, & Crosley, 1959), life changes (Jacobs, Spilken, & Norman, 1969), social instability and lack of resources (Kasl et al., 1979), moods (Luborsky, Mintz, Brightman, & Katcher, 1976), and family patterns (Meyer & Haggerty, 1962) have been examined. Although many of these studies link or correlate psychosocial factors with subsequent illness to determine causality or at least to help us start to understand the process, immunocompetence was not measured during the progression of the disorders. To achieve an understanding of the process that the immune system goes through during such stressors, immunological changes need to be monitored. Immunological parameters that have been measured under psychosocial stress include: lymphocyte count and reactivity and hematological/immunological factors during spaceflight (Fischer et al., 1972; Kimzey, 1975; Kimzey, Johnson, Ritzman, & Mengel, 1976), S-lgA levels during exposure to positive film stimuli (McClelland & Kirshnit, 1984), interferon-producing capacity and phagocytosis (Palmblad et al., 1976), blood coagulation and fibrinolysis (Palmblad et al., 1977), and ego strength and antibody titer (Roessler, Cate, Lester, & Couch, 1979). That psychosocial factors may affect or moderate stress immune response before (Kasl et al., 1979) or after a stressful event occurs (Dillon, Minchoff, & Baker, 1985; Kiecolt-Glaser et al., 1985; Locke et al., 1984) suggests that behavioral intervention for immune system disorders may be undertaken at various stages of illness or may be done preventatively. However, specific immunocompetence must be understood before the observed outcome of such interventions can be attributed to immunoenhancement rather than to other factors or mediators.

Unfortunately, the need to show care as well as to receive care is often lacking in psychotic individuals, and this need for reciprocity and its health consequences has been reported (Henderson et al., 1978; Horowitz, Schaefer, Hiroto, Wilner, & Levin, 1977; Lin, Ensel, Simeone, & Kuo, 1979; Mueller, 1980; Pattison, DeFrancisco, Wood, Frazier, & Crowder, 1975; Tolsdorf, 1976). Social networks of people who have psychiatric illnesses often differ from the networks of others (Heller, 1978; Henderson et al., 1978)—that is, psychotic individuals have a very small primary network of family members and few or no friends.

Degrees of psychiatric illness may be related to network size and quality of exchanges, including the ability to participate in reciprocal care-giving relationships (Froland et al., 1979; Sokolovsky, Cohen, Berger, & Geiger, 1978). It has been postulated that the reality of our world is affirmed and validated through our conversations and social interactions. Mental illness often involves the substitute of a pseudocommunity to fill these needs, often manifested in grand delusions and hallucinations.

How can social support contribute to health? Three theories have been postulated by Pilisuk and Parks (1986): (1) *the buffer theory* proposes that social contacts serve as filters and moderate the meaning of a stressful event; a *compensation theory* suggests that social contacts provide a means of coping with stress; (2) *the direct effect theory* proposes that the benefits of social support can be observed without any obvious stressful stimuli and that the individual's attitude or coping style may best determine the immunological consequences of everyday living (Andrews & Tennant, 1978; Dean & Lin, 1977; Meyers, Lindenthal, & Pepper, 1975; Turner, 1982); and (3) *the cognitive-dissonance theory* (cognitive interpretation—function and meaning) postulates a need to be positively connected and active in a social group whose values and interaction fit into the individual's view of reality. In McClelland and Kirshnit's study (1984), students exposed to a film about Mother Teresa's work of loving care had measurably higher levels of S-lgA than when they were exposed to other films. A positive and stable connection to a larger social group or to humanity/nature may improve resistance because a person can give and receive, can care and love. The complex interaction of stress and coping occurs inextricably within the larger context of social support. While the complexity of analyzing such a system in terms of factors may tax even the most creative researchers, it cannot be dismissed or ignored.

PEOPLE, PETS, AND PSYCHONEUROIMMUNOLOGY

Psychosocial research on humans is supported by psychosocial experiments with animals. When "cage mates" were familiar, animals subjected to stressful situations were more able to cope with hypertension (Henry & Cassel, 1976), neoplasms (Gross, 1973), noxious stimuli (Liddell, 1950), and maternal separation (Bowlby, 1973; Harlow & Harlow, 1962). This animal research reaffirms some continuity in social mechanisms that may have evolved to sustain health. A closer look at the specific social structures of species that are used as models might also give us insight into the dynamics of social support and psychosocial factors in other species.

Not all social relationships are supportive, and the quality of the relationship may determine the health consequences. Within Western culture, kinship bonds and traditional family units are more difficult to cultivate, and individuals sometimes find other support to supplement traditional support systems. Close and supportive relationships with other living things often creates strong and enduring bonds. The health benefits of the human-animal relationship and bonding have been reported for a variety of specific illnesses (Arehart-Treichel, 1982; Holden, 1981). Arkow (1984) and McCulloch (1981, 1982) have reviewed and discussed the beneficial nature of human-animal interactions during medical interventions. Since human-animal bonds are specifically emotional in nature, and given that emotions and neuropeptides may be linked, possible health consequences from these interactions are comprehensible. Psychological and physical changes of humans during the human-animal bonding process include: decreased blood pressure (Baun, Baun, Thoma, Langston, & Bergstrom, 1983; Friedman, Katcher, Lynch, & Thomas, 1982; Friedman, Katcher, Thomas, Lynch, & Messent, 1983; Grossberg & Alf, 1984; Jenkins, 1984; Katcher, 1981) and decreased anxiety in cancer patients (Muschel, 1984). Other studies focused on the effect of pets on psychotherapeutic interventions (Corson & O'Leary Corson, 1979; Corson, O'Leary Corson, Gwynne, & Arnold, 1975, 1977; Corson, et al., 1976; Glasser, 1965; Mugford & McComisky, 1975), on autism and neurological disorders (Smith, 1982), and on therapy on staff (Shaheen, 1986). Suggested mechanisms for the positive health effects of human-animal interactions include the use of nonverbal and tactile communication skills, increased attentiveness and caring, responsibility by patients, emotional bonds, and an increase in social connectedness. The value of interaction with other living organisms, besides humans, has only recently been recognized. Specific guidelines with respect to disorders and personality traits should be elaborated for the use of this potentially valuable social and behavioral intervention for health.

INTERACTIONS: IMMUNE SYSTEM, NERVOUS SYSTEM, AND SOCIAL MIND

Rather than focusing on the function of either the immunological, neurological, or psychological system, current research converges on the interaction *between* these three systems. Each individual system is constantly being challenged to respond to external and internal stimuli.

Likewise, each receives and communicates information to other systems. Reviews of this interaction are provided by Pert (1986), Besedovsky et al., (1983), and Cunningham (1981). This literature review demonstrates that the processes underlying these three systems have common elements:

1. All three systems defend and adapt. The immune system recognizes "self" from "nonself" and tries to rid the body of the "invader." The nervous system protects via psychological defense mechanisms. The social mind tries to conform and connect with society, with humanity, and with nature.

2. All three systems learn from experience and have a mechanism of memory. The immune system develops new antibodies after exposure to a new antigen and can also be conditioned by experience (Ader & Cohen, 1975; Gorczpynski et al., 1982). The nervous system learns to discriminate neural signals and can show physical dendritic growth through a behaviorally enriched environment. The social mind interacts with the environment and can go through great transformations during life.

3. All three systems show similar processes of analogous functions and are involved in information transfer. Their mechanisms of signal processing may be different, but they show evidence of interaction between systems. That the immune system is directly affected by social factors links the translation of information from the environment, through the mind, to the immune system, probably via emotion. It is the translation of this information that relates the "invading stressors" as friend or foe, positive or negative, and evocative or nonevocative of memory or emotionally related experience. Since all three systems show analogous properties of defense and adaption, experience and memory, and information transfer, each individual system should be able to translate across the others. When the immune system is defending against an invader, the brain should recognize the concept of defense and simultaneously or supportively induce defensive mechanisms. If this system is biochemical, then the brain can communicate or "entrain" the immune system into adaption or defensive maneuvers. Whether the translation of signals is mediated by a language of neuropeptides, by an emergent quality of the neuropeptides, or by the system itself remains unclear. Whether the direct nervous system connection fibers function in this regard is also unclear. However, it seems that the chain of physiological events that transpire and the individual's disease resistance can be affected by the highest integrating system of the body-human consciousness.

Understanding this higher cognitive control will open the door to greater control of our health and resistance to illness.

BIOLOGICAL DETECTION OF SUBTLE SIGNALS IN PSYCHONEUROIMMUNOLOGY

In 1872, Darwin (1965) was one of the first to note the many functions and expressions of human and animal emotion. Subtle cues and signaling play a very important role in human, animal, and human-animal communication (Hinde, 1972). Although such cues necessitate cautious approaches to avoid the misinterpretations created by the "clever Hans phenomena" in the early 20th century (Hediger, 1981; Orne, 1981), these cues may be critical to understanding the dynamics of complex communication systems. As in all communication systems, there is a subtlety involved in social support systems. Revenson, Wollman, and Felton (1983) discuss the importance of intent that is conveyed by body language, tone of voice, and the context of relationships from the giver to the receiver of social support. Often an unmeasurable variable may be an important one in the individual interpretation of the message of caring. These nuances of an exchange have been difficult to measure, but techniques for discerning discrete emotional and information states exist in the areas of verbal and nonverbal communication of humans and animals.

The mind-body system seems capable of interpreting subtle features on a cognitive level. How the subtle cues are interpreted in the greater cognitive complex of an individual mind may determine ultimate behavior or immune reactions. Studies of nonverbal cues, such as facial action coding (Ekman, 1982, 1984), rhythms in speech (Byers, 1973), and work with neuromuscular expression and perception of emotions of human communication (Clynes, 1973), suggest that many emotions have discrete formulas that are recognizable and interpretable as discrete emotional states (Hurley, 1983; Wallbott & Scherer, 1986). Ekman (1982) discusses the potential of using facial action coding to evoke specific emotions as well as to monitor them. If humans detect, recognize, and emotionally translate such subtle cues, it seems possible that such emotionally evocative messages might start a sequence of hormonal and immunological changes, but the detailed mechanism remains unknown.

Hemispheric lateralization of emotions is well documented (Ley, 1983; Silberman & Weingartner, 1986) and may point to a source of potential immunomodulation via conscious or unconscious activation of hemispheres or their related functions. This research demonstrated that the left hemisphere is involved in the processing of positive emotions and in the stimulation of the immune system. Conversely, the right hemisphere seems to be involved in the processing of negative emotions and in the suppression of the immune system, either directly or by mediating and/or inhibiting the activity of the left. The late Norman Geshwind and his colleagues (Geschwind & Behan, 1982) reported the relationship between brain lateralization and immunological disease. Left-handed people are more susceptible to autoimmune disorders, and mathematically gifted and learning-disabled individuals are more prone to developing allergies. Both of these populations have anomalies in brain symmetry that may disrupt the balanced regulation of the immune system. Renoux (Wechsler, 1987) has even postulated that patients who exercise the right hemisphere during imagery practices may "distract" the right hemisphere from suppressing the immune system. Comprehending these neurophysiological mechanisms of cognitive activation and control will be critical to understanding immunological competence.

Research on the selective activation of hemispheres during meditation indicates that right-hemisphere activation may be induced through control of attention, visual imagery, and selective thought (Earle, 1981). These data suggest that selective hemispheric activation and emotional states, and subsequently emotions and their concomitant neuropeptides, may be consciously controlled. Subtle interaction between mind and self also are reported in mindfulness meditation (Forte, Brown, & Dysart, 1984), during which subjects experience changes in basic physical perceptions as well as in inner awareness of functions. There is an extensive ongoing database development of over 3,600 documented instances of spontaneous remission (Kent, Coates, & Pelletier, 1987). Medically unexplainable remission of disease states has been documented, but it is in an area of controversy and needs more documentation. Whether the "faith" element of such remissions is mediated unconsciously through neuropeptide pathways or whether direct CNS pathways are utilized remains unclear. Placebo research (Evans, 1984; Ney, Collins, & Spensor, 1986; O'Regan & Hurley, 1985), which shows that belief of the action of a nondrug shows physical effects, is another gray area. Conscious or unconscious control may be evident during placebo treatment, but immunological measures have not been followed during placebo response.

Possibly the best example of self-deception and personality correlates with immune parameters exists in the research literature on multiple personalities (Braun, 1983). There is evidence that electroencephalographic recordings are as statistically different between personalities as they are between two different individuals. Furthermore, in one personality an individual may be allergic to cats or food, and in another personality the same individual will not show allergic reactions. Such shifts demonstrate that allergic responses are capable of being triggered by changes in personality, just as shifts in allergic reaction can be brought on through hypnotic induction. It is interesting to note that most multiple-personality individuals experience childhood trauma, usually of an emotional and physical nature. Many researchers theorize that the formation of alternate personalities is a defense mechanism during abusive situations. Given the ability of the immune system to be behaviorally conditioned through experience, it is possible that the mechanism for subsequent retention for multiple personalities and their concomitant immune responses may involve such learning.

Subtle cues and their interpretation also are determined by the larger context, by the relationship between interacting individuals, and by the individually determined meaning of the message (Moles, 1963; Smith, 1977). Emotional messages may concomitantly activate moods via neuropeptides, suggesting that there may be an extremely important and complex language of subtle signals that needs to be decoded to elucidate neuropeptide activity. The detection of subtleties can be deceptive, even to the self (Jamner & Schwartz, 1986; Sackeim & Gur, 1978; Schwartz, 1983). Measures of affective arousal states and "inattention to distress" have been reported in subjects whose physiological records showed signs of alarm. Schwartz (1983) has speculated that a repressive style may activate the right hemisphere. Whether this activates the right hemisphere's ability to suppress the immune system or to evoke negative emotions and their subsequent neuropeptides, or whether it "distracts" the right hemisphere from the suppression or retention of immune-system balance is unknown. These different strategies of coping with information, raising or not raising them to levels of awareness, could be critical in determining ultimate health competence.

Asthmatics evidencing repressive defense styles are unable to detect subtle changes in airway obstruction, which suggests that cognitive mechanisms override physiological perception (Steiner, Higgs, Fritz, Laszlo, & Harvey, 1987). The asthmatic-prone personality is generally described as depressed, hostile, introverted, covertly aggressive, and defiant; however, the only trait for which there is clear evidence is that of heightened dependency. Although a clear personality dimension in asthma remains unproven, asthma should prove amenable to PNI investigation, since both bronchospasm and mast cell mediation of the immune response are likely sites of involvement. To date, one research project failed to demonstrate the ability of asthmatic patients to influence their mast cell mediation of antigen response through a combination of relaxation and specific visualizations (Polonsky et al., 1985). Associative conditioning of single sensory neurons also has been suggestive of a cellular mechanism for learning (Walters & Byrne, 1983). Both of these aspects, along with evidence from the multiple-personality research, suggest that cognitive control and learning can take place at a very elementary level—the cellular one—but can be perceived, repressed, or encouraged on a cognitive level. The mind seems to perceive itself, like the immune system, as self or nonself, and its choice is determined by subtle signals perceived and interpreted in a larger social context.

Some help in elucidating specific processes of the mind may come from the application of modern technology to the questions of subtle energy. As Pert's (1987) evidence suggests, all neuropeptides may be made up of one molecule; it is the changes in the configuration of this molecule that define different neuropeptides from each other. What factors determine the change from one configuration to another? If we could apply our technology to the problem of observing this process of transformation, we might discover what cellular, biochemical, or neural factors govern such changes. Another possible application of technology might be in the area of imagery. Finke (1986) suggests that imagery may involve the same kinds of internal neural processes as perception; thus imagery is subject to similar activation of information processing on higher levels. One controversial example of modern technology and subtle energy detection is in the area of homeopathy. Mechanisms of action of homeopathic remedies that do not contain any of the original molecules of substance (microdoses) have been speculated on by various researchers (Boyd, 1954; Callinan, 1985). Recently, Reilly, Taylor, McSharry, and Aitchison (1986) reported no evidence to support the idea that placebo action fully explains positive clinical responses to homeopathic remedies. Barnard (1965) and Barnard and Stephenson (1967) proposed that the solvent functioned as the carrier of molecular configuration information. Applications of nuclear magnetic resonance (NMR) analysis on the changes of the water structure of the remedy revealed a configurational change in the hydrogen-oxygen bond of the water molecules (Young, 1975). Although not definitive in its conclusions about the actual mechanism of homeopathic action, this study is an example of possible applications of technologies such as NMR to subtle energy interventions whose mechanisms remain unknown. Perhaps, subtle influences on neuropeptides, water molecule configurations, emotions, thoughts, and subjective imagery can exert a leveraging influence upon health and disease. Unfortunately, as in most clinical trials, these subtle interventions are first undertaken with the most severe conditions. Another equally viable approach would be the systematic, longitudinal application of such interventions for health maintenance or applying them at early stages of evident risk factors or immediately upon diagnosis, when such interventions may be most efficacious in exerting a fulcrum effect.

A MODEL OF MIND-BODY INTERACTION—CRITICAL ISSUES

General Observations

1. At the present time, research data in the numerous areas of stress and coping, PNI, psychosocial support, hemispheric specialization with particular reference to the lateralization of immunological influences, neuroendocrinology, and related areas appear to point toward a unified field theory of mind-body-psychosocial interaction. However, the specialized nature of the operational definitions, of research designs, and of data analysis and the lack of adequate cross-referencing among studies leaves more confusion than cohesion at the present time.

2. The data suggest the existence of an interactive system linking psychological, neurological, physiological, immunological, endocrine, and biochemical internal events with the external psychosocial and physical environment of both people and animals. Since the research areas of stress and PNI ultimately address these issues, and since they constitute a large and growing area of data, these areas merit more focused consideration.

3. Given the preliminary but promising nature of the data in these disparate areas, it seems to be prudent to develop a synthesis of the known data into a more coherent, testable model with specific falsifiable hypotheses. Generating more specialized research will not resolve this problem. Collaborative research publications, as well as further collaborative literature reviews, would be extremely useful.

4. Basic insights from quantum physics regarding the Heisenberg principle of uncertainty, complementarity, unified field theory, and even the postulation of the unifying "superstrings" of astrophysics, could be considered as having analogous principles or applications in the mind-body area.

5. Whatever the nature of mind-body interaction is, it clearly involves subtle energy or subtle information exchange. In fact, there may be no difference between energy states and information in such a system. Or it may be that information is encoded in the energy, as it is in most other communication systems, and is decoded and recognized from patterns of information via changes in patterns of modulation in such aspects as frequencies, amplitudes, and time patterns. Clearly, these are more than semantic considerations, and terms need to be clarified and defined before progress can be made.

6. Applications of medical-imaging technologies have the potential to link observable activity within the brain in a relatively unobtrusive manner during normal, human, psychological tasks. These imaging technologies detect subtle energies and may provide clarification of precisely which neurophysiological regions of the brain are involved in the complex operations of human consciousness and their subsequent interactions with the biochemistry of the body and interaction with the environment. Precise tracking of psychological events through multiple levels of organization may begin to clarify the conflicting data of the mediating pathways in the mind-body system.

7. Imaging techniques—including the use of electromagnetic energy in x-rays, in CAT (computerized axial tomography), in PETT (positron emission transaxial tomography), and in SQUID (subquantum interference detector), and the use of magnetic energy in NMR (nuclear magnetic resonance)—and ultrasound diagnostic techniques demonstrate the sophisticated detection capabilities of the imaging technologies. The diagnostic uses of such subtle energy technology are accompanied by the effects of such energies on the physical, hormonal, and behavioral aspects of living organisms. The subtle biological effects of electromagnetic radiation, ultrasound, pulsed ultrasound, oxygen and radiation of DNA, and enzymes on living systems have been reported. The benefits of these diagnostic procedures may presently outweigh the risks. Such subtle energies have been harnessed to produce positive changes; for example, electromagnetic energy has been used in regeneration of nerve tissues. However, the manipulation of subtle magnetic fields also has resulted in negative behavioral changes, such as increased aggressive behavior. That mammalian organs perceive and react to such energies, which then elicit biological response, is not surprising. But a specific theoretical framework to explain the action of these subtle energies is lacking.

8. The mind-body model that emerges from the field of PNI should incorporate a systems approach in defining the role of consciousness of the individual or social mind. The study of analogous processes of the psychological, neurological, and immune systems in conjunction with the emergent properties of higher cognitive functions may provide a working model in the application and interventions of a behavioral nature.

Stress-Psychoneuroimmunology Linkage

1. Despite the large number of studies that reported links between both generalized and specific stressor effects and subsequent organic disease, the linkage is not definitive. Whether this effect is a direct or

indirect one still remains to be assessed. Within the life stress index literature, the correlation between life events and subsequent illness is often markedly low. When more objective measures are utilized, it is also evident that only a small number of individuals actually develop organic disease.

2. Virtually all PNI research studies have lacked adequate experimental control groups or conditions. At minimum, the control groups need to be matched by age, gender, life stress levels, and social support indicators, since these have been demonstrated to be significant variables.

3. Since most of the research developed from earlier stress research, PNI has done little to clearly define the nature of the stressor in terms of validity or reliability. Assumptions as to the nature of stress abound, but only three areas of study (examinations, bereavement, and sleep deprivation) are based on standardized stress inducements.

4. Both the experimental stressor and clarification of the specific psychological assessments of those stressors are essential, given recent evidence indicating that individual responses and coping styles may be more important than the challenge itself in determining the subsequent neurophysiological and immunological responses.

5. Most of the PNI studies actually document a correlation rather than the causal relationship between stress, psychological states, immunological changes, and subsequent health and disease status. Clearly, longitudinal studies of more stringent design are necessary.

Immunological Variables

1. Without establishment of more precise immunological norms, the data indicating changes in immunological parameters are difficult to assess in terms of significance. Statistically significant results were within normal laboratory values, so the issue of the "clinical" significance of the change is questionable at best. To restate a familiar homily: statistical significance does not necessarily equal clinical significance.

2. It follows from this first observation that even a statistically significant change in immunological parameters cannot be judged as negative ("impaired," "detrimental") or as positive ("improved," "enhanced," "beneficial") until the links between the variable and subsequent health or disease are established. Such assignments of clinical value or significance need to be suspended given the present objective studies. Statistical significance is not necessarily clinically significant in PNI nor in any other research area.

3. Regarding immunological indices, the effect of stress on components of the immune system, such as NK cell activity, total lymphocyte

count, total B-lymphocytes, IgA, granulocyte activity, and total monocytes, is inconsistent and may be elucidated through clarification of antecedent stressors and modifying responses, as well as through more
sensitive norms for these parameters per se. Three immunological indices that appear to be unaffected as dependent variables in the data to
date are total T-lymphocytes, T-suppressor cells, and T-helper cells.

4. According to the excellent methodological critique of Workman
and La Via (1987), the most promising immunological indices are responses to the antigens phytohemaglutinin (PHA) and concanavalin A
(Con A). Since these two mitogens activate T-lymphocytes, these findings indicate that stress is likely to influence the functional effectiveness
of the cellular activation process itself. It appears that future research
should concentrate on mitogen responsiveness as a primary dependent
variable and should employ lipopolysaccharide and pokeweed mitogens
to determine the potential function of B-cell blastogenesis in reactions to
stress.

5. Immunologists have been successful in defining the cellular components and functions of the immune system and, to some degree, how
they interact in a subtle communications model of receptor sights. However, what regulates the collective functions has not been determined.
Among the possible regulators of the immune system, the role of human
consciousness needs to be given prominent consideration.

Psychosocial Factors

1. Although most of the studies on the relationship of psychosocial
factors and immunity have focused on stress-induced states, there is a
growing literature on enhancing immunity through positive interventions of a social nature. Though these social factors can also have negative consequences, the individual's coping mechanisms and social
stability play a major role in health outcomes. Understanding the mechanisms at work and how social support gets "into" the immune system
should be prioritized.

2. Another growing field of inquiry is that of social interaction with
pets and other living organisms. The generally fragmented state of Western society increases the need to find supplemental and supportive relationships outside of traditional family ties. This fact, combined with the
growing evidence of physiological and psychological effects on humans
during human-animal interactions, suggests that new behavioral interventions for disease prevention and modification should be considered.

3. Our general perceptions of the world and exposure to positive or
negative stimuli may directly affect our immune systems. This observation

is borne out most clearly by the McClelland and Kirshnit (1984) study of positive film stimuli and increased S-IgA levels. Regardless of whether the individual verbally supported the content of the film, his or her immune system reacted in a positively enhancing way. The need for specific immunological measures during psychosocial interventions should be given primary consideration.

Clinical-Experimental Implications

1. Clinical-experimental studies need to be conducted on a longitudinal basis in order to make the assumed linkage between PNI changes and subsequent health and disease status more explicit. Studies monitoring the psychological, neurophysiological, immunological, and neuroendocrine markers during behavioral interventions (e.g., stress management techniques) will be of major significance in guiding the efficacy of such interventions in psychosomatic disorders, coronary heart disease, alcohol and substance abuse, autoimmune disorders, chronic obstructive pulmonary disease, and in related disorders in which behavioral medicine has preliminary evidence of effectiveness.

2. Although extensive evidence links psychological factors (e.g., various stressors and depression) with subsequent morbidity and mortality, it is not certain that these same stressors or psychological disorders are the same as those that are linked to immunosuppression. One of a few explicit linkages between the two realms of research is a finding by Levy and her colleagues (Levy, Lippman, & Terry, 1980) involving breast cancer patients. Patients with higher NK cell activity had fewer positive lymph nodes and thus a more optimistic prognosis. More research needs to be undertaken linking an explicit stressor, immunological responses, and subsequent clinical outcome significance.

3. One extremely important area of clinical-experimental work is that of AIDS. Given the role of mind-body interaction in influencing immunity, consideration needs to be given to the effects of stress upon seropositive HIV findings and on subsequent development of AIDS-related conditions (ARC). The efficacy of stress management and psychosocial interventions need to be evaluated as a tool for possibly preventing HIV progression. Finally, the impact of the disease itself on psychological and behavioral functioning needs to be considered, given the bidirectional communication in the mind-body system.

4. Meditation and relaxation therapies, such as autogenic training and clinical biofeedback, have been demonstrated to be effective in stress management and have been documented to manifest neurophysiological

and biochemical changes characteristic of deep relaxation response. Future research in PNI may serve to make such interventions more precise. There might be a new generation of biofeedback instrumentation that not only feeds back patterns of neurophysiological responses but also integrates a hematological analysis, so that individuals might learn to govern their antibody or other immunological responses.

CONCLUDING REMARKS

Data from the emerging field of PNI and related disciplines increasingly indicate a mind-body continuum and discredit the anachronistic split of Cartesian dualism. Concepts and models from quantum physics, as well as theoretical speculations from key researchers, indicate that human consciousness is not only reducible to neural or biochemical events but may, in fact, exert a superordinate organizing function over these biological functions. While the precise means by which this organizing function occurs is far from explicable at the present time, it is far more complex than the current attempts to reduce human consciousness to random protoplasm suggest. At the forefront of developing this model is PNI, since the subtlety of the systemic interactions between the mind-body and environment is so critical and unequivocal. An alternative to the biological determinism or even the quantum mechanics models of the mind is that aspects of human consciousness (e.g., "will," "decision," "beliefs," and "values") may emerge as ineliminatable, irreducible, organizational, and causal principles of the mind-body system. The biological substrates and lawful determinism of brain function are fully acknowledged, but human consciousness may not be limited to those laws. This critical review has taken tentative steps toward suggesting the components of such a paradigm in present research, while documenting the major shortcomings of present research design, methodology, data analysis, and subsequent hypotheses. Speculations concerning the ultimate role of beliefs, positive emotions, and spiritual values in organizing and transcending biological determinism would seem to be philosophical speculation if the answers to these questions were not so critical to our survival as a species.

References

Ader, R. (1981). *Psychoneuroimmunology.* New York: Academic Press.

Ader, R. (1983). Developmental psychoneuroimmunology. *Developmental Psychobiology, 16*(4), 251–267.

Ader, R., & Cohen, N. (1975). Behaviorally conditioned immunosuppression. *Psychosomatic Medicine, 37,* 333–340.

Ader, R., & Cohen, N. (1981). Conditioned immunopharmacologic effects. In R. Ader (Ed.), *Psychoneuroimmunology* (pp. 281–319). New York: Academic Press.

Ahlquist, J. (1981). Hormonal influences on immunologic and related phenomena. In R. Ader (Ed.), *Psychoneuroimmunology* (pp. 355–403). New York: Academic Press.

Amkraut, A. A., Solomon, G. F., & Kraemer, H. C. (1971). Stress, early experience and adjuvant-induced arthritis in the rat. *Psychosomatic Medicine, 33,* 203–214.

Andrews, G., & Tennant, C. (1978). Life event stress, social support, coping style and the risk of psychological impairment. *Journal of Nervous and Mental Disease, 166*(7), 605–612.

Arehart-Treichel, J. (1982). Pets: The health benefits. *Science News, 121,* 220–224.

Arkow, P. (1984). *Dynamic relationships in practice: Animals in the helping professions.* Alameda, CA: Latham Foundation.

Arnetz, B. B., Wasserman, J., Petrini, B., Brenner, S. O., Levi, L., Eneroth, P., Salovaara, H., Hjelm, R., Salovaara, L., Theorell, T., & Petterson, I. L. (1987). Immune function in unemployed women. *Psychosomatic Medicine, 49*(1), 3–12.

Barnard, G. P. (1965). Microdose paradox—A new concept. *Journal of the American Institute of Homeopathy, 58,* 205–212.

Barnard, G. P., & Stephenson, J. H. (1967). Microdose paradox: A new biological concept. *Journal of the American Institute of Homeopathy, 60,* 277–286.

Bartrop, R. W., Lazarus, L., Luckhurst, E., Kiloh, L. G., & Penny, R. (1977). Depressed lymphocyte function after bereavement. *Lancet, 1,* 834–836.

Baun, M. M., Baun, D. N., Thoma, L., Langston, N., & Bergstrom, N. (1983). Effects of bonding vs. non-bonding on the physiological effects of petting. *Proceedings of the Conferences on the Human-Animal Bond.* University of Minnesota, June 13–14, 1983, and University of California, June 17–18, 1983.

Berkman, L., & Syme, L. (1978). Social networks, host resistance and mortality: A nine year follow-up study of Alameda County residents. *American Journal of Epidemiology, 109*(2), 186–204.

Bertalanffy, L. (1968). *General system theory: Foundations, development, applications.* New York: Braziller.

Besedovsky, H. O., del Rey, A. E., & Sorkin, E. (1983). What do the immune system and the brain know about each other? *Immunology Today, 4*(12), 342–346.

Besedovsky, H. O., Felix, D., & Haas, H. (1977). Hypothalamic changes during immune response. *European Journal of Immunology, 7*(5), 323–325.

Bishopric, M. J., Cohen, H. J., & Lefkowitz, R. J. (1980). Beta-adrenergic receptors in lymphocyte subpopulations. *Journal of Allergy and Clinical Immunology, 65,* 29–33.

Black, S. (1963). Inhibition of immediate-type hypersensitivity response by direct suggestion under hypnosis. *British Medical Journal, 6,* 925–929.

Black, S., Humphrey, J. H., & Niven, J. S. (1963). Inhibition of Mantoux reaction by direct suggestion under hypnosis. *British Medical Journal, 6,* 1649–1652.

Blank, H., & Brody, M. W. (1950). Recurrent herpes simplex. *Psychosomatic Medicine, 12,* 254–260.

Bloom, B., Asher, S., & White, S. (1978). Marital disruption as a stressor: A review and analysis. *Psychological Bulletin, 85*(6), 867–894.

Bohm, D. (1980). *Wholeness and the implicate order.* London: Routledge and Kegan Paul.

Borysenko, M. (1987). *Area review: Psychoneuroimmunology. Annals of Behavioral Medicine, 9*(2), 3–10.

Borysenko, M., & Borysenko, J. (1982). Stress, behavior, and immunity: Animal models and mediating mechanisms. *General Hospital Psychiatry, 4,* 59–67.

Bovbjerg, D., Ader, R., & Cohen, N. (1984). Aquisition and extinction of conditioned suppression of a graft-vs-host response in the rat. *Journal of Immunology, 132,* 111–113.

Bowers, K. S., & Kelly, P. (1979). Stress, disease, psychotherapy, and hypnosis. *Journal of Abnormal Psychology, 85,* 490–505.

Bowlby, J. (1973). *Separation.* New York: Basic Books.

Boyce, W. T., Jensen, E. W., Cassel, J. C., Collier, A. M., Smith, A. H., & Ramey, C. T. (1977). Influence of life events and family routines on childhood respiratory tract illness. *Pediatrics, 60,* 609–615.

Boyd, W. E. (1954). Biochemical and biological evidence of the activity of high potencies. *British Homeopathy Journal, 44,* 6–44.

Braun, B. (1983). Psychophysiologic phenomena in multiple personality and hypnosis. *American Journal of Clinical Hypnosis, 26*(2), 124–137.

Brayton, A. R., & Brain, P. F. (1975). Effects of differential housing and glucocorticoid administration on immune responses to sheep red blood cells in albino TO strain mice. *Journal of Endocrinology, 54*(1), 4–5.

Brown, G. W., Bhrolchaim, M. N., & Harris, T. (1975). Social class and psychiatric disturbance among women in an urban population. *Sociology, 9,* 225–254.

Brown, G. W., Davidson, S., & Harris, T. (1977). Psychiatric disorder in London and North Ulster. *Social Science and Medicine, 11,* 367–377.

Brown, G. W., & Harris, T. (1978). *Social origins of depression: A study of psychiatric disorder.* New York: Free Press.

Bulloch, K., & Moore, R. Y. (1981). Innervation of the thymus gland by brainstem and spinal cord in mouse and rat. *American Journal of Anatomy, 162,* 157–166.

Byers, P. (1973). Biological rhythms as information channels in interpersonal communication behavior. In P. P. G. Bateson & P. H. Klopler (Eds.), *Perspective in ethology* (Vol. 2, pp. 135–164). New York: Plenum.

Callinan, P. (1985). The mechanism of action of homeopathic remedies— Towards a definitive model. Section C: Mode of action. *Journal of Complementary Medicine, 1,* 35–56.

Cannon, W. B. (1926). The emergency function of the adrenal medulla in pain and the major emotions. *American Journal of Physiology, 33,* 356–372.

Canter, A. (1972). Changes in mood during incubation of acute febrile disease and the effects of pre-exposure psychological status. *Psychosomatic Medicine, 34,* 424–425.

Canter, A., Cluff, L. E., & Imboden, J. B. (1972). Hypersensitive reactions to immunization inoculations and antecedent psychological vulnerability. *Journal of Psychosomatic Research, 16,* 99–101.

Cassel, J., & Tyroler, H. A. (1961). Epidemiological studies of culture change: Health status and recency of industrialization. *Archives of Environmental Health, 3,* 25–33.

Chen, E., & Cobb, S. (1960). Family structure in relation to health and disease. *Journal of Chronic Disease, 12,* 544–567.

Claman, H. M. (1972). Corticosteroids and lymphoid cells. *New England Journal of Medicine, 287,* 388–397.

Clarkson, A. K. (1937). The nervous factor in juvenile asthma. *British Medical Journal, 2,* 845–850.

Clynes, M. (1973). Sentography: Dynamic forms of communication of emotion and qualities. *Computers in Biology and Medicine, 3,* 119–130.

Coates, T. J., & Greenblatt, R. M. (1986, 1987). Behavioral change using intervention at the community level. In K. K. Holmes (Ed.), *Sexually transmitted diseases.* New York: McGraw-Hill.

Cobb, S., Kasl, S. V., French, J., & Norstebo, G. (1969). The intrafamilial transmission of rhematoid arthritis: Why do wives with rheumatoid arthritis have husbands with peptic ulcer? *Journal of Chronic Disease, 22,* 279–293.

Cohen-Cole, S., Cogen, R., Stevens, A., Kirk, K., Gaitan, E., Hain, J., & Freeman, A. (1981). Psychosocial, endocrine, and immune factors in acute necrotizing ulcerative gingivitis ("trenchmouth"). *Psychosomatic Medicine, 43,* 91 (Abstract).

Corson, S. A., & O'Leary Corson, E. (1979). Pet animals as nonverbal communication mediators in psychotherapy in institutional settings. In *Ethology and nonverbal communication in mental health; An interdisciplinary biopsychosocial exploration* (pp. 83–110). Oxford: Pergamon.

Corson, S. A., O'Leary Corson, E., Dettass, D., Gunsett, R., Gwynne, P. H., Arnold, L. E., & Corson, C. N. (1976). *The socializing role of pet animals in nursing homes; An experiment in non-verbal communication therapy.* Oxford: Oxford University Press.

Corson, S. A., O'Leary Corson, E., Gwynne, P., & Arnold, L. (1975). Pet-faciliated psychotherapy in a hospital setting. In J. H. Masserman (Ed.), *Current psychiatric therapies* (Vol. 15).

Corson, S. A., O'Leary Corson, E., Gwynne, P., & Arnold, L. (1977). Pet dogs as non-verbal communication links in hospital psychiatry. *Comprehensive Psychiatry, 18,* 61–72.

Cousins, N. (1981). *Anatomy of an illness as perceived by the patient.* New York: Bantam.

Crary, B., Borysenko, M., Sutherland, D. C., Kutz, I., Borysenko, J. Z., & Benson, H. (1983). Decrease in mitogen responsiveness of mononuclear cells from peripheral blood after epineprine administration in humans. *Journal of Immunology, 130,* 694–697.

Crary, B., Hauser, S. L., Borysenko, M., Kutz, I., Hoban, C., Ault, K. A., Weiner, H. L., & Benson, H. (1983). Epinephrine-induced changes in the distribution of lymphocyte subsets in peripheral blood of humans. *Journal of Immunology, 131,* 1178–1181.

Cunningham, A. J. (1981). Mind, body, and immune response. In R. Ader (Ed.), *Psychoneuroimmunology* (pp. 609–617). New York: Academic Press.

Cunningham, A. J. (1986). Information and health in the many levels of man: Towards a more comprehensive theory of health and disease. *Advances, 3*(1), 32–45.

Darwin, C. (1965). *The expression of the emotions in man and animals.* Chicago: University of Chicago Press.

Davis, D. E., & Read, C. P. (1958). Effect of behavior on development of resistance in trichinosis. *Proceedings of the Society for Experimental Biology and Medicine, 99,* 269–272.

Dean, A., & Lin, N. (1977). The stress buffering role of social support. *Journal of Nervous and Mental Disease, 165,* 403–417.

Derogatis, L., Abeloff, M., & Melisaratos, N. (1979). Psychobiological coping mechanisms and survival time in metastatic breast cancer. *Journal of the American Medical Association, 242,* 1504–1508.

Dillon, K. M., Minchoff, B., & Baker, K. H. (1985). Positive emotional states and enhancement of the immune system. *International Journal of Psychiatry in Medicine, 15,* 13–17.

Dirks, J. F., Robinson, S. K., & Dirks, D. L. (1981). Alexithymia and the psychomaintenance of bronchial asthma. *Psychotherapy and Psychosomatics, 36,* 63–71.

Dohrenwend, B. S., & Dohrenwend, B. P. (1974). *Stressful life events: Their nature and effects.* New York: Wiley.

Dorian, B. J., Keystone, E., Garfinkel, P. E., & Brown, G. M. (1982). Aberrations in lymphocyte subpopulations and functions during psychological stress. *Clinical and Experimental Immunology, 50,* 132–138.

Earle, J. B. B. (1981). Cerebral laterality and meditation: A review of the literature. *Journal of Transpersonal Psychology, 13*(2), 155–173.

Edwards, E. A., & Dean, L. M. (1977). Effects of crowding of mice on humoral antibody formation and protection to lethal antigenic challenge. *Psychosomatic Medicine, 39,* 19–24.

Edwards, E. A., Rahe, R. H., Stephens, P. M., & Henry, J. P. (1980). Antibody response to bovine serum albumin in mice: The effects of psychosocial environmental change. *Proceedings of the Society for Experimental Biology and Medicine, 164*, 478–481.

Ekman, P. (1982). *Emotion in the human face*. Cambridge: Cambridge University Press.

Ekman, P. (1984). Expression and the nature of emotion. In K. R. Scherer & P. Ekman (Eds.), *Approaches to emotion* (pp. 319–344). London: Erlbaum.

Evans, F. J. (1984). Unravelling placebo effects. *Advances, 1*(3), 11–20.

Fauci, A. S. (1978). Mechanisms of the immunosuppressive and anti-inflammatory effects of glucocorticosteroids. *Journal of Immunopharmacology, 9*, 1–25.

Finke, R. A. (1986). Mental imagery and the visual system. *Scientific American, 254*(3), 88–95.

Fischer, C. L., Daniels, J. C., Levin, S. L., Kimzey, S. L., Cobb, E. K., & Ritzman, W. E. (1972). Effects of the spaceflight environment on man's immune system: II. Lymphocyte counts and reactivity. *Aerospace Medicine, 43*, 1122–1125.

Forte, M., Brown, D., & Dysart, M. (1984). Through the looking glass: Phenomenological reports of advanced meditators at visual threshold. *Imagination, Cognition and Personality, 4*(4), 323–338.

Fox, B. (1981). Psychosocial factors and the immune system in human cancer. In R. Ader (Ed.), *Psychoneuroimmunology* (pp. 103–182). New York: Academic Press.

Frey, B. M., Walker, C., Frey, J., & de Weck, A. L. (1984). Pharmacokinetics and pharmacodynamics of three different prednisolone prodrugs: Effect on circulating lymphocyte subsets and function. *Journal of Immunology, 133*, 2479–2487.

Friedman, R., & Rosenman, R. H. (1974). *Type A behavior and your heart*. New York: Fawcett.

Friedmann, E., Katcher, A. H., Lynch, J. J., & Thomas, S. A. (1982). Animal companions and one-year survival of patients after discharge from a coronary care unit. *California Veterinarian, 8*, 45–50.

Friedmann, E., Katcher, A. H., Thomas, S. A., Lynch, J. J., & Messent, P. R. (1983). Social interaction and blood pressure: Influence of animal companions. *Journal of Nervous and Mental Disease, 171*(8), 461–465.

Froland, C., Brodsky, G., Olson, M., & Stewart, L. (1979). Social support and social adjustment: Implications for mental health professionals. *Community Mental Health Journal, 15*(2), 82–93.

Fujiwara, M., Muryobayashi, T., & Shimamoto, K. (1966). Histochemical demonstration of monoamines in the thymus of rats. *Japanese Journal of Pharmacology, 16*, 493–494.

Gallup, G. G. Jr. (1985). Do minds exist in species other than our own? *Neuroscience and Biobehavioral Reviews, 9*, 631–641.

Geschwind, N. & Behan, P. (1982). Left-handedness: Association with immune disease, migraine, and developmental learning disorder. *Proceedings of the National Academy of Sciences, USA, 79*, 5097–5100.

Gilman, S. C., Schwartz, J. M., Milner, R. J., Bloom, F. E., & Feldman, J. D. (1982). Beta-endorphin enhances lymphocyte proliferative responses. *Proceedings of the National Academy of Sciences, USA, 79*, 4226–4230.

Glasser, W. (1965). *Reality Therapy: A New Approach to Psychiatry.* New York: Harper & Row.

Goodkin, K., Antoni, M. H., & Blaney, P. H. (1986). Stress and hopelessness in the promotion of cervical intraepithelial neoplasia to invasive squamous cell carcinoma of the cervix. *Journal of Psychosomatic Research, 30*(1), 67–76.

Gorczynski, R. M., Macrae, S., & Kennedy, M. (1982). Conditioned immune response associated with allogeneic skin grafts in mice. *Journal of Immunology, 129*, 704–709.

Greenfield, N. S., Roessler, R., & Crosley, A. P. (1959). Ego strength and length of recovery from infectious mononucleosis. *Journal of Nervous and Mental Disease, 128*, 125–128.

Gross, W. (1973). Stressor effects of initial bacterial exposure of chickens as determined by subsequent challenge exposure. *American Journal of Veterinary Research, 35*(9), 1225–1228.

Grossberg, J. M., & Alf, E. F. (1984). Interaction with pet dogs: Effect on human blood pressure. *Presented at the 92nd Annual Convention of the American Medical Association,* Toronto, Canada.

Hall, H., Longo, S., & Dixon, R. (1981). Hypnosis and the immune system: The effect of hypnosis on T and B cell function. Paper presented at the 33rd Annual Workshop and Scientific Meeting of the Society for Clinical and Experimental Hypnosis, Portland, OR.

Hall, H. R. (1983). Hypnosis and the immune system: A review with implications for cancer and the psychology of healing. *American Journal of Clinical Hypnosis, 25*(2–3), 92–103.

Hamilton, D. R. (1974). Immunosuppressive effects of predator induced stress in mice with acquired immunity to hymenolepsis nana. *Journal of Psychosomatic Research, 18*, 143–150.

Hammer, M. (1963). Influence of small social networks as factors on mental hospital admissions. *Human Organizations, 22*, 243–251.

Harburg, E., Erfurt, J. C., & Chape, C. (1973). Socio-ecological stressor areas and black-white blood pressure. *Journal of Chronic Disease, 26*, 595–611.

Harlow, H., & Harlow, M. (1962). Social deprivation in monkeys. *Scientific American, 207*(5), 136.

Hazum, E., Chang, K. J., & Cuatrecasas, P. (1979). Specific nonopiate receptors for beta-endorphin. *Science, 205*, 1033–1035.

Hediger, H. K. P. (1981). The clever Hans phenomenon from an animal psychologist's point of view. In T. A. Sebeok & R. Rosenthal (Eds.), *The clever Hans phenomenon: Communication with horses, whales, apes and people* (pp. 1–17).

Heller, K. (1978). The effects of social support: Prevention and treatment implications. In A. P. Goldstein & F. H. Kanfer (Eds.), *Maximizing treatment gains:*

Transfer enhancement in psychotherapy (pp. 353–382). New York: Academic Press.

Henderson, S., Byrne, D., Duncan-Jones, P., Adcock, S., Scott, R., & Steele, G. (1978). Social bonds in the epidemiology of neurosis: A preliminary communication. *British Journal of Psychiatry, 132,* 463–466.

Henry, J., & Cassel, J. (1976). Psychosocial factors in essential hypertension: Recent epidemiological and animal experimental evidence. *American Journal of Epidemiology, 104*(1), 1–8.

Hinde, R. A. (1972). *Non-verbal communication.* Cambridge: Cambridge University Press.

Holden, C. (1981). Human-animal relationship under scrutiny. *Science, 214,* 418–420.

Holmes, T. H., Hawkins, N. G., Bowerman, C. E., Clarke, E. R., & Joffe, J. R. (1957). Psychosocial and physiological studies of tuberculosis. *Psychosomatic Medicine, 19,* 134–143.

Horowitz, M., Schaefer, C., Hiroto, D., Wilner, N., & Levin, B. (1977). Life events questionnaires for measuring presumptive stress. *Psychosomatic Medicine, 39*(6), 413–431.

Hurley, P. M. (1983). Communication variables and voice analysis of marital conflict stress. *Nursing Research, 32*(3), 164–169.

Ikemi, Y., & Nakagawa, S. (1962). A psychosomatic study of contagious dermatitis. *Kyushu Journal of Medical Science, 13,* 335–350.

Ishigami, T. (1919). The influence of psychic acts on the progress of pulmonary tuberculosis. *American Review of Tuberculosis, 2,* 470–484.

Jackson, G. G., Dowling, H. F., Anderson, T. O., Riff, L., Saporta, J., & Turck, M. (1960). Susceptibility and immunity to common upper respiratory viral infections—The common cold. *Annals of Internal Medicine, 53,* 719–738.

Jacobs, M. A., Spilken, A., & Norman, M. (1969). Relationship of life change, maladaptive aggression, and upper respiratory infection in male college students. *Psychosomatic Medicine, 31,* 31–44.

Jamner, L. D., & Schwartz, G. E. (1986). Self-deception predicts self-report and endurance of pain. *Psychosomatic Medicine, 48*(3/4), 211–223.

Jemmott, J. B., III, Borysenko, M., Borysenko, J., McClelland, D. C., Chapman, R., Meyer, D., & Benson, H. (1982). Academic stress, power motivation, and immunity. Unpublished manuscript, Princeton University, Department of Psychology, Princeton, NJ.

Jemmott, J. B., Borysenko, J. Z., Borysenko, M., McClelland, D. C., Chapman, R., Meyer, D., & Benson, H. (1983). Academic stress, power motivation, and decrease in salivary immunoglobulin A secretion rate. *Lancet, 1,* 1400–1402.

Jemmott, J. B., & Locke, S. E. (1984). Psychosocial factors, immunologic mediation, and human susceptibility to infectious disease: How much do we know? *Psychological Bulletin, 95,* 78–108.

Jenkins, J. (1984). *Physiological effects of petting a companion animal.* Unpublished master's thesis, San Francisco State University, San Francisco, CA.

Jennings, J. L. (1985). The fallacious origin of the mind-body problem: A reconsideration of Descartes' method and results. *The Journal of Mind and Behavior,* 6(3), 357–372.

Jensen, M. M., & Rasmussen, A. F., Jr. (1963). Stress and susceptibility to viral infections. II. Sound Stress and susceptibility to vesicular stomatitis virus. *Journal of Immunology, 90,* 21–23.

Jensen, M. R. (1984). *Psychobiological factors in the prognosis and treatment of neoplastic disorders.* Unpublished doctoral dissertation, Yale University, New Haven, CT.

Joasoo, A., & McKenzie, J. M. (1976). Stress and the immune response in rats. *International Archives of Allergy and Applied Immunology, 50,* 659–663.

Kaneko, Z., & Takaishi, N. (1963). Psychosomatic studies on chronic uriticaria. *Folia Psychiatrica et Neurologica Japonica, 17,* 16–24.

Kasl, S. V., Evans, A. S., & Neiderman, J. C. (1979). Psychosocial risk factors in the development of infectious mononucleosis. *Psychosomatic Medicine, 41,* 445–466.

Katcher, A. (1981). Interactions between people and their pets—Form and function. In B. Fogle (Ed.), *Interrelations between people and pets.* Springfield, IL: Thomas.

Katcher, A. H., Brightman, V., Luborsky, L., & Ship, I. (1973). Prediction of the incidence of recurrent herpes labiales and systemic illness from psychological measurements. *Journal of Dental Research, 52,* 49–58.

Kent, J., Coates, T., & Pelletier, K. R. (1989). Spontaneous remission. Manuscript in preparation. University of California at San Francisco Medical School, Department of General Internal Medicine.

Kiecolt-Glaser, J. K., Fisher, L. D., Ogrocki, P., Stout, J. C., Speicher, C. E., & Glaser, R. (1987). Marital quality, marital disruption, and immune function. *Psychosomatic Medicine, 49*(1), 13–34.

Kiecolt-Glaser, J., Garner, W., Speicher, C., Penn, G., Holliday, J., & Glaser, R. (1984). Psychosocial modifiers of immunocompetence in medical students. *Psychosomatic Medicine, 46*(1), 7–14.

Kiecolt-Glaser, J. K., Glaser, R., Williger, D., Stout, J. C., Tarr, K. L., Holliday, J. E., & Speicher, C. E. (1985). Psychosocial enhancement of immunocompetence in a geriatric population. *Health Psychology, 4,* 25–41.

Kimzey, S. L. (1975). The effects of extended spaceflight on hematologic and immunologic systems. *Journal of American Medical Women's Association, 30*(5), 218–232.

Kimzey, S. L., Johnson, P.C., Ritzman, S. E., & Mengel, C. E. (1976). Hematology and immunology studies: The second manned Skylab mission. *Aviation, Space, and Environmental Medicine,* Vol. V, 383–390.

Kissen, D. M. (1967). Psychosocial factors, personality and lung cancer in men aged 55–64. *British Journal of Medial Psychology, 40,* 29–43.

Kleiger, J. H., & Kinsman, R. A. (1980). The development of an MMPI alexithymia scale. *Psychotherapy and Psychosomatic*, 34(1), 17–24.

Kobasa, S. C. (1982). The hardy personality: Toward a social psychology of stress and health. In G. S. Sanders & J. Suls (Eds.), *Social psychology of health and illness*. Hillsdale, NJ: Erlbaum.

Kraus, A., & Lilienfeld, A. (1959). Some epidemiological aspects of the high mortality rate in the young widowed group. *Journal of Chronic Disease, 10*, 207–217.

Kraus, L. J., Locke, S. E., & Kutz, I. (1984). Effect of norepinephrine infusion on human natural killer cell activity. *Proceedings of the First International Workshop on Neuroimmunomodulation*, Bethesda, MD.

Laudenslager, M. L., Reite, M., & Harbeck, R. (1982). Suppressed immune response in infant monkeys associated with maternal separation. *Behavioral and Neural Biology, 36*, 40–48.

Laudenslager, M. L., Ryan, S. M., Drugan, R. C., Hyson, R. L., & Maier, S. F. (1983). Coping and immunosuppression: Inescapable but not escapable shock suppresses lymphocyte proliferation. *Science, 221*, 568–570.

Lazarus, R. S. (1970). Cognitive and personality factors underlying stress and coping. In S. Levine & N. Scotch (Eds.), *Social stress*. Chicago: Aldine.

Lazarus, R. S. & Folkman, S. (1984). *Stress, appraisal, and coping*. New York: Springer.

Levy, S., Lippman, M., & Terry, W. (1980). Emotional response to breast cancer and its treatment. *NCI–NIH Protocol*, 80-C-49.

Lewis, J. W., Schavit, Y., Terman, G. W., Nelson, L. R., Gayle, R. P., & Liebeskind, J. C. (1983). Apparent involvement of opioid peptides in stress-induced enhancement of tumor growth. *Peptides, 4*(5), 635–638.

Ley, R. G. (1983). Cerebral laterality and imagery. In A. A. Sheikh (Ed.), *Imagery: Current theory, research, and application* (pp. 69–86). New York: Wiley.

Libet, B. (1985). Unconscious cerebral initiative and the role of conscious will in voluntary action. *The Behavioral and Brain Sciences, 8*, 529–566.

Liddell, H. (1950). Some specific factors that modify tolerance for environmental stress. *Proceedings of Academic Research in Nervous and Mental Disorders, 29*, 155–159.

Lin, N., Ensel, W., Simeone, R., & Kuo, W. (1979). Social support, stressful life events and illness. A model and an empirical test. *Journal of Health and Social Behavior, 20*, 108–119.

Linn, B. S., Linn, M. W., & Jensen, J. (1982). Degree of depression and immune responsiveness. *Psychosomatic Medicine, 44*, 128–129.

Locke, S. E., Kraus, L., Leserman, J., Hurst, M. W., Heisel, S., & Williams, R. M. (1984). Life change stress, psychiatric symptoms, and natural killer cell activity. *Psychosomatic Medicine, 46*, 441–453.

Lowenthal, M. F., & Haven, C. (1968). Interaction and adaptation: Intimacy as a critical variable. In B. Neugarten (Ed.), *Middle age and aging* (pp. 390–400). Chicago: University of Chicago Press.

Luborsky, L., Mintz, J., Brightman, V. J., & Katcher, A. H. (1976). Herpes simplex virus and moods: A longitudinal study. *Psychosomatic Research, 20,* 543–548.

Maslow, A. (1943). Dynamics of personality organization. *Psychological Review, 50,* 514–558.

Mason, A. A. (1952). A case of congenital ichthyosiform erythrodermia of Brocq treated by hypnosis. *British Medical Journal, 2,* 422–423.

Mason, A. A. (1961). *Hypnotism for medical and dental practitioners.* London: Secker and Warburg.

Mason, A. A., & Black, S. (1958). Allergic skin responses abolished under treatment of asthma and hayfever by hypnosis. *Lancet, 1,* 877–880.

McClelland, D. C., Alexander, C., & Marks, E. (1982). The need for power, stress, immune function, and illness among male prisoners. *Journal of Abnormal Psychology, 91,* 61–70.

McClelland, D. C., Floor, E., Davidson, R. J., & Saron, C. (1980). Stressed power motivation, sympathetic activation, immune function, and illness. *Journal of Human Stress, 6*(2), 11–19.

McClelland, D. C., & Jemmott, J. B., III. (1980). Power motivation, stress, and physical illness. *Journal of Human Stress, 6*(4), 6–15.

McClelland, D. C., & Kirshnit, C. (1984). *The effect of motivational arousal through films on salivary immune function.* Unpublished paper. Harvard University, Department of Psychology and Social Relations, Cambridge, MA.

McClelland, D. C., Locke, S. E., Williams, R. M., & Hurst, M. W. (1978). *Power motivation, distress, and immune function.* Unpublished manuscript, Harvard University, Department of Psychology and Social Relations, Cambridge, MA.

McCulloch, M. (1981). The pet as prosthesis: Defining criteria for the adjunctive use of companion animals in the treatment of medically ill, depressed outpatients. In B. Fogle (Ed.), *Interrelations between people and pets.* Springfield, IL: Thomas.

McCulloch, M. (1982). Animal facilitated therapy: Overview and future direction. *California Veterinarian, 8,* 13–24.

Mechanic, D. (1977). Illness behavior, social adaptation, and the management of illness: A comparison of educational and medical models. *Journal of Nervous and Mental Disease, 165,* 79–87.

Meyer, R. J., & Haggerty, R. J. (1962). Streptococcal infections in families. *Pediatrics, 29,* 539–549.

Meyers, J., Lindenthal, J., & Pepper, M. (1975). Life events, social integration psychiatric symptomatology. *Journal of Health and Social Behavior, 16,* 421–429.

Michaut, R. J., Dechambre, R. P., Doumerc, S., Lesourd, B., Devillechabrolle, A., & Moulias, R. (1981). Influence of early maternal deprivation on adult humoral immune response in mice. *Physiology Behavior, 26,* 189–191.

Mishler, E. & Scotch, N. (1963). Sociocultural factors in the epidemiology of schizophrenia: A review. *Psychiatry, 26,* 315–351.

Mohamed, M. A., and Hanson, R. P. (1980). Effect of social stress on Newcastle disease virus (LaSota) infection. *Avian Diseases, 24*, 908–915.

Moles, A. (1963). Animal language and information theory. In R. G. Busnel (Ed.), *Acoustic behavior of animals*. Amsterdam, New York: Elsevier.

Monjan, A. (1981). Stress and immunologic competence: Studies in animals. In R. Ader (Ed.), *Psychoneuroimmunology* (pp. 185–227). New York: Academic Press.

Moos, R. H., & Solomon, G. F. (1964). Personality correlates of the rapidity of progression of rheumatoid arthritis. *Annals of Rheumatic Disease, 23*, 145–151.

Mueller, D. P. (1980). Social networks: A promising direction for research on the relationships of the social environment to psychiatric disorder. *Social Science and Medicine, 14*a, 147–161.

Mugford, R. A., & McComisky, J. G. (1975). Some recent work on the psychotherapeutic value of caged birds with old people. In R. S. Anderson (Ed.), *Pet animals and society*. London: Bailliere Tindall.

Mumford, E., Schlesinger, H., & Glass, G. (1982). The effects of psychological intervention on recovery from surgery and heart attacks: An analysis of the literature. *American Journal of Public Health, 72*(2), 141–151.

Murray, H. A. (1939). *Explorations in personality*. New York: Oxford University Press.

Muschel, I. J. (1984). Pet therapy with terminal cancer patients. *Journal of Contemporary Social Work*, 451–458.

Ney, P. G., Collins, C., & Spensor, C. (1986). Double blind: Double talk or are there ways to do better research. *Medical Hypnosis, 21*, 119–126.

O'Regan, B., & Hurley, T. J. III. (1985). Placebo. *Investigations*, Institute of Noetic Sciences, 2(1).

Orne, M. T. (1981). The significance of unwitting cues for experimental outcomes: Toward a pragmatic approach. In T. A. Sebeok & R. Rosenthal (Eds.), *The clever Hans phenomenon: Communication with horses, whales, apes and people* (pp. 152–159). *Annals of the New York Academy of Sciences*.

Ornstein, R., & Sobel, D. (1987, March). The healing brain. *Psychology Today*, pp. 48–52.

Palmblad, J. (1981). Stress and immunologic competence: Studies in man. In R. Ader (Ed.), *Psychoneuroimmunology* New York: Academic Press.

Palmblad, J., Blomback, M., Egberg, N., Froberg, J., Karlsson, C., & Levi, L. (1977). Experimentally induced stress in man: Effects on blood coagulation and fibrinolysis. *Journal of Psychosomatic Research, 21*, 87–92.

Palmblad, J. Cantell, K., Strander, H., Froberg, J., Karlsson, C., Levi, L., Gronstrom, M., & Unger, P. (1976). Stressor exposure and immunological response in man: Interferon-producing capacity and phagocytosis. *Journal of Psychosomatic Research, 20*, 193–199.

Palmblad, J., Petrini, B., Wasserman, J., & Akerstedt, T. (1979). Lymphocyte and granulocyte reactions during sleep deprivation. *Psychosomatic Medicine, 41*, 273–278.

Parkes, C. M., Benjamin, B., & Fitzgerald, R. G. (1969). Broken heart: A study of increased mortality among widowers. *British Medical Journal, 1,* 740–743.

Pattison, E. M., DeFrancisco, D., Wood, P., Frazier, H., & Crowder, J. A. (1975). Psychosocial kinship model for family therapy. *American Journal of Psychiatry, 132,* 1246–1251.

Pelletier, K. R. (1977). *Mind as healer, mind as slayer: A holistic approach to preventing stress disorders.* New York: Delacorte Press/Seymour Lawrence.

Pelletier, K. R. (1979). *Holistic medicine: From stress to optimum health.* New York: Delacorte Press/Seymour Lawrence.

Pelletier, K. R., & Herzing, D. L. (1988). Psychoneuroimmunology: Toward a mindbody model. *Advances, 5*(1), 27–56.

Pelletier, K. R., & Peper, E. (1977). Alpha EEG feedback as a means for pain control. *Journal of Clinical and Experimental Hypnosis, 25*(41), 361–371.

Perloff, M. M., & Spiegelman, J. (1973). Hypnosis in the treatment of a child's allergy to dogs. *American Journal of Clinical Hypnosis, 15,* 269–272.

Pert, C. B. (1986). The wisdom of the receptors: Neuropeptides, the emotions, and bodymind. *Advances, 3*(3), 8–16.

Pert, C. B. (1987). Neuropeptides: The emotions and bodymind. *Noetic Sciences Review, 2,* 13–18.

Pettingale, K. W., Greer, S., & Tee, D. E. H. (1977). Serum Ig-A and emotional expression in breast cancer patients. *Journal of Psychosomatic Research, 21,* 395–399.

Pettingale, K. W., Morris, T., & Greer, S. (1985). Mental attitudes to cancer: An additional prognostic factor. *Lancet, 1,* 750.

Phillips, R. (1975). Role of lifestyle and dietary habits in risk of cancer among seventh-day adventists. *Cancer Research, 34,* 3513–3522.

Pilisuk, M., & Parks, S. H. (1986). *The healing web: Social networks and human survival.* City: University Press of New England.

Plato (1929). *Timaeus* (R. G. Bury, Trans.). London: Loeb Classical Library.

Polonsky, W. H., Knapp, P. H., Brown, E. L., & Schwartz, G. E. (1985). Psychological factors, immunologic function, and bronchial asthma. *Psychosomatic Medicine, 47,* 114.

Pribram, K. (in press). *A holonomic brain theory.*

Prigogine, I., & Stengers, I. (1984). *Order out of chaos: Man's new dialogue with nature.* New York: Bantam.

Raphael, B. (1977). Preventive intervention with the recently bereaved. *Archives of General Psychiatry, 34,* 1450–1457.

Reilly, D. T., Taylor, M. A., McSharry, C., & Aitchison, T. (1986). Is homeopathy a placebo response? Controlled trial of homeopathic potency with pollen in hayfever as model. *Lancet, 2,* (8512), 881–886.

Reite, M., Harbeck, R., & Hoffman, A. (1981). Altered cellular immune response following peer separation. *Life Sciences, 29,* 1133–1136.

Revenson, T. A., Wollman, C. A., & Felton, B. J. (1983). Social supports as stress buffers for adult cancer patients. *Psychosomatic Medicine, 40*(4), 321–332.

Riley, V. (1981). Psychoneuroendocrine influences on immunocompetence and neoplasia. *Science, 212,* 1100–1109.

Roark, G. E. (1971). Psychosomatic factors in the epidemiology of infectious mononucleosis. *Psychosomatics, 12,* 402–411.

Roessler, R., Cate, T. R., Lester, J. W., & Couch, R. B. (1979). *Ego strength, life events, and antibody titer.* Paper presented at the 36th Annual meeting of the Psychosomatic Society, Dallas, TX.

Rogentine, G. N., Jr., van Kammen, D. P., Fox, B. H., Docherty, J. P., Rosenblatt, J. E., Boyd, S. C., & Bunney, W. E. (1979). Psychological factors in the prognosis of malignant melanoma: A prospective study. *Psychosomatic Medicine, 41,* 647–655.

Rogers, M. P., Dubey, D., & Reich, P. (1979). The influence of the psyche and the brain on immunity and disease susceptibility: A critical review. *Psychosomatic Medicine, 41,* 147–164.

Russell, M., Dark, K. A., Cummins, R. W., Ellman, G., Callaway, E. & Peeke, H. V. S. (1984). Learned histamine-release. *Science, 225,* 733–734.

Sachar, E. J., Fishman, J. R., & Mason, J. W. (1965). Influence of the hypnotic trance on plasma 17-hydroxycorticosteroid concentration. *Psychosomatic Medicine, 27,* 330–341.

Sachar, E. J., Cobb, J. C., & Shor, R. E. (1966). Plasma cortisol changes during hypnotic trance. *Archives of General Psychiatry, 14,* 482–490.

Sackeim, H. A., & Gur, R. C. (1978). Self-deception, self-confrontation, and consciousness. In G. E. Schwartz & D. Shapiro (Eds.), *Consciousness and self-regulation* (pp. 139–197). New York: Plenum.

Scherer, K. R. (1979). Nonlinguistic vocal indicators of emotion and psychopathology. In C. E. Izard (Ed.), *Emotions in personality and psychopathology.* New York: Plenum.

Scherer, K. R. (1982). Methods of research on vocal communication: paradigms and parameters. In K. R. Scherer and P. Ekman (Eds.). *Handbook of methods in nonverbal behavior research.* Cambridge University Press: pp. 136–189.

Schleifer, S., Keller, S., Cammerino, M., Thornton, J., & Stein, M. (1983). Suppression of lymphocyte stimulation following bereavement. *Journal of the American Medical Association, 250*(3), 374–377.

Schleifer, S., Keller, S. E., Meyerson, A. T., Raskin, M. J., Davis, K. L., & Stein, M. (1984). Lymphocyte function in major depressive disorders. *Archives of General Psychiatry, 41,* 484–486.

Schwartz, G. E. (1983). Disregulation theory and disease: Applications to the repression/cerebral disconnection/cardiovascular disorder hypothesis. *International Review of Applied Psychology, 32,* 95–118.

Seligman, M. E. P. (1975). *Helplessness: On depression, development, and death.* San Francisco: Freeman.

Selye, H. (1950). *The physiology and pathology of exposure to stress.* Montreal: Acta.

Shaheen, C. M. (1986). *Animals on the health care unit.* Unpublished master's thesis, San Francisco State University, San Francisco, CA.

Shavit, Y., & Martin, F. C. (1987). Opiates, stress, and immunity: Animal studies. *Annals of Behavioral Medicine, 9*(2), 11–14.

Shekelle, R. B., Raynor, W. J., Ostfeld, A. M., Garron, D. C., Bieliauskas, L., Liu, S. C., Maliza, C., & Paul, O. (1981). Psychological depression and 17-year risk of death from cancer. *Psychosomatic Medicine, 43,* 117–125.

Silberman, E. K., & Weingartner, H. (1986). Hemispheric lateralization of functions related to emotion. *Brain and Cognition, 5,* 322–353.

Simonton, D. C., Matthews-Simonton, S., & Creighton, J. L. (1978). *Getting well again.* Los Angeles: Tarcher-St. Martins.

Sklar, L. S., & Anisman, H. (1980). Social stress influences tumor growth. *Psychosomatic Medicine, 42,* 347–365.

Smith, B. (1982). Project Inreach: A program to explore the ability of Atlantic bottlenose dolphins to elicit communication responses from autistic children. In A. Katcher & A. Beck (Eds.), *New perspectives on our life with companion animals.* Philadelphia: University of Pennsylvania Press.

Smith, G. R., McKenzie, J. M., Marmer, D. J., & Steele, R. W. (1985). Psychologic modulation of the human immune response to varicella zoster, *Archives of Internal Medicine, 145,* 2110–2112.

Smith, W. J. (1977). *The behavior of communicating: An ethological approach.* Cambridge: Harvard University Press.

Sokolovsky, J., Cohen, C., Berger, D., & Geiger, J. (1978). Personal networks of ex-mental patients in a Manhattan SRO hotel. *Human Organization, 37,* 5–15.

Solomon, G. F. (1981). Emotional and personality factors in the onset and course of autoimmune disease, particularly rheumatoid arthritis. In R. Ader (Ed.), *Psychoneuroimmunology.* New York: Academic Press.

Solomon, G. F., & Amkraut, A. A. (1981). Psychoneuroendocrinological effects of the immune response. *Annual Review of Microbiology, 35,* 155–184.

Solomon, G. F., Levine, S., & Kraft, J. K. (1968). Early experience and immunity. *Nature* (London), *220,* 821–822.

Solomon, G. F., & Moos, R. H. (1965). Psychologic aspects of response to treatment in rheumatoid arthritis. *General Psychiatry, 114,* 113–119.

Sperry, R. (1986). The new mentalist paradigm and ultimate concern. *Perspectives in Biology and Medicine, 29*(3), 413–422.

Steiner, H., Higgs, C. M. B., Fritz, G. K., Laszlo, G., & Harvey, J. E. (1987). Defense style and the perception of asthma. *Psychosomatic Medicine, 49*(1), 35–44.

Surman, O. S., Gottlieb, S. H., Hackett, T. P., & Silverberg, E. L. (1973). Hypnosis in the treatment of warts. *Archives of General Psychiatry, 28,* 439–441.

Syme, S. L. (1982, July/August). People need people. *American Health,* pp. 49–51.

Tecoma, E. S., & Huey, L. Y. (1985). Psychic distress and the immune response. *Life Sciences, 36*(19), 1799–1812.

Temoshok, L., & Fox, B. H. (1984). Coping styles and other psychosocial factors related to medial status and to prognosis in patients with cutaneous malignant melanoma. In B. H. Fox and B. H. Newberry (Eds.), *Impact of psychoendocrine systems in cancer and immunity.* New York: Hogrefe.

Thomas, C. B., Krush, A. J., Brown, C. H., Shaffer, J. W., & Duszynski, K. R. (1982). Cancer in families of former medical students followed to mid-life— Prevalence in relatives of subjects with and without major cancer. *Johns Hopkins Medical Report, 151*(5), 193–202.

Tolsdorf, C. (1976). Social networks, support and coping: An exploratory study. *Family Relations, 5*(4), 407–418.

Totman, R. G., & Kiff, J. (1979). Life stress and susceptibility to colds. In D. J. Osborne, M. M. Gruneberg, & J. R. Eiser (Eds.), *Research in psychology and medicine* (Vol. 1, pp. 141–149). New York: Academic Press.

Turner, R. J. (1982). Social support as a contingency in psychological well being. *Journal of Health and Social Behavior, 22,* 357–387.

Wallbott, G. F., & Scherer, K. R. (1986). Cues and channels in emotion recognition. *Journal of Personality and Social Psychology, 51*(4), 690–699.

Walters, E. T., & Byrne, J. H. (1983). Associative conditioning of single sensory neurons suggests a cellular mechanism for learning. *Science, 219,* 405–407.

Wechsler, R. (1987, February). A new prescription: Mind over malady. *Discover, February 1987,* pp. 51–61.

Weinberger, D. A., Schwartz, G. E., & Davidson, R. J. (1979). Low-anxious, high-anxious, and repressive coping style: psychometric patterns and behavioral and physiological responses to stress. *Journal of Abnormal Psychology, 88,* 369–380.

Williams, J. M., Petersen, R. G., Shea, P. A., Schmedtje, J. F., Bauer, D. C., & Felten, D. (1981). Sympathetic innervation of murine thymus and spleen: Evidence for a functional link between the nervous and immune systems. *Brain Research Bulletin, 6,* 83–94.

Workman, E. A., & La Via, M. F. (1987). Immunological effects of psychological stressors: A review of the literature. *International Journal of Psychosomatics, 34*(1), 35–40.

Wybran, J., Appelboom, T., Famaey, J. P., & Govaerts, A. (1979). Suggestive evidence for receptors for morphine and methionine-enkephalin on normal human blood T lymphocytes. *Journal of Immunology, 123,* 1068–1070.

Young, T. M. (1975). Nuclear magnetic resonance studies of succussed solutions. *Journal of the American Institute of Homeopathy, 68,* 8–16.

Zukav, G. (1979). *The dancing Wu Li masters.* New York: Morrow.

14

The Importance of Modern Physics for Modern Medicine

LARRY DOSSEY

The old gods are dead or dying and people everywhere are searching, asking: What is the new mythology to be, the mythology of this unified earth as one harmonious being?

> Joseph Campbell, *The Inner Reaches of Outer Space: Metaphor and Myth as Religion*

INTRODUCTION: WHY MODERN PHYSICS?

Does modern physics hold any relevance for today's medicine? On the surface the answer might appear to be no. For instance, a quick survey of the curricula of modern medical schools reveals that physics—classical or modern—simply is not taught; even at the undergraduate level the only exposure premedical students have to physics is to the classical or traditional type. It is quite likely that a physician today can complete his or her training in medicine or surgery without any exposure whatsoever to the body of knowledge of modern physics. It is difficult for any physician to fully implement the art of medicine in the 20th

395

century without a genuine awareness of the central messages from modern physics. To try to do so would be as difficult as trying to practice medicine without the use of modern devices, such as drugs or x-rays.

The failure to appreciate the crucial insights of the physics of this century has led to a constricted vision of human function, which in some ways has been disastrous in the actual clinical approach to illness. It has led—in ways we shall explore—to a medicine that has a hollow ring to our patients. The fact that few are happy with this state of affairs today in medicine, whether patients or physicians, has resulted in periodic excoriations of the profession. This is ironic, since in many respects medicine has never been more powerful, never able to do more. Thus, rather than occupying a position of respect and admiration, physicians now find themselves frequent objects of scorn—physicians are perceived to be uncaring, overpaid, and underregulated, with many believing that a physician's activity should be dictated by bureaus and agencies that can be more sensitive to the welfare of patients than physicians are considered to be.

These observations may seem hyperbolic and might appear to have nothing to do with the relationship between modern physics and medicine. But as we shall see, they flow at least in part from the failure of the profession to implement a coherent and up-to-date world view. It is not widely appreciated that physicians and patients cannot interact without invoking a world view, but world views are a vital part of medical practice. It is the business of physics to provide us with world views, which are simply broad, general visions of how the world operates. The very meanings of illness and health, the body, the will, therapies of all sorts and how to use them—all these issues depend on a world view for their meanings. Thus it is never a matter of whether or not the physician or patient will invoke a world view, but rather which world view it is to be.

Any discussion of the relevance of modern physics to medicine is bound to be limited for several reasons. First, physics is a dynamic science. As a body of knowledge it is not fixed; it is always changing and evolving. No matter how comforting it is for us to believe that today's science has had the last word, it cannot be so. Future generations may well smile at many of our beliefs, just as we now know that many of the "unchallengeable" tenets of earlier science were incomplete or wrong. Thus any relevance for medicine we might find in present-day physics must be tempered by the recognition that this relevance may take on a different meaning for those who come after us, as they will have access to a better science.

It is also important to realize that there simply is no consensus, even among experts, about the meanings contained in many areas of modern physics. The interpretation of many of the points that seem crucial for medicine are hotly disputed. This does not mean that the factual content of these areas is in dispute, but there are central questions of *meaning* that remain. For example, what is the role of the observer in how reality unfolds or comes about? What does it really mean to say that distant events in the universe are correlated? What does it mean to say that if the universe were only slightly different than it is, life could not exist? Does this suggest it was "designed" for life? Physicists draw a wide variety of meanings from such observations—meanings that are by no means trivial, for they have enormous philosophical implications for all persons.

Whose meanings shall we then employ? Shall we believe the modern interpreters who deny that consciousness matters in the way reality unfolds, or will we believe those physicists who claim that the human mind is the key to the creation and continued existence of the universe? Because there is no consensus in these and many other important points in modern physics, any discussion of the relevance of physics to medicine must be qualified from the start. Thus I wish to offer a disclaimer: although we must be consistent if possible with the great science of physics, there comes a point where physics cannot go, whether the physics is that of Newton or of our own time. At this point, medicine must "go it alone." This is generally when factors such as feelings, emotional states, spiritual values, and matters of consciousness in general become involved in the body's responses. But before that point is reached, we should attempt to rest the art of healing on the most accurate science we can find, which is that of modern physics—recognizing all the while, however, that physics will not, it cannot, provide us with all the directives we require in dealing with the health and illness of human beings.

Why should medicine look to physics of whatever kind? Do not physicians get along today just fine by confining their attention to livers, spleens, hearts, and lungs? Why bring in physics? The answer is obvious if we consider the definition of physics—that is, the study of matter and energy and their interrelations. Are not human bodies made of matter, and do they not require energy for their activities? How can healers *not* be concerned with physics? But which physics should physicians look to? Here the realization surfaces that there is no homogenous body of knowledge that can be called "physics." For within the field there are the two broad divisions of classical physics (traditional, Newtonian) and modern physics. And within modern physics (as within classical physics) there are also many divisions, the most fundamental of which are quantum mechanics and relativity theory. Only a general appreciation of the broad differences between traditional and modern physics is necessary for the reader to understand the following discussion. However, a more detailed analysis of these differences can be found in Herbert (1986), Pagels (1982), and Wolf (1981).

The Body

It is in the most fundamental domain of medicine—the body itself—that modern physics casts a gigantic fly in the classical ointment. It does so by asking what it is we mean by a body in the first place. Raising this question is by no means absurd. What is a human body? What is it that provides the physician with complaints and with a history of an illness? What is it that the physician then examines? What is it that the surgeon resects? What is it that the pathologist examines under the microscope? As long as we confine ourselves to the see-touch-feel world of the senses, the world of common, everyday ordinariness, we *know* what bodies are, and there is no need to raise the questions. But it is the business of modern physics to look beyond the world of the senses, to abandon the domain of common sense happenings; at this point human bodies are not what they seem.

In contrast to what we see at the macroscopic level (which is describable by traditional physics), physical bodies at the level of the atom are mostly nothing but thin air. The amount of actual "material" inside an atom is roughly that of a baseball inside the Astrodome. This fact stands in stark contrast to the sensory experience of the doctor who experiences the body as a substantial concrete entity.

But physicians see a body that is made up of "things"—organ systems such as the cardiovascular system; specific organs such as the liver; individual cells that comprise the organs; intracellular components such as the ribosomes and mitochondria; different molecules such as the DNA; and atoms and subatomic particles that comprise the molecules. Summing all these "things," the physician arrives at a definition of the body. This is the "classical body"—a concrete entity that occupies a particular position in space, a thing that is confined to a point in time, an entity that endures for a particular span of time, the behavior of which can be described as obeying the common sense laws of cause and effect. And why not view the body this way? The view works well and has endured for centuries. Patently, it is said, the body can be viewed as a classical macroscopic object, just like Newton's falling apple.

The paradox is that at the most elemental level the picture is very different. From the point of view of modern physics, the body is mostly nothing: it is almost total emptiness. There are no hard elemental particles, no separate bits that are assembled in ever-increasing complexity to finally add up to a body; there are only evanescent phenomena that cannot be pinned down at points in space and time as billiard balls might be. In the body's microworld, there are strange happenings. "Particles" are smeared across space, showing only "tendencies" to exist more at one point than another; these "particles" have no definable position until the observer actually looks for them. And what is more, the "particles" can be shown to be either particles or waves, depending on the whim of the observer and owing to how he or she decides to arrange the experimental apparatus with which he or she is looking. Moreover, these "particles" may suddenly disappear by vanishing into the void—all of which is shielded from the physician's awareness.

Yet it is obvious that all this can be ignored. Both physicians and patients can go blithely along believing that the body is a classical, concrete, here-and-now object. But this deeply held belief—that the body is made up of individual, elemental particles—breaks down in the light of modern physics.

Let us observe for now that almost everyone cherishes a false view of the body. There simply are no bits from which it is made, only endlessly changing patterns of energy and matter. The "concrete" body is a contradiction in terms. Furthermore, ordinary awareness tells us that the body is relatively stable during its sojourn between birth and death. But again, this classical view is not true, for the body is astonishingly dynamic. It has been shown beyond doubt that the body is being constantly replaced. All its tissues are in motion, coming and going, albeit at different rates. Some tissues, such as bone, are extremely dynamic and replaced rapidly. Even major organs, such as the stomach and liver, are entirely replaced every few weeks. The skin, the lining of the gastrointestinal tract, and many other tissues are also currently on the move with rapid turnover rates. Although other tissues (e.g., the supporting structures in the brain) are relatively resistant to being replaced, by the end of a year 98% of the matter in the body is totally replaced, and after 5 years 100% of the body has been totally renewed. Thus the reader can know with certainty that 5 years ago his or her current body did not exist and that five years hence a new one will take its place.

This kind of dynamism is not apparent through the focusing lens of classical physics. Seen from the classical perspective, the body seems static, adynamic, and fixed. But when we examine the domain of the very small, the world of the atom that has been opened up by modern physics, a different picture awaits us. It is a dancing, rhythmic, dynamic body we see—a body that is constantly being renewed.

Modern physics allows us to realize that the ordinary view of the body is wrong. It is not substantiated with facts. This ordinary view neglects the dynamic shuffling of the "stuff" of the body, the endless interchange with the outside world, and it also misinterprets the nature of the "stuff." Having started out with a misconception of what a body is and how it behaves, it is not surprising that our classically based therapies, which are actually applied to the erroneously conceived body, are themselves sometimes inaccurate in major ways. Flawed images *of* the body lead to flawed therapies *for* the body.

The strangeness surrounding the body multiplies when we observe that bodies interchange not only with the outside world, but with each other. For example, it has been shown that there is a constant intermixing of bodies. At any given moment, each human body may contain numerous molecules of oxygen that have been breathed in the past month by millions of other humans on the earth (let alone the other respiring mammals). Each breath contains the mobile, shuttling part of other bodies still alive as well as those no longer living. Thus bodies can be seen as chains, stretching out through time and space, by virtue of the sharing of actual constituent parts—a point of view that is obscured by the traditional view of the body as a concrete, enduring, unchanging object.

These observations may strike some as trivial curiosities; however, they point to a fact that contains potentially important ethical, moral, and spiritual ramifications. These observations show an inherent nonlocal character to the body—that is, in the strictest sense, there are no isolated bodies, there is only Body. All bodies interact, not just in "psychological" ways but in actual physical ways. Ethicists and moralists have been exceedingly slow to notice these facts, due in large part to their own classical world views. How does the relevance to ethical, moral, and spiritual concerns arise? If I really believe my body is nonlocal, that it cannot be confined in space and time, that it is part of yours as yours is part of mine, I might be moved to treat you differently. Our concept of "self" might be considerably renovated and expanded, and the earth-threatening specter of selfishness might be lessened. There might also arise a greater tolerance to the spiritual traditions that have always spoken of an essential unity of human beings. All of these prospects could flow from a more accurate view of what bodies are, as revealed through the modern physical world view.

It may be that the most significant part of the legacy of modern physics to medicine will be the destruction of a rigidly local view of human beings. Locality—the idea that something is fixed at a particular point in time and space—fails at the level of the atom, and it fails also at the large-scale level of human bodies when they are viewed with pinpoint accuracy. A modern view of the body implies an unmistakable connectedness between all bodies, an intrinsic nonlocality that is part of the life process. This quality cannot be found in the classical view of bodies or of living things: It is one of the most profound differences separating the medicine of the past and that of the future.

Connectedness

The general process of connectedness, so apparent at the level of the body, also makes itself known at the remote subatomic level. Here the idea of isolated, particulate matter has evaporated, to be replaced by the concept of fields of interaction. Particles, including those of the body, can no longer be seen as idealized billiard balls caroming off each other. Rather, they are described by physicists as processes that overlap in never-ending webs of interaction. Physicists have often resorted to metaphor and symbols to describe these events. Sir Arthur Eddington, for example, lent his poetic imagination to the task by stating that when the electron vibrates, the universe shakes—suggesting that the universe is a single fabric and an unbroken whole.

It is frequently stated, however, that nothing of this subatomic picture is relevant to the macroscopic level of the human body. These events are simply too remote to make a difference. And they are predictable only by applying statistical descriptions to large ensembles of them; only through the laws of probability can their random, quirkish behavior be anticipated. Human bodies contain unimaginably large numbers of single subatomic events, and by the time one reaches this large-scale level, the effects of the unpredictable single particles have been "washed out." Thus human bodies behave classically and predictably, and follow all the familiar laws of cause and effect. They share nothing of the character of the randomly behaving subatomic processes. Thus any "connectedness" one might find at the level of the atom cannot be superimposed onto the macroscopic human body; and if human bodies do connect, the connectedness is of a different kind and for a different reason than what is seen among the subatomic particles.

We should acknowledge that amid the flurry of recent articles and books on "new age physics," there have been flagrant abuses of language and stretching of comparisons. For example, if electrons have "fields," then so do humans; if the particles are intimately connected, then so are we; if the behavior of electrons are not determined, then neither is the behavior of humans determined, and—presto—proof of freedom of the will is at hand. Sometimes this reasoning is based on nothing more than accidental correlations of the language, as physicist Jeremy Bernstein (1978) has pointed out. At other times, it rests on abuses of logic called category errors, as in saying that the "unity" that is experienced by human beings is the same as the "unity" that one sees among the sub-atomic particles. This is shoddy reasoning. Both levels do express a unity of sorts, but to conjoin the two as if one accounted for the other is specious. Thus we should always beware of these kinds of traps.

We are justified, however, in talking about general principles that seem to manifest themselves at distant levels in nature. And a decidedly important lesson that medicine might take from modern physics is contained in a principle that seems to operate throughout the natural world, whether one is concerned with atoms, human bodies, or stars. This principle is that the observer is inseparable from what is observed. It reaches into the small-scale domain; it touches our own level of human bodies; and it extends even into the astronomical world of stars, moons, and planets. True, each of these levels is vastly separated from those above or below. But modern physics has confirmed that this principle of connectedness between the observer and the observed is not confined to any particular level. And within this principle lies great importance for medicine.

But can we go farther? Can we extend this principle to our level, where patients and physicians interact? Indeed there are reasons why we can. First, these quantum-sized effects to which the physicist Werner Heisenberg refers do have relevance for our macroscopic world. As science philosopher Jacob Bronowski (1978) stated, "these small events are not by any means unimportant [at our level]. They are just the sorts of events which go on in the nerves and the brain and in the giant molecules which determine the qualities we inherit" (p. 68). The tiny quantum-sized events do make a difference for us. In fact, we may owe our very existence as a species to them, for they are responsible for the genetic mutations that provide the biological variations that fuel the evolutionary process of natural selection. Were it not for quantum-sized events occurring deep within chromosomes, there would not be an evolutionary process as we know it (Davenport, 1979). The great physicist Niels Bohr may have had this in mind when he predicted, decades ago, that the eventual application of biological concepts to quantum mechanics was a foregone conclusion (Green & Weinstein, 1981, p. 27).

The principle of interconnectedness, so obvious in the quantum domain, also announces itself at the largest scale we know—that is, in the cosmos itself. Here the connecting principle between the observer and the observed continue to hold true. Observers and "things" go together. For in the world of the very large, where gigantic distances and enormous time scales are involved, the role of the observer is crucial just as it is at the level of the atom, though for different reasons. As Bronowski (1978) put it, "[At a certain point] it turns out that time and space, which

Newton thought absolute, cannot be given physical meaning without the observer: that is the relationship which Einstein saw as the fundamental unit in physics. Relativity is the understanding of the world not as events, but as relations" (p. 103). Whitehead (1968) also saw this relationship as fundamental at all levels of nature, particularly our own. As he put it, "our whole experience is composed out of our relationships to the rest of things" (p. 31).

Modern physics has revealed many astonishing insights into the world, but among the most profound is the principle of relatedness. We cannot step outside nature. In a sense, any picture we have of the world reflects our own actions. We are part of the picture. Any hope of a totally remote observership—whether as a particle physicist interacting with electrons, an astronomer viewing a distant galaxy, or a physician examining a patient—is misconstrued. The world does not allow this hoped-for remoteness, which has heretofore guided and informed our vision of an "objective" medicine. Later we will see how this principle of connectedness surfaces clinically in health and illness.

Bits and Pieces

One of the central features of classical physics is that nature can be "atomized"—that is, it can be divided into units that are ultimately indivisible and separate. This feature of separateness cannot be found in modern atomic physics. Here the idea of separately existing particles has been impossible to demonstrate, as we have seen. But in addition to the notion of interacting, interpenetrating fields by which "particles" are now understood, and in addition to the inseparability of the observer and the events being observed, the element of connectedness surfaces in modern physics in a particularly dramatic way. In what has become popularly known as Bell's theorem, a facet of nature has been revealed that has stirred the imagination of physicists and laypeople alike. Physicist John S. Bell showed that if the statistical predictions of quantum mechanics are true (they have never been proved false), then an objective universe is incompatible with the law of local causes. In other words, if quantum mechanics "works" and if we want to hang on to the idea of a world that does not exist entirely in our own minds, then we must give up the idea of locality. Now, locality, as physicists use the term, means that things happen locally, in the sense that signals cannot travel faster than the speed of light. Nonlocality, on the other hand, refers to instantaneous transfer of signals—faster than the speed of light—which is expressly forbidden by Einstein's special relativity theory, one of the sacred canons of contemporary physics. But Bell showed that locality could be violated; when Bell's theorem was put to the test, it was indeed shown that the long-distance, faster-than-light connections do appear to take place. As strange as it may seem, the experimental results of recent tests indicate that even if particles that have once been in contact are separated, no matter how far apart, when one is changed the other also undergoes change instantly and to the same degree. Moreover, it is generally understood that nothing mediates this change and that no "signal" is involved in the sense of some energy transfer. For the speed of any signal would, according to Einstein's special theory, be limited by the speed of light and would also diminish in strength with increasing spatial separation. So far, the experimental results seem firm: given prior contact, separated particles seem to "know" what each other are "doing," and they respond in kind.

Bell's theorem points to a quality of the world that was absent from the classical view—that of interdependence among the elements of the world. In the old view, interaction was of a bumptious sort with atoms caroming and ricocheting off each other following collision. By comparison, the modern view contains an unmistakable delicateness. In it change occurs almost eerily, depending on events in the farthest reaches of the universe. The violence of collision is bypassed in favor of a principle of connectedness that does not lend itself easily to verbal description (Davies & Brown, 1986).

Complementarity

A further feature of the physics of this century that sets it apart from classical physics is the idea of complementarity. This view is due to the insights chiefly of the Danish physicist Niels Bohr, who was one of the founding architects of modern physics. Bohr's view came about on the heels of a troubling situation. In attempting to study the behavior of electrons, one could design an experiment that showed the electron to be a wave, while it was possible to demonstrate with equal rigor in another experiment that the electron is a particle. But how could it be both? Common sense held that it must be one or the other, either a wave or a particle. Bohr reasoned that common sense in this instance was misleading. He held that the electron was indeed both, behaving as a particle on one occasion and as a wave on another, neither of which was "false" behavior. He maintained that these patterns were complementary—that is, they were both necessary to give a complete account of the nature of the electron even though they were mutually exclusive. Bohr's principle of complementarity is one of the most vivid ways in which the modern vision of the world violates common sense and stretches intuition to the limits. It teaches us that, in investigating the world through the tools of modern physics, we must leave all "shoulds" and "oughts" behind in interpreting the results.

Bohr frequently spoke of his belief that the general notion of complementarity extended far beyond atomic physics into the level of everyday experience. India's eminent physicist D. S. Kothari commented on the extension of this idea:

> The Principle of Complementarity . . . is perhaps the most significant and revolutionary concept of modern physics. The complementarity approach can enable people to see that seemingly irreconcilable points of view need not be contradictory. These, on deeper understanding, may be found to be complementary and mutually illuminating—the two opposing contradictory aspects being parts of a "totality," seen from different perspectives. It allows the possibility of accommodating widely divergent human experiences into an underlying harmony, and bringing to light new social and ethical vistas for exploration and for alleviation of human suffering. Bohr fervently hoped that one day complementarity would be an integral part of everyone's education and provide guidance in the problems and challenges of life. (Kothari, 1985, p. 325)

An immediate application of Bohr's idea of complementarity in medicine can be made in regard to two of life's everyday events: health and illness. They seem to be mutually exclusive, irreconcilable opposites. Yet a strong case can be made that they are both necessary for human life to endure, that health itself would be unknowable without some degree of experience of "nonhealth," and that only by combining these contradictory experiences can we glean a more complete understanding of the totality of health. These views were extensively elaborated in an earlier work, *Beyond Illness* (Dossey, 1984).

Indeterminacy

Another striking difference between the physics of classical science and that of our own day concerns the degree of knowability that is contained in the world. Before this century, there was enormous faith in our ability to know. Given enough effort and steady scientific enthusiasm, nature would yield her secrets. Indeed, at the turn of the century, it was assumed by many physicists that the answers were either in the bag or nearly so. Lord Kelvin, speaking to London's Royal Society, the most prestigious group of scientists in the world, frankly advised young scientists to seek a field other than physics, for the work of physics, in his view, was nearly done. There only remained three little clouds of ignorance to be cleared up, he stated, and then the great secrets of nature could be laid to rest. It is a matter of history that he was monumentally mistaken.

Modern physics challenges the concept of an unlimited knowability in nature. The most dramatic expression of this idea came through the work of Werner Heisenberg; it came to be called the uncertainty principle. Heisenberg saw that in order to know something of the behavior of the electron, one must make a choice in what one will look for. For example, one may determine either the position or the velocity of the electron, but not both; for in determining the velocity, the position is disturbed, and in determining the position, the velocity is changed— and by an unpredictable amount. What is crucial to Heisenberg's insight is that this unknowability is essential. It is inherent and built in; it does not enter as a consequence of the clumsiness of the experimenter or the experimental apparatus. The problem is here to stay as part of nature. This recognition is a refutation of the Baconian ideal of putting nature "on the rack" and through ingenious means forcing her, eventually, to yield her secrets. The experimenter must be more humble than Bacon realized; even the best efforts will never be enough to reveal all the experimenter seeks. This is not because the job is difficult and intricate; it is because all the secrets will *never* yield, no matter how ingenious the scientists may be.

Time

Of all the ways in which classical physics differs from the new, it is perhaps in the view of time that these differences achieve their most striking proportion. Newton viewed time as one looking through the spectacles of common sense—as linear, as divisible into a past, present, and future. Newton's time was external and had an existence of its own. It depended in no way on a human observer. Moreover, it was everywhere, and it was eternal. It was describable by two common metaphors: (1) as a river that flows without end, passing by all events and objects, or (2) as a body of water through which the things and events themselves flowed. In one picture, it is time that moves; in the other, it is the things and events that move against the backdrop of time. In either case, time is something external and provides the world with an absolute past, present, and future.

Modern physics has reshaped this view. Gone is the external quality of time; gone is any concept of flow; gone is the notion that time is the same for everyone; gone is the idea that time stands alone, unaffected by other aspects of the universe's behavior. In modern physics, time may be different for each observer, depending on his or her state of motion, and it is not external to an observer. According to the great physicist Erwin Schrödinger, "time no longer appears to us as a gigantic, world-dominating [force], nor as a primitive entity, but as something derived from phenomena themselves. It is a figment of my thinking" (Schrödinger, 1954, p. 341). Gone, too, is the concept of an absolute past, present, and future, for it can clearly be shown that the future of one observer is the past or present of another; and as there is no observer who is privileged to maintain that his or her time is the "right" time, the absoluteness of time evaporates.

Nothing about time is today regarded as "flowing." And what is more, time is now known to be allied with space, a concept made famous in Einstein's well-known space-time continuum. The perception of space or time is not possible without a concomitant perception of the other. In addition, time is elastic: it slows or speeds depending on other factors, such as gravity and mass. It is known that as one approaches the speed of light, time slows, and at the speed of light, time is predicted to stop altogether. Gravitation affects time as well. Clocks at sea level run slower than clocks atop mountains or in orbiting satellites. All these observations add up to a view of time that is radically different from the view of classical physics.

What Is Real?

If we survey the differences between the traditional and the modern physical view of reality from the widest possible perspective, the most fundamental and sweeping contrast might be this: In the new view, humankind is part of the picture of what is "real." The world cannot be given a meaning without taking into account an observer or, at a bare minimum, the measuring instrument belonging to an observer. (We are not making here any claims about ultimate reality, for that is not the business of physics; it is the role of physics to focus on the observable, not on what may be behind the scenes. Reality, as Morris Raphael Cohen once put it, belongs to the category of religion, not science.) Traditional physicists believed they could describe nature "as it is." But now, we have no hope of such an ability. As we have seen, there are too many ways in which the "what is" is linked to the actions of an observer who must "shatter the glass" and "reach in," as the physicist John Archibald Wheeler (1981) has stated, thereby entering the picture that is perceived in an inextricable way. This linking of the observer and the observed leads to what Wheeler calls a "participatory reality"—a concept to which the classicists would not have been hospitable.

RELEVANCE FOR MEDICINE

The Disappearance of Separate, Isolated Units in Nature

For 300 years, medicine has measured its component parts just as in classical physics. For the physicists, there were isolated units of building blocks; the early physicians, wishing to embody the same accuracy as the physicists, saw similar patterns. But today in medicine, just as in physics, the individual units have disappeared as the intrinsic connections between them have come to light.

This principle of connectedness, so apparent in physics today, is highly relevant for medicine. Just as modern physics cannot be understood through the concept of a billiard ball world, so too medicine cannot be understood in terms of separate bodies, organs, or even molecules.

We have already seen how no precise definition of the boundary of the body can be given. Radionuclide studies of the turnover rate of atoms clearly show that the human body is not fixed in time and space, just as the physicists' particles are not fixed. Studies show that after 5 years, every single atom of the body is replaced. At the clinical level where illness is actually expressed, "parts thinking" cannot account for the origins of health and illness. This is because their roots are simply not traceable in every case to breakdowns or malfunctions at the level of cells, molecules, or atoms.

This is particularly obvious when examining the behavior of the immune processes in the body. For example, it has been shown that, following the death of a spouse, the T-cells and B-cells of the immune system stop working; they cannot be made to work even if extracted from the blood and exposed in test tubes to chemicals that ordinarily stimulate them (Schleifer, Keller, Carmerino, Thornton, & Stein, 1983). Here the origin of illness does not seem to have its roots within body parts. Try as one might to find the initiating disturbance causing the immune failure in the bereaved, depressed, and grieving person, it cannot be done. Rather, it is the fieldlike, interlocking connections between persons that appear to be the key. Only by enlarging the concept of illness to go beyond the idea of "person" and "parts" can a full account of the malfunction be achieved. Here the ideal of physical reductionism—that is, of defining all behavior by what the parts are doing—breaks down.

This does not mean that a physical reduction approach to understanding medical problems is not wise. Drugs have been developed to help the immune system when it fails, using the approach of material reductionism, and the drugs do work. There is in our time too much hostility to this approach (usually from people in good health and who have not needed the fruits of a materially based medicine). It is easy to forget the fact that humans can be described, to a point, materially and reductionistically, just as atoms can be described to a point in the same way. Indeed, the physicists' approach using this method worked for 200 years, and in their day-to-day work physicists still overwhelmingly rely on classical physics. Ingeniously effective therapies can also be devised that are based on the classical approach. The fact that they are incomplete does not mean that these therapies are wrong or that they are "bad" in some moral sense. Indeed, there is nothing "bad" about Newton's physics, nor did classical physics cease to work when Einstein and Planck developed their theories. The achievements of traditional physics were great and remain great to this day, as Bronowski puts it. In the same way, the achievements of materialistic medicine have been and remain great. So let us retain a certain gratefulness to the fruits of materialistic medicine; for if anything is "bad" perhaps it is the arrogance that comes when new knowledge is gained. It is too easy to forget that our current insights rest on those of the past.

In cardiovascular disease, the primary cause of death in industrialized societies, it is necessary to view human beings transpersonally to account for what we observe. The expressions of the disease cannot be understood by focusing on parts of individuals or even on separate persons. For example, the incidence of angina pectoris, the pain associated with coronary artery disease, has its origins without as well as within the person. If a man with the disease has a loving, supportive spouse, the rate of anginal attacks is reduced by 50% (Medalie & Goldbourt, 1976). Here the disease leapfrogs the single person to envelop others. The same is true in the development of malignant, life-threatening arrhythmias (disorders of the heartbeat). When persons admitted to coronary care units for treatment of severe, potentially fatal arrhythmias are surveyed, a high percentage have been shown to have undergone severely traumatic emotional upsets in the 24 to 48 hours prior to the onset of the arrhythmia (Reich, DeSilva, Lown, & Murawski, 1981). Similarly, Engel (1971) has described the influence of severe emotional shock on persons who "drop dead." As he points out, these accounts seem more likely to be an example of folk wisdom than folklore.

Modern insights into the connections between the brain, the sensory organs, and the heart are making clearer how these morbid events take place. Lynch (1985) has shown that hypertension (high blood pressure) may be due at least in part to problems of interpersonal communication. When a person merely speaks to another, the blood pressure rises; and when one has difficulty being heard or understood, the event is even more pronounced. Interestingly, this rise does not occur if one merely reads to oneself; and it is blocked if a person holds a pet in his or her lap.

A survey in the state of Massachusetts showed that the most important risk factor in the development of coronary heart disease was job dissatisfaction, not high blood pressure, diabetes mellitus, hypercholesterolemia, or cigarette smoking as was commonly believed (*Work in America*, 1973). As another example, men with high cholesterol levels have demonstrated marked reductions if they sit quietly and clear their minds for 15 minutes twice daily (Cooper & Aygen, 1978). Studies in animals have shown that if they are regularly touched, held, and petted that atherosclerosis can be reduced by 60% compared to control animals, when both groups are fed a diet rich in fat and cholesterol (Nerem, Levesque, & Cornhill, 1980).

These kinds of observations assume potentially stunning importance when we realize that the majority of persons who suffer their first heart attack in this country have none of the commonly recognized risk factors for heart disease (Jenkins, 1971). In other words, the traditional risk factor approach, as valuable as it is in predicting heart disease in persons who in fact do possess these risk factors, cannot account for even a simple majority of new heart attacks. It is obvious that something is being left out in our accounting of the most common cause of death in our society.

Heart disease cannot be understood by confining our scrutiny to single persons or to body parts, just as the quantum world cannot be understood by looking for parts. Transpersonal events such as misperceptions of meanings, job dissatisfaction, lack of communication between individuals, and lack of love and trust are capable of setting this disease in motion. Not only are these factors causative of illness, they can ameliorate it too, as is demonstrated by the reduction in angina in men with heart disease who have loving wives (Medalie & Goldbourt, 1976).

In sum, these observations demonstrate that the roots of illness cannot be found only in molecules and atoms, nor even in single organs or in individual persons. Just as physicists cannot "atomize" their domain into discrete entities, neither can physicians. The entities in both cases—whether electrons or human beings—behave more like processes and fields than self-contained, isolated objects. Thus a fieldlike approach is needed to account for the spectrum of illness in human beings—not that the "fields" that physicians are concerned with are the same as those with which the physicists deal, but only that the metaphor applies in both cases. In both domains, when we try to concern ourselves with bits and pieces, our attempts to precisely account for our observations fail.

Causality

The view of nature in which isolated parts are replaced by interacting fields or spheres of influence poses great difficulties for the common notions of causality. Put simply, if there are no discrete parts, how can we speak of a single "thing" causing another "thing" to occur, if individual "things" do not in fact exist? If fields overlap and interact, with no specific boundaries between them, how can specific causes be assigned? Does it make sense to even speak of "a" cause? This problem for physics was described by Sir James Jeans (1981) in a well-known book, *Physics and Philosophy:*

> There is no scientific justification for dividing the happenings of the world into detached events, and still less for supposing that they are strung in pairs, like a row of dominoes, each being the cause of the event which follows and at the same time the effect of that which precedes. The changes in the world are too continuous in their nature, and also too closely interwoven, for any such procedure to be valid. . . . Any effect is seen to be connected to previous events by an endless succession of strings of events all of which meet in effect. . . . If we suppose that the happenings of nature are governed by a causal law, we must suppose that the cause of any effect is the whole previous state of the world, so that every effect has an infinite number of causes. . . . The mere formulation of the law of causality presupposes the existence of an isolated objective system which an isolated observer can observe without disturbing it. . . . But if there is no sharp distinction between observer and observed, this becomes meaningless since any observation he makes must influence the future course of the system. (pp. 103, 144)

And the new view of time in modern physics also creates problems for the traditional notion of causality. According to Jeans, "the question of causality has assumed a new aspect. We can no longer say that the past creates the present; past and present no longer have any objective meanings, since the four-dimensional continuum can no longer be sharply divided into past, present and future" (p. 119).

In medicine, we are wedded to strict causal concepts. How could we possibly give up our beloved concept of a rigid causal interpretation of the origin of illness when it has worked so well in the past? Perhaps the acausality described by modern physicists applies only to the small domain of the atom, not to human bodies. But medicine, like modern physics, has encountered similar problems of causality in chasing the origins of illness. We too find ourselves bedeviled when we look for strict stops and starts in the causal chain. The physician and philosopher Samuel Vaisrub (1979) describes the problems with causality that have surfaced in modern medicine:

> As various concepts of causality passed through the focusing prisms of medical philosophers, they underwent further changes to accommodate the need for understanding and treating diseases. Such accommodations resulted in the addition, among others, of such causes as macrocosm-microcosm, intrinsic, contributory, predisposing, and necessary. Newer cybernetic mechanisms have added further complexities to understanding causality in human physiology. Cause and effect no longer bear a straight linear relationship to each other. Circular mechanisms of positive and negative feedbacks have taken over in the operational depths of homeostasis. The chain of causation is fast dissolving before our eyes to be replaced by some form of invariable association that does not lend itself readily to a graphic, mathematical, or any other representation. (p. 830)

This is not to say that there is a direct homology between the reasons why the causal chain evaporates in modern physics and in clinical medicine, only that it effectively does so in each case. And if physicists have had difficulty establishing a precise causal chain, perhaps we in medicine can learn to be more at ease with less-than-distinct chains of causation also. There is no harm in doing so: The discipline of physics did not evaporate with the recognition that a strict causality cannot be invoked, nor will medicine. Physics goes on, it endures, it "works" in the absence of a precisely identifiable cause for every phenomenon; and medicine will endure and flourish as well.

In giving up the illusion of strict causality, much is gained. For instance, the concept of illness is enriched and broadened as a result. We no longer need to delude ourselves as in saying that the specific cause of "strep throat" is the streptococcus. As long as we rely on the illusion of strictly caused events, that is indeed the conclusion to which we are attracted, sometimes to the extent of being blinded to other factors. By doggedly insisting on a strict causal chain and an origination point where the illness abruptly begins, we tend to overlook the fact that many persons who harbor the streptococcus do not come down with "strep throat." Some persons become mere carriers of the organism and experience no discernible illness. Others develop only mild symptoms, while others undergo a profound illness. Still others develop strep-related problems later, such as rheumatic fever, meningitis, or pneumonia.

There may well be as yet unknown expressions and nuances of the illness that we will be able to see when we allow a certain ambiguity to engage us—as when we become willing to entertain the effects that emotions, attitudes, and perceived meanings have on the function of the immune system. Here we quickly see that the spectrum of streptococcal disease does not begin with "strep" bacteria. It may include, if we examine the issue with pinpoint accuracy, "the whole previous state of the world," as Sir James Jeans put it.

Not that we need to be this precise in dealing with illness, for we do not; streptococci will respond to penicillin even if we are ignorant of all the world's prior history. But our picture of human illness and health will be considerably enriched and more accurate if we can relax our insistence on strict beginnings of illnesses, for they do not exist. They can be defended only out of a kind of clinical or therapeutic convenience. In effect, we detract from our role as participants in the universe when we install the "strep" bacterium as the sole progenitor of disease in this case. This is a bad habit not only in this illness, but in all illnesses. It denies the richness of the world; it erases the majestic colors and hues with which the canvas of illness is always painted; and it installs simplicities where a greater complexity always reigns.

If we find the prospect of endless causal chains to be bewildering, perhaps it is only because we have sold short our own majestic involvement in the world. Perhaps we are intimidated because we have too long thought ourselves to be lowly creatures, the outcome of mere accidents and mutations, the playthings of natural forces beyond our control, the children of chance and necessity. But bewilderment need not be our response to the discovery of endless causal chains in health and illness. It is equally appropriate to be moved with awe, wonder, and gratitude to find that we are an intrinsic part of the causal web of the world.

Interaction of the Observer and the Observed

Modern physics shows that it is impossible to gain information at the smallest levels of the physical world without paying a price. As we have seen, to know nature's ways at the level of the atom and below is to disturb it. One cannot remain uninvolved or aloof. Therefore, the picture that one derives from looking into nature includes oneself. This situation has great relevance for medicine.

The importance of "observer effects" in medicine in modern times has been vastly underrated. By and large these kinds of effects are eschewed. The old clinicians, however, in the eras before our technological age, felt differently. They were keenly aware of the "disturbances" they created in patients by interacting with them—in touching the patient, in being in his or her presence, in glancing, remarking, or alluding, in being at the bedside. They knew that these influences, these "observer effects," were of profound importance in bringing about curing or healing, and having far fewer techniques at hand than physicians have today, they made much of these effects and cultivated them to a high degree.

Today, however, we have come to view these effects in a different way. They are frequently viewed as nuisances, something to be eliminated. This is especially true in the setting of clinical research. We want our therapies to be "clean," in which all "placebo" effects are weeded out. If the doctor creates effects in the patient by "mere" words or actions, these interfere with the assessment of the therapy being scrutinized. Therefore, these effects have come to be regarded by many physicians as somehow less substantial or less "real" than the effects of drugs or surgery. They can be left out, and one can get on with the business of curing with "real" techniques.

Perhaps it is true that the elimination of "observer effects" is desirable at a certain phase in the experimental, clinical trials of various therapies. But the problem is that this tendency is carried too far. Students of medicine acquire the habit of assigning these effects to a stepchild category, and they are almost never trained in how to use them. The delicate and powerful nuances of the doctor-patient relationship are neglected, mainly because their professors have themselves forgot them or have never learned them. The end result is predictable: Medicine becomes equated with technology, drugs, surgery, transplanted organs, and so forth. The tragedy is that medicine has amputated much of its healing power as these participatory or observer effects have been forgotten. This unfortunate development has been accompanied by a backlash from patients who sense the resultant fallibility and loss of power of their physicians. An unmistakable sense of remoteness and inhumanity is now perceived by patients as physicians have neglected these powerful healing forces. Patients simply are not consoled by the knowledge that medicine has never been more powerful. For it is not only power that ailing human beings want, but healing, love, and care. It is quite remarkable how difficult it seems for many modern physicians to grasp this extraordinarily simple fact. People in need of healing do not desire "clean" therapies, no matter how aesthetically appealing they might be to the physician. Patients want the "contaminating" influences of the physician's touch, words, caring, and love.

Given the potency of the doctor-patient interaction at the clinical level, we must ask ourselves seriously why we would want to eliminate the effects of interaction. The situation in modern physics suggests that some degree of interaction with one's subject is an ineradicable fact and that the effort to purge this feature from the world is doomed in principle. This awareness might provide a firm nudge to physicians not to attempt to cleanse therapy of such phenomena, but to recognize them as an ineradicable part of the therapeutic process and to make the most of them. Acknowledging that this aspect of the world is fundamental might allow us to recover something that has always been contained in the word "healer."

Time

A revision of the view of time in modern medicine, consistent with the view contained in modern physics, would lead to sweeping changes in many commonly held views. We acknowledge once again, however, that there is no single, unanimous attitude toward time in modern physics. However, there is common agreement that time does not flow; that it is not some external, substantial "thing;" that it is not independent of factors such as mass and gravity and space; and that it is not the same for all observers. Despite this common agreement, however, none of these facets of time are recognized in medicine today, a vivid example that medicine is still embedded in classical physical views.

If asked, "What is the most important mission of medicine?" most patients and physicians would likely answer that it is to forestall death, the end to our existence. But if we view death through the modern view of nonlinear, nonflowing time, something changes. Our ordinary view is that death is tragic because it is final. But an event is a finality only if lodged in a flowing, one-way, linear time, which is precisely the sort of time that cannot be proved to exist in modern physics.

Then what happens to death? Does it cease to exist with the new view of time? To claim that death has been banished as a result of modern physics is absurd. But because modern physics implies that absolute finalities are misconstrued because there is no one-way time, death becomes much less grotesque than we have believed. So it is the meaning of death that is changed, if not its existence. This is quite an odd turn of events. Most persons view science as the enemy of spiritual concepts and religious comforts; however, it appears that by demonstrating that death may not be final, science has somehow become the ally of religion instead of its enemy. For it is linear time that is man's devourer, his scourge; and it is linear time that has itself been scourged by modern physics.

And what of birth? Birth, like death, is a "signpost" we erect at one end of life to demarcate the passage of time. Birth and death are the absolute boundaries of life, the beginning and ending. But birth suffers the same fate as death in the new view: it is redefined. Just as death cannot be said to be final outside of linear time, birth cannot be given an absolute status for the same reason: beginnings, like endings, have no absolute status outside linear time.

The goal of medicine, then, which is to extend life to the fullest extent possible, must be rethought. Physicians can still work to relieve suffering and to forestall death; but with this effort comes a new understanding, an awareness that there is something much less grim about the "Grim Reaper" than we have heretofore imagined. There is, of course, nothing new in this recognition: many traditions have long held the view that death is not final. But what is new is that this belief can now be defended against the background of modern science.

The task of healers is considerably modified against the backdrop of the modern physical view of time. As stated previously in *Space, Time and Medicine*, it can be summarized in a new way:

> The most hideous aspects of illness are the distortions in spacetime that sick persons experience. These distortions accentuate pain, suffering, and anguish. The spacetime view of health and disease tells us that a vital part of the goal of every therapist is to help the sick person toward a reordering of his world view. We must help him realize that he is a *process* in spacetime, not an isolated entity who is fragmented from the world of the healthy and who is adrift in flowing time, moving slowly toward extermination.
>
> To the extent that we accomplish this task we are healers. (Dossey, 1982, p. 176)

The Interrelation of Mass and Energy

If medicine were to take quite literally the new knowledge that mass and energy are interconvertible, our ideas about our own body might be considerably broadened. Modern physics has conclusively demonstrated that the old idea that the universe consists of nothing but matter on the one hand and a dead, empty void on the other is wrong. The "void" is hardly empty. It contains the energy that spawns the substance out of which the world is made, as one can easily see in any physicist's cloud chamber where particles erupt from the void and disappear back into it. In medicine, however, we strongly counterpose the idea of matter with utter nothingness. This is expressed most strongly in our idea of death which, we say, is the equivalent of an empty, black, sterile void. This nothingness will eventually swallow everyone and will be the end of the matter that is ourselves. Yet there is nothing contained in the whole of modern physics that justifies this attitude toward the void. Rather, the void is seen to be hopping with about-to-happen events of an invisible sort. This view contrasts mightily with the deadness we ordinarily associate with the void. Matter *cannot* come to nothing, as we suppose; it can only be transmuted into energy and vice-versa. Thus there can never really be an end to ourselves, only a transmutation, as various religious traditions have maintained.

What Modern Physics Does *Not* Say to Modern Medicine

Amid the flurry of interest that now surrounds the "new physics," it is as important to realize what physics does not say about our medical approaches as what it does say. For instance, the egregious extensions of speculative areas of modern physics to medicine, in my opinion, are quite unjustified. These have mainly to do with the role of mind and consciousness.

Today there is an enormous interest in the development of a medical science that is more humane and "person oriented" than the cold, technological medicine with which we are all so familiar. There is a great emphasis today on treating the "whole person." We wish to make allowances for not only the body, but also for the mind and spirit. These latter factors have been felt to be relatively unimportant in health and illness in our century. Science has no tolerance for entities such as the spirit, and even the mind has been largely viewed as a by-product of the brain, merely a consequence of its anatomy and biochemistry. No matter that these views are unsatisfying to patients and many physicians, an objective science simply has not been able to make a place for them.

Enter the "new physics," with its talk of the importance of "the observer." Of all the marvelous revelations of the new physical outlook, the role of conscious observers has captivated the common mind more than any other. If an observer is required to "collapse the wave function" and bring the myriad quantum possibilities into reality, then, it is surmised by those who believed all along that "the mind matters," this is proof that consciousness can change the physical body. This is the evidence we've been looking for! For a decade interested onlookers have seen in the new physics a corroboration of a variety of ideas requiring a potency of the mind.

The use of the new physics as a justification for a mind-oriented, holistic medicine is a distortion of the worst kind. Not only is it a disservice to physics, it is a shameless distortion of medical science as well. Most persons who jump on the bandwagon of new physics to justify a role for the mind in medicine seem to have little feel for the intricacies of modern physics and even less awareness of the emerging data of modern medicine, which, in fact, offer a more solid kind of proof than anything that can currently be found in physics.

The debate over a role for the mind in modern physics theory is just that—a debate. There simply is no consensus on this matter. Physicists cannot agree even on what it is that is required for the act of observation in an experimental set-up. Is a mind required to do the looking? Will an unconscious machine do as well? In view of these uncertainties, it is not reasonable to equate "observer" with a conscious, sentient being. For many physicists, "observing" can be done by a machine—a Geiger counter or a sensitive photographic plate, either of which can bring about the irreversible act of amplification that is required for quantum events to become known. Still other physicists believe the act of observation is not complete until the event is cognized, until it has entered the mind of a conscious being or perhaps a group of them.

One of the most eloquent and brilliant physicists writing about the principle of "observership" today is John Archibald Wheeler, who stated that "Quantum theory says that no elementary phenomenon is a phenomenon until it is an observed phenomenon" (Wheeler, 1981, p. 87). This is hardly a sanction for the mind. For in the same breath Wheeler states, "Let us not invoke either 'consciousness' or 'observer' as prerequisite for what in quantum mechanics we call the elementary act of observation" (Wheeler, 1981, p. 97).

Niels Bohr, with whom Wheeler studied, was one of the great architects of quantum physics. He was also wary of imputing a primary role for human consciousness. In fact, he rejected the word "consciousness" in defining what is meant by an elemental act of observation (Wheeler, 1981, p. 94). A machine, Bohr contended, was an adequate observer. But could a machine be conscious? Interestingly, Bohr, in his typical fashion, complicated and extended the debate about consciousness by refusing to restrict certain mental qualities to human beings. He acknowledged that machines might demonstrate attributes we generally reserve for ourselves. In his words, "I am absolutely prepared to talk of the spiritual life of an electronic computer to state that it is reflecting or that it is in a bad mood. . . . The question whether the machine really feels or ponders, or whether it merely looks as though it did, is of course absolutely meaningless" (Wheeler, 1981, p. 94). In effect, Bohr threw a monkey wrench into the debate. For if he is right, the fact that sentience may be required in the act of observation is no proof that humans are needed, for machines may be sentient as well.

Physicist David Bohm, who has been widely embraced by the holistic health community for his adventuresome idea of the "implicate" and "explicate" orders, is generally cited by mind-oriented holists as a supporter of a role for human consciousness in physics. Yet this is a distortion of Bohm's views. In fact, he has bluntly stated, "I don't think [the mind] has a significant effect on atoms" (Bohm, 1986, p. 120).

We always want to know, what did Einstein say? Einstein, as is widely known, believed in a reality that existed independently of the mind of the observer. As such, he was not cordial to the idea that mind is crucial for the elaboration of physical reality. As he put it, "It is difficult to believe such a description [as offered in quantum theory] is complete. It seems to make the world quite nebulous unless someone, like a mouse, is looking at it" (Wheeler, 1981, p. 91).

In view of thee comments, it may appear that physicists unanimously reject a prominent role for the mind in the way reality unfolds. But this is hardly so: It is not hard to find representatives for the other side. One of the enthusiasts for a role for the human mind in modern physics is Nobelist Eugene Wigner. Wigner (1969) believes that "an observation is only then an observation when it becomes part of 'the consciousness of the observer'" (p. 97). And while this point of view is in the minority, its critics can offer no persuasive, final counterarguments—which is to say that the debate over the role of the mind in quantum mechanics is unsettled, to put it mildly.

It is healthy to realize how tentative the positions of these physicists really are. Words are bandied about by all of them without clear meaning—words like "mind," "consciousness," and "observation." Those who believe physics has had the last word on how things work in our universe can be taken in by the phrases and terms that are used and can assume that physicists are closer to real knowledge than they actually are. Physicist John S. Bell, who is credited with providing physics with Bell's theorem described earlier in this chapter, explains this dilemma in plain language: "I think that—when you analyze this language that the physicists have fallen into, that physics is about the results of observations—you find that on analysis it evaporates, and nothing very clear is being said" (Bell, 1986, p. 48).

The point may be this: If eminent physicists cannot agree on the role of the mind in the world, it is outrageously dishonest for anyone to appropriate a single point of view from physics as if it represented a consensus. There is no consensus in physics about the role of the mind.

An equally important and overlooked point is that this unsettled state of affairs does not mean that the mind is not a crucial factor in health and illness. The best data for a role from the mind are not to be found in physics laboratories, but in the macroscopic world of the living. To know if the mind matters, you must study living creatures, not quarks or subatomic forces. You must look to the clinic, not to the cloud chamber. You must go to hospital, not to the superconducting supercollider.

The "physics envy" that has so embraced holistically oriented medicine has in many ways fogged our vision, not cleared it, and it is time we looked to our own turf instead of that of others for evidence of what the mind can do. When we do so, we shall find that our definitions of "mind" and "consciousness" may indeed be no clearer than those of the physicists. Yet this impediment can be offset in a major way by the vast amount of data—some of which we have alluded to in this chapter— showing that the mind, however we may choose to define it, is an important and ineradicable factor in health and illness.

Perhaps our flirtation in medicine with "new physics" can temporarily be set aside, at least until the physicists make up their minds about key issues that interest us. We should realize that there are lessons we can glean from this important area of science other than those having to do with the role of the mind. For instance, we can learn to think of ourselves in new ways, ways that hinge on the new views of mass, energy, causation, space, and time. Above all, let us recognize what physics can, and cannot tell us. Physicist John Archibald Wheeler once remarked, "Until we understand the true constitution of the world, I think we have to depend much more on what wise men of the past have told us about the subject of religion than on anything that science shows us" (Gliedman, 1984, p. 34ff). The lesson for medicine and its attempt to understand what the mind can do is, I feel, much the same: Until physicians and patients know more clearly the way the world works, we have to depend more on our own observations, those that are anchored in the world of the living, than on what "new physics" can currently tell us.

CONCLUDING REMARKS

It is odd that medicine, which considers itself to be scientific in the most modern sense, utilizes a set of assumptions about the workings of the world that completely ignore many of the insights of the physics of this century. This has led to a situation that is in many ways schizophrenic. While one group of scientists (modern physicists) are well informed of the new world view and employ it when necessary, another group of scientists (physicians, physiologists, and bioscientists of almost every stripe) invoke a very different world view (that of traditional, classical physics) and are virtually ignorant of the essential messages of the most accurate science of this century. To be sure, these perspectives are not mutually exclusive by any means and can be used in tandem in medicine, just as they are used together in physics.

The picture of the world that classical and modern physics gives us is radically different, and the question is, is there any reason why medicine should take the new world view seriously in the day-to-day implementation of the healing art? There are at least two good reasons why one set of scientific beliefs should be replaced by another: (1) if one set fails to account for what is observed or (2) if it is less powerful in predicting future happenings. There are reasons to believe that the explanatory power of the traditional view of the human body, and of health and illness, breaks down in ways we have examined above and that greater predictive power may lie in the direction of the modern physical view of the world.

The classical view of nature has led us to view our own bodies as isolated objects completely disconnected from the power of our own mind and consciousness and from the rest of the world at large. The body, our "life" sciences tell us, is wholly governed by the "blind laws of matter." Even our consciousness is nothing but an elaborate expression of those same laws, ultimately explainable by the brain's anatomy, chemistry, and physiology. The situation that has resulted is one of ethical, moral, and spiritual disaster, and is expressed well by the nuclear physicist and author, Jeremy Hayward (1984):

> [We have lost] our health-giving connection with the earth. We live as if we existed in dead, empty space; therefore, all our energy and insight must come from within, and we constantly feel overcome with anxiety lest our energy run out. We live as if time did indeed flow from past to future; therefore we do not rest in this moment at all. (p. 67)

We have assumed that the classical view of the world is the only one that is needed to apply to living beings, such as ourselves, and that the alternative, relativistic, quantum mechanical ideas are fit only for unimaginably small objects, such as electrons, or for stupendously large objects, such as stars. Indeed, modern physics does apply to these worlds that border us on either side. But why should it spare us in the middle world?

The likely answer is that it does not spare us. Yet it is for us to determine how we are affected—what the new lessons are and the extent to which they apply. And we must go carefully, never forgetting that classical descriptions do work and that they have been enormously successful—up to a point. But just as physicists discovered situations in nature where Newton's physics failed, we are finding areas in medicine where our traditional world view breaks down.

We are discovering that it is not just bodies that falter and need healing from time to time; world views can also break down and can need healing too. Today it is our medical world view that is in need of such healing. Let the healing begin!

References

Bell, J. (1986). Interview in P. C. W. Davies & J. R. Brown (Eds.), *The ghost in the atom*. New York: Cambridge University Press.

Bernstein, J. (1978). A cosmic flow. *American Scholar, 48*, 8.

Bohm, D. (1986). Interview in P. C. W. Davies & J. R. Brown (Eds.), *The ghost in the atom*. New York: Cambridge University Press.

Bronowski, J. (1978). *The common sense of science*. Cambridge: Harvard University Press.

Cooper, M., & Aygen, M. (1978). Effect of meditation on blood cholesterol and blood pressure. *Journal of the American Medical Association, 95*, 1.

Davenport, R. (1979). *An outline of animal development*. Reading, MA: Addison Wesley.

Davies, C. W., & Brown, J. R. (1986). *The ghost in the atom*. New York: Cambridge University Press.

Dossey, L. (1982). *Space, time and medicine*. Boston: New Science Library.

Dossey, L. (1984). *Beyond illness*. Boston: New Science Library.

Engel, G. L. (1971). Sudden and rapid death during psychological stress: Folklore or wisdom? *Annals of Internal Medicine, 74*, 771–782.

Gliedman, J. (1984). Turning Einstein upside down. *Science Digest*, p. 34ff.

Green, J. P., & Weinstein, H. (1981, September). Quantum mechanics can account for the affinities of drugs and receptors. *The Sciences*, p. 27.

Hayward, J. (1984). *Perceiving ordinary magic*. Boston: New Science Library.

Herbert, N. (1986). *Quantum reality*. New York: Doubleday.

Jeans, J. (1981). *Physics and philosophy*. New York: Dover.

Jenkins, C. D. (1971). Psychological and social precursors of coronary artery disease. *The New England Journal of Medicine, 284*, 244–255.

Kothari, D. S. (1985). Complementarity principle and syadvada. In A. P. French & P. J. Kennedy (Eds.), *Niels Bohr volume*. Cambridge: Harvard University Press.

Lynch, J. J. (1985). *The language of the heart: The body's response to human dialogue*. New York: Basic Books.

Medalie, J. H., & Goldbourt, U. (1976). Angina pectoris among 10,000 men II: Psychosocial and other risk factors as evidenced by a multivariate analysis of five-year incidence study. *American Journal of Medicine, 60*, 910–921.

Nerem, R. M., Levesque, M. J., & Cornhill, J. F. (1980). Social environment as a factor in diet-induced atherosclerosis. *Science, 208,* 27 June 1980, pp. 1475–1476.

Pagels, H. R. (1982). *The cosmic code: Quantum physics as the language of nature.* New York: Simon & Schuster.

Reich, P., DeSilva, R. A., Lown, B., & Murawski, B. J. (1981). Acute psychological disturbances preceding life-threatening ventricular arrhythmias. *Journal of the American Medical Association, 246,* 233–235.

Schleifer, S. J., Keller, S. E., Carmerino, S. E., Thornton, J. C., & Stein, M. (1983). Suppression of lymphocyte stimulation following bereavement. *Journal of the American Medical Association, 250,* 374–377.

Schrödinger, E. (1954). The spirit of science. In J. Campbell (Ed.), *Spirit and nature* (Bollingen Series XXX, Vol. 1.). Princeton, NJ: Princeton University Press.

Vaisrub, S. (1979). Groping for causation. *Journal of the American Medical Association, 241,* 830.

Wheeler, J. A. (1981). Not consciousness but the distinction between the probe and the probed as central to the elemental quantum act of observation. In R. G. Jahn (Ed.), *The role of consciousness in the physical world.* Boulder: Westview Press.

Whitehead, A. N. (1968). *Modes of thought.* New York: Macmillan.

Wigner, E. P. (1969). Are we machines? *Proceedings of the American Philosophical Society, 113,* 2, April 1969, pp. 95–101.

Wolf, F. A. (1981). *Taking the quantum leap.* New York: Harper & Row.

Work in America: Report of a special task force to the secretary of health, education, and welfare. (1973) Cambridge: MIT Press.

TOWARD INTEGRATION

15

Meditation East and West

SUNDAR RAMASWAMI
ANEES A. SHEIKH

Those who seek the truth by means of intellect and learning only get further and further away from it. Not till your thoughts cease all their branching here and there, not till you abandon all thoughts of seeking for something, not till your mind is motionless as wood or stone, will you be on the right road to the Gate.

Huang Po

Those from the East have claimed that no Occidental mind can understand the inscrutable Eastern mystical tradition; conversely, Westerners have maintained that the Oriental mind cannot fathom the Western reflective tradition. However, it probably is more accurate to state that

mysticism is the same in all ages and all places, that timelessness and independent of history it has always been identical. East and West and other differences vanish here. Whether the flower of mysticism blooms in India or in China, in Persia or in the Rhine and in Erfurt its fruit is one.

Whether it clothes itself in the delicate Persian verse of Jelaleddin Rumi or in the beautiful middle German of a Meister Eckhart, in the scholarly Sanskrit of the Indian Sankara, or in the laconic riddles of the Sino-Japanese Zen school, these forms could always be exchanged one for the other. (Otto, 1970, p. 13)

The mystic impulse seems unaffected by geography or race. It is universal and immemorial. The ultimate good of the mystical impulse is the transformation of consciousness from normal everyday consciousness to the altered meditative state.

In this chapter, we shall first describe the nature of normal consciousness and the characteristics and functions of altered states of consciousness. Next, we shall explore the nature of the meditative state and its characteristic stages. Then we shall examine several representative Eastern and Western meditative systems to illustrate the different approaches used in the Orient and the Occident. The following sections will include an investigation of the psychophysiology of meditation, of its role in personality change, and of its relationship to the phenomenon known as deautomatization.

NORMAL CONSCIOUSNESS

When we examine our waking consciousness, we find it inhabited by a mélange of thoughts, ideas, ruminations, fantasies, and sensations. Objects, ideas, and people compete for attention. In addition, there are internal stimuli to be attended to—feelings of pain and pleasure, proprioceptive sensations, and so on. Also immense amounts of physical energy of the electromagnetic spectrum impinge on us continuously. We do not attend to all these stimuli that assault us; for that matter, we do not even have the sensory apparatus to receive the energies of the electromagnetic spectrum (Ornstein, 1975).

In relation to the wide array of possible stimuli, our consciousness is extremely limited. Ornstein (1975) suggested that personal consciousness cannot completely represent our internal or external worlds: It must of necessity present an abridged version of reality.

Our consciousness has so evolved as to make biological survival possible. Selective screening of sensory data admits certain stimuli and excludes others (Hall, 1966). "The survival-related stimuli that pass such a filtration form the building blocks for our personal construction, then each person can change his consciousness simply by *changing the way* he constructs it" (Ornstein, 1975, pp. 33–34).

For example, the visual process in humans filters out by means of the reticular activating system (RAS) the perceptions not attended to by the brain (White, 1972). White asserted that human beings are formed on the basis of evolutionally functional sensory repression and that survival of the species demands a selective deployment of attention. The visual process of the frog functions similarly (Lettvin, Maturana, McCulloch, & Pitts, 1965). One experiment illustrated that the retina of the frog, which is similar to that of the human eye, responds only to four kinds of messages. Of the myriad colors, shapes, and movements that could be presented, the frog's eye discards all but the following four patterns: sustained-contrast detectors (SC), moving-edge detectors (ME), net-dimming detectors (ND), and net-convexity detectors (NC). SC detectors offer a hazy outline of the visual field, ME detectors are sensitive to moving shadows, ND detectors are sensitive to sudden decreases in light, and NC detectors respond to small, dark, bug-like objects (Matturana, Lettvin, McCulloch, & Pitts, 1960). Thus the retina of the frog is ideally "wired" to detect its natural prey—small, moving bugs.

A similar arrangement occurs in the human visual cortex. The Nobel Prize–winning work of Hubel and Wiesel (1965, 1968) indicates that the human visual cortex is similarly wired to respond to specific properties of the visual world. Presumably, the visual cortex ignores many other features "irrelevant" to the biological system.

Most of the work on information processing has been done on vision; however, one may infer that selective screening goes on in other sensory systems as well. Not only do these systems distinguish between survival-related and irrelevant stimuli, but they also respond to changes in the sensory field (Groves & Schlesinger, 1979). This brings us to habituation, which is a decrease in response to a repetitive stimulus and therefore may be considered as the organism's way of ignoring trivial, repetitive environmental stimuli. Habituation, or nonassociative learning (Kupferman, 1975), is an elementary form of learning that occurs in the spinal cord. It has been extensively investigated in isolated spinal preparations (Thompson & Spencer, 1966), but it is also well known in intact organisms.

When learning a skill, such as driving or skiing, we pay close attention to the minute details. But after the skill has become "automatic," the hundreds of separate movements do not enter the consciousness. Habituation also explains why we do not "see" the familiar pictures on the wall, "tune out" the buzz of the refrigerator, or the ticking of the clock.

Pribram (1969) recounted an astonishing twist to the habituation response. At a particular time each night, a noisy train rumbled along the elevated tracks on Third Avenue in New York. After the tracks were torn down, the police reported receiving calls from the neighbors complaining of strange noises reportedly occurring at around the time the train used to pass by. Pribram has called this fascinating phenomenon the "Bowery El effect."

As we shall see later, meditation and other altered states of consciousness affect a startling reversal of the automation that underlies our daily actions.

Our normal consciousness, then, is a highly selective, evolutionally adaptive filter that ensures species survival. But is this the only type of consciousness accessible to us? Or is it "but one special type of consciousness, whilst all about it, parted from it by the filmiest of screens, there lie potential forms of consciousness entirely different" (James, 1902, p. 378).

ALTERED STATES OF CONSCIOUSNESS

The nature, function, and manifestations of this realm have not been systematically explored. Altered states of consciousness (ASC) include daydreaming and dream states, hypnosis, sensory deprivation, hysterical states of depersonalization and dissociation, and meditative states. An altered state of consciousness is any mental state

> induced by various physiological, psychological, or pharmacological maneuvers or agents, which can be recognized subjectively by the individual himself . . . as representing a sufficient deviation in subjective experience or psychological functioning from certain general norms for that individual during alert, waking consciousness. This sufficient deviation may be represented by a greater preoccupation than usual with internal sensations or mental processes, changes in the formal characteristics of thought, and impairment of reality testing to various degrees. (Ludwig, 1969, pp. 9–10)

Production of ASC

ASC, including the meditative states, can be produced by techniques that interfere with the normal flow of sensory or proprioceptive stimuli or with the normal flow of cognitive processes (Ludwig, 1969). Levels of stimulation above or below the optimal range of enteroceptive stimulation necessary to maintain waking consciousness may produce ASC (Lindsey, 1961). Dramatic reductions in sensory input as well as continuous exposure to repetitive and monotonous stimulation are important contributing factors. Thus ASC are associated not only with meditation but also with solitary confinement, prolonged stimulus deprivation at sea (Anderson, 1942), and sensory deprivation states (Lilly, 1956). An increase in enteroceptic stimulation as a result of memory overload, emotional arousal, or physical activity also may be contributing factors. Examples of ASC thus produced are: mental states produced by brainwashing (Sargant, 1957), religious conversion (LaBarre, 1962), spirit possession states (Sargant, 1957), shamanistic trance states (Murphy, 1964), and the trance states of the "whirling" dervishes during their "devr" dance (Williams, 1958). Also they have been noted in fugues, amnesias, traumatic neuroses, depersonalization, panic states, and in rage reactions (Ludwig, 1969), prayer (Bowers, 1959), and intense absorption in a mental task.

ASC also occur in conditions of decreased alertness. It is under these conditions that mystic states usually arise. The states of *satori, samadhi,* or *Nirvana* attained through meditation, profound aesthetic and creative experiences (Koestler, 1964), reading trance (Snyder, 1930), and mental states associated with deep muscular relaxation may be grouped in this category.

Alterations in body chemistry also bring about certain ASC (Hinkle, 1961). Thus hypoglycemia, dehydration, sleep deprivation (West, Janszen, Lester, & Comelisoon, 1962), and hyperventilation serve to induce ASC.

Common Features of ASC

ASC have many common characteristics, and their differences in outward manifestations usually are due to cultural expectations (Wallace, 1959), role playing, demand characteristics (Orne, 1962), or individual frame of mind.

1. *Alterations in thought.* Disturbances in concentration, attention, and memory are commonly found (Ludwig, 1969). Primary process thinking is present, reality testing is impaired, and reflective awareness (Rapaport, 1951) is reduced.

2. *Disturbed time sense.* The sense of time is distorted; subjective feelings of timelessness, of time coming to a stop, have been reported (Ludwig, 1969).

3. *Perceptual alterations.* In many ASC, perceptual aberrations, such as hallucinations, illusions, and visual imagery, are common. The context of these phenomena is shaped by cultural and idiosyncratic factors, including wish fulfillment, fears, and repressed material (Ludwig, 1969).

4. *Changes in body image.* Distortions in body image occur frequently in ASC. Generally a sense of depersonalization, a merging of the self with the universe is reported. Many mystics speak of the feeling of "oneness" or an "oceanic feeling."

5. *Loss of control.* ASC are accompanied by subjective feelings of loss of control. However, subjects often gain greater control: For example, hypnotized subjects vicariously identify with the power of the hypnotist (Kubie & Margolin, 1944). In mystical states, individuals surrender personal volition in order to experience cosmic consciousness.

6. *Sense of the ineffable.* Persons who experience transcendental states express an inability to communicate their experience to those who have not shared the experience. What is experienced seems inexpressible. Julian of Norwich (1966, p. 76), a 14th-century English mystic, attempted to communicate the incommunicable experience:

> All this was shown to me in three ways, in actual vision, in imaginative understanding, and in spiritual sight. This last I cannot, and may not disclose as openly and fully as I should like to. But I trust that God almighty will of his goodness and love enable you to savour its spirit and sweetness more than my feeble efforts permit.

7. *Noesis.* The individual who has undergone an ASC feels that he or she has experienced a union with a divine power (Linn, 1967) and that a tremendous illumination has occurred, that he or she has plumbed the depths of the universe.

Functions of ASC

Do meditative and other ASC perform any useful psychological functions for human beings? Mystical and aesthetic experiences are supremely uplifting and enable human beings to transcend both the boundaries of language and the barriers of their everyday minds. Huxley (1954) was an eloquent spokesman for this view. Each one of us, he said, is potentially "Mind At Large":

> But insofar as we are animals, our business is at all costs to survive. To make biological survival possible, Mind At Large has to be funneled through the reducing valve of the brain and nervous system. What comes out at the other end is a measly trickle of the kind of consciousness which will help us to stay alive on the surface of this particular planet. To formulate and express the contents of this reduced awareness, man has invented

and endlessly elaborated those symbol-systems and implicit philosophies that we call languages. Every individual is at once the beneficiary and the victim of the linguistic tradition into which he has been born—the beneficiary inasmuch as language gives access to the accumulated records of other peoples' experience, the victim insofar as it confirms him in the belief that reduced awareness is the only awareness and as it bedevils his sense of reality, so that he is all too apt to take his concepts for data, his words for actual things. That which, in the language of religion, is called "this world" is the universe of reduced awareness expressed, and, as it were, petrified by language. The various "other worlds" with which human beings erratically make contact, are so many elements of the totality of awareness belonging to Mind At Large. Most people most of the time know only what comes through the reducing valve and is consecrated as genuinely real by their local language. Certain persons, however, seem to be born with a kind of bypass that circumvents the reducing valve. In others temporary bypasses may be acquired either spontaneously or as a result of deliberate "spiritual exercises" or through hypnosis or by means of drugs. Through these permanent or temporary bypasses there flows . . . something more than, and above all something different from, the carefully selected, utilitarian material which our narrow, individual minds regard as a complete, or at least sufficient, picture of reality. (pp. 22–24)

This elusive "something" that is so different from our everyday reality may be a higher knowledge, divine inspiration, or a sudden illumination. Throughout history, individuals have used meditation and prayer in creating the temporary bypass, in "opening new realms of experience, reaffirming moral values, resolving emotional conflicts, and often enabling him to cope better with his human predicament and the world about him" (Ludwig, 1969, p. 20).

Koestler (1964) suggested other uses of ASC. Creativity and problem solving are enhanced in ASC, such as trance, meditation, and drowsiness. For example, the English poet Coleridge wrote his fabulous poem *Kubla Khan* in a drug-induced trance.

From time immemorial, ASC have been a key ingredient in the healing arts. Shamans went into a trance to diagnose ailments (Murphy, 1964). The Egyptian practice of "incubation" in the sleep temple, the cures at Lourdes, exorcism, magnetic treatment, and modern hypotherapy illustrate the role of ASC in therapy (Ludwig, 1964). ASC produced by drugs, such as ether, LSD-25, and amytal, have been used in psychiatry (Sargant, 1957).

Finally, ASC seem to satisfy certain social needs. Spirit possession states win absolution from responsibility for one's actions. Consequently, they are a useful and socially acceptable way of expressing aggression and sexual conflicts (Mischel & Mischel, 1958). Group themes, such as death and cultural taboos, also can be expressed in ritualized ways (Belo, 1960; Deren, 1952; Ravenscroft, 1965). In summary, the existence of "such practices represents an excellent example of how society creates modes of reducing frustrations, stress and loneliness through group action" (Ludwig, 1969, p. 21).

MEDITATION

Of the many ways to induce an altered state of consciousness, none is more celebrated than meditation. No other aspect of Eastern psychology is as misunderstood as meditation. The moment meditation is mentioned, one thinks of sitting in a strange posture in some cave or desert, totally self-absorbed and oblivious to the rest of the world. Such an image both repels and attracts. It is either dismissed as alien to the Western ethos or practiced with zeal. Its votaries ascribe miraculous properties to meditation; its detractors see in it a catatonic withdrawal from life itself. To add to the prevailing confusion, there seem to be different kinds of meditations.

What, exactly, is meditation? Sufi dervishes dance in circles, Buddhists are attentive to their breaths, Yogis chant *mantras* or gaze at the tip of their noses, Wall Street brokers "meditate" on what stocks to buy. It is this last meaning of meditation that is most familiar to Westerners. Consequently, Eastern claims that meditation leads to *Nirvana* or emptiness or a state of "no mind" seem silly. How can reasoning lead to emptiness (Koestler, 1960)?

In the West, meditation also is used to describe a set of techniques designed to alter our normal mode of consciousness and bring about a harmonious reintegration of the human personality (Russell, 1986). This aspect of meditation is concerned with the development of an attitude, a presence that expresses itself in every situation, transforming whatever it embraces.

> If its medium is movement, it will turn into dance; if stillness, into living sculpture; if thinking, into the higher reaches of intuition; if sensing, into a merging with the miracle of being; if feeling, into love; if singing, into sacred utterance; if speaking, into prayer or poetry; if doing the things of ordinary life, into a ritual in the name of God or a celebration of existence. (Naranjo & Ornstein, 1971, p. 8)

This is the transformation of an ordinary individual into a *zaddik* or saint. It is the emergence of a New Person who relates to the world not covetously but receptively, lovingly, who acts skillfully and mindfully in every circumstance of life.

Meditation is perhaps as old as humankind. Surely, human beings have from time to time found themselves transported to the point of abandonment, reflective to the point of absorption. Only recently, however, has meditation been promoted along with jogging and vitamin C as a panacea for the 40-hour week.

The central fact of the meditative experience in both Eastern and Western traditions is an overwhelming and compelling consciousness of the soul's oneness with God or the Divine Ground. The Sanskrit formula, *"Tat Tvam Asi"* ("Thou Art That"), expresses this feeling most accurately. The totally illuminated human being knows that God is present in the deepest and most central part of his or her own soul. "Me is God nor do I recognize any other me except my God himself," said Saint Catherine of Genoa. This same thought was expressed by the noted 14th-century Catholic mystic Ruysbroeck, "The spirit possesses God essentially in naked nature and God the spirit" (as cited in Huxley, 1970, p. 12). In the Eastern tradition, Jallal-Uddin Rumi agrees: "The Beloved is all in all, the lover merely veils him; the Beloved is all that lives, the lover a dead thing" (Rumi, 1898, p. 27). In the meditative experience, personal category is transcended. Thus we have Plotinus in raptures over the "Bare Pure One" and Kabir listening to the "rhythmic music of reality."

Neither the Eastern nor the Western mystic is concerned with knowledge. They long for salvation. They aspire to be delivered from "separate self-hood in time and into eternity as realized in the unitive knowledge of the Divine Ground" (Huxley, 1970, p. 202). Salvation is deliverance from evil, which is an epi-phenomenon of separate self-hood; heaven is not a posthumous condition, but freedom from death.

Both Eastern and Western mystics are firmly anchored in theism. For example, Shankara displayed a passion for a personal God, Ishvara (Huxley, 1970); in the Western mystical tradition, Eckhart, St. Theresa, and others were moved by visions of the saviour. Shankara distinguished between the lower and higher knowledge: The lower knowledge of a personal world-controlling God disappears when the higher knowledge of the Divine Ground enters. The Catholic mystics, on the other hand, maintained a clear relationship between their mysticism and their orthodox religion; their mysticism is permeated by Christianity. Love and light play a permanent role in both traditions. "By love he may be gotten and holding, by thought never," says the unknown author of the *Cloud of Unknowing* (1961). Kabir exclaims, "The middle region of the sky wherein the spirit dwelleth is radiant with the music of light" (as cited in

Underhill, 1960, p. 16). Thus a mood of humble and loving receptivity is a prerequisite for the mystic experience.

Mortification is another theme that permeates both traditions. This mortification is called "purgation" in the Christian tradition. False ways of thinking and feeling have to be broken up. The monastic rules of poverty, chastity, and obedience—which are common to both traditions—aim at the eradication of self-centered desires and attachments. "He who no longer craves for personal possessions, pleasures or pressures is very near to perfect liberty. His attention is freed from its usual concentration on the self's immediate interest and at once he sees the Universe in a new, more valid, because disinterested light" (Underhill, 1960, p. 13). The "perfect charity in life surrendered" is an important trait of the mystic. The means by which this is attained is asceticism, the gymnastics of the soul. That austerities can be hindrances was aptly remarked upon by Jacopone da Todi (cited in Huxley, 1970), who said that his austerities resulted chiefly in indigestion and insomnia. While austerity is preferable to indulgence, perfect inward detachment is not incongruous with a normal life; true asceticism is one of the mind involving watchfulness and charity.

The mystic experience has invariably been attended by certain byproducts: divine visions and occult powers. Most mystics have warned against relying too much on such favors and have denied that they mediated a valid spiritual experience. The Sufis regard miracles as veils between God and the soul. The Hindu Yogis warned their disciples that the *Siddhis*, or occult powers, were obstacles to deliverance. Jean Pierre Camus elegantly summed up the mystics's attitude to such phenomena: "One ounce of santifying grace is worth more than a hundred weight of those graces which theologians call gratuitous, among which is the gift of miracles. It is possible to receive such gifts and yet be in mortal sin; nor are they necessary for salvation" (as cited in Huxley, 1970, p. 260).

The path to salvation is succintly expressed by the phrase, "Our Kingdom Go" which is the natural corollary to the Christian prayer "Thy Kingdom Come." The Divine Ground can be realized only by losing the impulse of egocentric wishing, thinking, and feeling. Practices that encourage a deliberate dying to the self are enjoined by both Eastern and Western traditions. However, these practices are never an end in themselves. The great spiritual teachers in all traditions have conceded that such practices may confer psychic powers; however, they have maintained that such powers have nothing to do with liberation. If valued highly, they become obstacles to the path. "When thou did give thyself up to physical mortification, thou was great, thou was admired." So writes Suso of his own experiences—experiences that led him to give up

his course of bodily penance (Huxley, 1970, p. 100). The best mortification of all, "a holy indifference," is also the most difficult. When Saint
Ignatius of Loyola was asked how he would feel if the Pope disbanded
the Society of Jesus, he replied, "A quarter of an hour of prayer and I
should think no more about it." In the Eastern tradition, Chuang Tzu
states this idea eloquently: "By a man without passions I mean one that
does not permit good or evil to disturb his inward economy but rather
falls in with what happens and does not add to the sum of his mortality"
(as cited in Huxley, 1970, p. 103).

Mystics have been charged with indulging in mere personal satisfactions of no value to humanity. While it is true that the essence of the
mystic's experience is a solitary communion with the Divine Ground, it is
inaccurate to say that it has not enriched humanity. Mystics, like artists,
mediate between the beauty and truth to which they have access and
those who cannot discern without special assistance. Mystics see reality
in its immeasurable aspect and attempt, like other artists, to reveal it to a
phenomenal world. Having heard the music of the inner life, the mystic
weaves it into melodies that other humans can understand. The mystic
and the artist reveal to us an entirely new order of experience. Our
spiritual world—that is, the symbols, ideas, and images we hold—is the
result of the topography revealed by mystics. They have done this by
descriptions addressed to the discriminating intellect and suggestion to
the imagination. "At one end of the scale is the vivid, prismatic imagery
of the Christian apocalypse, at the other the fluid, ecstatic poetry of
some of the Sufi saints" (Underhill, 1960, pp. 68–69).

According to Willis (1979), meditation is characterized by four stages:
preparation, attention, reception, and higher consciousness.

Preparation

Meditative traditions do not always agree on the kinds of preparation
a meditator requires (Goleman, 1977). Some kind of purification—
through fasting, ascetic practices, or monastic training—is often considered a prerequisite, although some gurus, notably Maharishi Mahesh
Yogi and J. Krishnamurti, dismiss it as irrelevant.

Religious doctrine finds a place in almost every spiritual tradition. In
the Christian tradition, the "discursive prayer, a thoughtful ruminating
over the truths of sacred scriptures and the exemplary lives of saintly
predecessors, serves as the aspirant's access ramp to the road of the
'higher' meditative states" (Willis, 1979, p. 97).

In most systems, the novice attaches himself or herself to a guru, but
this practice is denounced by the contemporary mystic, Krishnamurti.

Attention

LeShan (1974) discerns four types of instruments of meditative attention: the body, the intellect, the emotions, and action.

Methods that involve the body include Yoga and the Sufi dance of the dervish. An ancient Hasidic story offers a beautiful illustration of the healing nature of bodily movement:

> A great rabbi was coming to visit a small town in Russia. It was a very great event for the Jews in the town and each thought long and hard about what questions they would ask the wise man. When he finally arrived, all were gathered in the largest room and each was deeply concerned with the questions they had for him. The Rabbi came into the room and felt the great tension in it. For a time he said nothing and then he began to hum softly a Hasidic tune. Presently all there were humming with him. He then began to sing the song and soon all present were singing with him. Then he began to dance and soon all were deeply involved in the dance, all fully committed to it, all just dancing and nothing else. In this way, each one became whole with himself, each healed the splits within himself which kept him from understanding. After the dance went on for some time, the Rabbi gradually slowed to a stop, looked at the group, and said, "I trust that I have answered all your questions." (LeShan, 1974, pp. 36–37)

The use of the intellect as a tool for meditation is best exemplified in Western meditative traditions. "The prayerful consideration of sacred revelation and tradition as well as the quiet recognition of one's own finite condition have been principal methods for unlocking the mediator's affections and directing his attention toward God" (Willis, 1979, p. 98). Eastern traditions, too, use the intellect to great effect: *Mantra* Yoga of Hinduism and *vipassana* (mindfulness meditation) of Buddhism are good examples.

> Whatever the intellectual method, however, the goals remain identical: through discursive reasoning or impossible mental task, through monotonous repetition or minute awareness, the mediator's intellect eventually is quieted, is without object, and is thus left behind for the world of nonintellectual awareness. (Willis, 1979, p. 98)

The use of the emotions to achieve a loving union with God was commended by many, including the 14th-century English mystic who wrote *The Cloud of Unknowing* (1961). He cautioned against an intellectual approach to God who, he asserted, can be apprehended by love alone.

Love of the infinite is ignited in many ways: In Ingatian contemplation by entering imaginatively into the loving, saving actions of Christ; in *Bhakti* (devotion) Yoga through attentive devotion to the images of the infinite; in Christian Hesychasm by the continual repetition of the "Jesus Prayer" ("Lord Jesus, Son of God, have mercy on me, a sinner"). . . . Instead of intellectual reasoning, concentration, or mindfulness, meditative attention means the loving attentiveness of an awakened heart. (Willis, 1979, p. 99)

The path of action, on the other hand, demands loving attention to the task in the immediate present. Thus Hindus invest every action with a spiritual grace, accepting it as God's will, and Zen Buddhists give undivided attention to the mundane and the insignificant. Attentive living banishes egotistic desires and vain imaginings; it heals the split between thought and affect and informs the current moment with a benevolent presence. The supreme importance of singular attention is aptly illustrated in this story:

> One day a man of the people said to Zen master Ikkyu:
>
> "Master, will you please write for me some maxims of the highest wisdom?"
>
> Ikkyu immediately took his brush and wrote the word "Attention."
>
> "Is that all?" asked the man. "Will you not add something more?"
>
> Ikkyu then wrote twice running: "Attention. Attention."
>
> "Well," remarked the man rather irritably, "I really don't see much depth or subtlety in what you have just written."
>
> Then Ikkyu wrote the same word three times running: "Attention. Attention. Attention."
>
> Half-angered, the man demanded: "What does that word 'Attention' mean anyway?"
>
> And Ikkyu answered gently: "Attention means attention."
>
> (Adapted from Kapleau, 1967, pp. 10–11)

No wonder the wise raja (king) in Huxley's mythical *Island* (1962, p. 6) populated his kingdom with mynah birds that insisted, "Attention, attention. Here and now, boys; here and now, boys."

Reception

The real activity of meditation is a nonactive, passive awareness, which Krishnamurti (1954) calls "choiceless awareness." The devices considered so far—the preparatory and attentive phases—are mere orienting or centering techniques that pave the way to the supremely transcendent experience that is true meditation. The centering techniques are not meditation (Carrington, 1977). If the mere physiological quieting that accompanies the preparatory and attentive phases is taken to be meditation, then meditation may become indistinguishable from progressive relaxation or bidfeedback.

The difference lies in the presence or absence of what Willis (1979) has termed "active reception." The phase of receptivity is characterized by three distinct qualities. First, there is a heightened inner awareness. Meditators are intensely aware even though the physiological state may suggest drowsiness or sleep. Second, there is a psychological and physiological quieting. The turbulent waves of the mind become ripples, and metabolic activities slow to a crawl. Third, there is a potent mix of passive volition and energy. "The Bhagavad Gita tells us to work without coveting the fruits of our labor. In other words, we want the fruit but we don't strive and strain to attain it. In a sense we don't want it at all, and we are wholly detached. This is an example of passive volition" (Johnston, 1974, pp. 111–112). Associated with the mood of passive volition is a core of passive energy that belongs to the intuitive and nondiscursive way of thinking.

Higher Consciousness

Finally, ordinary consciousness is transformed by union with the divine, by seeing into the void of the mind, or by the "blowing out" of *Nirvana*. This experience is almost always considered ineffable. The Western mystic interprets this experience in theistic terms; in Eastern tradition, it is not Grace that transforms, rather it is the individual's own potential for growth and fulfillment. The Buddhist believes that each one of us has a Buddha nature buried like a lotus in the mud (Prince, 1978). The practice of mindfulness awakens our Buddha nature and propels us into a *jhanic* state. Mindfulness shatters the comfortable illusions of continuity that form the fabric of mental life. We realize suddenly the "random units of mind stuff" from which we make up reality. From this realization comes a series of insights culminating in *Nirvana* (Goleman, 1977).

THE CHRISTIAN MYSTICAL TRADITION

The formative period for Christian mystical theology was the Patristic period, which extended into the late fifth century. It began with Plato's search for Being in the *Phaedo;* for the Good in the *Republic;* for Beauty, in the *Symposium* and *Phaedrus;* and for the One in the *Philebus.* In all his works, the object of the search finally becomes the Eternal that transcends the Phenomenal world. Plato did not merely continue the search of the pre-Socratics for an understanding of the nature of the world; he articulated the religious urges of human beings. He postulated the realm of the Forms as the Divine World. The human soul can know the Forms because it, too, is divine, and due to its nature, it seeks to return to the divine realm. The path of this return is described in Plato's allegory of the Cave in the seventh book of the *Republic.*

Plato does not propose any concept of God; but with Middle Platonism, the concept of God emerges and is best enunciated by Philo. Philo's God is the God of Isaac and Abraham. He is essentially unknowable by humans because they are in a creaturely state. In Philo, we find for the first time the vocabulary of mysticism—initiation, greater and lesser mysteries. The soul seeks God because it has known God; in fact, the ultimate goal of existence is the soul's knowledge of God. Philo speaks of this knowledge in terms of ecstacy, *"sortie de soi."* However, the soul's capacity to know God is God given.

Philo's tentative attempts at mythical theology find supreme expression in Plotinus. In him "converge almost all the main currents of thought that come down from eight hundred years of Greek speculation: out of it there issues a new current destined to fertilize minds as different as those of Augustine, Boethius, Dante, and Meister Eckhart, Coleridge, Bergson and T. S. Eliot" (Dodds, 1973, p. 126).

Origen states that the soul's ascent to God is made possible by Christ. "The mystical life is the working out, the realizing of Christ's union with the soul effected in baptism and is a communion, a dialogue between Christ and the soul" (as cited in Louth, 1981, p. 53). It was Origen who first outlined the three stages of the mystical life: purificatory, illuminative, and unitive. For Origen, the Songs of Songs represented the zenith of mystical life, the union of the soul with God.

The Council of Nicaea, in 325 A.D., a watershed in Christian thought, inhibited mystical theology for some time. It set forth the doctrine of *creatio nihilo*—that is, the soul is created out of nothing. According to this creed, there is an ontological gulf between God and the soul. Contemplation cannot divinize the soul; divinization is an act of grace. Since there is no point of contact between God and the soul, God is totally unknowable except if he, through an act of grace, chooses to reveal himself.

The mystical and antimystical strands come together in the fourth and fifth centuries in the monastic tradition. For those who went into the desert, the so-called Desert Fathers, life was a continual combat with demons tempting them to sin. They divided the way of the soul into three stages: *pratike* is the stage when the soul practices virtue; *physike* is the stage of contemplation; and *theologia* is the knowledge, or *gnosis*, of the Holy Trinity. They can be summarized as effort, knowledge, and prayer. "The way to seek the experience of grace is through prayer, perseverance in prayer, night and day lamenting one's sinful state and beseeching God" (Louth, 1981, p. 122).

A number of prominent men of the church stressed the mystical aspect. For St. Augustine the soul's ascent to God is made possible by introspection. Gregory the Great, who was pope from 590 to his death in 604, stressed that the capacity for mystical apprehension is trained within the world of asceticism. To him asceticism was a form of spiritual training that made man fit to receive the divine presence. In the 12th century, Bernard of Clairvaux gave the next thrust to Christian mysticism, maintaining that many of the most profound truths are accessible only through personal mystical experience. His interiorization of religion was expressed in the language of love and courtship (Capps & Wright, 1978).

However, the full flowering of Christian mysticism occurred in the 14th century. Richard Rolle was the most well known of the medieval mystics. In *Melos Contemplativorum* and *Incendium Amoris,* Rolle outlines his concept of the mystical life. He claims to have experienced the heat, song, and sweetness of mystical ecstasy, which remained with him intimately for the rest of his life. He proposes a number of prerequisites for the mystical life: "A man must be truly turned to Him and in his innermost mind turn away from all visible things before he can express the sweetness of Divine Love" (as cited in Knowles, 1961, p. 59). The beginner, he says, must practice severe austerities, such as continuous prayer and meditation. He adds that mystical ecstasy is a gift from God and that the highest love of Christ consists of fire, song, and sweetness.

The unknown author of the *The Cloud of Unknowing* (1961), on the other hand, insists on "naked faith, the restriction of the highest and purest contemplation to an incommunicable and indescribable experience without any eternal manifestations" (as cited in Knowles, 1961, p. 77). There are three aspects to his teaching. First, it is addressed to those who are ascetically inclined; second, it is an exercise of the will, of the love of God; and third, it rests upon the premise that between the soul and God there is a Cloud of Unknowing.

Julian of Norwich is an "unlettered" mystic who desired three favors of God: the bodily sight of the Passion, a bodily sickness in order to be purified, and three wounds—sorrow, suffering, and longing for God. She did fall seriously ill and even as she lay dying, she had the vision of the Passion. The "shewings," as she called her mystical experiences, quickly followed. At the time of this grave illness, 14 visions were impressed upon her soul. Central to these was the unfolding meaning of the Passion of Christ. The message was that the love of God redeems what is unredeemable.

The greatest figure in the 14th-century Christian mystical movement was Meister Eckhart (1260–1327). His concept of the soul was the most unique aspect of his teaching. He believed that man's soul is of the same nature as God. "This spark is none other than a spark of the Divine Nature, a Divine light, a ray of Divinity" (as cited in Jones, 1971, p. 74). He affirmed that the soul carried the capacity to receive the fullness of God. For Eckhart, the birth of God within the soul is that decisive early event within interior consciousness. From that event, the soul is compelled toward the Godhead. Eckhart's glimpse of the Godhead as the Source comes close to Hindu notions of Brahman as the Source.

Suso (1300–1366) characterized the search for the Ground as love for eternal wisdom. Tauler (1300–1361) urged that the "inner man" must guide the outer man. To make it possible, a deep humility is required. Tauler proposed that five prisons enslave us: love of creatures, of self, of reason, attachment to experiences, and self-will. By breaking through these, one enters the mystic way,

> a way strewn with joy but also darkened by painful interior purgings through which the sufferer must pass in faith, hope and humility in order to arrive at last at the innermost part of the soul where God dwells. Here in this hidden darkness, this wild desert, one encounters the marvelous Unity in which all multiplicity is lost. (as cited in Capps & Wright, 1978, p. 123)

In the 16th century, Spain produced a number of contemplatives who enriched the mystical tradition. Teresa of Avila explored the interior life with resolute care and emotional intensity. According to her, the goal of human life is the vision of God. In the *Interior Castle,* Teresa describes the soul's journey to God, a journey that demands perpetual interior cleansing, prayer, humility, and the grace of God. John of the Cross provided "an anatomy or grammar of the interior life that has been consulted by practitioners of religious sensitivity from the sixteenth century to the modern era" (Capps & Wright, 1978, p. 187). His central statement is that the soul must travel through darkness if it is to unite with God. The journey involves a stripping away of impurities and imperfections. "And as the soul travels through the process of purification, it penetrates evermore deeply through separating screens to the core of reality" (as cited in Capps & Wright, 1978, p. 188). According to John, divine grace ignites the soul like fire does wood. "God strips one of everything contrary, faculties, feelings and affections, leaving the understanding dark, the will dry, the memory empty, and affections in deep affliction" (as cited in Capps & Wright, 1978, p. 188).

The Christian contemplative tradition involves meditation on the scriptures and on the life of Christ. This aspect distinguishes it from the passive Buddhist/Hindu techniques. The initial prayer is the discursive prayer of the three powers of the soul (memory, understanding, and will); then begins the affective prayer in which one performs acts of love and gratitude to God. The prayer of simplicity consists of the Jesus Prayer, which involves invoking the mercy of Christ. This prayer is the bridge to silent contemplation, the *silentium mysticum*, in which one remains tranquil in God. This silence is also called the "cloud of unknowing." The mystic is in a cloud and unable to see clearly, since discursive reasoning is suspended (Johnston, 1970). All thoughts, all desires, all hopes, all fears, all ambitions must be stamped out. Then there will be a stirring of love that will possess one's whole being, and the self will die.

Another bridge to silent prayer is the chanting of "Abba." The Christian mystics also have used the expression "Jubilatio," which is a form of speaking or singing with no conceptual meaning, somewhat like the yodeling of Swiss shepherds. Both are affective in transcending systematic reasoning and thinking.

In the Christian tradition, no prayer can be performed without grace. St. Paul declares that no one can even call on Jesus without divine assistance. Thus, it is grace that stirs up love of God.

JEWISH MYSTICISM

The Kabbalah is the mystical branch of Judaism. The word "Kabbalah" comes from the Hebrew expression meaning "to receive." It contains metaphysical discourses as well as specific techniques to aid in transcending a mundane frame of mind. The Kabbalah dates back to the Merkabah or Chariot Epoch, which extended from the 1st century B.C. to the 10th century A.D. There are two branches to the Kabbalah, the Ma'aseh Bereshit (act of creation), which dealt with the creation of the world, and the Ma'aseh Merkabah (an act of the divine chariot), which elaborated on our connection to the Godhead. Those who pursued the study of the Kabbalah were called the "Yorde Merkabah" (those who descend in the chariot), because they were thought to descend into the depths of their own minds. In the so-called Heikhalot (heavenly hall writings), the Jewish sages describe the inner journey.

The most important development of the Kabbalah occurred in 1175, when the *Sefer Bahir* (Book of Brilliance) first appeared. Its anonymous author proclaimed the existence of a higher consciousness beyond everyday reality. One of the methods of raising consciousness was channeling life energy—a notion similar to the Hindu concept of awakening the Kundalini. The most important Kabbalist of this period was Abraham Ben Samuel Abulafia (c. 1240) who set forth methods for altering consciousness. Abulafia suggested specific body postures, breathing exercises, solitary contemplation, and fasting as paths to the divine.

The next development in the Kabbalah came in the form of a remarkable volume called the *Zohar* (Book of Splendor), published by Moses de Leon (1250–1305). The most important premise of the *Zohar* is the assertion that action must be coupled with contemplation to achieve salvation. Like the *Tantra* of Buddhism, it affirmed that sexual intercourse is a method for achieving illumination. The *Zohar* is also replete with nondualistic concepts (Hoffman, 1981).

The Jewish expulsion from Spain in 1492 gave a fresh impetus to Kabbalism. The town of Safed in Palestine became a center for Kabbalistic study. Moses Cordovero (1522–1570), a Safed Kabbalist, wrote the *Pardes Rimmonim* (Orchard of Pomegranates) in which he urged an ethical approach to the Godhead. He drew up a list of moral precepts for daily life, much like those found in the *Vinaya* of Buddhism. These precepts included: never become angry, always be truthful, mentally review one's actions during the day before gong to sleep at night, and so on. Another Safed Kabbalist, Isaac Luria (1534–1572), experienced visions as a result of Kabbalist practices that utilized complicated visualization techniques. He wrote copiously on reincarnations, dreams, and meditations.

But the Kabbalah rose to its greatest influence under the charismatic leadership of Israel Ben Eliezer (1698–1760), who founded the movement known as Hasidism, or the Devout (Hoffman, 1981). He urged prayer and meditation for attaining higher consciousness. Every action, if carried out with the right intention or Kavvanah, "helps in the redemption of the cosmos from darkness and confusion" (Hoffman, 1981, p. 20). One of Ben Eliezer's disciples, Rabi Schneur Zalman of Liady (1747–1812), thought that the human goal was to seek union with the divine. Another, Rabi Nachman of Bratslav (1772–1810), wrote about dreams, altered states of consciousness, and the mind-body relationship. Convinced of the survival of human consciousness after death, he preached that the time of physical death is crucial in determining the course of one's consciousness after death.

According to the Kabbalah, we have several levels of consciousness. The lowest levels, Nefesh and Ruach, concern instinctual needs.

Neshamah is the higher consciousness associated with the transcendent self. There is a constant interplay between these forces as the higher consciousness struggles to assert itself. Like the Buddhists, the Kabbalists maintain that thought, speech, and action are the doorways of sin. The doorway to transcendent consciousness is meditation, which leads to the Devekuth, or the cleaving to the divine.

The Kabbalists prescribed meditative exercises to achieve transcendence. Physical well-being was regarded as a prerequisite to mental well-being. Many of the Kabbalists, such as Rabbi Akiva, were outdoor laborers much like the Zen masters. Although the Kabbalah frowns on asceticism, fasting was recommended for cleansing the body. Another technique involved subjecting the body to extreme temperatures, which is practiced also by the Tibetan Buddhists. The third involved Kavvanah or one-pointed attention.

Jewish meditative exercises can be grouped under three headings. Concentration exercises involved visual symbols and chants that help in focusing attention. Ego-annihilating techniques involve a deliberate dying of the personality. One ego-annihilating technique consists of meditation on one emotional trait at a time until it withers. After various aspects of one's personality have been taken care of, this exercise destroys one's separate identity. The third technique pertains to sound as a spiritual force. The Kabbalists believed that every sonance has a spiritual effect and that various hymns and chants help to induce higher states of consciousness.

These Kabbalist techniques conferred paranormal abilities on the practitioner. But, like their Buddhist and Hindu counterparts, the Jewish sages downplayed the importance of psychic powers.

Like other Eastern disciplines, the Kabbalah maintained that death is a step in evolution, that the frame of mind at the time of death is crucial for spiritual transcendence. Hence, the Rabbi Schmelke, for example, is reported to have spent his final moments "sitting erect in his chair with face serene and vision undimmed" (Newman, 1975, p. 71). On his deathbed, Rabbi Bunam remarked to his crying wife, "Why do you weep? All my life was given merely that I might learn how to die" (as cited in Newman, 1975, p. 70). Gehinnom, or the Jewish purgatory, is a realm where the soul can cleanse itself in order to evolve into a divine state. After the cleansing, the soul gravitates to its own level, determined by the individual's frame of mind during his or her earthly life. Each soul is free to create its heaven or hell. There are infinite possibilities, infinite realms, depending on the soul's spiritual texture. In a striking parallel with the Bodhisattva ideal of Buddhism, the Kabbalah asserts that a few perfectly evolved beings return to earth in order to elevate their fellow human beings.

Thus, according to both the Christian and the Jewish mystical traditions, our purpose on earth is a return to the Divine Ground; hence, we must recognize the illusory nature of everyday reality and take steps to awaken to our full potential.

THE HINDU AND BUDDHIST TRADITIONS

Meditation techniques based on concentration antedate the Buddha and probably were devised by the Upanishadic philosophers and the wandering *samanas* (Hindu ascetics). Patanjali's Yoga Sutras are a quintessential example of concentrative meditation (Prabhavananda & Isherwood, 1969). Objects of concentrative meditation, whether visual symbols or verbal chants/formulas, share certain characteristics. The lotus as well as the cross evoke the idea of a center. This center is conceived not only as a point of balance but also as a source of emanation— fire and light emit energy, plant symbols emit growth, so do the cross and the *mandala* (Naranjo & Ornstein, 1971). The center of the lotus or the *mandala* also evokes notions of supreme emptiness—death defying as well as death affirming. The *kasina* (an object of meditation) and the *mandala* also express order and lawfulness. Naranjo and Ornstein (1971) saw the *mandala* also as an expression of conformity to God's will or surrender to *Dharma* (Universal Law). The idea of a center as a source of growth and emanation, whose intrinsic quality is emptiness, expresses the innermost core of our being.

A different concentration exercise was employed by the Hindu saint Ramana Maharishi to penetrate the fog of ignorance surrounding the self. His disciples used the question, "Who am I?" somewhat as a koan to break through to a new understanding of their essential nature. Concentration on the "I" thought and tracing its source to its most subtle beginnings eventually leads to *samadhi*, the subtle state of consciousness of the *jivan-mukta*, the liberated being.

A concentrative exercise used in Yoga is the chanting of *mantras*. A *mantra* is a "combination of sacred syllables which forms a nucleus of spiritual energy" (Radha, 1980, p. 3). The chanting and repetition of the *mantra* supposedly activates a creative spiritual current. According to Radha, every *mantra* has five aspects: a *rishi*, or sage, who revealed the *mantra* as a channel for the flow of grace; the *raga*, or melody (a sequence of sounds); the *devata*, or presiding deity of the *mantra*; the *bija*, which is the seed and essence of the *mantra*; and the *kilaka* (pillar), which is the steadfastness needed by the adept when uttering the *mantra*.

Mantras are passed down from *guru* to disciple, a specific *mantra* for each individual. A specific time is set aside for reciting the *mantra*. It is done in any one of four ways: When the *mantra* is uttered loudly, it is called *Vaikhasi japa;* when whispered, it is *Uparusu japa;* when repeated mentally, *Manasika japa;* when written, *Likhita japa.* The goal is to concentrate on the *mantra* to the exclusion of everything else.

The cosmic sound *"OM,"* the supposed origin of all other sounds, is the most famous of *mantras.* The repetition of a divine name is also considered efficacious. In the West, the chant *"Hare Krishna, Hare Krishna, Krishna Krishna, Hare Hare, Hare Rama, Hare Ramam Rama Rama, Hare Hare"* has been made familiar by the disciples of Swami Prabhupada. The *Hare Krishna* group stems from the orthodox *bhakti* tradition of Hinduism, which prescribes that the object of devotion should become one's central thought. The *Bhagavat Gita,* a sacred book of the Hindus, recommends the chanting of Lord Krishna's name as the method par excellence; however, one may choose any divine being as a devotional object. One must then strive to maintain the name or thought of the deity in one's mind at all times. This practice, called *japa,* may be aided by a rosary, linking recitation to breathing, etc. The goal is one-pointedness of mind wherein one thought alone invades and consumes every corner of the mind.

The silent repetition of a *mantra* in order to achieve one-pointedness of mind is also the basis of the transcendental meditation technique made famous by Maharishi Mahesh Yogi. He described the focal narrowing of attention on a meditation object and the later transcendence of this object as "turning the attention inward towards the subtler levels of a thought until the mind transcends the experience of the subtlest state of the thought and arrives at the source of thought" (Maharishi, 1969, p. 470).

Arya (1981) pointed out a *mantric* tradition within the Quran. Sufism, the mystic tradition within Islam, has close affinities to the *bhakti* tradition of Hinduism. Certainly some of the chants of the Sufis have much in common with *Mantra* Yoga. The *Zikr,* the repetition of the divine name, is an important meditative technique in Sufism. The *Zikr* involves rhythmic breathing, music, and dance. "The dance opens a door in the soul to divine influences," said the Sultan Walad, Rumi's son, "the dance is good when it arises from remembrance of the Beloved" (as cited in Rice, 1964, p. 101). In repetitive physical movements such as the Yogic *mudras* (Vyas-Dev, 1970) and the Sufi dances of the dervishes (Trimingham, 1971), attention is centered on the movements. The process of attending to postures and gestures is similar to focusing on visual images or chanting.

The Buddha practiced these concentrative Yogic exercises, but *Nirvana* still eluded him. Hence, he devised *vipassana* (insight) meditation, which utilizes attention and vigilance and leads to full liberation of mind, to *Nirvana*. *Vipassana* has been called the light that reveals the truth of the impermanence, impersonality, and painfulness of all aspects of phenomenal existence (Nyanatiloka, 1950). In its essence, *vipassana* consists of attending to all experiences and states under the aspect of their impermanence, impersonality, and painfulness. Hence, even after attaining the *jhanas* (trance states), the meditator should understand through *vipassana* introspection that the *jhanic* states are not completely free of *samsaric* (literally, wheel of birth and death) qualities. "The trance mode, rapt away from the flux of ordinary consciousness, as a 'peaceful abiding' may seem to the meditator to be *Nibbanic* realization itself. Therefore the *vipassana* method must be applied to the *jhanic* experience *especially*" (King, 1980, p. 95). In the classic Buddhist meditational structure, *vipassana* understanding of all body-mind experiences, "including the *jhanic*, as impermanent, painful and impersonal, is to be directly applied to the *jhanic* states subsequent to their attainment. And the *jhanic* and *vipassanic* progressions together lead on to the crowning attainment of cessation" (King, 1980, p. 116).

Since *vipassana* understanding—that everything, including *jhanic* states, is impersonal, impermanent, and sorrowful—alone provides the liberating wisdom leading to *Nirvana*, *vipassana* methods by themselves, without *jhanic* practices, are considered sufficient for enlightenment. In fact, several prominent Buddhist meditation centers today use *vipassana* techniques alone.

In actual meditative practice, *vipassana* understanding may be applied to any ongoing body-mind activity. In the *Satipatthana Sutta* (Discourse on Mindfulness; see King, 1980), the Buddha instructed the meditator to attend to the impermanence, impersonality, and painfulness of bodily movements, feelings, thought processes, breathing, and tactile sensations. This mindfulness meditation should always be contextualized by the *vipassana* understanding of impersonality, impermanence, and sorrow. Used thus, mindfulness meditation is a dynamic *vipassana* method leading directly to enlightenment (Kutz, Borysenko, & Benson, 1985).

PSYCHOPHYSIOLOGY OF THE MEDITATIVE STATE

One problem that bedevils the researcher is the rarity of occurrence of the genuine mystical experience. Not only are authentic mystics a rare species, but the mystical experience is also transient, often lasting only minutes (Bucke, 1901). Consequently, the psychophysiological studies of meditation draw heavily upon experimental studies of meditation in normal subjects (most of the studies on transcendental meditation come under this category), in yogis, and in practitioners of Zen, who may be experiencing an ASC less profound than authentic mystical experience. Nevertheless, there are pillars of convergence in the accounts of mystics as well as experimental subjects. Presumably the two experiences share certain characteristics. However, a caveat is in order: The physiological correlates of the true mystical experience may well differ from those of the meditative experience that is accessible to scientific scrutiny.

Davidson (1976), Woolfolk (1975), and Delmonte (1985) offered excellent reviews of the psychophysiological effects of meditation. These effects are reviewed next.

Cardiopulmonary Responses

Significant decreases in respiration, heart rate, oxygen consumption and carbon dioxide elimination, arterial blood lactate titer and minute volume have been recorded in meditators (Davidson, 1976).

The earliest recorded measurements of the meditative state were conducted in 1935 by the French cardiologist Therese Brosse (cited in Pelletier & Garfield, 1976). But systematic investigation into the physiological correlates of meditation was launched more than 20 years later when Bagchi and Wenger (1957) reported on the autonomic functions of yogis. They found a lowering of the rate of respiration during meditation. In a later study, Wenger and Bagchi (1961) found the respiration rate to be lower during meditation than during relaxation. Anand, Chinna, and Singh (1961b) observed significant decreases in oxygen consumption during meditation in an airtight box.

Nevertheless, the oft-quoted studies by Wenger, Bagchi, and Anand (1961, 1963) did not find consistent changes in heart rate among meditating yogis. Despite their claims, the yogis were unable to stop the heart; however, they were able to slow their hearts by means of the so-called Valsalva maneuver (expiratory movement with the glottis closed and consequent reduction in venous return to the cardiac chambers) (Anand & Chinna, 1961).

It must be mentioned that such conscious control of the heart rate and blood pressure is well known to biofeedback researchers, who explained it in terms of operant conditioning of the autonomic nervous system (ANS) control of cardiac function (Obrist, Webb, Sutterer, & Howard, 1970).

The studies of Wenger et al. (1961, 1963) on meditating yogis showed a reduced respiratory frequency but bound no consistent changes in heart rate or blood pressure. The authors of the studies concluded that

(1) the control of autonomic functions is probably through voluntary mechanisms and (2) that meditation is a deep relaxation of the ANS.

In a study of Zen monks, Sugi and Akutsu (1968) noted a 20% decrease in oxygen consumption during meditation. This finding is supported by Akishige (1968) and Hirai (1960).

A dramatic drop in respiration rate—a 50% reduction—relative to a basal rate, recorded while the subject was watching television, was observed by Allison (1970) in a one-subject study involving transcendental meditation (TM). Wallace (1970) noted a 20% decrease in oxygen consumption in his TM subjects. But, the statistical analysis of his findings is inadequate. In a later study (Wallace, Benson, & Wilson, 1971), the subjects served as their own controls. The results showed marginally significant decreases in oxygen consumption and respiration rate during meditation.

The findings of Wallace et al. (1971) are summarized below:

1. There was a decrease in total oxygen consumption.
2. Cardiac output showed a mean decrease of 25%.
3. Brain wave patterns suggested a state of restful alertness.
4. There was an increase in galvanic skin response (GSR) (which is inversely related to stress).
5. There was a decrease in lactate ion concentration (increases in lactate ion concentration suggest fatigue).

Based on these findings, Wallace et al. asserted that the physiological changes in TM are different from those occurring in dream, sleep, and waking states. Wallace et al. contended that, during meditation, their subjects entered the fourth major state of consciousness—transcendental consciousness.

However, the lack of valid controls and the inadequacy of the statistical analyses cast doubt on their claims. Wallace conceded the difficulties in the selection and measurement of yogic subjects (Pelletier & Garfield, 1976). This factor alone could account for the conflicting results in the research into the psychophysiology of meditation.

Electrodermal Changes

Changes in skin resistance have been linked to stress (Mundy-Castle & McKiever, 1953). Bagchi and Wenger (1957) reported that palmar skin resistance increased during periods of meditation. In a later study, Wenger and Bagchi (1961) compared the response of yoga practitioners during meditation with responses taken during a relaxation period. The palmar skin resistance was greater during meditation. Woolfolk (1975) proposed that these findings are not reliable since postural differences were involved. During meditation, the subjects sat in the lotus position; during the relaxation periods, they reclined. Karambelkar, Vinekar, and Bhole (1968) failed to confirm differences between meditating yogis and controls on measures of skin resistance.

In his study of Zen monks, Akishige (1968) found a decrease in spontaneous skin conductance during *zazen*. Wallace (1970), in his study of TM practitioners, observed a significant increase in palmar skin resistance during TM. Wallace et al. (1971) confirmed these findings. Orme-Johnson (1973) cited two studies that investigated the stability of skin resistance as an effect of TM. In the first study, GSR habituation to aversive auditory stimuli was noted in both meditators and controls. However, the GSR habituated faster in meditators. Also, in a test of GSR stability, meditators had fewer spontaneous GSR fluctuations during meditation than did controls during rest. The second Orme-Johnson study replicated these findings: The GSR of meditators was more stable during meditation than that of resting controls. West (1979) found that his meditating subjects showed a significant decrease in spontaneous skin conductance responses. Together, these findings suggest greater behavioral stability.

Electroencephalographic Effects

Electroencephalographic (EEG) changes during meditation were reported by Anand, Chinna, and Singh (1961a), Das and Gastaut (1955), and Kasamatsu and Hirai (1966). Wallace et al. (1971) offered a scanty report on EEG changes in TM practitioners. Banquet (1973) wrote a detailed report complete with spectral analysis.

The most common findings include changes in the incidence of the alpha wave (8–13 Hz). The highest incidence of alpha is found in the waking state, when recordings are made from occipital leads when the subject sits quietly with eyes closed (Davidson, 1976). Lynch, Paskewitz, and Orne (1974) claimed that further increases are not possible even with biofeedback training involving alpha. The processes yielding high alpha presumably are similar in both meditation and biofeedback—that is, the processes disinhibit stimuli that block alpha frequencies. Banquet (1973) found that the alpha produced during meditation extended to the eyes-open postmeditation situation. Akishige (1968, 1970) reported increased alpha in all regions of the scalp where EEG measurements were taken. He also found increases in the amplitude of alpha and a decrease in the frequency of alpha.

Anand et al. (1961a) measured the scalp EEG of yogis during the state of *samadhi* (transcendence). All the yogis studied showed prominent alpha patterns in their resting EEGs. In deep meditation the alpha wave became persistent with increase in amplitude. External alpha-blocking stimulation—strong light, banging noise, tuning fork, and touching with a hot glass tube—was presented before and during meditation, and the effect on the EEG was recorded. When the yogis were not meditating, the external stimulation blocked alpha, changing it to low-voltage fast activity. But, when the yogis were in *samadhi*, the stimuli did not block the alpha pattern.

The appearance of the theta waves (4–7 Hz) has been reported by Wallace et al. (1971), Kasamatsu and Hirai (1966), and Banquet (1973). In Zen monks, the theta train appeared only in long-term practitioners (15–20 years). In an attempt to ascertain if the EEG recordings reflected changes in consciousness, Banquet tried to correlate the EEG data with subjective changes as reported by his subjects. His subjects were instructed to signal changes in consciousness by pressing a button, using a predetermined code to distinguish between the occurrence of bodily sensations, visual imagery, deep meditation, and the state of transcendence. The signaling of the last two stages was correlated with generalized fast frequencies of beta. Das and Gastaut (1955) reported similar findings in yogis. The fast patterns were of high amplitude in one who claimed to have reached the state of *samadhi.*

In the study by Kasamatsu and Hirai (1966), the EEG was recorded continuously before, during, and after *zazen.* Throughout, the meditators had their eyes open. The subjects—48 in all—were Zen masters and disciples of both Soto and Rinzai sects. They varied in age from 24 to 72 years. They were classified as disciples or priests according to the number of years spent in Zen training. The controls—22 in all—had no experience in Zen; their EEGs also were recorded with eyes open.

In Zen masters (priests with over 20 years of training) alpha waves of 40–50 MV, 11–12 seconds, appeared within 50 seconds. After 8 minutes and 20 seconds, the amplitude increased to 60–70 MV; after 27 minutes and 10 seconds, rhythmical waves of 7–8 seconds appeared for 2 seconds. Twenty seconds later, theta trains (70–90 MV, 6–7 seconds) made their appearance. The alpha waves persisted for 2 minutes after meditation ended. No such changes were seen in the EEG of controls.

This pattern of EEG changes was not present in all Zen students. Kasamatsu and Hirai (1966) classified the EEG changes in Zen meditation into four stages:

Stage 1: appearance of alpha despite open eyes

Stage 2: increase in amplitude of alpha

Stage 3: decrease in alpha frequency

Stage 4: appearance of rhythmical theta (this does not always appear)

The more years spent in Zen training, the more the EEG changed. There was also a close relationship between the degree of EEG changes and the Zen master's rating of his disciples' mental status. Kasamatsu and Hirai (1966) asserted that the EEG changes in Zen meditation are different from those observed in hypnosis and sleep.

The pattern of alpha in Zen meditation suggested lowered vigilance (Mundy-Castle, 1958; Mundy-Castle & McKiever, 1953). Alpha waves seem to reflect hypofunction of the brain (Lindsley, 1952). Zen meditation may well lead to a decrease in metabolism, which may in turn alter the EEG. The decrease in respiration, total volume, and oxygen consumption during Zen meditation seems consistent with the hypothesis of decrease in energy metabolism (Hirai, 1960; Sugi & Akutsu, 1968).

Woolfolk (1975) offered a balanced summary of the existing research. According to Woolfolk,

> [The various studies] have thus far failed to verify an easily replicable, special "state" of meditation with physiological concomitants that are consistent across the various esoteric traditions. This is not surprising in view of the fact that extra-technical factors inherent in the training of meditators and laboratory situational factors have tended to be quite diverse. These problems are particularly evident in studies of Indian Yoga, while the research on TM and Zen has yielded a much more consistent picture. This research indicates meditation to be associated with a slowing and increased synchronization of electrocortical rhythms, an increased or more stable SR, and slower rate of respiration. These changes are all in the direction of lowered arousal and suggest a diminishing of energy metabolism. (p. 1331)

MEDITATION AND PERSONALITY CHANGE

Maupin (1965) made one of the first attempts to ascertain the psychological correlates of meditation. His subjects practiced *zazen* for 45 minutes daily for 3 weeks. At the conclusion of every session, each subject reported his or her experience, and this response to *zazen* was rated as low, moderate, or high. The responses were correlated with premeditation measures of digitspan, tolerance for unrealistic experience (determined by using Rorschach), and capacity for adaptive regression (also determined by using Rorschach). The term "adaptive regression" is used to describe the psychodynamic mechanisms through which people tap their unconscious experience of the inner self.

Significant correlations were found between tolerance for unrealistic experience and the capacity for adaptive regression as measured by the Rorschach test and by the responses of subjects to *zazen*. Maupin (1965) concluded that the practice of meditation may facilitate adaptive regression. A study by Curtin (1973) showing that TM increases one's capacity for adaptive regression lent some support to Maupin's conclusion.

Orme-Johnson's (1971) study showed that TM practitioners are less irritable than nonmeditators. When a sudden stressor is presented, the amplitude of the galvanic skin response (GSR) decreases sharply for a few seconds and then returns to basal levels. Habituation occurs as a result of repeated presentations. Orme-Johnson's study showed that when meditators and nonmeditators were subjected repeatedly to loud noises, the meditators ceased reacting earlier than did nonmeditators. When the nonmeditators who had shown the largest number of GSR fluctuations were instructed in TM, their rate of fluctuation dropped.

Shapiro (1975) investigated the effect of TM on measures of negative personality characteristics (e.g., depression and neuroticism), anxiety, and self-actualization. Using the Northridge Developmental Scale (NDS) and the State-Trait Anxiety Inventory (STAI) A-Trait Scale, Shapiro found: (1) a highly significant change in the direction of greater self-actualization for the whole group; (2) significant changes on all NDS scales measuring negative personality characteristics, such as aggression, depression, and neuroticism; and (3) a highly significant reduction in anxiety as measured by the STAI.

The phenomenological experience of Zen meditators has been investigated through the use of structured interviews with 10 highly persistent meditators between the ages of 25 and 35 who were not taking drugs, were not in therapy, and had never been hospitalized for psychiatric reasons (Kirschner, 1975). Results indicated that subjects attributed several important life changes to the practice of *zazen:* They claimed to be more intimate with and less fearful of people; they stated that they had more energy for work, were more relaxed, and less susceptible to depression; and they reported that they had become more conscious of diet, exercise, and posture, and hence had giving up smoking, drinking, and the use of drugs since the beginning of their practice.

That the regular practice of meditation might eliminate the cigarette-smoking habit was suggested by Ottens (1974). He assigned subjects randomly to one of three groups: transcendental meditation (TM) ($n = 18$); self-control (SC) ($n = 18$); and no treatment ($n = 18$). The TM group practiced meditation daily; the SC group members were given information relating to smoking and participated in a group session designed to break the habit. Both the TM and the SC groups significantly reduced their cigarette consumption, but the differences between the two groups were so small that it was impossible to conclude that one treatment was more effective than the other. Hence Ottens recommended TM as an alternative strategy for modifying the cigarette-smoking habit.

Using the Tennessee Self-Concept Scale (TSCS) and the State-Trait Anxiety Inventory (revised form), Berkowitz (1977) assessed the effect of TM on self-concept and trait anxiety. He found that meditators showed a significant reduction in anxiety as well as improvements (short of significance) in self-concept. Significant positive changes in self-concept have been reported by Valois (1975) and Kongtawng (1977). Kongtawng's subjects—20 in the experimental group, 20 controls—were administered the TSCS twice over a 2-month period. The meditators, who practiced *vipassana* meditation, showed significantly greater positive change in self-concept than the nonmeditators.

Further confirmation of these results was obtained from Willis's (1979) study of the effect of TM on self-concept. Analysis of data on the TSCS was accomplished by a series of groups-by-trials and analysis of variance in which group membership was based on type of treatment (control or experimental), while trial was based on time of testing (pretest and posttest).

A significant difference between groups was found on net conflict, total positive, self-satisfaction, moral-ethical self, family self, social self, general maladjustment, personality disorder, psychosis, personality integration, and a number of deviant sign scales. A significant difference between trials was found on total positive, self-satisfaction, personal self, family self, variability, defensive positive, personality disorder, and neurosis scale. A significant group-by-trials interaction was found in a number of deviant sign scales.

Meditation seems to provide worthwhile and valuable changes in self-actualizing values (Blanz, 1973; Polowniak, 1973; Riddle, 1979) and also to promote an internal locus of control (Dice, 1979). Dick (1973) offered tentative support for the view that the practice of meditation may enhance the university counselee's sense of well-being as revealed in perception of locus of control.

Meditation has also been found to reduce state anxiety (Marron, 1973; Delmonte, 1986), trait anxiety (Rios, 1979), and test anxiety (Comer, 1977; Diner, 1978). However, it should be mentioned that several authors (Rogers & Livingston, 1977; Williams, Francis, & Durham, 1976) have reported that those attracted to meditation are significantly more anxious and neurotic than the normal population in the first place.

From an integrative "meta-analysis," involving 50 experimental studies with a total of 9,700 subjects and 400 outcome findings, Ferguson (1980) concluded that the treatment effects of TM produce a moderate effect outcome in both clinical and academic settings. These effects are consistent in highly controlled experimental conditions. Other meditation techniques produce marginal treatment effects.

Theory and research suggest that during meditative states of consciousness, change and transformation are experienced as basic features of reality. Hence meditators might be expected to show less death anxiety than nonmeditators. Support for this hypothesis comes from a study by Curtis (1980). Curtis's recommendation that mediation might be efficacious in reducing death anxiety in the aged and dying seems to have been taken to heart by Carson (1974). Eighteen elderly subjects (60 to 86 years of age) were taught *zazen* for 6 weeks in an effort to determine the effects of meditation on death anxiety, depression, physical symptomatology, and decreased ability to process perceptual input—all common problems of the elderly. Carson concluded that increased relaxation, increased ability to contend with threatening environmental events, and increased interest in inner psychic events are the benefits of *zazen* in the elderly.

Meditators also may show greater moral maturity than nonmeditators. Evidence for this was obtained by Nidich (1975) in an investigation of TM's relationship to Kohlberg's (1981) stages of moral reasoning. It was hypothesized that TM practitioners would score significantly higher than nonmeditators on Kohlberg's moral development scale, as determined by moral maturity and stage scores; that long-term meditators would score higher on Kohlberg's scale than short-term meditators; and that there would be no significant difference between nonmeditators not predisposed to beginning TM and premeditators interested in immediately beginning TM.

Kohlberg's Moral Judgment Interview was administered to 20 nonmeditators, 10 premeditators, and 96 meditators. The meditators were divided into six subgroups according to the length of time they had practiced TM (which ranged from 1 to 3 1/2 years). All of the subjects, both males and females, were middle-class undergraduates between the ages of 18 and 24. All tests were sent to Harvard's Moral Development Center to be scored by an expert scorer.

Results showed that meditators' scores of moral maturity were significantly higher than those of nonmeditators. Meditators exhibited significantly less preconventional (Stage 2) thinking and significantly more conventional (Stage 4) thinking than nonmeditators. No significant differences were found between the six subgroups of meditators. No significant differences were found between nonmeditators and premeditators on moral maturity and stage scores. It was concluded that a positive relationship existed between the practice of TM and moral development, as measured by Kohlberg's scale.

Russie (1975) investigated the effectiveness of TM as a psychotherapeutic agent of positive mental health and self-actualization. He found that TM was an effective tool for

1. Changing an individual's time-orientation in the direction of living more in the "here and now"
2. Increasing the individual's behavioral motivation toward more inner-directedness
3. Developing sensitivity to one's own needs and feelings
4. Improving the individual's ability to express feelings spontaneously
5. Increasing self-acceptance
6. Raising the individual's level of self-actualization

Cowger (1973) reported the effects of *zazen* on selected dimensions of personal development among college students and confirmed Russie's findings:

1. Meditating college undergraduates became more present-oriented, independent, and self-supportive.
2. Meditation was an effective means of assisting individuals in dimensions of self-actualization.

Moles (1977) examined the effects of focused attention, as practiced in Zen meditation, on various ego functions: reality testing, impulse control, sense of reality of self and world, adaptive regression, defensive functions, thought processes, and synthetic-integrative functions. His results showed that Zen meditation led to a movement away from a normal conceptual-verbal mode of psychic function to one characterized as a passive-receptive mode based more on visual imagery. He attributed these changes to destablization and deautomatizations of ego functions due to a change in deployment of attention. His subjects—naïve college students—were divided into three groups: experimental Group 1 practiced *zazen* for 30 minutes for 4 weeks; experimental Control Group 2 sat upright but did not alter the normal model of attention deployment; Control Group 3 was not subjected to any treatment but took pretest and posttest measures.

Tests administered included the Free Association Text (to assess visual imagery in consciousness), the Holtzmann Inkblot Technique (to assess reality testing, impulse control, adaptive regression, defensive functions, and thought processes), and the Personal Orientation Inventory (to assess synthetic-integrative functions).

An adaptive regression score, a measure of ego strength, was computed for all subjects. The capacity for adaptive regression distinguished between subjects who were or were not able to allow for regression in the service of the ego. Subjects with a high adaptive regression score exhibited evidence of adaptive regression, while those with low scores did not. Moles (1977) interpreted his results to suggest that subjects go through an initial process in which they experience enhancement in awareness of body image and body boundaries, an ego-strengthening process that prepares the individual for regression. The results, he said, represent an opening to normally unconscious aspects of personality rather than the oscillating regression mentioned in psychoanalytic literature. No changes were apparent in reality testing, impulse control, defensive functions, and synthetic-integrative functions.

Finally, one other study of the effect of meditation on personality must be mentioned. Gaston de Grace (1976) investigated the effect of Zen meditation on personality and values. His subjects, 14 men and 14 women, were chosen from volunteers who were first-year students in the undergraduate psychology program at the University of Laval. These subjects had had no prior training in or exposure to meditation. Seven men and seven women were randomly assigned to the experimental group that was instructed in Zen meditation. The others were the control group and were taught meditation only after the experiment was concluded.

Two tests, the California Psychological Inventory, which is a measure of personality, and the Vos Tendances Personnelles (Allport, Vernon, & Shevenell, 1962), which is a measure of values, were used. An analysis of the results showed that the meditators became "less aggressive, less persistent, less manipulative, and verbal, less independent and playful than the nonmeditators. Furthermore, they also became less ambitious, less preoccupied with their future and less interested in the various aspects of social life than the Ss of the CG" (de Grace, 1976, p. 811). De Grace pointed out that these findings are in accord with the goals of Zen as outlined by Suzuki (1956):

Indeed, Zen strives to reduce distances that separate beings and that are the result of too strong an ego, a tendency to manipulate, difficulties in relating to others as a S and a too analytical and verbal mode of viewing and expressing reality; these distances are also the result of too great an importance attached to personal history and desires and a refusal to accept that things change as well as an inability to live fully in the here and now. (de Grace, 1976, p. 811)

MEDITATION AS DEAUTOMATIZATION

Meditative states generally have been explained in terms of regression. Franz Alexander (1931) described meditation as the withdrawal of libido from the world. Freud (1961) stated that the "oceanic feeling" is the memory of an undifferentiated infantile ego state. More recently, meditation has been explained as a turning off of awareness and a process of deautomatization. Whether a symbol is used, or a *mantra*, or body movement, or mental contemplation, thee is a concerted attempt to restrict awareness. Naranjo and Ornstein (1971) saw this as an attempt to recycle the same routine in the nervous system.

Experimental work on stablized images and the *ganzfield* show that when an image is focused steadily on the retina, it disappears. Ganzfield subjects report an experience of "not seeing" after only 15 minutes of exposure (Cohen, 1957; Pritchard, Heron, & Hebb, 1960).

Hartmann (1958) first used the word *"automatization"* to describe the phenomenon that in the formation of perceptual and motor habits considerable amounts of attentional energy are required at first, but subsequently the process becomes automatic and results in savings in energy.

Deikman (1963, 1966a) used the concept to explain perceptual changes described by subjects of experimental meditation. He explained mystic states from the point of view of attentional mechanisms in perception and cognition. According to Deikman (1966b), mystic phenomena are the result of deautomatization of psychological processes that organize, select, and interpret perceptual stimuli.

There are two attentional strategies in meditation that can be explained in terms of alterations in attentional mechanisms. During concentration, the turning off of awareness is accomplished by holding a specific mental device while at the same time excluding every other thought, image, and perception. It is this attentional retraining that produces the meditation-induced altered states whose cardinal feature is the total banishment from awareness of normal acts of perception and cognition (Goleman, 1976). Mindfulness is the next attentional strategy that is deployed during meditation. It involves noting each mental context or event dispassionately. Whenever a reaction arises to any mental content, this, too, is noted but neither pursued nor rejected.

Thus mindfulness serves as a powerful tool for dishabituation of habitual and stereotyped response patterns.

Deautomatization also involves a movement toward a more primitive cognitive organization. Werner (1957) has described primitive imagery—the perceptual and cognitive functioning of people in primitive societies—as (1) more vivid and sensuous, (2) syncretic, (3) animated, (4) dedifferentiated with respect to the distinctions between self and object, and (5) characterized by a dedifferentiation and fusion of sense modalities (as cited in Deikman, 1969).

It will immediately strike the reader that the experience of unity so frequently mentioned in mystic literature is actually a dedifferentiation of self and the world. The impression that the world and its contents are more vivid and sensorily rich is a prominent feature of mystic experience. Zen masters talk of seeing the world as if for the first time: The grass greener, the rose prettier. William James (1902, p. 244) quoted Bray, "I was like a new man in a new world." In the immortal words of Blake, the doors of perception are cleansed.

The meditation experiments of Deikman (1963) met Werner's criteria. His subjects described their reaction to the blue vase—the percept—as: (1) increased vividness and richness, (2) animation in the base, (3) decrease in self-object distinction, and (4) syncretic thought and an alteration of ordinary perceptual modes. The evidence appears to bear out Deikman's claim that contemplative meditation produces deautomatization.

This deautomatization is aided by acts of renunciation. By adopting vows of poverty, chastity, and isolation, the anchorite excludes from awareness worldly objects and desires. This exclusion of distracting stimuli from awareness tends to weaken normal perceptual and cognitive structures (Rapaport, 1951). Deikman's (1963) subjects became less responsive to distracting stimuli as their meditation proceeded. EEG studies of Zen masters show that they are minimally affected by distracting stimuli (Kasamatsu & Hirai, 1966). Sensory isolation experiments show that deprivation of a class of stimuli causes changes in the functions established to deal with those stimuli (Schultz, 1965). Thus renunciation aids in deautomatization.

CONCLUDING REMARKS

The research discussed so far strongly suggests that the meditative state is an altered state of consciousness that is attended by unique psychological and psychophysical effects. These effects are in the direction of reduced energy metabolism, greater cortical alertness, limbic inhibition, and a deautomatization of the attentional mechanisms involved in perception and cognition. Do these effects represent, as Alexander (1931) eloquently proclaimed, a libidinal, narcissistic turning inward, a sort of artificial schizophrenia? Or is mystical repose something quite different? "Mystical ecstasy may seem to be repose, but it is a repose like that of a locomotive standing in a station under a head of steam. Such a person has the capacity to help effect a change in humanity" (Michaelson, 1975, p. 8). This capacity is the product of a fully self-actualized life that flowers from an understanding of the ways of the self. To know the self is to be free of it. Such self-knowing is a *sine qua non* for actualizing our full potential. In losing the self, one gains a universe of possibilities. Such a transcendental expression of our full humanity is a verifiable return to an innocent Eden. Meditation systems, then, help us regain our unsullied nature, a state of grace that is in complete harmony with the Divine Ground of all substance (Goldstein & Kornfield, 1987; Goleman, 1988).

References

Akishige, Y. (Ed.). (1968). Psychological studies on Zen. *Bulletin of Faculty Literature of Kyrushu University, 5 & 11*. Fukuoka, Japan.

Akishige, Y. (Ed.). (1970). *Psychological studies on Zen*. Tokyo: Zen Institute of Komazawa University.

Alexander, F. (1931). Buddhist training as an artificial catatonia. *Psychoanalytic Review, 18*, 129–145.

Allison, J. (1970). Respiration changes during transcendental meditation. *Lancet, 1*, 833–834.

Allport, G., Vernon, P., & Shevenell, R. (1962). *Vos tendancies personnelles*. Ottawa, Canada: Presses de l'Universite de'Ottawa.

Anand, B. K., & Chinna, A. (1961). Investigation on yogis' claiming to stop their hearts. *Indian Journal of Medical Research, 49*, 90–94.

Anand, B. K., Chinna, G. S., & Singh, B. (1961a). Some aspects of electroencephalographic studies in yogis. *Electroencephalography and Clinical Neurophysiology, 13*, 452–456.

Anand, B. K., Chinna, G. S., & Singh, B. (1961b). Studies on Sri Ramanand Yogi during his stay in an airtight box. *Indian Journal of Medical Research, 49*, 82–89.

Anderson, E. (1942). Abnormal mental states in survivors, with special reference to collective hallucinations. *Journal of the Royal Navy Medical Service, 28*, 361–377.

Arya, U. (1981). *Mantra and meditation*. Honesdale, PA: Himalayan International Institute.

Bagchi, B. K., & Wenger, M. A. (1957). Electrophysiological correlates of some yogi exercises. *Journal of Electroencephalography and Clinical Neurophysiology*, 7, 132–149.

Banquet, J. P. (1973). Spectral analysis of the EEG in meditation. *Electroencephalography and Clinical Neurophysiology*, 35, 143–151.

Belo, J. (1960). *The trance in Bali.* New York: Columbia University Press.

Berkowitz, A. H. (1977). The effect of transcendental meditation on trait anxiety and self-esteem (Doctoral dissertation, University of Colorado at Boulder, 1977). *Dissertation Abstracts International*, 38, 2353B–2354B.

Blanz, L. T. (1973). Personality changes as a function of two different meditative techniques (Doctoral dissertation, University of Tennessee, 1973). *Dissertation Abstracts International*, 34, 7035A–7036A.

Bowers, M. (1959). Friend or traitor. Hypnosis in the service of religion. *International Journal of Clinical and Experimental Hypnosis*, 7, 205–217.

Bucke, R. M. (1901). *Cosmic consciousness.* Philadelphia: Dutton Books.

Capps, W. H., & Wright, W. M. (Eds.). (1978). *Silent fire: An invitation to western mysticism.* San Francisco: Harper & Row.

Carrington, P. (1977). *Freedom in meditation.* Garden City, NY: Doubleday.

Carson, L. G. (1974). Zen meditation in the elderly (Doctoral dissertation, University of Nevada, 1974). *Dissertation Abstracts International*, 36, 903B–904B.

The cloud of unknowing. (1961). (C. Wolters, Trans.). Baltimore: Penguin Books.

Cohen, W. (1957). Spatial and textural characteristics of the ganzfield. *American Journal of Psychology*, 70, 403–410.

Coleridge, S. T. (1972). Kubla Khan. In W. Empson & D. Pirie (Eds.), *Coleridge's verse: A selection.* London: Faber & Faber.

Comer, J. F., Jr. (1977). Meditation and progressive relaxation in the treatment of test anxiety (Doctoral dissertation, University of Kansas, 1977). *Dissertation Abstracts International*, 38, 6142B–6143B.

Cowger, E. L. Jr. (1973). The effects of meditation (zazen) upon selected dimensions of personal development (Doctoral dissertation, University of Georgia, 1973). *Dissertation Abstracts International*, 34, 4734A.

Curtin, T. G., (1973). The relationship between transcendental meditation and adaptive regression (Doctoral dissertation, Boston University, 1973). *Dissertation Abstracts International*, 34, 1696A.

Curtis, M. J. (1980). The relationship between bimodal consciousness, meditation and two levels of death anxiety (Doctoral dissertation, California School of Professional Psychology, Los Angeles, 1980). *Dissertation Abstracts International*, 41, 2314B.

Das, H., & Gastaut, H. (1955). Variations de l'activite electrique du cerveau, du couer et des muscles squelettiques an cours de la meditation et de l'extase Yogique. *Electroencephalography and Clinical Neurophysiology*, (Suppl. 6), 211–219.

Davidson, J. M. (1976). The physiology of meditation and mystical states of consciousness. *Perspectives in Biology and Medicine, 19*(3), 345–379.

de Grace, G. (1976). Effects of meditation on personality and values. *Journal of Clinical Psychology, 32*(4), 809–813.

Deikman, A. J. (1963). Experimental meditation. *Journal of Nervous and Mental Diseases, 136*(4), 392–473.

Deikman, A. J. (1966a). Deautomatization and the mystic experience. *Psychiatry, 29*, 324–338.

Deikman, A. J. (1966b). Implications of experimentally induced contemplative meditation. *Journal of Nervous and Mental Diseases, 142*(2), 101–116.

Deikman, A. J. (1969). Deautomatization and the mystic experience. In C. Tart (Ed.), *Altered states of consciousness*. New York: Wiley.

Delmonte, M. M. (1985). Biochemical indices associated with meditation practice: A literature review. *Neuroscience and Biobehavioral Reviews, 9*(4), 557–561.

Delmonte, M. M. (1986). Meditation as a clinical intervention strategy: A brief review. *International Journal of Psychsomatics, 33*(3), 9–12.

Deren, M. (1952). Religion and magic in Haiti. In E. Garrett (Ed.), *Beyond the five senses*. New York: Lippincott.

Dice, M. L., Jr. (1979). The effectiveness of meditation on selected measures of self-actualization (Doctoral dissertation, St. Louis University, 1979). *Dissertation Abstracts International, 40*, 2534A.

Dick, L. D. (1973). A study of meditation in the service of counseling (Doctoral dissertation, University of Oklahoma, 1973). *Dissertation Abstracts International, 34*, 4037B.

Diner, M. D. (1978). The differential effects of meditation and systematic desensitization on specific and general anxiety (Doctoral dissertation, Temple University, 1978). *Dissertation Abstracts International, 39*, 1950B.

Dodds, E. R. (1973). Tradition and personal achievement in the philosophy of Plotinus. In E. R. Dodds (Ed.), *The ancient concept of progress*. London: Oxford University Press.

Ferguson, P. C. (1980). An integrative meta-analysis of psychological studies investigating the treatment outcomes of meditation techniques (Doctoral dissertation, University of Colorado at Boulder, 1980). *Dissertation Abstracts International, 42*, 1547A.

Freud, S. (1961). *Standard edition of the complete psychological works* (Vol. 21). London: Hogarth Press.

Goldstein, J., & Kornfield, J. (1987). *Seeking the heart of wisdom: The path of insight meditation*. Boston: Shambhala.

Goleman, D. (1976). Meditation and consciousness: An Asian approach to mental health. *American Journal of Psychotherapy, 30*(1), 41–54.

Goleman, D. (1977). *The varieties of the meditative experience*. New York: Dutton.

Goleman, D. (1988). *The meditative mind*. Los Angeles: Tarcher.

Groves, P., & Schlesinger, K. (1979). *Introduction to biological psychology.* Dubuque, IA: William Brown.

Hall, E. T. (1966). *The hidden dimension.* New York: Doubleday.

Hartmann, H. (1958). *Ego psychology and the problem of adaptation.* New York: International University Press.

Hinkle, L. (1961). The physiological state of the interrogation subject as it affects brain function. In A. Biderman & H. Zimmer (Eds.), *The manipulation of human behavior.* New York: Wiley.

Hirai, T. (1960). Electroencephalographic study on the Zen meditation. *Folio Psychiatrica and Neurologica Japanica, 62,* 76–105.

Hoffman, E. (1981). *The way of splendour: Jewish mysticism and modern psychology.* Boulder, CO: Shambhala.

Hubel, D. H., & Wiesel, T. N. (1965). Receptive fields and functional architecture in two nonstriate visual areas (18 and 19) of the cat. *Journal of Neurophysiology, 28,* 229–289.

Hubel, D. H., & Wiesel, T. N. (1968). Receptive fields and functional architecture of the monkey striate cortex. *Journal of Physiology* (London), *195,* 215–243.

Huxley, A. (1954). *The doors of perception and heaven and hell.* New York: Harper & Row.

Huxley, A. (1962). *Island.* New York: Harper & Row.

Huxley, A. (1970). *The perennial philosophy.* New York: Harper & Row.

James, W. (1902). *The varieties of religious experience.* New York: The Modern Library, Random House.

Johnston, W. (1970). *The still point.* New York: Fordham University Press.

Johnston, W. (1974). *Silent music.* New York: Harper & Row.

Jones, R. M. (1971). *The flowing of mysticism.* New York: Hafner.

Julian of Norwich. (1966). *Revelations of divine love* (C. Wolters, Trans.). Baltimore: Penguin Books.

Kapleau, P. (1967). *The three pillars of Zen.* Boston: Beacon Press.

Karambelkar, P. V., Vinekar, S. L., & Bhole, M. V. (1968). Studies on human subjects staying in an airtight pit. *Indian Journal of Medical Research, 56,* 1282–1288.

Kasamatsu, A., & Hirai, T. (1966). An electroencephalographic study of the zen meditation (zazen). *Folio Psychiatria and Neurological Japanica, 20,* 315–336.

King, W. L. (1980). *Theravada meditation.* University Park: Pennsylvania State University Press.

Kirschner, S. (1975). Zen mediators: A clinical study (Doctoral dissertation, Adelphi University, 1975). *Dissertation Abstracts International, 36,* 3613B–3614B.

Knowles, D. (1961). *The English mystical tradition.* London: Burns & Oates.

Koestler, A. (1960). *The lotus and the robot.* New York: Harper & Row.

Koestler, A. (1964). *The act of creation.* New York: Macmillan.

Kohlberg, L. (1981). *The philosophy of moral development: Moral stages and the idea of justice.* San Francisco: Harper & Row.

Kongtawng, T. (1977). Effects of meditation on self-concept (Doctoral dissertation, Memphis State University, 1977). *Dissertation Abstracts International, 38,* 1230A.

Krishnamurti, J. (1954). *The first and last freedom.* London: Gollancz.

Kubie, L., & Margolin, S. (1944). The process of hypnotism and the nature of hypnotic state. *American Journal of Psychiatry, 100,* 611–622.

Kupferman, I. (1975). Neurophysiology of learning. *Annual Review of Psychology, 26,* 367–391.

Kutz, I., Borysenko, J. Z., & Benson, H. (1985). Meditation and psychotherapy: A rationale for the integration of dynamic psychotherapy, the relaxation response, and mindfulness meditation. *American Journal of Psychiatry, 142*(1), 1–8.

LaBarre, W. (1962). *They shall take up serpents.* Minneapolis: University Press.

LeShan, L. (1974). *How to meditate.* Boston: Little, Brown.

Lettvin, J. Y., Maturana, H. R., McCulloch, W. S., & Pitts, W. H. (1965). What the frog's eye tells the frog's brain. In W. S. McCulloch (Ed.), *Embodiments of mind.* Cambridge: M.I.T. Press. (Reprinted from *Proceedings of the Institute of Radio Engineers,* 1959, 47, 140–151).

Lilly, J. (1956). Discussion. In *Illustrative strategies on psychopathology in mental health, Symposium No. 2.* New York: Group for the Advancement of Psychiatry.

Lindsey, D. (1961). Common factors in sensory deprivation, sensory distortion, and sensory overload. In P. Solomon et al. (Eds.), *Sensory deprivation.* Cambridge: Harvard University Press.

Lindsley, D. (1952). Psychological phenomena and the electroencephalogram. *Electroencephalography and Clinical Neurophysiology, 4,* 443–456.

Linn, L. (1967). Clinical manifestations of psychiatric disorders. In A. M. Freedman & H. I. Kaplan (Eds.), *Comprehensive textbook of psychiatry.* Baltimore: Williams & Wilkins.

Louth, A. (1981). *The origins of the Christian mystical tradition.* Oxford: Clarendon Press.

Ludwig, A. (1964). An historical survey of the early roots of mesmerism. *International Journal of Clinical and Experimental Hypnosis, 12,* 205–217.

Ludwig, A. M. (1969). Altered states of consciousness. In C. Tart (Ed.), *Altered states of consciousness.* New York: Wiley.

Lynch, J. J., Paskewitz, D. A., & Orne, M. T. (1974). Some factors in the feedback control of human alpha rhythm. *Psychosomatic Medicine, 36*(5), 399–410.

Maharishi, M. Y. (1969). *On the Bhagavad Gita.* Baltimore: Penguin Books.

Marron, J. P. (1973). Transcendental meditation: A clinical evaluation (Doctoral dissertation, Colorado State University, 1973). *Dissertation Abstracts International, 34,* 4051B.

Matturana, H. R., Lettvin, J. Y., McCulloch, W. S., & Pitts, W. H. (1960). Anatomy and physiology of vision in the frog (*rana pipiens*). *Journal of General Physiology, 43,* 129–175.

Maupin, E. (1965). Individual differences in response to a Zen meditation exercise. *Journal of Consulting Psychology, 29,* 139–145.

Michaelson, R. S. (1975). *The American search for soul.* Baton Rouge: Louisiana State University Press.

Mischel, W., & Mischel, F. (1958). Psychological aspects of spirit possession. *American Anthropology, 60,* 249–260.

Moles, E. A., (1977). Zen meditation. A study of regression in service of the ego (Doctoral dissertation, California School of Professional Psychology, Berkeley, 1977). *Dissertation Abstracts International, 38,* 2871B–2872B.

Mundy-Castle, A. (1958). An appraisal of electroencephalography in relation to psychology. *Journal of the National Institute for Personnel Research,* (Suppl. 2), 1–43.

Mundy-Castle, A., & McKiever, B. (1953). The psychophysiological significance of the galvanic skin response. *Journal of Experimental Psychology, 45,* 15–24.

Murphy, J. (1964). Psychotherapeutic aspects of shamanism on St. Lawrence Island, Alaska. In A. Kiev (Ed.), *Magic, faith and healing.* New York: Free Press.

Naranjo, C., & Ornstein, R. (1971). *On the psychology of meditation.* New York: Viking Press.

Newman, L. I. (1975). *Hasidic anthology.* New York: Schocken.

Nidich, S. I. (1975). A study of the relationship of transcendental meditation to Kohlberg's stages of moral reasoning (Doctoral dissertation, University of Cincinnati, 1975). *Dissertation Abstracts International, 36,* 4361A.

Nyanatiloka, M. (1950). *Buddhist dictionary.* Columbia: Island Hermitage Publication, Frewin & Co.

Obrist, P. A., Webb, R. A., Sutterer, J. R., & Howard, J. L. (1970). The cardiac-somatic relationship: Some reformulations. *Psychophysiology, 6*(5), 569–587.

Orme-Johnson, D. W. (1971, August). *Transcendental meditation and autonomic liability.* Paper presented at the meeting of the First International Symposium on the Science of Creative Intelligence, Arcata, CA.

Orme-Johnson, D. W. (1973). Autonomic stability and transcendental meditation. *Psychosomatic Medicine, 35*(4), 341–349.

Orne, M. (1962). On the social psychology of the psychological experiment with particular reference to demand characteristics and their implications. *American Psychology, 17,* 776–783.

Ornstein, R. (1975). *The psychology of consciousness.* New York: Pelican Books.

Ottens, A. J. (1974). The effect of transcendental meditation upon modifying the cigarette smoking habit. *Dissertation Abstracts International, 35,* 7131A.

Otto, R. (1970). *Mysticism East and West.* New York: Macmillan.

Pelletier, K. R., & Garfield, C. (1976). *Consciousness East and West.* New York: Harper & Row.

Polowniak, W. A. (1973). The meditation-encounter-growth group (Doctoral dissertation, U. S. International University, 1973). *Dissertation Abstracts International, 34,* 1732B.

Prabhavananda, S., & Isherwood, C. (1969). *How to know God: Yoga aphorism of Patanjali.* New York: Signet.

Pribram, K. H. (1969, January). The neurophysiology of remembering. *Scientific American,* pp. 73–86.

Prince, R. (1978). Meditation: Some psychological speculation. *The Psychiatric Journal of the University of Ottawa, 3*(3), 202–209.

Pritchard, R. M., Heron, W., & Hebb, D. O. (1960). Visual perception approached by the method of stabilized images. *Canadian Journal of Psychology, 14,* 67–77.

Radha, S. S. (1980). *Mantras: Words of power.* Porthill, ID: Timeless Books.

Rapaport, D. (1951). The autonomy of the ego. *Bulletin of the Menninger Clinic, 15,* 113–123.

Ravenscroft, K. (1965). Voodoo possession: A natural experiment in hypnosis. *International Journal of Clinical and Experimental Hypnosis, 13,* 157–182.

Rice, C. (1964). *The Persian sufis.* London: Allen & Unwin.

Riddle, A. G. (1979). Effects of selected elements of meditation on self-actualization, locus of control, and trait anxiety (Doctoral dissertation, University of South Carolina, 1979). *Dissertation Abstracts International, 40,* 3419B.

Rios, R. J. (1979). The affect of hypnosis and meditation on state and trait anxiety and locus of control (Doctoral dissertation, Texas A&M University, 1979). *Dissertation Abstracts International, 40,* 5209A–6210A.

Rogers, C. A., & Livingston, D. D. (1977). Accumulative effects of periodic relaxation. *Perceptual and Motor Skills, 44,* 690.

Rumi, J. (1898). *Masnavi* (E. H. Whinfield, Trans.). London: Clarendon Press.

Russell, E. W. (1986). Consciousness and the unconscious: Eastern meditative and western psychotherapeutic approaches. *Journal of Transpersonal Psychology, 18*(1), 51–72.

Russie, R. E. (1975). The influence of transcendental meditation on positive mental health and self-actualization; and the role of expectation, rigidity, and self-control in the achievement of these benefits (Doctoral dissertation, California School of Professional Psychology, Los Angeles, 1975). *Dissertation Abstracts International, 36,* 5816B.

Sargant, W. (1957). *Battle for the mind.* Garden City, NY: Doubleday.

Schultz, D. (1965). *Sensory restriction: Effects on behavior.* New York: Academic Press.

Shapiro, J. S. (1975). The relationship of selected characteristics of transcendental meditation to measures of self-actualization, negative personality characteristics, and anxiety (Doctoral dissertation, University of Southern California, 1975). *Dissertation Abstracts International, 36,* 137A.

Snyder, E. (1930). *Hypnotic poetry.* Philadelphia: University of Pennsylvania Press.

Sugi, Y., & Akutsu, K. (1968). Studies on respiration and energy metabolism during sitting in zazen. *Research Journal of Physical Education, 12,* 190.

Suzuki, D. T. (1956). *Zen Buddhism.* Garden City, NY: Anchor Books, Doubleday.

Thompson, R. F., & Spencer, W. A. (1966). Habituation: A model phenomenon for the study of neuronal substrates of behavior. *Psychological Review, 173,* 16–43.

Trimingham, J. S. (1971). *Sufi orders in Islam.* Oxford: Clarendon Press.

Underhill, E. (1960). *The essentials of mysticism.* New York: Dutton.

Valois, M. G. (1975). The effects of transcendental meditation on the self-concept as measured by the Tennessee Self-Concept Scale (Doctoral dissertation, University of Kansas, 1975). *Dissertation Abstracts International, 37,* 208A.

Vyas-Dev, S. (1970). *First steps to higher yoga.* Gangotri, India: Yoga Niketan Trust.

Wallace, R. K. (1970). Physiological effects of transcendental meditation. *Science, 167,* 1751–1754.

Wallace, R. K., Benson, H., & Wilson, A. F. (1971). A wakeful hypometabolic physiologic state. *American Journal of Physiology, 221*(3), 795–799.

Wenger, M. A., & Bagchi, B. K. (1961). Studies of autonomic functions in practitioners of yoga in India. *Behavioral Science, 6,* 312–323.

Wenger, M. A., Bagchi, B. K., & Anand, B. K. (1961). Experiments in India on voluntary control of the heart and pulse. *Circulation, 24,* 1319–1325.

Wenger, M. A., Bagchi, B. K., & Anand, B. K. (1963). Voluntary heart and pulse control by yoga methods. *International Journal of Parapsychology, 5,* 25–41.

Werner, H. (1957). *Comparative psychology of mental development.* New York: International University Press.

West, L., Janszen, H., Lester, B., & Comelisoon, F. (1962). The psychosis of sleep deprivation. *Annals of the New York Academy of Science, 96,* 66–70.

West, M. A. (1979). Physiological effects of meditation: A longitudinal study. *British Journal of Social and Clinical Psychology, 18,* 219.

White, J. (1972). *The highest state of consciousness.* New York: Doubleday.

Williams, G. (1958). Hypnosis in perspective. In L. LeCron (Ed.), *Experimental hypnosis.* New York: Macmillan.

Williams, P., Francis, A., & Durham, R. (1976). Personality and meditation. *Perceptual and Motor Skills, 43,* 787.

Willis, R. J. (1979). Meditation to fit the person: Psychology and the meditative way. *Journal of Religion and Health, 18*(2), 93–119.

Woolfolk, R. L. (1975). Psychophysiological correlates of meditation. *Archives of General Psychiatry, 32,* 1326–1333.

16

Healing Images: From Ancient Wisdom to Modern Science

ANEES A. SHEIKH
ROBERT G. KUNZENDORF
KATHARINA S. SHEIKH

In the early days of the Meiji era, there lived a well-known wrestler called O-nami, Great Waves. O-nami was immensely strong and knew the art of wrestling. In his private bouts, he defeated even his teacher, but in public he was so bashful that his own pupils threw him.

O-nami felt he should go to a Zen master for help. Hakuju, a wandering teacher, was stopping in a little temple nearby, so O-nami went to see him and told him his trouble. "Great Waves is your name," the teacher advised, "so stay in this temple tonight. Imagine that you are those billows. You are no longer a wrestler who is afraid. You are those huge waves sweeping everything before them, swallowing all in their path. Do this and you will be the greatest wrestler in the land."

The teacher retired. O-nami sat in meditation trying to imagine himself as waves. He thought of many different things. Then gradually he turned more and more to the feeling of the waves. As the night advanced the waves became larger and larger. They swept away the flowers in their vases. Even the Buddha in the shrine was inundated. Before dawn the temple was nothing but the ebb and flow of an immense sea.

In the morning the teacher found O-nami meditating, a faint smile on his face. He patted the wrestler's shoulder. "Now nothing can disturb you," he said. "You are those waves. You will sweep everything before you."

The same day O-nami entered the wrestling contests and won. After that, no one in Japan was able to defeat him.

Zen Flesh, Zen Bones,
Compiled by P. Reps, 1957, pp. 25–26

The ancient literature of numerous cultures abounds with accounts of spectacular cures resulting from the imaging process. These accounts are now being corroborated by a growing body of clinical and experimental evidence. The effectiveness of mental imagery in the treatment of a wide variety of problems has been documented (Sheikh, 1983). These include: obesity (Bornstein & Sipprelle, 1973), insomnia (Sheikh, 1976), phobias and anxieties (Habeck & Sheikh, 1984; Meichenbaum, 1977; Singer, 1974), depression (Schultz, 1984), sexual malfunctions (Singer & Switzer, 1980), chronic pain (Jaffe & Bresler, 1980; Korn & Johnson, 1983), fibroid tumors (Pickett, 1987–1988), cancer (Hall, 1984), and a host of other ailments (Sheikh, 1984).

This chapter will outline the use of imagery in various ancient traditions, as well as in Western medical practice; it will review current imagery-based therapeutic approaches; it will summarize some of the most significant recent scientific research on the physiological consequences of the imaging process; and it will conclude with some observations about the role of imagery in healing.

HEALING IMAGES: ANCIENT WISDOM

Many believe that in the beginning our universe was completely sacred and that humans were an integral part of it (Eliade, 1959; Samuels & Samuels, 1975). Their existence consisted of participating in the endless dance of creation, carefully examining its steps, resonating with its rhythm, and exploring its many meanings. Humans sought solitude to contemplate the multiple facets of the self and they also sought companionship. They intuitively understood that humans and all other aspects of the universe, the animals, plants, minerals, and stars, issued from the same spring and were one. They knew life and death but did not distinguish between them. Consciousness was not restricted to the self but echoed the heartbeat of the entire universe. Within this context, health consisted simply of being in harmony with creation (Scholem, 1961).

Over time, this sense of unity with the universe was lost; the feeling of the interrelation and interdependence of all things faded from human consciousness. There now was an abyss separating individuals from God, or, in Judeo-Christian terms, they had been driven from the Garden of Eden. They experienced loneliness and anxiety; their quest for a return to the state of grace is called "mysticism" (Scholem, 1961).

The basic means that mystics have used to regain the state of unity and to experience the ecstasy produced by it are ascetic practices and visualization. Shamanism is an ancient form of mysticism.

Shamanism and Imagery

Shaman is derived from the Russian *saman*, which means "ascetic." The concept of the shaman, which encompasses the notions of priest, healer, and magician, is at least 20,000 years old and is found among the people of all continents. Also, shamanistic practices are remarkably similar across cultures (Achterberg, 1985). Basically they consist of healing by imagination or, more specifically, by using visualization to bridge the gulf between the individual and the universe. Eliade (1964) has called the shaman "the great master of ecstasy" and has defined shamanism as the "technique of ecstasy."

In primitive societies, where shamanism flourished, sacred and secular aspects of life were thoroughly integrated. Hence the shamans were equally involved with such diverse affairs as raising crops, waging war, performing marriages, and providing spiritual guidance. In short, they used their power to assist the community in whatever area a need arose.

The shamans were both priest and doctor. They were concerned both with the spirit and with the body because they considered the two to be aspects of one integrated organism. Obviously the current dominant belief among Western physicians that mind and body are separate entities stands in radical opposition to the shamanic stance. Modern scientists generally look upon the body independently of the spirit. Disease is an external agent, something against which one should protect oneself; failing that, disease is something that should be removed or destroyed through technological intervention. The shamans not only knew of no reason to isolate the spirit from the body, but they even recognized the danger of doing so. In their view, the primary problem was not the pathological change in the body but the decrease in personal power that led to the intrusion of disease. In other words, disease was a concrete manifestation of a spiritual crisis. Hence the shamans' first course of treatment for all ailments consisted of an attempt to build up the patient's power; only then would they begin to deal with the bodily symptoms. For instance, among the Navaho Indians, elaborate concrete visualizations are used to bolster the patient's spiritual resources. This rite, in which a number of people participate, encourages the patient to visualize himself or herself as healthy, and it aids the healer to visualize the patient regaining a harmonious place (Achterberg, 1985; Samuels & Samuels, 1975).

The shamans' primary focus was not bodily well-being but spiritual health. They were not primarily concerned with prolonging life, but rather with improving its quality by restoring harmony. Their interest in disease sprang from their belief that illness pointed to a spiritual crisis. If it was handled incompetently, it could be destructive; however, it also could become the springboard for personal growth and vision. According to shamanic tradition, a person's reason for being is to be initiated into the realm of the spirit and thereafter to live in harmony with the rest of the universe. The ultimate disaster is the loss of one's soul, for it robs life of all meaning forevermore (Achterberg, 1985; Grossinger, 1980; La Barre, 1938, 1979).

The shamans' primary mission was to nurture the soul and to protect it from going astray; thus they often described their role in the health process as making an imaginary journey in quest of the sick person's soul, finding it, and returning it to its owner. Although the shamans were active in many facets, their own cultures rated them primarily on their skill as "technicians of the sacred" (Rothenberg, 1968).

A closer look at some shamanic healing procedures would be appropriate. Spiritualistic methods predominated, but a variety of other approaches also were used widely, and many of these were imagery based. A four-step training process developed by the Kahuna healers of Polynesia and described by King (1983) will serve as our example. It involves (1) awareness of thoughts (ike), (2) establishing goals (makia), (3) changing (kala), and (4) directing energy (manawa).

The Kahunas maintain that before you can proceed to change attitudes and assumptions, you must be aware of the ones you have (ike). Therefore, the Kahuna may begin by encouraging the patient to note habitual patterns of speech, internal dialogue, and imagery themes. A patient who is accustomed to suppressing negative thoughts often requires considerable help to bring them to consciousness. Toward this end, the Kahuna attempts to stimulate *makahu* imagination, which is spontaneous or stimulated imagination that reveals belief patterns; the means is guided imagery. Sometimes the mere awareness of the counter-productive habits of thought or speech suffices to bring about immediate changes in attitude, but generally awareness alone does not lead to any change. The Kahunas feel that this is so because all current experience is supported by habits, and their way of dealing with a bad habit is replacing it with another desirable habit. This leads to the next step, *makia* (establishing goals).

Goals would include adopting new beliefs and habits and making plans for the future. The Kahuna nudges the patient toward clear ideas of his or her target state of health, personality, and environment and toward the realization of what he or she will need to do to achieve the goals. An important technique used in *makia* is *pa laulele* ("see and be"). It consists of clearly visualizing a desired circumstance and then adding oneself to the picture with all one's senses. In other words, one is aiming for the mind set of a mime during his or her act. This exercise pretrains the subconscious and the body in preparation for the new experience. Another technique in *makia* is the repetition of short, emotionally laden affirmations. These must be chosen with care in order to ensure that they are fostering the desired condition and not merely suppressing unwanted material. Affirmations that are believable are generally more effective than those that are not. Maintaining "I am healthy" when one is ill, is effective with only a few.

Many patients display considerable subconscious resistance to change. This will prompt the Kahuna to proceed to the next step, *kala* (changing). The word *kala* means "release, freedom, and forgiveness," and also "changing one's path" (King, 1983, p. 127). In order to be successful in this phase, the patient must recognize his or her inner conflict with respect to the negative habit, and he or she must be consciously willing to relinquish old ways and adopt new ones. The Kahuna will encourage the patient to replace the undesirable thought, feeling, or action with a desirable one, stressing replacement rather than suppression followed by substitution. To facilitate the task, the healer may use a variety of techniques. The Kahuna may instruct the patient in muscle relaxation, since negative thoughts and emotions do not develop in a relaxed state. The healer may decide to lead the patient in an exploration of his or her memory with the aim of reinterpreting or even altering past experiences. But the Kahuna's main technique for dealing with negative habits is *laulele*, or deliberate imagination. It is an imagery pattern to direct thoughts, emotions, and actions into new directions. With practice, this pattern becomes a habit. This process involves the step of *manawa* (directing energy).

The word *manawa* means "directing *mana*" (energy, life force). *Manawa* involves the establishment and maintenance of positive habits, and this can be accomplished only through practice. The patient may use anything that contributes to reinforcing target habits, such as reading material, symbolic pictures and objects, rituals, physical surroundings, and the company of role models.

The Kahunas stress the final step. They maintain that ideas are ineffective unless they are part of the *Ku* mind (the subconscious). Knowledge that is merely intellectual is just an opinion, and, as such, is incapable of affecting the individual's life. Hence another Huna word for enlightenment is *na' auao*, which means "gut knowledge."

This is a very cursory outline of some shamanic healing practices involving imagination. A closer look would reveal their intricacies and sophistication.

Imagery in Judaism, Christianity, and Islam

The ecstasy states and the powers that accompany them, which have been described by the shamans, were echoed by the disciples of the evolving religions of India, the Middle East, and Europe. As the modern religions of Judaism, Christianity, and Islam developed, they became more institutionalized—that is, they elaborated doctrines and policies that were based on reason and emphasized the authority of the institution. Also they established priests as mediators between the individual and God, thus curtailing direct experience of God (Samuels & Samuels, 1975).

But visualization continued to play a role in these institutionalized religions. It could not be otherwise, for all religions involve the notion of a spiritual universe that cannot be verified in the physical world. Biblical Jews rejected idols, which are externalizations of inner images, but the Old Testament and the New Testament are replete with visions and dreams. These visions are unique in that they come and go unbidden, often are extremely vivid, and generally exert a profound effect. A familiar example is the dream of the Egyptian pharaoh of seven fat cows being devoured by seven gaunt cows, and seven full ears of corn being swallowed up by seven thin ears. Joseph's interpretation that 7 years of plenty would be followed by 7 years of famine proved to be correct.

In addition to textual examples of visualizations, the rituals of these religions rely heavily on imagery, for it has proven itself to be an effective technique in helping the faithful attain their spiritual goals. Visualization translates an abstract idea into a concrete experience and thus clarifies and intensifies it (Samuels & Samuels, 1975). The Christian Communion service is an eminent example. As participants in the ceremony partake of bread and wine, they visualize the Last Supper, which Christ shared with his disciples, and are purified by it. Furthermore, Roman Catholics believe that the bread and wine *become* the body and blood of Christ, that they are transmuted, transubstantiated in the ceremony. We read in I Corinthians 11:23–25:

> The Lord Jesus the same night in which he was betrayed took bread: And when he had given thanks, he brake it, and said, "Take, eat: this is my body, which is broken for you: this do in remembrance of me." After the same manner also he took the cup, when he had supped, saying, "This cup is the new testament in my blood: this do ye, as oft as ye drink it, in remembrance of me."

Throughout history, many rich mystical traditions have coexisted with the institutionalized forms of Judaism, Christianity, and Islam. The mystics sought a personal experience of God, or ecstatic states, and their methods to achieve their goal generally involved visualization.

Kabbalah is a Jewish mystical tradition that began in Biblical times and is still alive today. In early times, it was regarded to be heretical by mainstream Judaism, and hence its teachings were spread secretly (Scholem, 1961).

Kabbalistic mysticism involves the use of symbolic doctrines, magic, and ascetic rites. The latter relied heavily on visualization. The practice of the Kabbalistic mystics of the period between the 1st century B.C. and the 10th century A.D. will serve as an example. They aspired to the ascent of their soul from earth, past hostile rulers of the cosmos, to its ultimate home in God's light. To bring about this ascent, the devoted fasted, whispered hymns, and sat with their heads between their knees. Then they visualized the seven palaces of the hostile rulers and entered one after the other. They saw the rulers of the palaces and used armor, weapons, or secret names to pass through. Then they experienced the burning of their body, and finally they came into the presence of God. This visualization may not have originated with the Kabbalistic mystics, for it can be traced to Greek texts and to earlier papyri written in Egypt (Samuels & Samuels, 1975; Scholem, 1961).

The Christian Gnostic tradition is very similar to the Kabbalistic one. The Christian mystics speak of detachment from external sensations, symbolism and magical rituals, intense concentration, visualizations of ascent and descent to other worlds, and direct experiences of God. A manual of spiritual exercises written in the first century A.D. by St.

Ignatius, one of the church fathers, illustrates the practices of this tradition. St. Ignatius instructs the reader to imagine a graded series of holy scenes leading up to a visualization of Christ, which fully absorbs the mind. St. Ignatius also wrote about personal mystical experiences: He reports that, upon one occasion, he distinctly saw the divine plan in the creation of the universe and that at another time he was allowed to contemplate, in images suited to man's feeble understanding, the mystery of the Holy Trinity (James, 1963; Jonas, 1958; Samuels & Samuels, 1975).

Another prominent example of the use of imagery within Christianity is provided by a relatively recent development. In the late 1800s, Mary Baker Eddy founded Christian Science, which rests on the concept that God is an infinite, divine mind. Disease is essentially a human product, and deep prayer causes the power of the Divine Mind to focus on the disease and to bring about healing. Mary Baker Eddy (1934) described this procedure: in the

> To prevent disease or to cure it, the power of Truth, of divine Spirit, must break the dream of the material senses. To heal by argument, find the type of the ailment, get its name, and array your mental plea against the physical. Argue at first mentally, not audibly, that the patient has no disease, and conform the argument so as to destroy the evidence of disease. Mentally insist that harmony is the fact, and that sickness is a temporal dream. Realize the presence of health and the fact of harmonious being, until the body corresponds with the normal conditions of health and harmony. (p. 412)

The importance of imagination has been recognized also in Sufism, the mysticism of Islam (Corbin, 1970). There are several Sufi meditative techniques in which imagery inevitably plays a role. These include: (1) *zekr*, a contemplation on the 99 names or attributes of God; (2) *takhliya*, a meditation aimed at obviating one's moral weaknesses; and (3) *tahliya*, a meditation designed to strengthen one's virtues so that vices become weak and ultimately die (Ajmal, 1986). For further details about Sufism, the reader is referred to Chapter 6.

Imagery in the Hindu/Buddhist Tradition

Although most of the religions of the world employ imagery techniques for healing and spiritual growth, the Hindu/Buddhist traditions—in particular the Indian Yogic practices and the Tibetan Buddhist medical systems—display the most highly developed forms.

Imagery in Yoga.   Indian yogic practices have included visualization for thousands of years. Although the *Yoga Sutras* of Patanjali was written approximately 200 B.C., the ascetic practices it contains had been in use in India for millennia. Some of the main yogic practices described are *dharana*, or riveting one's attention on a specific place inside or outside the body; *dhayana*, or sustained focus of attention supported by helpful suggestions; and *samadhi*, or the union of the object of concentration and the person focusing upon it. According to the *Yoga Sutra*, when an individual achieves this union, he or she grasps the truth of the object and attains a state of bliss (Eliade, 1958, 1976; Mishra, 1973).

Tantric yoga is the most sophisticated system of holding images in the mind for a specific purpose. *Tantra* means "that which extends knowledge." It arose in India and Tibet around 600 A.D., and it became a dominant religious and philosophical force because it provided an answer to the current belief that humans had lost direct contact with truth. Tantra offered a series of complex methods by which the individual could attain truth once more (Samuels & Samuels, 1975).

Like other religions, Tantra distinguishes between the ephemeral world of matter and the real world of the spirit. According to Tantra, the entire cosmos is *maya*, or cosmic illusion—that is, the physical world of the senses as well as the mental realm of thoughts and dreams are *maya*. Beyond matter and mind lies absolute reality, which is eternal and permanent. A primary goal of Tantrism is liberation from the illusion that the physical world, as perceived by the senses and the mind, is real (Eliade, 1958).

In order to achieve this goal, the aspirant must transcend the ego, that is, both the "I" of the conscious reality of the senses and the "I" of subconscious tendencies and realities. He or she must stop regarding himself or herself as matter and learn to identify with the absolute (Samuels & Samuels, 1975).

This is accomplished not by means of theoretical learning but through personal experience or, more precisely, by learning to concentrate, to control the mind, and to ignore the distractions offered by the senses. The basic techniques for changing the focus from the physical world to the spiritual realm are visualization and meditation. The master may instruct the yogi to visualize a certain god or an object, and the yogi will focus repeatedly upon this image until it is very clear, which may take years (Eliade, 1958).

After the yogi has succeeded in developing a vivid image of the deity, the master may direct him or her to identify himself or herself with this deity. This technique of visualization and identification is not just a mental exercise, it serves to awaken the divine nature within the practitioner and thus helps him or her to go beyond *maya* to ultimate reality (Samuels & Samuels, 1975).

In the book, *Tibetan Yoga and Secret Doctrines*, Evans-Wentz (1967) includes a number of visualizations taken from ancient Tantric texts. One example follows:

> Imagine thyself to be the Divine Devotee Vajra-Yogini (a goddess of intellect and energy); . . . the right hand holding aloft a brilliantly gleaming curved knife and flourishing it overhead, cutting off completely all mentally disturbing thought-processes; the left hand holding against her breast a human skull filled with blood (symbolizing renunciation of the world) . . . with a tiara of five dried human skulls (symbolizing highest spiritual discernment) on her head; wearing a necklace of fifty blood-dripping human heads (symbolizing severance from the round of death and re-birth); her adornments, five of the Six Symbolic Adornments (the tiara of human skulls, the necklace of human heads, armlets and wristlets, anklets, the breastplate Mirror of Karma), the cemetery-dust ointment (symbolizing renunciation of the world and conquest of fear over death) being lacking, holding in the bend of her arm, the long staff, symbolizing the Divine Father, the Heruka (the male power); nude, and in the full bloom of virginity, at the sixteenth year of her age (unsullied by the world); dancing, with the right leg bent and foot uplifted, and the left foot treading upon the breast of a prostrate human form (treading upon ignorance and illusion); and flames of wisdom forming a halo about her.

> (Visualize her as being thyself), eternally in the shape of a deity, and internally altogether vacuous like the inside of an empty sheath, transparent and uncloudedly radiant; vacuous even to the fingertips, like an empty tent of red silk, or like a filmy tube distended with breath. (pp. 173–175)

In other visualization exercises commonly used by Tantric yogis, a mandala is the concentration device. A mandala is a complex circular design composed of concentric geometric forms that may contain images of deities or objects. The contents symbolize principles of the universe, such as tension, action, receptivity, and wholeness, as well as Tantric doctrines, such as the eradication of ignorance. Concentration upon the mandala, again, is not just a mental discipline; it eventually leads to identification with the principles depicted (Mookerjee, 1971).

Healing and salvation also are promoted by *mantras*, or mystic syllables. The energy of the body produces vibrations. The vibrations of the diseased body produce a discordant sound, but the recitation of *mantras* can restore harmony.

Tantric yogic practices involving visualization were extensively incorporated and developed by the Tibetan Buddhist medical tradition.

Imagery in Tibetan Buddhist Medicine. Religion, mysticism, psychology, and scientific medicine have come together in Buddhist Tibetan medicine to produce a highly complex tradition. To the Westerner steeped in scientific materialism, the study of this product of an ancient and sacred culture is baffling but also richly rewarding. It offers carefully elaborated and relevant models of holistic medicine, of psychosomatic medicine, of mental and psychic healing, of the role of the healer, and of the use of illness to develop wisdom. Tibetan medicine, like most traditional systems, is holistic. It recognizes the link between mind and body and also between humans and the cosmos. The Tibetan approach also shares with other ancient medical systems the view that health is a matter of balance; however, the Tibetans have presented the most refined version of this concept. They propose that illness is brought on by imbalance or disharmony within the microcosm or between the latter and the macrocosm. The root cause is the delusion of the ego's self-existence; thus the ultimate cure lies in enlightenment. The various aspects of Tibetan medicine are tightly integrated; however, in order to facilitate study, it is useful to separate them into three areas (Clifford, 1984).

1. *Somatic medicine* has its roots primarily in the Indian Ayurvedic system. It relies on naturopathy (e.g., massage and controlled diet), herbal medicines, acupuncture, and other techniques.

2. *Dharmic (or religious) medicine* utilizes spiritual and psychological practices, such as meditation, moral development, and prayer in order to fathom the nature of the mind and to control negative emotions.

3. *Tantric (or yogic) medicine* contains elements of both the mental and the physical approach. It relies on psychophysical practices to direct the body's energy toward healing.

Both the dharmic and the tantric aspects of Tibetan medicine utilize meditation and visualization extensively. One widely used visualization involves the mandala of the medicine Buddha. At the center of the mandala, a radiant Buddha sits in lotus position on a 1,000-petaled lotus, which in turn is perched on a jeweled throne. In his right hand he is holding the myrobalan plant, and in his left hand a begging bowl filled with healing nectar. In this exercise, one imagines that one is sitting in a beautiful landscape and offering to the Buddha all that is precious. Now one asks him for his blessing and to sit on the top of one's head. Then one senses the Buddha's rays of brilliant light stream into the body, dissolving illness and suffering.

A variation is to visualize oneself as the medicine Buddha and the outer world as the outer part of the mandala. Thus one generates the healing light of the Buddha and thereby one's view of the self and of the world is purified.

The visualization of light plays a large part in tantric healing. One images brilliant light, generally white or blue, radiating from the deity and flowing through one's being, purifying it both mentally and physically. If the meditation is used for a personal ailment, the light is directed to the diseased area; if the exercise is used for the healing of others, the light is sent out into the universe. A variation of this exercise is to merge with the deity's light after it has entered one's being and to become light oneself. This light eradicates dualistic concepts; consequently, one enters a state of blissful emptiness. After coming out of this meditation, one is still identified with the deity and can focus one's healing light on disease in oneself or in someone else (Birnbaum, 1979).

Another healing meditation involves Buddha Vajrasattva, a deity of purification. He is white, sitting in lotus position, holding in his right hand a *vajra*, representing skillful means, and in his left hand a bell, representing wisdom. One imagines him to be sitting on the top of one's head and confesses one's transgressions to him. Then by the strength of one's promise to avoid further wrongdoing and due to Vajrasattva's vow to purify, his light streams into one's head and descends into the body illuminating it. All one's mental and physical ailments dissipate and exit one's being in the form of blood, pus, smoke, and insects.

Mantras are also widely utilized to promote well-being. They may be used alone but generally are used in combination with other techniques. One can visualize a healing *mantra* as a mandala. This mantric mandala can be imagined to be in one's own hand, conferring upon it a healing touch, or in the heart of the individual to be cured. Or one can repeat a *mantra* at the same time as one is doing the imagery of healing light (Clifford, 1984).

It is obvious that according to the Tibetan tradition disease originates in the spirit and thus the potential for recovery likewise lies in the spirit; cure cannot be wrought by mere external intervention. Unlike modern Western physicians, the Tibetan healer does not merely diagnose the ailment and prescribe treatment; he or she interacts with the patient and nurtures him or her back to health. Since this is a spiritual undertaking, the healer's moral quality is believed to play an important role in the cure. No matter which type of medicine the healer uses primarily, he or she also will be practicing some mystic healing exercises. Their potency is believed to be directly affected by the state of his or her consciousness—by the purity of intention and by the powers of concentration.

The ultimate goal of the healer is not to bring about relief from symptoms but to put the patient back on the path that leads to enlightenment—life's ultimate goal. Disease must be regarded as a blessing, for it lets the patient know that he or she is harboring a fundamental disharmony—that he or she is out of balance. This awareness is the first step in making necessary adjustments in life and thus progressing toward enlightenment (Blofeld, 1970; Burang, 1974; Clifford, 1984).

HEALING IMAGES: A HISTORICAL OUTLINE OF THEIR USE IN THE WESTERN MEDICAL TRADITION

To Westerners of the 20th century, it might appear that the use of imagination in healing is not part of our culture. Yet, this is untrue. In fact, the ethical code of honor accepted by all physicians today pays tribute to the mythical founding family of medicine who contributed a method for healing by the imagination. The oath begins: "I swear by Apollo, the Physician, by Asclepius, by Hygeia and Panacea and by all the Gods and Goddesses, making them my witnesses, that I will fulfill according to my ability and judgement this oath and this covenant."

As we have already noted, dreams and visions universally have been the most common method of diagnosis and treatment. But it was during the Grecian era, a time when the art of medicine flourished, that imagery-based diagnosis and therapy were systematized and incorporated into the standard approach to disease (Achterberg, 1985).

The figurehead of this movement was Asclepius. He probably was a mortal, but in the *Iliad*, Homer presents him as the son of Apollo who was brought into heaven by Zeus as a demigod. Asclepius's immediate family shared in his healing power. His wife, Epione, soothed pain; his daughters, Hygeia and Panacea, were regarded as deities of health and treatment; and his son, Telesphores, represented convalescence or rehabilitation.

Asclepius became the patron of healing for centuries, and his influence extended far beyond the borders of Greece. Asclepius seemed to satisfy the need for a personal, compassionate divinity; hence, wherever he was introduced, he replaced or merged with the local healing deity. The legend of Asclepius merged with that of the Egyptian god of healing, Imhotep, and with the god Serapis of the Ptolemics. Within Christianity, Saints Damian and Cosmos carried on the healing traditions of Asclepius (Lyons & Petrucelli, 1978).

A testimony to the influence of Asclepius is found in the over 200 temples, or Asclepia, which were built throughout Greece, Italy, and

Turkey both to pay tribute to him and to foster the practice of medicine. These Asclepia were the first holistic treatment centers. They were located in picturesque areas and contained baths, recreational facilities, and places of worship. All who sought treatment were admitted, regardless of their ability to pay, for Asclepius taught that a physician was primarily someone to whom anyone who was suffering could turn.

At the Asclepia, dream therapy or divine sleep, which later was renamed incubation sleep by Christian practitioners, was perfected as a diagnostic and therapeutic tool. Most of the patients who underwent this treatment were seriously ill and had not responded to other treatments. In preparation for dream therapy, the patient fasted for 1 day and did not consume wine for 3 days; thus attaining spiritual clarity to receive the divine message. Then the patient went to the temple to await the gods. Insight and consequently healing occurred during the state of consciousness immediately preceding sleep, when images appear unbidden. At this time, the image of Asclepius would emerge—a gentle but powerful healer, carrying a rustic staff entwined by a serpent—and he would either cure or prescribe treatment (Achterberg, 1985).

Many cures have been ascribed to Asclepian dream therapy: the blind, deaf, lame, impotent and barren, and those afflicted by innumerable other diseases have left stone images or written accounts of their cures on the temple walls.

Aristotle, Hippocrates, and even Galen have their roots in the Asclepian tradition and were convinced that imagination played a central role in health. Aristotle proposed "that the emotional system did not function in the absence of images. Images were formed by the sensations taken in and then worked upon by the *senses communis* or the 'collective sense.'" Also he felt that images of the dream state deserved special notice. In *Parva Naturalia*, he advises, "Even scientific physicians tell us that one should pay diligent attention to dreams, and to hold this view is reasonable also for those who are not practitioners but speculative philosophers" (see Achterberg, 1985, p. 56).

But it was Galen who was the first one to provide a detailed outline of the relationship between mind and body. He proposed that the patient's images or dreams provide valuable diagnostic information. For instance, images of loss, grief, or disgrace indicate an excess of melancholy (black bile), and images of fear or fighting reveal an excess of choler. Galen was aware of the vicious circle created by an excessive humor that produced corresponding images, which then exacerbated the humor; and he stressed that the cycle had to be broken in order to regain health (Binder, 1966; Osler, 1921).

The Asclepian tradition and the art of healing through imagination survived the gradual ascendancy of the Christian Church and its purge of pagan gods. Statues of the Asclepian family, the caduceus symbol, and the Hippocratic oath have endured perhaps because they stand for a value inherent in the art of medicine—respect for humanity. As Hippocrates said, "Where there is love for mankind, there is love for the art of healing" (see Achterberg, 1985, p. 57).

Within Christendom, however, the miracles of healing were no longer ascribed to the Asclepian family but rather to Saints Cosmos and Damian. These two men worked tirelessly to provide medical care until they became victims of the Diocletian persecution (278 A.D.). Churches dedicated to them were always open to the sick. The primary method of diagnosis and therapy in use was incubation sleep, a variation of the Asclepian divine sleep (Lyons & Petrucelli, 1978). During the state of drowsiness preceding sleep, the patient would have images of Saints Cosmos and Damian, who would offer a diagnosis and a cure (Achterberg, 1985).

Imagination continued to play an important role in the Western healing traditions well into the Renaissance. For instance, Paracelsus, a famous physician and the founder of modern chemistry, restated a theme common among the ancient Greeks—that is, the individual is comprised of three elements: the spiritual, the physical, and the mental. He reportedly said:

> Man has a visible and an invisible workshop. The visible one is his body, the invisible one is imagination (mind). . . . The imagination is the sun in the soul of man. . . . The spirit is the master, imagination the tool, and the body the plastic material. . . . The power of the imagination is a great factor in medicine. It may produce diseases . . . and it may cure them. . . . Ills of the body may be cured by physical remedies or by the power of the spirit acting through the soul. (Hartman, 1973, pp. 111–112)

Paracelsus also maintained, "Man is his own healer and finds proper healing herbs in his own garden, the physician is in ourselves, and in our own nature are all things that we need" (Stoddard, 1911, p. 231).

Physicians of the Renaissance still considered health to be a matter of equilibrium, and their therapy consisted of adjusting imbalance. Hence they prescribed arousing images for the phlegmatic personality and used joyful images to combat melancholy. Shakespeare reflects this view in the introduction to *The Taming of the Shrew.*

> For so your doctors hold it very meet:
> seeing too much sadness hath congeal'd your blood,

And melancholy is the nurse to frenzy:
Therefore, they thought it good you hear a play,
And frame your mind to mirth and merriment,
Which bars a thousand harms and lengthens life.
(Act I, Scene I)

This holistic approach prevailed until the 17th century when René Descartes (1596–1650) proposed a revolutionary view. He defined the mind as a separate entity. He maintained that the mind or soul, terms he used interchangeably, is "entirely distinct from the body . . . and would not itself cease to be all that it is, even should the body cease to exist" (McMahon & Sheikh, 1984, p. 13). This dualistic view, which gradually won over Western thinkers, quite radically changed the approach to disease.

Imagery in Pre- and Post-Cartesian Medicine: A Comparison.   In the pre-Cartesian period, no mind-body problem existed. Both mental and physical events had their roots in a common substrate, a biological soul. But Descartes proposed that mind and body are mutually exclusive entities. Therefore, mechanistic physiopathology became the dominant approach to disease (McMahon, 1976).

In the holistic era, imagination—a faculty of the biological soul—was considered to be a very significant psychophysiological variable. Aristotle had proposed, "The soul never thinks without a picture" (Yates, 1966, p. 32). He also felt that the emotions always were activated by imagery. Of course, the images were believed to provoke certain physical effects. That is, when the imagination conceived an image, spirits activated the brain and then aroused the heart, and the vividness and persistence of the image determined the extent of its impact on bodily functions. It is interesting to note that imagination was considered to be more powerful than sensations; therefore, dread of an event was viewed more harmful than the event itself. Images were considered sufficiently potent to be used to gain conscious control over autonomic or involuntary functions, and it was thought that images could even imprint traits on embryos in the womb. Charron stated in 1601, that imagery "marks and deforms, nay, sometimes kills embryos in the womb, hastens births, or causes abortions" (McMahon, 1976, p. 180).

The key to a correct evaluation of the role of the imagination in the pre-Cartesian period lies in realizing that imagery was regarded to be as much a physiological phenomenon as a psychological one. It was believed that a vivid and persistent negative image spread throughout the body and wrought its mischief, which soon became manifest in physical symptoms. Since healers of this period believed images to be capable of causing disease, it follows that they also looked to images for their therapies (McMahon & Sheikh, 1984; Sheikh, Richardson, & Moleski, 1979).

After Descartes's dualism had taken root in the Western mind, imagination was stripped of its role in disease and wellness. During the 18th and 19th centuries, several protests were voiced, but the dualistic trend prevailed.

HEALING IMAGES: PSYCHOTHERAPEUTIC USES

When psychology emerged as a separate science in the late 19th century, interest in the arousal function of imagery became apparent, and William James's theory of "ideo-motor action" was received very favorably. It seemed that the time was ripe for a renaissance of Aristotelian theory. But this was not the case. The behaviorists successfully eliminated all mentalistic concepts from the arena of serious research (McMahon & Sheikh, 1984). Watson (1913) regarded mental images as mere ghosts of sensations with no functional significance whatsoever. Klinger (1971) notes that from 1920 to 1960, there was a moratorium in North American psychology on the study of inner experience, and not even one book on the topic of mental imagery was published. However, in Europe the situation was not quite the same. European clinical psychologists and psychiatrists continued to evince significant sensitivity to the inner realm of imagery and were relatively unperturbed by the rapidly increasing influence of behaviorism in America. Several factors aided the continuation of this largely subjective approach to imagery in Europe: (1) many experimentalists left Europe during the two World Wars; (2) German and French phenomenology influenced European clinical and scientific systems; (3) the subjective approaches to the investigation of various aspects of the inner experience, proposed by Jung, affected many European practitioners; and (4) Europe had been influenced by subjective Eastern psychology (Jordan, 1979; McMahon & Sheikh, 1984; Sheikh & Jordan, 1983). It must be noted, however, that although European clinicians were successful in escaping the stranglehold of behavioristic formulations, until very recently, they were unable to elude the powerful influences of Cartesian dualism. Consequently, with a few exceptions, the use of imaginative skills was confined to the treatment of only the so-called psychological problems and was not applied to physical ones.

European Contributions in the 1900s

The notable contributions to the clinical use of images in the early 1900s include the work of Pierre Janet, Alfred Binet, Carl Happich, Eugene Caslant, Oscar Vogt, Johannes Schultz, Ludwig Frank, Sigmund Freud, and Carl Jung (see Sheikh & Jordan, 1983, for a review). Of all these, Jung's contribution played the most significant role in the imagery movement in psychotherapy. He regarded mental imagery as a creative process of our psyche to be employed for attaining greater individual, interpersonal, and spiritual integration (Jordan, 1979). Jung stated:

> The psyche consists essentially of images. It is a series of images in the truest sense, not an accidental juxtaposition or sequence but a structure that is throughout full of meaning and purpose; it is a picturing of vital activities and just as the material of the body that is ready for life has a need of the psyche in order to be capable of life, so the psyche presupposes the living body in order that its images may live. (Jung, 1960, pp. 325–326)

By recognizing the reciprocity of the psyche and the body, Jung indicated his belief in the mind-body unity as a life process and proposed that imagery is a vehicle of perceiving and experiencing this life process (Sheikh & Jordan, 1983). Jung remarked that when we "concentrate on a mental picture, it begins to stir, the image becomes enriched by details, it moves and develops . . . and so when we concentrate on inner pictures and when we are careful not to interrupt the natural flow of events, our unconscious will produce a series of images which makes a complete story" (Jung, 1976, p. 172). Jung's therapeutic use of imagery is best represented by the method he termed "active imagination." For details of the method, the reader is referred to other sources (Jung, 1960; Sawyer, 1986; Singer & Pope, 1978; Watkins, 1976).

More recently, several French, German, and Italian clinicians, all significantly influenced by Jung, have investigated the potential use of imagery as a method of psychotherapy. The most prominent of these approaches include Desoille's (1961, 1965) *Directed Daydream*, Fretigny and Virel's (1968) *Oneirodrama*, Leuner's (1977, 1978) *Guided Affective Imagery*, and Assagioli's (1965) *Psychosynthesis*. The first three of these four approaches have some basic similarities. The term "oneirotherapy" (from the Greek *oneiros* meaning "dream," hence also known as "dream therapy" or "waking-dream therapy") has been used to describe all three therapies (Much & Sheikh, 1986; Sheikh & Jordan, 1983).

1. All three oneirotherapies employ *extended* visual fantasies in *narrative* form to obtain data concerning the motivational system of

the client. These fantasies are generally preceded by an attempt to induce relaxation.

2. Products of visual imagination are used in conjunction with associations, discussion, and interpretation.

3. Generally, the client is presented with certain standard symbolic scenes as the starting images. These scenes are presumed to reflect common areas of conflict.

4. With respect to assumptions and interpretations, all oneirotherapeutic procedures are psychodynamic in nature. These methods rest on the belief that the symbolism inherent in visual imagery constitutes an affective language that expresses unconscious motives without fully imposing them on conscious recognition. Therefore, it is assumed that the participant will show less resistance to the expression of the underlying motives (Sheikh & Jordan, 1983).

In general, these methods have been reported to be effective in uncovering the structural details of the client's personality, in discovering the nature of the affective trauma, and in quickly ameliorating the symptoms. Fretigny and Virel (1968) mention a few other advantages of their use of imagery, which can be applied to all three approaches. They claim that: (1) mental imagery can be used with persons who find systematic reflection difficult due to their low level of sophistication; (2) the use of imagery circumvents the snares of rational thinking; (3) this approach discourages sterile rumination; and (4) mental imagery aims directly at the individual's affective experience (Sheikh & Jordan, 1983).

Compared to most European approaches, Assagioli's psychosynthesis is more holistic and eclectic. One of the goals of psychosynthesis is to enhance the personal and spiritualistic potential of the individual. To achieve this goal, Assagioli and his followers have employed Western analytic, behavioral, and humanistic procedures along with Eastern meditative techniques. In psychosynthesis, the human personality is considered to have a number of layers of awareness. The goal "is not only the explication of these various levels of awareness and the relief of personal difficulties. Rather, its goal is a thorough reconstruction of the total personality, exploration of the various levels of personality, and eventually the shift of personality to a new center through exploration of its fundamental core" (Singer, 1974, p. 109).

Mental imagery is only one of the many methods employed in psychosynthesis. Assagioli uses several imagery procedures that reflect the principles discussed by Jung, Desoille, and Leuner, along with conditioning and cognitive restructuring techniques. In interpreting the

images, accompanying verbal associations and other relevant information are utilized. Every element of the image is believed to represent, at
one level or another, a personality trait, albeit distorted, displaced, or
projected. Identification with all aspects of the image drama is regarded
as a means of assimilating repressed material in socialized form and
expanding the boundaries of the self (Sheikh & Jordan, 1983).

One must credit the European clinicians for not only keeping alive the
clinical use of images in the wake of behaviorism but also for providing a
rich heritage of therapeutic procedures, for keeping us in touch with the
unavoidable phenomenological nature of perception, and for building a
bridge between Eastern and Western approaches to the understanding of
the nature of human consciousness (Jordan, 1979; Panagiotou & Sheikh,
1977; Sheikh & Jordan, 1983).

Current American Approaches

During the last two decades, imagery has risen from a position of near
disgrace to become one of the hottest topics in both clinical and experimental cognitive psychology. Experimental and clinical psychologists of
varied persuasions have made imagery the subject of their inquiry, and
they have produced a considerable body of literature documenting that
images are indeed a powerful force.

Due to space limitation, it is not possible to present a detailed discussion
of various American imagery approaches to psychotherapy. Interested
readers are referred to other sources (Sheikh & Jordan, 1983; Singer, 1974;
Singer & Pope, 1978). However, it is possible to categorize the numerous
existing imagery approaches in America into the following six broad
groups.

1. A number of imagery approaches that are based largely on the
Pavlovian and Skinnerian models constitute the first group. They highlight the surface relationship between images and emotional responses
as well as the ability of images to act as powerful stimuli. These procedures consist of several variations of counterconditioning and emotional flooding (Sheikh & Panagiotou 1975; Sheikh & Jordan, 1983).
These procedures include systematic desensitization (Wolpe, 1969), im-
plosion therapy (Stampfl & Lewis, 1967), covert conditioning (Cautela,
1977), coping imagery and stress innoculation (Meichenbaum, 1977),
and many others.

2. The second category is composed of the procedures advanced by
a number of clinicians who believe that mental images effectively give
us a clear understanding of our perceptual and affective distortions.

Unlike the cognitive behavior therapists, proponents of these approaches do not resort to explanations in terms of conditioning principles. Beck (1970), for example, explains the conditioning effects of repetitive fantasy in cognitive terms. He states that the repetition of images provides important information and clarifies cognitive and affective distortion for the client. Gendlin and his associates (Gendlin, 1978; Gendlin & Olsen, 1970) employ "experiential focusing" to clearly comprehend all aspects of the feeling. They claim that emergence of an image frequently moves the client from a "global sense of feeling to a specific crux feeling." This image, "typically becomes quite stable as the feel of it is focused on and even refuses to change until one comes to know what the feeling it gives one is. Then one feels not only the characteristic release, but the image then changes" (Gendlin & Olson, 1970, p. 221). Morrison (1980) emphasizes "the value of retracing early developmental experiences in order to apply the adult's more adequate construct system" and thus to better understand those experiences (p. 313). In Morrison's emotive-reconstructive therapy, images are the primary therapeutic agent.

3. The third class includes a number of approaches that basically consist of imagery rehearsal of physical and psychological health. The client may be asked to image a malfunctioning organ becoming normal or to practice in imagination a healthy, interpersonal relationship. No complicated theories are offered except the assumption that sane imagination will eventually lead to sane reality (McMahon & Sheikh, 1984). No one can claim credit for developing these procedures, for, they have been around for centuries (Sheikh, 1984, 1986).

4. The fourth group consists of image therapies with a psychoanalytic orientation. Prominent among these approaches are "emergent uncovering" (Reyher, 1977) and "psycho-imagination therapy" (Shorr, 1978). Mardi Horowitz (1978) is another psychoanalytically oriented clinician who has made important contributions to the study of the role of mental images in clinical practice.

It is noteworthy that Freud was well aware of the spontaneous images experienced by his clients, and he apparently used imagery extensively prior to 1900. But he later abandoned it in favor of verbal free association. Yet, although Freud and his followers tended to avoid the explicit uses of mental images in therapy, several characteristics of the psychoanalytic setting encourage the production of imagery. These include: reclining in a restful position, low level of sensory stimulation, use of free association, and emphasis on dreams, fantasies, and childhood memories (Pope, 1977; Sheikh & Jordan, 1983; Singer & Pope, 1978).

5. The fifth class includes the "depth" imagery procedures in which emphasis is on healing through "magical" or "irrational" methods as opposed to rational or reflexive techniques. A prime example of this group is "eidetic psychotherapy" (Ahsen, 1968; Sheikh, 1978; Sheikh & Jordan, 1981), which relies on the elicitation and manipulation of eidetic images. Every significant event during our development is considered to implant an eidetic in the system. The eidetic is seen as a tridimensional unity. The visual component, the *image,* is always accompanied by a *somatic pattern*—a set of bodily feelings and tensions, including somatic correlations of emotions—and a cognitive or experiential *meaning.* This triadic unity is considered to display certain lawful tendencies toward change that are meaningfully related to psychological processes.

6. Recently, a sixth category of imagery approaches has been attracting increasing attention among health professionals. These approaches have resulted from the advent of the "third force," or humanistic psychology, and of the "fourth force," or transpersonal psychology. Both of these put emphasis on greater access to experience, on a variety of states of consciousness, and on increasing realization of our potentials. This orientation has led to the emergence of numerous novel imagery methods, which are derived from European oneirotherapies, psychosynthesis techniques, autogenic training, Jungian active imagination, and from Eastern meditative practices (Perls, 1970; Progoff, 1970; Sheikh & Jordan, 1983; Singer, 1974). These methods include taking an imaginary inventory of the body, having an imaginary dialogue with internal parts of oneself, creating and interacting with an inner advisor in one's imagery, dying in one's imagination, visualizing communication between the two hemispheres of the brain, crawling into various organs of the body for observatory or reparatory purposes, exorcising the parents from various parts of the body, and regressing into the "previous life" (Sheikh, 1986; Sheikh & Shaffer, 1979).

What Makes Images Clinically Effective

Researchers have ascribed the clinical efficacy of images to a variety of mechanisms. Singer (1974) believes that the effectiveness of imagery essentially depends on: (1) the client's clear discrimination of his or her ongoing fantasy processes; (2) clues provided by the therapist regarding alternate approaches to various situations; (3) awareness of usually avoided situations; (4) encouragement by the therapist to enter into covert rehearsal of alternate approaches; and (5) consequent decrease in fear of overtly approaching the avoided situations. Meichenbaum (1978) has suggested further simplification. He believes that the key to the effectiveness of the images lies in: (1) the feeling of control that the client gains from monitoring and rehearsing various images; (2) the modified meaning or changed internal dialogue that precedes, accompanies, and succeeds instances of maladaptive behavior; and, (3) the mental rehearsal of alternative responses that enhances coping skills (Sheikh & Jordan, 1983).

In addition to the processes outlined by Singer and Meichenbaum, numerous other characteristics of the imagery mode have been credited with contributing to its clinical effectiveness.

1. Experience in imagination can be viewed as psychologically equivalent, in many significant respects, to the actual experience; imagery and perception seem to be experientially and neurophysiologically similar processes (Klinger, 1980; Kosslyn, 1980; Richardson, 1969; Sheikh & Jordan, 1983).

2. Verbal logic is linear, whereas the image is a simultaneous representation. This trait of simultaneity gives imagery greater isomorphism with perception and, therefore, greater capacity for descriptive accuracy (Sheikh & Panagiotou, 1975).

3. The imagery system fosters a richer experience of a range of emotions (Singer, 1979).

4. Mental images lead to a variety of physiological changes (Richardson, 1984; Sheikh & Kunzendorf, 1984; White, 1978). More details of this issue are presented in the next section of this chapter.

5. Images are a source of details about past experiences (Sheikh & Panagiotou, 1975).

6. Imagery readily provides access to significant memories of early childhood when language was not yet predominant (Kepecs, 1954).

7. Imagery appears to be very effective in bypassing defenses and resistances (Klinger, 1980; Reyher, 1963; Singer, 1974).

8. Imagery frequently opens up new avenues for exploration, after therapy has come to an impasse (Sheikh & Jordan, 1983).

9. Images are less likely than linguistic expression to be filtered through the conscious critical apparatus. Generally, words and phrases must be consciously understood before they are spoken—that is, they must pass through a rational censorship before they can assume a grammatical order. Perhaps imagery is not subject to this filtering process; therefore it may be a more direct expression of the unconscious (Panagiotou & Sheikh, 1977).

In the light of the foregoing characteristics of imagery, it seems reasonable to believe that images hold enormous potential for healing, and it is not surprising that extensive claims about the promise of imagery for therapeutic benefits have been made. A large body of recent scientific research on imagery indicates that these claims are justified. However, direct systematic research on the therapeutic outcome of imagery approaches with clients suffering from a variety of ailments is urgently needed.

HEALING IMAGES: MODERN SCIENCE

The results of controlled research corroborate the clinical evidence that imagery has a curative effect and refute the misguided "scientific" assumption that *mental* imagery cannot have any effect on the *physical* body. This misguided assumption, nevertheless, is historically important in the development of modern research on healing imagery.

In their historic endeavor to make psychology more physical and more "scientific," students of objective behavior and its physical causes dogmatically assumed that mental images and other conscious entities cannot causally affect behavioral responses (Pavlov, 1927; Skinner, 1974). Ironically, such an assumption implies that conscious images are not brain events—because if they were physical events in the brain, then they could regulate behavioral responses. Nonetheless, steadfast in their dogmatic denial of the efficacy of conscious imaging, behaviorists limited themselves to studying the effect of unconscious learning—Pavlovian conditioning and Skinnerian biofeedback—on health-related responses. Such studies, as the following discussion will show, eventually yielded evidence that both Pavlovian conditioning and biofeedback are mediated by mental imagery. Pursuant to the latter evidence, scientific studies finally focused on the bodily effects of mental imagery per se and successfully substantiated the many health-related effects reviewed below.

Pavlovian Conditioning and Mental Imagery

Prior to the "scientific" discoveries of Pavlov, Cartesian dogma attributed animal behavior to the instincts and reflexes of biological organisms, and human behavior to the reasoning and learning of human "souls." Pavlov's (1906) discovery that dogs' salivary reflexes can be conditioned to a bell—and the findings of his student Krasnogorski (1909) that childrens' eating behaviors can be similarly conditioned—put an end to

Cartesian dogma. In its stead, early behaviorist dogma asserted that the unconscious processes of Pavlovian conditioning applied to all animal and human responses (Watson, 1916, 1925)—including health-related responses, such as vasoconstriction and vasodilation (Menzies, 1937, 1941), heart-rate deceleration and heart-rate acceleration (Furedy & Poulous, 1976; Wegner & Zeaman, 1958), and suppressed immunoreaction and enhanced immunoreaction (Ader, 1985).

Several interpreters of Pavlovian conditioning have posited that conditioned responses are mediated by anticipatory images of the unconditioned stimulus—which are neurally similar to percepts of the unconditioned stimulus and, given sufficient similarity, are capable of evoking unconditioned responses (King, 1973, 1983; Konorski, 1967; Mowrer, 1960, 1977; Sheikh & Kunzendorf, 1984). One reason for positing such mediation is that Pavlovian conditioning is not successful for all subjects, just as mental imaging is not possible for all individuals. Indeed, individual differences in heart-rate conditioning are substantial, even within single experiments (Wegner & Zeaman, 1958), and Pavlovian conditioning of enhanced immunoreaction is possible for only half of all animal subjects (Gorczynski, Macrae, & Kennedy, 1982). Although Pavlov attributed unsuccessful conditioning to innate physiological inhibition, two studies with human subjects link conditioning differences to imaging differences. A study by Mangan (1974) found that the strength of appetitive GSR conditioning was positively correlated with the vividness of tactual imagery. Similarly, a study by Arabian and Furedy (1983) found that heart-rate-deceleration conditioning was stronger in a group of vivid imagers than in a group of poor imagers. Both studies measured vividness with the Questionnaire Upon Mental Imagery (Betts, 1909; Sheehan, 1967).

Thus recent evidence suggests that the Pavlovian conditioning of autonomic responses is mediated by mental imagery and demands that the autonomic effects of health-related imagery per se be studied. Consideration of such effects, as they have been studied to date, will follow consideration of the Skinnerian "science" of operant learning.

Biofeedback and Mental Imagery

In response to controlled studies of Eastern yogis trained in "voluntary" autonomic regulation (Green, Ferguson, Green, & Walters, 1970; Wenger & Bagchi, 1961), operant learning theorists developed and tested biofeedback as a "scientific" account of autonomic training. Although early tests indicated that heart rate and electrodermal activity could not be operantly conditioned with Skinnerian reinforcement (Harwood,

1962; Mandler, Preven, & Kuhlman, 1962), subsequent studies revealed that autonomic responses could be successfully conditioned with continuous reinforcement providing feedback about response magnitudes (Green, Walters, Green, & Murphy, 1969; Lisina, 1965; Miller, 1969). But as critical reviews of such successful studies indicate (King & Montgomery, 1980; Miller, 1978), biofeedback is not effective for all subjects.

Individual differences in the effectiveness of biofeedback, like individual differences in the effectiveness of Pavlovian conditioning, have been attributed to individual differences in imaging ability. Heart-rate biofeedback has produced greater heart-rate increases in biofeedback subjects with more vivid imagery, as measured by Betts's Questionnaire Upon Mental Imagery (Hirschman & Favaro, 1980). In addition, electrodermal biofeedback has produced greater electrodermal activity in subjects with "richer" imagery, as measured by the Sophian Scale of Imagery (Ikeda & Hirai, 1976) and greater electrodermal control in subjects with "more prevalent" imagery, as measured by Kunzendorf's (1981) Prevalence of Imagery Tests (Kunzendorf & Bradbury, 1983).

Moreover, the effectiveness of biofeedback has been linked not only to the ability to image, but also to the use of imagery during biofeedback. In biofeedback research with hypnotized subjects, Roberts, Kewman, and MacDonald (1973) noted that subjects who successfully altered their local skin temperature during biofeedback were subjects who spontaneously hallucinated such temperature alteration. In research without hypnosis, Schwartz (1975) found that subjects who successfully lowered their blood pressure in one feedback session and raised it in a different feedback session were subjects who spontaneously imaged emotional tranquillity in the former session and emotional agitation in the latter session. Similarly, Bell and Schwartz (1975), Schwartz (1975), Takahashi (1984), and White, Holmes, and Bennett (1977) reported that biofeedback subjects who successfully lowered and raised their heart rate were subjects who spontaneously imaged tranquillity and agitation. LaBouef and Wilson (1978) and Qualls and Sheehan (1979) confirmed that during biofeedback for relaxation subjects who successfully attenuated their electromyographic responses (EMGs) were also subjects who spontaneously imaged tranquillity.

Further research has explicitly compared the effectiveness of biofeedback alone, the effectiveness of biofeedback with imaging instructions, and the effectiveness of imaging instructions without biofeedback. In research on vasomotor control, Herzfeld and Taub (1980) and Ohkuma (1985) observed that biofeedback with instructions to image warmth produced greater skin temperature increases than biofeedback alone. Likewise in research on relaxation, Qualls and Sheehan (1981a) found that biofeedback with imaging instructions produced greater EMG decrements than biofeedback alone. However, Qualls and Sheehan (1981a, 1981b) also found that for some subjects biofeedback interfered with imaging. Thus, in Shea's (1985) study of heart-rate control, smaller heart-rate changes were produced by biofeedback than by emotional imaging without biofeedback and by hypnotic suggestion without biofeedback.

Collectively, the above studies suggest that many successful effects of biofeedback can be reduced to autonomic effects of mental imaging. Moreover, the last study raises the possibility that many autonomic effects of hypnotic suggestion also can be reduced to effects of mental imaging. Several psychosomatic studies of hypnosis and imagery address this possibility.

Psychosomatic Hypnosis and Mental Imagery

Psychosomatic hypnosis has a long history rooted in ancient ritual, Eastern medicine, and other "prescientific" paradigms of health psychology (Edmonston, 1986). Accordingly, biofeedback conditioning, Pavlovian conditioning, and other paradigms of "behavioral medicine" are historically set apart from hypnosis. But recently, controlled studies have shown that the autonomic effects of hypnotic suggestion are mediated by mental imagery (Barber, 1978, 1984) and thus are psychologically equivalent to the autonomic effects of behavioral conditioning.

Individual differences in the effectiveness of psychosomatic hypnosis, like individual differences in the effectiveness of behavioral conditioning, have been attributed to imaging ability in the only hypnotic study measuring such ability. Willard (1977) treated adult female clients who wanted to increase their breast size. The clients were instructed once a day to induce self-hypnosis, and "to visualize a wet, warm towel over their breasts and to allow this to produce a feeling of warmth" (p. 196). After 12 weeks of hypnotic visualizing, the increases in breast circumference averaged 1.37 inches, and correlated positively with the ability "to obtain visual imagery quickly, easily, and a large percent of the time" (p. 197).

Notwithstanding Willard's evidence that vivid imaging is necessary for bodily change, the more critical issue is whether hypnosis is also necessary. All case studies and experimental studies of psychosomatic hypnosis explicitly suggest that subjects imagine bodily change and thus implicitly assume that vivid imagery should produce such change. However, certain experiments (in addition to Shea's experiment) have shown that imagery is sufficient, and hypnosis is not necessary, for autonomic change. In one such experiment, Ikemi and Nakagawa (1962) found that poisonous leaves produced contact dermatitis when they were knowingly touched, but not when they were hypnotically imagined to be harmless and not when they were wakefully imagined to be harmless. Furthermore, Ikemi and Nakagawa found that harmless leaves produced contact dermatitis when they were hypnotically imagined to be poisonous and when they were wakefully imagined to be poisonous. In another experiment, Winer, Chauncey, and Barber (1965) found that salivary secretions increased when citric acid was applied to the tongue, but not when the citric acid was hypnotically imaged to be tasteless and not when the citric acid was wakefully imaged to be tasteless. In addition, Winer et al. (1965) found that salivary secretions increased when water was hypnotically imaged to be citric acid and when water was wakefully imaged to be citric acid. More recently, White (1978) found that such image-induced increases in salivary flow were positively correlated with "more vivid" imagery, as measured by Betts' Questionnaire Upon Mental Imagery (Betts, 1909; Sheehan, 1967).

Thus, in the studies by Winer et al. (1965), by Ikemi and Nakagawa (1962), and by Shea (1985), hypnotic images produced significant changes in bodily responses, and wakeful images produced equivalent or greater changes. All such changes are attributable to imagery, not to hypnosis, and are further reason for examining the health-related effects of imagery per se.

Mental Imagery and Physical Health

Mental images of particular events, without biofeedback and without hypnosis, have been shown to affect vasomotor responses in general, sexual responses, heart rate, blood pressure, EMGs, salivary responses, and immune responses. Moreover, in subjects who are vivid imagers, mental images have been shown to affect these bodily responses more strongly. All of these bodily responses to imagery will be reviewed. But for reasons both scientific and practical, the stronger bodily responses to vivid imagery will be given special consideration.

From a scientific standpoint, it is noteworthy that Watson's (1913) behavioristic argument against the efficacy of mental images was based on the empirical evidence in 1913, which contained no positive correlations between imagery vividness and memory ability. Although recent evidence continues to yield no significant correlations between imagery vividness and memory (Richardson, 1980), it yields many positive correlations between imagery vividness and autonomic responsiveness.

This correlational evidence for stronger autonomic responses to vivid images is even more important within the theoretical contexts, as opposed to the empirical contexts, of science. As noted earlier in this chapter, one of the theoretical assumptions adopted by most behavioral scientists is that mental images and other conscious entities cannot causally affect behavioral responses. But as Sheikh and Kunzendorf (1984) note, this behavioristic assumption implies that conscious images are not brain events—because if they were physical events in the brain, then they could regulate behavioral responses. The alternative assumption adopted by Sheikh and Kunzendorf (1984)—that specific mental images are particular brain states—implies that vivid imagers are better able to innervate particular neural states and are better able "to control whatever somatic effects are causally affected by those neural states" (p. 107). The remainder of this review focuses on these somatic effects of healing images, vivid images in particular, and does not attempt to describe the neural underpinnings of such images. Neurological models of imaging and their supporting data have been reviewed elsewhere (Bisiach & Berti, in press; Ehrlichman & Barrett, 1983; Farah, 1984; Kosslyn, 1987; Kunzendorf, in press; Ley, 1983; Marks, 1985; Sheikh & Kunzendorf, 1984; Starker, 1982).

Finally, from a practical perspective, it should be noted that individual differences in the vividness and effectiveness of healing images can unnecessarily hinder the clinical application of such images. For examples, practitioners of obstetrics tend to instruct all women in breathing techniques for the control of labor pain, even though imaging techniques work best in women with vivid imagery (Korn & Johnson, 1983). Ironically, to the extent that "attention to breathing" is just "anticipatory imaging of breathing" (Mowrer, 1977), future research on pain control might show that breathing techniques themselves—like biofeedback and Pavlovian conditioning—work best in vivid imagers. Indeed, past research has shown that attentional abilities outside the context of pain control are positively correlated with imaging abilities (Carey, 1915; Ernest & Paivio, 1971; Gur & Hilgard, 1975). Thus clinical applications of imagistic healing need not be hindered by individual differences any more than other applications of psychological healing are hindered. Rather, during clinical applications of the following findings, greater use should be made of Richardson and Patterson's (1986) procedures for increasing imagery vividness.

Imagery and Blood Flow. Vasoconstriction and vasodilation determine local blood flow and local skin temperature. Recently, four experimental studies demonstrated that vasomotor activity can be altered by imaging that specific skin regions feel colder or hotter (Dugan & Sheridan, 1976; Kunzendorf, 1981, 1984; Ohkuma, 1985). Moreover, Kunzendorf (1981) found that the magnitude of these image-induced alterations in skin temperature is positively correlated with "more prevalent" visual and tactual images, as measured by scores on Kunzendorf's Prevalence of Imagery Tests. Similarly, Kunzendorf (1984) found that the magnitude of image-induced alterations in skin temperature is positively correlated with "more intense" visual images, as measured by image-induced effects on subjects' electroretinograms.

Clinical studies of blood-flow control indicate that mental imagery can be used either to increase internal blood flow or to decrease external bleeding. In a previously described study, Willard (1977) showed that adult females can use vivid images of breast warmth to increase blood flow and breast growth. In contrast, Lucas (1965) showed that hemophilic dental patients can use images of inactivity to decrease external bleeding, and Chaves (1980) showed that normal dental patients can do the same. Although all three of these studies employed hypnosis as well as imagery, the above evidence indicates that images without hypnosis are sufficient to produce vasodilation and vasoconstriction.

Imagery and Sexual Response.   Penile engorgement and vaginal engorgement represent special cases of blood-flow control. Research by Laws and Rubin (1969) and Smith and Over (1987) showed that males' erotic images are sufficient to induce penile engorgement. Research by Stock and Geer (1982) showed that females' erotic images are sufficient to induce vaginal engorgement. In addition, Smith and Over (1987) reported that the degree of image-induced engorgement in penes is positively correlated with "more vivid" imagery, as measured by Betts' Questionnaire Upon Mental Imagery (Betts, 1909; Sheehan, 1967). Conversely, Stock and Geer (1982) reported that the degree of image-induced engorgement in vaginae is positively correlated with "more frequent" imagery, as measured by Singer and Antrobus's (1972) Imaginal Processes Inventory.

Applied research on erotic images confirms that such images arise during normal sexual behavior and that they enhance sexual responding. Over 65% of all women and over 75% of all men reportedly generate erotic images during sexual intercourse, either occasionally or frequently (Hariton & Singer, 1974; Lentz & Zeiss, 1983–1984; Pope, Singer, & Rosenberg, 1984). Furthermore, in normal women (Lentz & Zeiss, 1983–1984), the likelihood of attaining orgasm during intercourse is positively but insignificantly correlated with the frequency of erotic images during intercourse ($r = .19$, $p < .20$), and is significantly correlated with the frequency of erotic images during masturbation ($r = .30$, $p < .05$). Furthermore, for applications in a sex therapy context, erotic images induce consistent physiological arousal without any habituation, whereas, erotic pictures and x-rated films produce physiological arousal that gradually habituates (Smith & Over, 1987).

Imagery and Heart Rate. In the past 20 years, many studies obtained heart-rate increases in response to images of emotional and/or bodily arousal (Bauer & Craighead, 1979; Bell & Schwartz, 1975; Blizard, Cowings, & Miller, 1975; Boulougouris, Rabavilas, & Stefanis, 1977; Carroll, Baker, & Preston, 1979; Carroll, Marzillier, & Merian, 1982; Craig, 1968; Gottschalk, 1974; Grossberg & Wilson, 1968; Jones & Johnson, 1978, 1980; Jordan & Lenington, 1979; Lang, Kozak, Miller, Levin, & McLean, 1980; Marks & Huson, 1973; Marks, Marset, Boulougouris, & Huson, 1971; Marzillier, Carroll, & Newland, 1979; Roberts & Weerts, 1982; Schwartz, 1971; Schwartz, Weinberger, & Singer, 1981; Shea, 1985; Waters & McDonald, 1973). Moreover, five studies obtained heart-rate decreases in response to images of relaxation, especially relaxation in a supine position (Arabian, 1982; Bell & Schwartz, 1975; Furedy & Klajner, 1978; McCanne & Iennarella, 1980; Shea, 1985).

In the past 10 years, five heart-rate studies tested individual differences in imagery and found positive correlations with imaginal control of heart rate. Grossberg and Wilson (1968) and Lang, Kozak, Miller, Levin, and McLean (1980) found that subjects who exhibit greater heart-rate increases during "images of arousal" assign higher vividness ratings to those images. Carroll, Baker, and Preston (1979) found that subjects who exhibit greater heart-rate increases during "images of arousal" also assign higher vividness ratings to test images from the Vividness of Visual Imagery Questionnaire (Marks, 1973). Barbour (1981) found that subjects who show greater heart-rate change from "images of relaxation" to "images of arousal" assign higher vividness ratings to test images from the Questionnaire Upon Mental Imagery (Betts, 1909; Ashton & White, 1980). Kunzendorf (1984) found that subjects whose relaxing images and arousal images induce greater heart-rate change, controlling for breath-rate change, exhibit larger effects of visual imaging on the electroretinogram.

In applied research studies described by Lang, Kozak, Miller, Levin, and McLean (1980) and by Revland and Hirschman (1976), imagery training was successfully used to increase the imaginal control of heart rate in subjects with average imaging abilities. In clinical applications described by Engel (1979), biofeedback and imagery were successfully used to control the heart rate in patients with various arrhythmias.

Imagery and Blood Pressure. In experimental studies with normal subjects, Roberts and Weerts (1982) and Schwartz, Weinberger, and

Singer (1981) observed that diastolic blood pressure is raised by images of anger, but not by images of fear. However, both groups of experimenters reported that systolic blood pressure is raised by images of either anger or fear.

In applied research with chemotherapy patients, Burish and Lyles (1981) induced reductions in systolic blood pressure with relaxing images, which helped the patients to cope with fears of chemotherapy. In applied studies with hypertensive clients, Ahsen (1978) and Crowther (1983) induced long-lasting reductions in systolic and diastolic blood pressure with relaxing images, which presumably helped the clients to cope with various angers.

Imagery and EMGs. Electromyographs (EMGs) from the frontalis muscle provide one psychophysiological index of stress (Qualls, 1982–1983). In normal subjects, frontalis EMG activity and subjectively experienced tension have been increased with arousing images of stressful situations (Passchier & Helm-Hylkema, 1981). Conversely, in subjects with migraine headaches and muscle contraction headaches, frontalis EMGs and subjective tensions have been reduced with relaxing images (Thompson & Adams, 1984).

EMGs from other muscle locations provide covert indexes of imagistic thought related to those specific locations (McGuigan, 1978a, 1978b). For example, Lusebrink (1986–1987) found that visual images of a pencil are covertly accompanied by EMG activity in the right arm, whereas visual images of the letter "P" are covertly accompanied by EMG activity in the lip. Schwartz, Fair, Greenberg, Freedman, and Klerman (1974) found that images of sadness and images of happiness, respectively, elevate and reduce corrugator EMG activity—facial activity that is "not typically noticeable by either the casual observer or the subject himself" (Schwartz, 1975, p. 320). Findings such as these constitute strong support for James's (1890) ideo-motor theory of the relationship between imaged activity and real behavior: "We may then lay it down for certain that *every representation of a movement awakens in some degree the actual movement which is its object; and awakens it in a maximum degree whenever it is not kept from doing so by an antagonistic representation present simultaneously to the mind"* (p. 526).

Indeed, Schwartz (1975, 1978) noted that even when research subjects try to inhibit facial expression during sad and happy images covert changes in corrugator activity still differentiate the two images. Furthermore, in clinically applying James's ideo-motor theory, Quintyn and Cross (1986) noted that mental images of movement help to disinhibit the "frozen" body part in patients with Parkinson's disease.

Imagery and Electrodermal Activity.   Several research studies demonstrated that images of emotional and bodily arousal increase electrodermal activity in normal and abnormal subjects (Bauer & Craighead, 1979; Boulougouris, Rabavilas, & Stefanis, 1977; Drummond, White, & Ashton, 1978; Gottschalk, 1974; Haney & Euse, 1976; Jordan & Lenington, 1979; Marks, Marset, Boulougouris, & Huson, 1971; Passchier & Helm-Hylkema, 1981; Stern & Lewis, 1968; Waters & McDonald, 1973; Yaremko & Butler, 1975). In a study of individual differences in arousing images, Drummond, White, and Ashton (1978) showed that image-induced increases in galvanic skin response (GSR) are greater in subjects with "more vivid" imagery, as measured by Betts' (1909) Questionnaire Upon Mental Imagery. In an applied study of arousing images, Yaremko and Butler (1975) showed that 10 pretest images of electric shock produce faster electrodermal habituation to test shocks than 10 pretest shocks produce.

In applied research on images of relaxation, Thompson and Adams (1984) observed that such images reduce electrodermal responding in headache sufferers. In applied research on individual differences in lie detection, Kunzendorf and Bradbury (1983) observed that relaxing images attentuate lie-induced GSRs in those subjects with "more prevalent" images, as measured by Kunzendorf's (1981) Prevalence of Visual Imagery Test.

Imagery and Immune Responses.   Effects of mental images on immune response have been documented both in experimental research with healthy subjects and in clinical research with cancer patients. In healthy subjects, images of "white blood cells attacking germs" have been shown to produce greater immune responsiveness—in particular, greater neutrophil adherence (Schneider, Smith, Minning, Whitcher, & Hermanson, 1988) and higher lymphocyte counts (Hall, Longo, & Dixon, 1981). Also in healthy subjects, images of an unresponsive immune system have been shown to produce lower neutrophil adherence (Schneider et al., 1988) and less lymphocyte stimulation of immune response to the varicella zoster viral antigen (Smith, McKenzie, Marmer, & Steele, 1985). Both the image-induced increase in neutrophil adherence and the image-induced decrease in neutrophil adherence were positively correlated with the judged vividness of subjects' inducing images (Schneider et al., 1988, studies 7–8). Finally, in normal subjects, images of relaxation have been shown to reduce adrenal corticosteroids, the "stress hormones" that suppress immune function (Rider, Floyd, & Kirkpatrick, 1985).

In patients undergoing surgical and chemical treatments for cancer, mental images of "tumors being absorbed or attacked by white blood cells" have been shown to increase the likelihood of remission (Achterberg, Simonton, & Simonton, 1977; Pickett, 1987–1988; Simonton, Matthews-Simonton, & Sparks, 1980). Moreover, the likelihood of remission in these imaging patients has been found to correlate positively with their imaging abilities, as measured by Achtenberg and Lawlis's Image-CA scores (Achterberg, 1984; Achterberg & Lawlis, 1979; Achterberg, Lawlis, Simonton, & Matthews-Simonton, 1977).

CONCLUDING REMARKS

Although the healing images of ancient ritual and Eastern medicine have led to healing images in scientific research and Western medicine, the path is laden with historical detours and theoretical obstacles. As McMahon (1975) reminds us, Western doctors once refused to accept the fact that a soldier was frightened to death by a cannon ball breezing past his face, and instead they attributed his death to "the wind of the cannon ball" sucking all the air from his lungs. Of course, now many practitioners of medicine accept the evidence showing that mental variables such as fear and sadness can diminish physical health (Kunzendorf & Sheikh, in press) and even the evidence showing that behavioral treatments like biofeedback and Pavlovian conditioning can *improve* physical health. However, many practitioners still refuse to believe the evidence showing that mental images can improve physical health—perhaps, because healing images seem too ancient and Eastern to be "scientific." Nevertheless, we surmise that ancient wisdom regarding healing images, as supported by modern science, will prevail ultimately.

References

Achterberg, J. (1984). Imagery and medicine: Psychophysiological speculations. *Journal of Mental Imagery, 8,* 1–13.

Achterberg, J. (1985). *Imagery in healing.* Boston: Shambhala.

Achterberg, J., & Lawlis, G. F. (1979). A canonical analysis of blood chemistry variables related to psychological measures of cancer patients. *Multivariate Experimental Clinical Research, 4,* 1–10.

Achterberg, J., & Lawlis, G. F., Simonton, O. C., & Matthews-Simonton, S. (1977). Psychological factors and blood chemistries as disease outcome predictors for cancer patients. *Multivariate Experimental Clinical Research, 3,* 107–122.

Achterberg, J., Simonton, O. C., & Simonton, S. (1977). Psychology of the exceptional cancer patient: A description of patients who outlive predicted life expectancies. *Psychotherapy: Theory, Research, and Practice, 14,* 416–422.

Ader, R. (1985). Behaviorally conditioned modulation of immunity. In R. Guillemin, M. Cohn, & T. Melnechuk (Eds.), *Neural modulation of immunity* (pp. 55–66). New York: Raven Press.

Ahsen, A. (1968). *Basic concepts in eidetic psychotherapy.* New York: Brandon House.

Ahsen, A. (1978). Eidetics: Neural experiential growth potential for the treatment of accident traumas, debilitating stress conditions, and chronic emotional blocking. *Journal of Mental Imagery, 2,* 1–22.

Ajmal, M. (1986). *Muslim contributions to psychotherapy and other essays.* Islamabad, Pakistan: National Institute of Psychology.

Arabian, J. M. (1982). Imagery and Pavlovian heart rate decelerative conditioning. *Psychophysiology, 19,* 286–293.

Arabian, J. M., & Furedy, J. J. (1983). Individual differences in imagery ability and Pavlovian heart rate decelerative conditioning. *Psychophysiology, 20,* 325–331.

Ashton, R., & White, K. D. (1980). Sex differences in imagery vividness: An artefact of the test. *British Journal of Psychology, 71,* 35–38.

Assagioli, R. (1965). *Psychosynthesis: A collection of basic writings.* New York: Viking.

Barber, T. X. (1978). Hypnosis, suggestions, and psychosomatic phenomena: A new look from the standpoint of recent experimental studies. *American Journal of Clinical Hypnosis, 21,* 13-27.

Barber, T. X. (1984). Changing "unchangeable" bodily processes by (hypnotic) suggestions: A new look at hypnosis, cognitions, imagining, and the mind-body problem. In A. A. Sheikh (Ed.), *Imagination and healing* (pp. 69–158). Farmingdale, NY: Baywood.

Barbour, W. P. (1981). *Vividness of mental imagery and heart rate response to imagined anxiety evoking situations.* Unpublished honours thesis, University of Western Australia. (Summarized by Richardson, 1984)

Bauer, R. M., & Craighead, W. E. (1979). Psychophysiological responses to the imagination of fearful and neutral situations: The effects of imagery instructions. *Behavior Therapy, 10,* 389–403.

Beck, A. T. (1970). Role of fantasies in psychotherapy and psychopathology. *Journal of Nervous and Mental Diseases, 150,* 3–17.

Bell, I. R., & Schwartz, G. E. (1975). Voluntary control and reactivity of human heart rate. *Psychophysiology, 12,* 339–348.

Betts, G. H. (1909). *The distribution and functions of mental imagery.* New York: Teachers College, Columbia University.

Binder, G. A. (1966). *Great moments in medicine.* Detroit: Park-Davis.

Birnbaum, R. (1979). *The healing Buddha.* Boulder, CO: Shambhala.

Bisiach, E., & Berti, A. (in press). Waking images and neural activity. In R. G. Kunzendorf & A. A. Sheikh (Eds.), *The psychophysiology of mental imagery: Theory, research, and application.* Farmingdale, NY: Baywood.

Blizard, D. A., Cowings, P., & Miller, N. E. (1975). Visceral responses to opposite types of autogenic-training imagery. *Biological Psychology, 3,* 49–55.

Blofeld, J. (1970). *The Tantric mysticism of Tibet.* New York: Dutton.

Bornstein, P. H., & Sipprelle, C. N. (1973, April). Clinical applications of induced anxiety in the treatment of obesity. Paper presented at the Southeastern Psychological Association meeting.

Boulougouris, J. C., Rabavilas, D. D., & Stefanis, C. (1977). Psychophysiological responses in obsessive-compulsive patients. *Behaviour Research and Therapy, 15,* 221–230.

Burang, T. (1974). *The Tibetan art of healing.* London: Robinson and Watkins.

Burish, T. G., & Lyles, J. N. (1981). Effects of relaxation training in reducing adverse reactions to cancer chemotherapy. *Journal of Behavioral Medicine, 4,* 65–78.

Carey, N. (1915). Factors in the mental processes of school children: I. Visual and auditory imagery. *British Journal of Psychology, 7,* 453–490.

Carroll, D., Baker, J., & Preston, M. (1979). Individual differences in visual imaging and the voluntary control of heart rate. *British Journal of Psychology, 70,* 39–49.

Carroll, D., Marzillier, J. S., & Merian, S. (1982). Psychophysiological changes accompanying different types of arousing and relaxing imagery. *Psychophysiology, 19,* 75–82.

Cautela, J. R. (1977). Covert conditioning: Assumptions and procedures. *Journal of Mental Imagery, 1,* 53–64.

Chaves, J. F. (1980, September). Hypnotic control of surgical bleeding. Paper presented at Annual Meeting of the American Psychological Association, Montreal. (Summarized by Barber, 1984)

Clifford, T. (1984). *Tibetan Buddhist medicine and psychiatry.* New York: Samuel Weiser.

Corbin, H. (1970). *Creative imagination in the Sufism of Ibn 'Arabi* (R. Manheim, Trans.). London: Routledge & Kegan Paul.

Craig, K. D. (1968). Physiological arousal as a function of imagined, vicarious, and direct stress experience. *Journal of Abnormal Psychology, 73,* 513–520.

Crowther, J. H. (1983). Stress management training and relaxation imagery in the treatment of essential hypertension. *Journal of Behavioral Medicine, 6,* 169–187.

Desoille, R. (1961). *Theorie et pratique du rêve éveillé dirigé.* Geneva: Mont Blanc.

Desoille, R. (1965). *The directed daydream.* New York: Psychosynthesis Research Foundation.

Drummond, P., White, K., & Ashton, R. (1978). Imagery vividness affects habituation rate. *Psychophysiology, 15,* 193–195.

Dugan, M., & Sheridan, C. (1976). Effects of instructed imagery on temperature of hands. *Perceptual and Motor Skills, 42,* 14.

Eddy, M. B. (1934). *Science and health with key to the scriptures.* Boston: First Church of Christ Scientist.

Edmonston, W. E. (1986). *The induction of hypnosis.* New York: Wiley.

Ehrlichman, H., & Barrett, J. (1983). Right hemisphere specialization for mental imagery: A review of the evidence. *Brain and Cognition, 2,* 55–76.

Eliade, M. (1958). *Yoga: Immortality and freedom.* New York: Pantheon.

Eliade, M. (1959). *The sacred and the profane.* New York: Harper & Row.

Eliade, M. (1964). *Shamanism: Archaic techniques of ecstasy.* New York: Pantheon.

Eliade, M. (1976). *Patanjal and yoga.* New York: Schocken.

Engel, B. T. (1979). Behavioral applications in the treatment of patients with cardiovascular disorders. In J. V. Basmajian (Ed.), *Biofeedback: Principles and practices for clinicians.* Baltimore: Williams & Wilkins.

Ernest, C. H., & Paivio, A. (1971). Imagery and sex differences in incidental recall. *British Journal of Psychology, 62,* 67–72.

Evan-Wentz, W. Y. (1967). *Tibetan yoga and secret doctrine.* London: Oxford University Press.

Farah, M. J. (1984). The neurological basis of mental imagery: A componential analysis. In S. Pinker (Ed.), *Visual cognition* (pp. 245–271). Cambridge, MA: MIT Press.

Fretigny, R., & Virel. A (1968). *L'imageri mentale.* Geneva: Mont Blanc.

Furedy, J. J., & Klajner, F. (1978). Imaginational Pavlovian conditioning of large-magnitude cardiac decelerations with tilt as UCS. *Psychophysiology, 15,* 538–548.

Furedy, J. J., & Poulos, C. X. (1976). Heart-rate decelerative Pavlovian conditioning with tilt as UCS: Towards behavioral control of cardiac dysfunction. *Biological Psychology, 4,* 93–106.

Gendlin, E. T. (1978). *Focusing.* New York: Everest House.

Gendlin, E. T., & Olsen, L. (1970). The use of imagery in experiential focusing. *Psychotherapy: Theory, Research and Practice, 7,* 221–223.

Gorczynski, R. M., Macrae, S., & Kennedy, M. (1982). Conditioned immune response associated with allogeneic skin grafts in mice. *Journal of Immunology, 129,* 704–709.

Gottschalk, L. A. (1974). Self-induced visual imagery, affect arousal, and autonomic correlates. *Psychosomatics, 15,* 166–169.

Green, E. E., Ferguson, D., Green, A. M., & Walters, E. (1970). *Preliminary report on voluntary controls project: Swami Rama.* Topeka: Menninger Foundation.

Green, E. E., Walters, E., Green, A. M. & Murphy, G. (1969). Feedback technique for deep relaxation. *Psychophysiology, 6,* 371–377.

Grossberg, J. M., & Wilson, K. M. (1968). Physiological changes accompanying the visualization of fearful and neutral situations. *Journal of Personality and Social Psychology, 10,* 124–133.

Grossinger, R. (1980). *Planet medicine: From stone age shamanism to post-industrial healing.* New York: Doubleday.

Gur, R. C., & Hilgard, E. R. (1975). Visual imagery and the discrimination of differences between altered pictures simultaneously and successively presented. *British Journal of Psychology, 66,* 341–345.

Habeck, B. K., & Sheikh, A. A. (1984). Imagery and the treatment of phobic disorders. In A. A. Sheikh (Ed.), *Imagination and healing.* Farmingdale, NY: Baywood.

Hall, H. R. (1984). Imagery and cancer. In A. A. Sheikh (Ed.), *Imagination and healing* (pp. 159–169). Farmingdale, NY: Baywood.

Hall, H. R., Longo, S., & Dixon, R. (1981, October). *Hypnosis and the immune system: The effect of hypnosis on T and B cell function.* Paper presented at 33rd Annual Meeting for the Society for Clinical and Experiment Hypnosis, Portland, OR. (Summarized by Hall, 1984)

Haney, J. N., & Euse, F. J. (1976). Skin conductance and heart rate responses to neutral, positive, and negative imagery: Implications for covert behavior therapy procedures. *Behavior Therapy, 7,* 494–503.

Hariton, E. B., & Singer, J. L. (1974). Women's fantasies during sexual intercourse: Normative and theoretical implications. *Journal of Consulting and Clinical Psychology, 42,* 313–322.

Hartman, F. (1973). *Paracelsus: Life and prophecies.* Blauvelt, NY: Rudolf Steiner.

Harwood, C. W. (1962). Operant heart rate conditioning. *Psychological Record, 12,* 279–284.

Herzfeld, G. M., & Taub, E. (1980). Effect of slide projections and tape-recorded suggestions on thermal biofeedback training. *Biofeedback and Self-Regulation, 5,* 393–405.

Hirschman, R., & Favaro, L. (1980). Individual differences in imagery vividness and voluntary heart rate control. *Personality and Individual Differences, 1,* 129–133.

Horowitz, M. J. (1978). Controls of visual imagery and therapeutic intervention. In J. L. Singer & K. S. Pope (Eds.), *The power of human imagination.* New York: Plenum.

Ikeda, Y., & Hirai, H. (1976). Voluntary control of electrodermal activity in relation to imagery and internal perception scores. *Psychophysiology, 13,* 330–333.

Ikemi, Y., & Nakagawa, S. (1962). A psychosomatic study of contagious dermatitis. *Kyushu Journal of Medical Science, 13,* 335–350.

Jaffe, D. T., & Bresler, D. E. (1980). Guided imagery: Healing through the mind's eye. In J. E. Shorr, G. E, Sobel, P. Robin, & J. A. Connella, (Eds.), *Imagery: Its many dimensions and applications.* New York: Plenum.

James, W. (1890). *The principles of psychology* (Vol. 2). New York: Henry Holt.

James, W. (1963). *The varieties of religious experience.* New York: University Books.

Jonas, H. (1958). *The Gnostic religion.* Boston: Beacon Press.

Jones, G. E., & Johnson, H. J. (1978). Physiological responding during self-generated imagery of contextually complete stimuli. *Psychophysiology, 15,* 439–446.

Jones, G. E., & Johnson, H. J. (1980). Heart rate and somatic concomitants of mental imagery. *Psychophysiology, 17,* 339–347.

Jordan, C. S. (1979). Mental imagery and psychotherapy: European approaches. In A. A. Sheikh and J. T. Shaffer (Eds.), *The potential of fantasy and imagination.* New York: Brandon House.

Jordan, C. S., & Lenington, K. T. (1979). Physiological correlates of eidetic imagery and induced anxiety. *Journal of Mental Imagery, 3,* 31–42.

Jung, C. G. (1960). *The structure and dynamics of the psyche* (R. F. C. Hull, Trans.). (Collected works, Vol. 8). Princeton: Princeton University Press. (Original work published 1926)

Jung, C. G. (1976). *The symbolic life* (R. F. C. Hull, Trans. Collected works, Vol. 18). Princeton: Princeton University Press.

Kepecs, J. G. (1954). Observations on screens and barriers in the mind. *Psychoanalytic Quarterly, 23,* 62–77.

King, D. L. (1973). An image theory of classical conditioning. *Psychological Reports, 33,* 403–411.

King, D. L. (1983). Imagery theory of conditioning. In A. A. Sheikh (Ed.), *Imagery: Current theory, research, and application* (pp. 156–186). New York: Wiley.

King, N. J., & Montgomery, R. B. (1980). Biofeedback-induced control of human peripheral temperature: A critical review. *Psychological Bulletin, 88,* 738–752.

King, S. (1983). *Kahuna healing.* Wheaton, IL: Theosophical Publishing House.

Klinger, E. (1971). *The structure and function of fantasy.* New York: Wiley.

Klinger, E. (1980). Therapy and the flow of thought. In J. E. Shorr, G. E. Sobel, P. Robin, & J. A. Connella (Eds.), *Imagery: Its many dimensions and applications.* New York: Plenum.

Konorski, J. (1967). *Integrative activity of the brain.* Chicago: University of Chicago Press.

Korn, E. R., & Johnson, K. (1983). *Visualization: The uses of imagery in the health professions.* Homewood, IL: Dorsey.

Kosslyn, S. (1980). *Image and mind.* Cambridge: Harvard University Press.

Kosslyn, S. M. (1987). Seeing and imagery in the cerebral hemispheres: A computational approach. *Psychological Review, 94,* 148–175.

Krasnogorski, N. I. (1909). Uber die Bedingungsreflexe in Kindesalter. *Jahrburch für Kinderheilkunde und physische Erziehung, 69,* 1–24.

Kunzendorf, R. G. (1981). Individual differences in imagery and autonomic control. *Journal of Mental Imagery, 5,* 47–60.

Kunzendorf, R. G. (1984). Centrifugal effects of eidetic imaging on flash electroretinograms and autonomic responses. *Journal of Mental Imagery, 8,* 67–76.

Kunzendorf, R. G. (in press). Mind-brain identity theory: A materialistic foundation for the psychophysiology of mental imagery. In R. G. Kunzendorf & A. A. Sheikh (Eds.), *The psychophysiology of mental imagery: Theory, research, and application.* Farmingdale, NY: Baywood.

Kunzendorf, R. G., & Bradbury, J. L. (1983). Better liars have better imaginations. *Psychological Reports, 52,* 634.

Kunzendorf, R. G., & Sheikh, A. A. (in press). Imaging, image-monitoring, and health. In R. G. Kunzendorf & A. A. Sheikh (Eds.), *The psychophysiology of mental imagery: Theory, research, and application.* Farmingdale, NY: Baywood.

La Barre, W. (1938). *The peyote cult.* New Haven: Yale University Press.

La Barre, W. (1979). Shamanic origins of religion and medicine. *Journal of Psychedelic Drugs, 1-2,* 7–11.

Lang, P. J., Kozak, M. J., Miller, G. A., Levin, D. N., & McLean, A. (1980). Emotional imagery: Conceptual structure and pattern of somato-visceral response. *Psychophysiology, 17,* 179–192.

Laws, D. R., & Rubin, H. B. (1969). Instructional control of an autonomic sexual response. *Journal of Applied Behavior Analysis, 2,* 93–99.

LeBouef, A., & Wilson, C. (1978). The importance of imagery in maintenance of feedback-assisted relaxation over extinction trials. *Perceptual and Motor Skills, 47,* 824–826.

Lentz, S. L., & Zeiss, A. M. (1983–1984). Fantasy and sexual arousal in college women: An empirical investigation. *Imagination, Cognition, and Personality, 3,* 185–202.

Leuner, H. (1977). Guided affective imagery: An account of its development. *Journal of Mental Imagery, 1,* 73–92.

Leuner, H. (1978). Basic principles and therapeutic efficacy of guided affective imagery. In J. L. Singer & K. S. Pope (Eds.), *The power of human imagination.* New York: Plenum.

Ley, R. G. (1983). Cerebral laterality and imagery. In A. A. Sheikh (Ed.), *Imagery: Current theory, research, and application* (pp. 252–287). New York: Wiley.

Lisina, M. I. (1965). The role of orientation in the transformation of involuntary reactions into voluntary ones. In L. Veronin, A. Leontiev, A. Luria, C. Sokolov, & O. Vinogradova (Eds.), *Orienting reflex and exploratory behavior.* Washington, DC: American Institute of Biological Sciences.

Lucas, O. (1965). Dental extractions in the hemophiliac: Control of the emotional factors by hypnosis. *American Journal of Clinical Hypnosis, 7,* 301–307.

Lusebrink, V. B. (1986–1987). Visual imagery: Its psychophysiological components and levels of information processing. *Imagination, Cognition, and Personality, 6,* 205–218.

Lyons, A. S., & Petrucelli, R. J. (1978). *Medicine: An illustrated history.* New York: Abrams.

Mandler, G., Preven, D. W., & Kuhlman, C. K. (1962). Effects of operant reinforcement on the GSR. *Journal of the Experimental Analysis of Behavior, 62,* 552–559.

Mangan, G. L. (1974). Personality and conditioning: Some personality, cognitive and psychophysiological parameters of classical appetitive (sexual) GSR conditioning. *Pavlovian Journal of Biological Sciences, 9,* 125–135.

Marks, D. F. (1973). Visual imagery differences in the recall of pictures. *British Journal of Psychology, 64,* 17–14.

Marks, D. F. (1985). The neuropsychology of imagery. In D. F. Marks (Ed.), *Theories of image formation.* New York: Brandon House.

Marks, I., & Huson, J. (1973). Physiological aspects of neutral and phobic imagery: Further observations. *British Journal of Psychiatry, 122,* 567–572.

Marks, I., Marset, P., Boulougouris, J., & Huson, J. (1971). Physiological accompaniments of neutral and phobic imagery. *Psychological Medicine, 1,* 299–307.

Marzillier, J. S., Carroll, D., Newland, J. R. (1979). Self-report and physiological changes accompanying repeated imaging of a phobic scene. *Behavior Research and Therapy, 17,* 71–77.

McCanne, T. R., & Iennarella, R. S. (1980). Cognitive and somatic events associated with discriminative changes in heart rate. *Psychophysiology, 17,* 18–28.

McGuigan, F. J. (1978a). *Cognitive psychophysiology.* Englewood Cliffs, NJ: Prentice-Hall.

McGuigan, F. J. (1978b). Imagery and thinking: Covert functioning of the motor system. In G. E. Schwartz & D. Shapiro (Eds.), *Consciousness and self-regulation: Advances in research and theory* (Vol. 2, pp. 37–100). New York: Plenum.

McMahon, C. E. (1975). The wind of the cannon ball. *Psychotherapy and Psychosomatics, 26,* 125–131.

McMahon, C. E. (1976). The role of imagination in the disease process: Pre-Cartesian history. *Psychological Medicine, 6,* 179–184.

McMahon, C. E., & Sheikh, A. A. (1984). Imagination in disease and healing processes: A historical perspective. In A. A. Sheikh (Ed.), *Imagination and healing.* Farmingdale, NY: Baywood.

Meichenbaum, D. (1977). *Cognitive-behavior modification: An integrative approach.* New York: Plenum.

Meichenbaum, D. (1978). Why does using imagery in psychotherapy lead to change? In J. L. Singer & K. S. Pope (Eds.), *The power of human imagination.* New York: Plenum.

Menzies, R. (1937). Conditioned vasomotor responses in human subjects. *Journal of Psychology, 4,* 75–120.

Menzies, R. (1941). Further studies of conditioned vasomotor responses in human subjects. *Journal of Experimental Psychology, 29,* 457–482.

Miller, N. E. (1969). Learning of visceral and glandular responses. *Science, 163,* 434–445.

Miller, N. E. (1978). Biofeedback and visceral learning. *Annual Review of Psychology, 29,* 373–404.

Mishra, R. (1973). *Yoga stuvas.* Garden City, NY: Anchor Press.

Mookerjee, A. (1971). *Tantra art.* Paris: Ravi Kumar.

Morrison, J. K. (1980). Emotive-reconstructive therapy: A short-term psychotherapeutic use of mental imagery. In J. E. Shorr, G. E. Sobel, P. Robin, & J. A. Connella (Eds.), *Imagery: Its many dimensions and applications.* New York: Plenum.

Mowrer, O. H. (1960). *Learning theory and the symbolic processes.* New York: Wiley.

Mowrer, O. H. (1977). Mental imagery: An indispensable psychological concept. *Journal of Mental Imagery, 2,* 303–326.

Much, N. C., & Sheikh, A. A. (1986). The oneirotherapics. In A. A. Sheikh (Ed.), *Anthology of imagery techniques.* Milwaukee, WI: American Imagery Institute.

Ohkuma, Y. (1985). Effects of evoking imagery on the control of peripheral skin temperature. *Japanese Journal of Psychology, 54,* 88–94. (English abstract)

Osler, W. (1921). *The evolution of modern medicine.* New Haven: Yale University Press.

Panagiotou, N., & Sheikh, A. A. (1977). The image and the unconscious. *International Journal of Social Psychiatry, 23,* 169–186.

Passchier, J., & Helm-Hylkema, H. (1981). The effect of stress imagery on arousal and its implications for biofeedback of the frontalis muscles. *Biofeedback and Self-Regulation, 6,* 295–303.

Pavlov, I. (1906). The scientific investigation of the psychical faculties or processes in the higher animals. *Science, 24,* 613–619.

Pavlov, I. (1927). *Conditioned reflexes: An investigation of the physiological activity of the cerebral cortex.* London: Oxford University Press.

Perls, F. (1970). *Gestalt therapy verbatim.* New York: Bantam.

Pickett, E. (1987–1988). Fibroid tumors and response to guided imagery and music: Two case studies. *Imagination, Cognition, and Personality, 7,* 165–176.

Pope, K. S. (1977). The flow of consciousness. Unpublished doctoral dissertation, Yale University, Cambridge.

Pope, K. S., Singer, J. L., & Rosenberg, L. C. (1984). Sex, fantasy and imagination: Scientific research and clinical applications. In A. A. Sheikh (Ed.), *Imagination and healing* (pp. 197–209). Farmingdale, NY: Baywood.

Progoff, I. (1970). Waking dream and living myth. In J. Campbell (Ed.), *Myths, dreams and religion.* New York: Dutton.

Qualls, P. J. (1982–1983). The physiological measurement of imagery: An overview. *Imagination, Cognition, and Personality, 2,* 89–101.

Qualls, P. J., & Sheehan, P. W. (1979). Capacity for absorption and relaxation during electromyograph biofeedback and no-feedback conditions. *Journal of Abnormal Psychology, 88,* 652–662.

Qualls, P. J., & Sheehan, P. W. (1981a). Imagery encouragement, absorption capacity, and relaxation during electromyograph biofeedback. *Journal of Personality and Social Psychology, 41,* 370–379.

Qualls, P. J., & Sheehan, P. W. (1981b). Role of the feedback signal in electromyograph biofeedback: The relevance of attention. *Journal of Experimental Psychology: General, 110,* 204–216.

Quintyn, M., & Cross, E. (1986). Factors affecting the ability to initiate movement in Parkinson's disease. *Physical and Occupational Therapy in Geriatrics, 4,* 51–60.

Reps, P. (Compiler). (1957). *Zen flesh, Zen bones.* Rutland, VT: Tuttle.

Revland, P., & Hirschman, R. (1976). Imagery training and visual biofeedback *Psychophysiology, 13,* 186–187.

Reyher, J. (1963). Free imagery, an uncovering procedure. *Journal of Clinical Psychology, 19,* 454–459.

Reyher, J. (1977). Spontaneous visual imagery: Implications for psychoanalysis, psychopathology, and psychotherapy. *Journal of Mental Imagery, 2,* 253–274.

Richardson, A. (1969). *Mental imagery.* New York: Springer.

Richardson, A. (1984). Strengthening the theoretical links between imaged stimuli and physiological responses. *Journal of Mental Imagery, 8,* 113–126.

Richardson, A., & Patterson, Y. (1986). An evaluation of three procedures for increasing imagery vividness. *International Review of Mental Imagery, 2,* 166–191.

Richardson, J. T. E. (1980). *Mental imagery and human memory.* New York: St. Martins.

Rider, M. S., Floyd, J. W., & Kirkpatrick, J. (1985). The effect of music, imagery, and relaxation on adrenal corticosteroids and the reentrainment of circadian rhythms. *Journal of Music Therapy, 22,* 46–58.

Roberts, A. H., Kewman, D. G., & MacDonald, H. (1973). Voluntary control of skin temperatures: Unilateral changes using hypnosis and feedback. *Journal of Abnormal Psychology, 82,* 163–168.

Roberts, R. J., & Weerts, T. C. (1982). Cardiovascular responding during anger and fear imagery. *Psychological Reports, 50,* 219–230.

Rothenberg, J. (Ed.). (1968). *Technicians of the soul.* Garden City, NY: Doubleday.

Samuels, M., & Samuels, N. (1975). *Seeing with the mind's eye.* New York: Random House.

Sawyer, D. (1986). How Jungians work with images. In A. A. Sheikh (Ed.), *Anthology of imagery techniques.* Milwaukee, WI: American Imagery Institute.

Schneider, J., Smith, C. W., Minning, C., Whitcher, S., & Hermanson, J. (1988, June). *Psychological factors influencing immune system function in normal subjects: A summary of research findings and implications for the use of guided imagery.* Paper presented at the Tenth Annual Conference of the American Association for the Study of Mental Imagery, New Haven, CT.

Scholem, G. (1961). *Jewish mysticism.* New York: Schocken.

Schultz, K. D. (1984). The use of imagery in alleviating depression. In A. A. Sheikh (Ed.), *Imagination and healing.* Farmingdale, NY: Baywood.

Schwartz, G. E. (1971). Cardiac responses to self-induced thoughts. *Psychophysiology, 8,* 462–467.

Schwartz, G. E. (1975). Biofeedback, self-regulation, and the patterning of physiological processes. *American Scientist, 63,* 314–324.

Schwartz, G. E. (1978). Psychobiological foundations of psychotherapy and behavior change. In S. Garfield & A. Bergin (Eds.), *Handbook of psychotherapy and behavior change* (pp. 63–99). New York: Wiley.

Schwartz, G. E., Fair, P. L., Greenberg, P. S., Freedman, M., & Klerman, J. L. (1974). Facial electromyography in assessment of emotion. *Psychophysiology, 11,* 237.

Schwartz, G. E., Weinberger, D. A., & Singer, J. A. (1981). Cardiovascular differentiation of happiness, sadness, anger, and fear following imagery and exercise. *Psychosomatic Medicine, 43,* 343–364.

Shea, J. D. (1985). Effects of absorption and instructions on heart rate control. *Journal of Mental Imagery, 9,* 87–100.

Sheehan, P. W. (1967). A shortened form of Betts' Questionnaire Upon Mental Imagery. *Journal of Clinical Psychology, 23,* 386–389.

Sheikh, A. A. (1976). Treatment of insomnia through eidetic imagery: A new technique. *Perceptual and Motor Skills, 43,* 994.

Sheikh, A. A. (1978). Eidetic psychotherapy. In J. L. Singer & K. S. Pope (Eds.), *The power of human imagination.* New York: Plenum.

Sheikh, A. A. (Ed.). (1983). *Imagery: Current theory, research and application.* New York: Wiley.

Sheikh, A. A. (Ed.). (1984). *Imagination and healing.* Farmingdale, NY: Baywood.

Sheikh, A. A. (Ed.). (1986). *Anthology of imagery techniques.* Milwaukee, WI: American Imagery Institute.

Sheikh, A. A., & Jordan, C. S. (1981). Eidetic psychotherapy. In R. J. Corsini (Ed.), *Handbook of innovative psychotherapies.* New York: Wiley.

Sheikh, A. A., & Jordan, C. S. (1983). Clinical uses of mental imagery. In A. A. Sheikh (Ed.), *Imagery: Current theory, research, and application.* New York: Wiley.

Sheikh, A. A., & Kunzendorf, R. G. (1984). Imagery, physiology, and psychosomatic illness. *International Review of Mental Imagery, 1,* 95–138.

Sheikh, A. A., & Panagiotou, N. C. (1975). Use of mental imagery in psychotherapy: A critical review. *Perceptual and Motor Skills, 41,* 555–585.

Sheikh, A. A., & Shaffer, J. T. (Eds.). (1979). *The potential of fantasy and imagination.* New York: Brandon House.

Sheikh, A. A., Richardson, P., & Moleski, L. M. (1979). Psychosomatics and mental imagery: A brief view. In A. A. Sheikh and J. T. Shaffer (Eds.), *The potential of fantasy and imagination.* New York: Brandon House.

Shorr, J. E. (1978). Clinical use of categories of therapeutic imagery. In J. L. Singer & K. S. Pope (Eds.), *The power of human imagination.* New York: Plenum.

Simonton, O. C., Matthews-Simonton, S., & Sparks, T. F. (1980). Psychological intervention in the treatment of cancer. *Psychosomatics, 21,* 226–227.

Singer, J. L. (1974). *Imagery and daydream methods in psychotherapy and behavior modification.* New York: Academic Press.

Singer, J. L. (1979). Imagery and affect psychotherapy: Elaborating private scripts and generating contexts. In A. A. Sheikh & J. T. Shaffer (Eds.), *The potential of fantasy and imagination.* New York: Brandon House.

Singer, J. L., & Antrobus, J. S. (1972). Daydreaming, imaginal processes, and personality: A normative study. In P. Sheehan (Ed.), *The function and nature of imagery* (pp. 175–202). New York: Academic Press.

Singer, J. L., & Pope, K. S. (1978). The use of imagery and fantasy techniques in psychotherapy. In J. L. Singer & K. S. Pope (Eds.), *The power of human imagination.* New York: Plenum.

Singer, J. L., & Switzer, E. (1980). *Mind play: The creative uses of imagery.* Englewood Cliffs, NJ: Prentice-Hall.

Skinner, B. F. (1974). *About behaviorism.* New York: Knopf.

Smith, D., & Over, R. (1987). Does fantasy-induced sexual arousal habituate? *Behaviour Research and Therapy, 25,* 477–485.

Smith, G. R., McKenzie, J. M., Marmer, D. J., & Steele, R. W. (1985). Psychologic modulation of the human immune response to varicella zoster. *Archives of Internal Medicine, 145,* 2110–2112.

Stampfl, T., & Lewis, D. (1967). Essentials of therapy: A learning theory–based psychodynamic behavioral therapy. *Journal of Abnormal Psychology, 72,* 496–503.

Starker, S. (1982). Toward a psychophysiology of waking fantasy: EEG studies *Perceptual and Motor Skills, 55,* 891–902.

Stern, R. M., & Lewis, N. L. (1968). Ability of actors to control their GSRs and express emotions. *Psychophysiology, 4,* 294–299.

Stock, W. E., & Geer, J. H. (1982). A study of fantasy-based sexual arousal in women. *Archives of Sexual Behavior, 11,* 33–47.

Stoddard, A. M. (1911). *Life of Paracelsus.* London.

Takahashi, H. (1984). Experimental study on self-control of heart rate: Experiment for a biofeedback treatment of anxiety state. *Journal of Mental Health, 31,* 109–125. (English abstract)

Thompson, J. K., & Adams, H. E. (1984). Psychophysiological characteristics of headache patients. *Pain, 18,* 41–52.

Waters, W. F., & McDonald, D. G. (1973). Autonomic response to auditory, visual and imagined stimuli in a systematic desensitization context. *Behaviour Research and Therapy, 11,* 577–585.

Watkins, M. J. (1976). *Waking dreams.* New York: Harper.

Watson, J. B. (1913). Image and affection in behavior. *Journal of Philosophy, Psychology, and Scientific Methods, 10,* 421–428.

Watson, J. B. (1916). The place of the conditioned reflex in psychology. *Psychological Review, 23,* 89–116.

Watson, J. B. (1925). *Behaviorism.* New York: Norton.

Wegner, N., & Zeaman, D. (1958). Strength of cardiac conditioned responses with varying unconditioned stimulus durations. *Psychological Review, 65,* 238–241.

Wenger, M. A., & Bagchi, B. K. (1961). Studies of autonomic functions in practitioners of Yoga in India. *Behavioral Science, 6,* 312–323.

White, K. D. (1978). Salivation: The significance of imagery in its voluntary control. *Psychophysiology, 15,* 196–203.

White, T., Holmes, D., & Bennett, D. (1977). Effects of instructions, biofeedback, and cognitive activities on heart rate control. *Journal of Experimental Psychology: Human Learning and Memory, 3,* 477–484.

Willard, R. D. (1977). Breast enlargement through visual imagery and hypnosis. *American Journal of Clinical Hypnosis, 19,* 195–200.

Winer, R. A., Chauncey, H. H., & Barber, T. X. (1965). The influence of verbal or symbolic stimuli on salivary gland secretion. *Annals of the New York Academy of Sciences, 131,* 874–883.

Wolpe, J. (1969). *The practice of behavior therapy.* New York: Pergamon.

Yaremko, R. M., & Butler, M. C. (1975). Imaginal experience and attenuation of the galvanic skin response to shock. *Bulletin of the Psychonomic Society, 5,* 317–318.

Yates, F. A. (1966). *The art of memory.* London: Routledge & Kagan Paul.

17

Transcultural Psychotherapy

SOHAN L. SHARMA

Like a potter molding clay, culture molds the person. Trans-cultural consciousness/awareness can liberate the individual from the mold.

Haider Minza (1499–1551), author of
Ta'rikh-i-Rashidi, written between 1541–47

Many definitions of culture are presented in the literature. For our purposes, however, we may define culture as a shared social-psychological nexus of beliefs and values, which provides guidelines for one's actions and gives meaning to their actions. It is learned through imitation, identification with significant others, incorporation of their values, and educational and cultural media. A culture exists, essentially, as it is embodied in living people (Abel, Metraux, & Roll, 1987) and is manifested in behavior and actions. Some writers, therefore, have focused on behavior rather than on customs and institutions in the definition of culture (LeVine & Padilla, 1980).

In view of this, transcultural therapy may be defined as a relationship and a process in which the therapist and the client belong to different cultures, in which multiple value systems and diverse assumptions of normality and psychopathology come into play, and in which procedure,

516

goals, and parameters of the process have to be adopted to suit the cultural context of the client.

MENTAL ILLNESS AND THE SIGNIFICANCE OF CULTURE

Culture, implicitly and explicitly, defines social psychological reality for its members. It is against such reality that one's behavior is judged as acceptable or unacceptable. When a member's conduct is perceived as unacceptable, deviant, disturbed, or disturbing to others, it requires some form of control or management. A first step in the process is to categorize it and then attach various labels to the unacceptable behavior (e.g., sinful, immoral, deviant, criminal, possessed, or mentally ill). For instance, during the Middle Ages in Europe the deviant, the disturbed, and disturbing behaviors were labeled as "possessed by the devil." Since the mid-19th century, for a variety of reasons, similar behaviors have been labeled "mentally ill." Illustrating this point, Marsella (1985) states,

> [If] cultures vary with regards to their conception of reality, disorders which are based on reality contact also vary. For example, psychotic disorders are by definition a function of loss of contact with reality. In western psychiatry, there are three general classes of psychotic disorders: schizophrenia, manic-depressive disorders, and paranoid states. The central feature of these disorders is a loss of contact with reality, characterized by delusions, hallucinations, disorientation for time, place, and person, and general confusion.
>
> But among the non-western cultural groups, reality boundaries are not so rigidly fixed as they are in the west. Mystical states, depersonalization, visions and deviant belief systems are tolerated far more, especially if no one is physically harmed by the individual's behavior. For example, among the rural Philipinos with whom I worked, seeing visions, speaking with saints or dead relatives, beliefs in supernatural forces including witches, are all accepted as normal. (pp. 302–303)

Since culture defines the limits of unacceptable or deviant behaviors (mental illness), it also points the direction in which explanation and/or the causes of the deviant behavior may be sought (Erikson, 1966). Such direction may take various forms.

Some cultures attribute disturbed and deviant behaviors to the genetic background or the biochemical imbalance within the individual, as the present-day culture of the United States does. In patriarchal cultures, explanation may be sought in bad "parental modeling." Some find its causes in the supernatural or in the evil spirits, as the rural Hindu culture does. Still other cultures find causes in the deficient diet, as is frequently the case in underdeveloped countries. Some may point to the existing socioeconomic conditions (e.g., social oppression, economic exploitation, and lack of personal freedom) as the causes of the disturbed behavior, as the women's liberation movement does.

As the socioeconomic conditions and the *weltanschauung* of a culture changes, so does the explanation of the disturbed behavior or mental illness change. Hence the presumed cause and explanation of mental illness may vary, from time to time, within the same culture. For example, in the United States during the period of "moral treatment," between 1817 and 1865, superintendents of mental hospitals sought causes and explanation of the disturbed behavior (the term "mental illness" had not come in vogue yet) in the immoral life or background of the inmates (e.g., intemperance, overwork, greed, vulgar language, impious thoughts, etc.) (Bockoven, 1963, Grob, 1975). Today, however, this is explained as biochemical imbalance.

CULTURAL INFLUENCES ON THERAPY

When a behavior is deemed deviant or disturbed, the interventions or therapy required for its rectification are vaguely suggested by the culture. Generally, suggestions for treatment or therapy are in accord with the presumed causation of mental illness. For example, during the period of "moral treatment" in the United States, when the causes of the disturbed behavior was assumed to be immoral life, the proposed remedy was regular church attendance, thinking pious thoughts, hard work, abstinence from alcohol, and so on. Similarly, in the present culture of the United States, since a biochemical explanation of the disturbed behavior, or mental illness, is in vogue, suggested remedies are drugs, pills, and electroshock. In many villages of India, mental disturbances are attributed to sorcery or evil spirits. Hence the recommended therapy is to place the individual under the tutelage of a "spiritual" individual who can exorcise the evil spirits. Cultures designate or appoint certain individuals to perform such remedial, therapeutic functions and proffer on them a certain degree of power and prestige to execute their prescribed role.

The culturally provided explanation of the disturbed behavior (or mental illness) is, at least, partially accepted by the individual. For instance, it is not unusual these days for an American, middle-class individual to say that he or she is suffering from a biochemical imbalance, rather than to say that he or she is depressed.

If the client and the therapist belong to the same culture or ethnic group, many of the aforementioned problems may not be too difficult to manage in therapy, for they share similar social-psychological realities, similar value structures, and similar explanations and interpretations of the disturbed behavior. However, when the participants in a therapeutic situation have different racial and ethnic backgrounds, communication problems become complex and sometimes confusing (Sue, 1981). Reasons for this seem to be that due to racial and ethnic differences between the therapist and the client, the attributed cause(s) of mental illness may differ. The validity of the symptoms of mental illness may be questioned by one of the participants; their attitudes toward mental illness may differ; and their expectations of therapy may differ.

Littlewood and Lipsedge (1982), for example, describe such a situation in some of the psychiatric wards of English hospitals. "A not uncommon situation is the Indian (from India) junior psychiatrist attempting to interpret the experience of an Eastern European patient to a white British consultant on the basis of reports made by Malaysian or West Indian nurses." In this situation, all members of the staff work in the same setting and in the same country; however, because of the differences in beliefs about and explanation of the causes of mental illness, confusion and contradictions abound so that it becomes difficult to help the client in any form of psychotherapy. Other forms of treatments are resorted to (e.g., drugs, pills, etc.).

EXPECTATIONS IN THERAPY

When a client goes to therapy he or she has certain expectations of therapy and the therapist. It is important to understand clients' expectations because they either facilitate or retard the progress of therapy. Expectations are determined, in a major way, by the conditions and circumstances that bring the client to therapy and by the prevailing cultural beliefs about the causes and treatment of the disturbance.

Some ethnic clients, because of their cultural background, expect herbs and potions for their troubles; some expect the therapist to be an authoritarian who should tell them what to do about their troubles. Immigrant clients from the subcontinent of India, especially the middle class, expect the therapist to engage in semipersonal and semiphilosophical discussion with them. They also expect that the therapist will talk to their family members, whom they are likely to bring along with them. Length of therapy, therefore, depends upon the expectations of the client. If the client expects herbs, pills, or advice, therapy is likely to last only a few sessions. If clients expect some form of self-exploration, then it is likely to last longer.

Some of the clients' expectations are mentioned cryptically; some are raised as rhetorical questions; some are mentioned directly; and some are kept secret, mentioned only to other members of the ethnic group. Generally, ethnic clients are reticent and shy about stating their expectations to therapists of different ethnicity. However, it is the therapist's task to support and encourage the client to express his or her expectations.

A therapist also has certain expectations in therapy. For instance, he or she expects the client to follow the implicit role relations in therapy—namely, that the therapist is the expert and the client is the help seeker; that in his or her life, outside therapy, the client should follow or practice what has been discussed or prescribed in therapy. Some therapists expect to see the client only, and no one else; others may expect to see the spouse and other family members, along with the client. Therapists do not expect to go to the client's home to do therapy. A therapist should make these expectations clear to the client. If this is not done, then the possibility of misunderstanding and miscommunication emerges early in therapy. Initiate a dialogue. This will remove the mystical aspects of therapy.

DIAGNOSIS

Therapists are expected to make a diagnosis of their clients. Therapists generally believe that

> [A] diagnosis rendered should clarify the nature and extent of psychological distress that initially gives rise to help-seeking behavior and should also structure the path of psychotherapeutic treatment and subsequent follow-up efforts to facilitate readjustment with the community setting. (Malgady, Rogler, & Constantino, 1987)

On many counts, however, making a diagnosis of an ethnic client is fraught with problems that every transcultural therapist should be aware of. First, a satisfactory level of intrapsychiatrist agreement exists only for three categories—organic brain syndrome, mental retardation, and alcoholism. Agreement is only fair for diagnosis of psychosis and schizophrenia and is fairly poor for all other categories (King, 1978).* Thus the reliability of psychiatric diagnosis is quite low.

---

*For various reasons, which are not germane to our discussion, the reported reliability of diagnostic categories based on DSM-III is higher than those reported by King.

Second, generally, the accuracy of psychodiagnosis decreases as the sociocultural distance between the clinician and the patient increases (Gross, Knatterud, & Donner, 1969). Even when a diagnosis is made on the basis of psychological tests, such as MMPI, similar biases and errors emerge (Jones & Thorne, 1987; Koh & Upshaw, 1987; Olmedo, 1981; Sue & Sue, 1987).

Third, the cultural background of the diagnostician influences the approaches used for diagnosis. Li-Repac (1980) asked five Caucasians and five Chinese-American therapists to rate Chinese and Caucasian clients during a videotaped interview. Caucasian clinicians rated Chinese clients as anxious, awkward, confused, nervous, and reserved, whereas Chinese clinicians rated the same clients as adaptable, alert, dependable, friendly, and practical. In rating Caucasian clients, the Caucasian clinicians rated them as affectionate, adventurous, and capable; Chinese clinicians rated the Caucasian clients as active, aggressive, and rebellious. Caucasian clinicians saw Chinese clients as more depressed and inhibited, less socially poised, and having less capacity for interpersonal relationships than did the Chinese-American clinicians. Chinese-American clinicians rated Caucasian clients as more seriously disturbed than did Caucasian clinicians.

Perhaps the most important problem in making a diagnosis of the ethnic client is language. Many ethnic clients are not proficient in the language of the diagnostician, or they are bilingual. Psychiatric diagnosis is generally made on the basis of an interview(s), which relies heavily on the use of language. Serious bias, prejudices, and errors are likely to creep into the diagnosis of a client who is not fluent in the interviewer's language. LeVine and Padilla (1980), summarizing a number of studies on diagnosis of Spanish-speaking and bilingual clients, state, "concepts of mental illness may vary among Hispanics depending on whether English or Spanish is spoken. Bilingual patients were judged to be more pathological when they responded in English . . . than when they responded in Spanish" (p. 54).

Inference about the degree and type of psychopathology, (i.e., the assigned diagnosis) is made on the basis of the use of language. If the language used by the client does not convey clear meanings, is tangential or circumstantial, or has implied surplus meanings, a diagnostician is likely to interpret the client's behavior as more seriously disturbed (Malgady et al., 1987).

Diagnosis of schizophrenia is a case in point. Disturbance of language and thought (i.e., tangential, circumstantial language, and/or inappropriate use of words and language) is deemed a primary symptom of schizophrenia. The language problem increases the likelihood of an ethnic client being diagnosed as schizophrenic. Some writers, therefore, have stated that "an individual's social class and racial background corresponds with the severity of diagnosis given, what treatment is offered, by whom, where, length of hospitalization, dropout rate, and outcome of therapy" (Bulhan, 1985, p. 302).

Finally, studies suggest that the premorbid personality of the client is a good predictor of improvement in therapy (Draguns & Phillips, 1971; Frank, 1975). Therefore, the clinician must learn about the ethnic client's premorbid personality—his or her achievements, strengths, problems, and confusions—rather than put all the emphasis on a diagnosis, which is likely to be flawed or misapplied.

The task of a transcultural therapist is complicated. He or she must be sensitive to the expectations of the client, must be aware of the issues of ethnicity and social class (for they become inextricably intertwined in the process of therapy), must be aware of the diagnostic bias, and must take into account the imprecise or idiosyncratic use of the client's language. The therapist must then chart the course of therapy accordingly.

UNDERUTILIZATION AND DROPPING OUT OF THERAPY

By now it is well known that ethnic clients (especially the minority clients in England and the United States) underutilize the existing mental health services (Gordon, 1965; Karno & Edgerton, 1969; Mayo, 1974; Sue, 1977; Sue & McKinney, 1975). Many reasons have been given for this. The geographical location of the mental health facilities contributes to it as centers are often located outside the ethnic groups' residential areas. The cost of transportation and the lack of child care facilities discourages them from traveling to these centers (LeVine & Padilla, 1980). Some believe there is a lack of knowledge among the ethnic minorities about the existing mental health facilities (Mokuau, 1985). Some believe that shame and stigma associated with emotional difficulties is much greater among ethnic groups, which acts as a deterrent to seeking therapy (Sato, 1975; Yamamoto & Acosta, 1982).

Some maintain that the ethnic clients show preferences for sources other than Western mental health facilities. In the Philippines, "Whereas modern health services were preferred for treatment of physical symptoms, religious or traditional sources of help were often preferred for mental symptoms" (Church, 1987, p. 284).

In a survey of Hawaiian ethnic groups—Chinese, Japanese, Filipino, and Samoan—Prizzia and Villanueva-King (1977) found that they sought help from the family first. Seeking help outside the family was still tied to the cultural community; outside the family, priests were approached first, then public sources, then psychiatrists last. Such findings have been supported by other studies, which used clients whose ethnic origin was different from those used in Prizzia and Villanueva-King's studies (Nishio & Bilmas, 1987).

Sue and Sue (1987), on the basis of review of existing studies conclude "that Asian Americans seek treatment only when the disorders are relatively severe and that those with milder disturbances do not turn to mental health services" (p. 480).

Sue and Zane (1987), after an extensive review of literature conclude that the "single most important explanation for the problems in service delivery involves the inability of the therapist to provide culturally responsive form of treatment" (p. 37).

Others believe that the Asian-Americans' pattern of mental health utilization in the United States does not necessarily reflect a lack of need for it. On the basis of existing studies, Root (1985) concludes that Asian-Americans tend to experience stress psychosomatically. Nishio and Bilmas (1987) observe that "Among Asians, many psychological problems are expressed as somatic complaints. . . . Many southeast Asian refugees believe that the health of the body and mind are inseparable. Illness of the mind, then, is treated by attending to the body" (p. 343). For these reasons they search for organic or physiological explanations of their psychological troubles (e.g., headaches, stomach upsets, etc.). Hence they seek medical help rather than psychotherapeutic help.*

DROPPING OUT

Studies show that the dropout rate of the ethnic clients is higher than that of the Anglo clients (Sue, 1977). Some reasons for this include: majority therapists hold a stereotypical view of the ethnic client (Bloombaum, Yamamoto, & Evan, 1968; Crosby, Bromley, & Saxe, 1980); ethnic clients

---

*It should be brought to the reader's attention that initially the native-born Anglo clients also seek an organic explanation of their psychological troubles—about 60% of the time (Sharma, 1986). Nishio and Bilmas (1987) report that "More than 60% of Southeast Asian clients who brought physical complaints to a community health center in San Diego, California were diagnosed as having psychological problems" (Egawa & Tashima, 1981). Thus the limited number of existing studies would not support the prevailing belief that ethnic clients are more prone to somatization of their psychological problems. This author is not aware of any study that directly compares the initial rate of somatization of the ethnic and the Anglo client.

perceive Anglo therapists as cold and insincere (Kline, 1969) and feel alienated from and poorly understood by them (Warren, Jackson, Nugarai, & Farley, 1973). There may be difficulties of communication between the ethnic client and the therapist; therapist may feel baffled or diffident, as he or she may not fully comprehend the psychological context and/or depth of the ethnic client's conflicts. Hence ethnic clients, as compared to the Anglo clients, are less frequently referred for psychotherapy and are more frequently put on ataractic drugs (Cole & Pilisuk, 1976; Sharma, 1986) and given electroshock.

Sue and Zane (1987), after reviewing studies on this issue, state:

> We doubt that an ethnic minority client prematurely terminates solely because he or she may be ashamed of seeking help or is unfamiliar with psychotherapy. He or she leaves after a series of frustrations, misunderstandings, disappointments, and defensive reactions on his or her part that combine to create a poor response to treatment. For many ethnic clients, language problems, ambiguities, misinterpretations of behavior, differences in priorities of treatment, and so forth occur in conjunction with one another to produce a rapidly accelerating negative process in therapy. (p. 44)

These observations and findings should alert every transcultural therapist to the attitudes and behaviors that are likely to contribute to the dropping out of an ethnic client.

BEGINNING OF THERAPY

For many reasons, the beginning phase of therapy—the first two or three sessions—is particularly important with ethnic clients. First, a therapist must earn the client's trust and establish his or her own credibility with the client. Second, the therapist must avoid many of the pitfalls that await him or her in therapy. Third, he or she may have to critically examine the existing theoretical model(s) of therapy; or, in some cases, he or she may have to evolve a more appropriate model for the ethnic client. Finally, the therapist will have to learn to use the cultural themes, patterns, and dynamics of the ethnic client in therapy. These factors reinforce each other during the course of therapy, but for schematic purposes we shall discuss them separately.

Trust

Establishing trust in therapy and in the therapist is an elusive and difficult issue, especially when working with ethnic clients. A therapist must earn it by manifesting certain attitudes: warmth, genuiness, and acceptance of the client as he or she is (Rogers, 1967). These attitudes of the therapist help alleviate some of the client's anxiety, indirectly reinforce positive aspects of the clients's self-concept, and assist in building trust in the therapist (Sharma, 1986).

Differences in ethnic background can also be used to generate trust in the therapist. For example, Thomas and Dansby (1985), in discussing psychotherapy with black clients state:

> Although there are those who propose treating black clients as though color blind, that is, treating them the same way that they treat whites and not initiating discussion on race or racial issues, we propose as does Griffith (1977) that race be discussed in the initial session, whether or not the therapist is white, black, Asian, Hispanic, or another race. Being black holds such a central place in the identity of the blacks that not to discuss it is to deny a significant part of client's self-image. If the race of the client and the therapist are different, the therapist should point out that fact and ask the client how he or she feels about it. This provides a role model of openness upon which trust in therapeutic relationship can be built. (p. 401)

Although the aforementioned suggestion seems to be effective in generating trust, every transcultural therapist must be sensitive to the fact that many clients, for whatever reason, do not wish to discuss the ethnic differences between themselves and the therapist; nor are they eager to open up their ethnic background for discussion. Wishes of such clients must be respected.

Credibility

Credibility refers to the client's perception of the therapist as an effective and trustworthy helper (Sue & Zane, 1987). It is somewhat difficult to say what enhances a therapist's credibility; it is easier to define what reduces credibility.

According to Sue and Zane (1987), three aspects of a therapist's behavior are likely to reduce therapist's credibility.

1. "Conceptualization of the problem. If the client's problems are conceptualized in a manner that is incongruent with the client's belief systems, the credibility of the therapist is diminished" (p. 41). For example, if an Asiatic or Middle Eastern client complains of having sexual difficulties with his wife, and the therapist infers or implies that it may have something to do with the client's sexual feelings toward his mother, it

would destroy the therapist's credibility, since in the client's perception this would be a cultural impossibility.

2. "Means for problem resolution. If the therapist requires from the client responses that are culturally incompatible or unacceptable, the achieved credibility of the therapist is diminished" (p. 41). For example, in working with a depressed Asiatic or Middle Eastern client, a therapist may formulate that the client's problems stem from his or her aggressive feelings turned inward or from a lack of direct expression of anger toward parents or in-laws. The therapist may then encourage the client to express such feelings directly, which is likely to be antithetical to the client's value structure.

3. "Goals for treatment. If the definition of goals are discrepant between therapist and the client, credibility of the therapist will be diminished" (p. 41). For example, a client from India may go to therapy complaining that his living arrangement within the joint family system is replete with bickering and petty quarrels, which affects his work and outside relationships. The therapist may formulate the goal of therapy to be the client's moving out on his own. The client would not view this as compatible with his goals, since within the client's cultural context this may cause more friction and bickering within the family members, and his goal is to alleviate that friction.

To *enhance* credibility, the therapist should be sure that the client obtains some kind of meaningful gain or relief or a clearer perception of his or her troubles and conflicts early in therapy (Sue & Zane, 1987). For some clients it may be clarifying confusions; for others it may be relief from anxiety; for still others instilling hope. For some clients it may be "normalization"—that is, a realization by clients "that their thoughts, feelings, or experiences are common, and that many individuals encounter similar experiences—it is intended to reassure clients, who may magnify problems and who are unable to place their experiences in a proper context because of a reluctance to share thoughts with others" (Sue and Zane, 1987, p. 42). If a therapist is able to help the client achieve any of these goals, his or her credibility is likely to increase.

THE PITFALLS

The pitfalls a therapist must circumvent in therapy with an ethnic client are built into what has been called "the structural aspects of psychotherapy." It is essential that these pitfalls be avoided in the beginning of therapy; however, the importance of avoiding them in no way diminishes at any stage of therapy.

Conventional psychotherapy is given a structure by adumbrating certain implicit and explicit rules for the participants. These include: (1) the client should be seen in therapy for a specified period of time, generally one hour, which should be fixed in advance, although the client could be seen more than once a week; (2) the client should not "drop in" without making prior arrangements; (3) the client should go to therapist's office; the therapist should not go to client's home to do psychotherapy; (4) the therapist should not make telephone calls, in between the sessions, to inquire about the client's welfare; (5) offerings of beverages or cigarettes during any phase of the meeting should be discouraged; and (6) the therapist's charges and payment expectations should be delineated.

When working with an ethnic client, most of these structural parameters must become more flexible. First, the ethnic client expects to be received in a cordial manner. Offering of beverages and cigarettes is a demonstration of hospitality. Otherwise, to the client therapy becomes a business-like, impersonal transaction. In such an atmosphere the ethnic client will not expose his or her personal and private life.

Second, an ethnic client believes that when troubles and torments of one's life are discussed, the soul is bared. Anyone who professes to be an ally and a sympathetic listener would not cut the client off because "time is up." Arbitrarily set time limits do not take precedence over the bearing of one's soul. In such situations, the concept of time becomes fluid for the client, and he or she expects the therapist to reciprocate. Further, the ethnic client expects that a therapist who is sympathetic and caring would inquire from time to time about that client's welfare; or, at least, the client should be able to call the therapist if necessary.

Third, many ethnic clients, especially the seriously disturbed ones, expect that on some occasions the therapist will come to their home for conducting therapy. The rigid adherence to the office visits is seen as a gesture of distance and haughtiness on the part of the therapist.

Fourth, the language used by the participants is an important factor in therapy with ethnic clients. Certainly, it would be a great boon if the therapist was bilingual, but that is not often the case. Insistence on the use of the therapist's language in which the client may not be proficient makes the client feel restricted and hesitant to express emotions. Clients should be encouraged to use their native language whenever they wish to. If the therapist does not understand it, he or she should ask the client to translate it. This gives the client a feeling of freedom, acceptance, and equality.

Fifth, the attitude of many ethnic clients toward money is lax. Not paying bills on time may not be viewed as a serious dereliction. If the therapist insists on payments in a certain way, at a certain date, it may be viewed as crass materialism. Some form of negotiations that allows a certain flexibility in manner and time of payment is advisable.

Such implicit expectations of the ethnic client run counter to the rules of conventional therapy. If a therapist is not comfortable in bending them, it would be difficult to establish some form of working alliance for any length of time.

THEORETICAL MODEL—THE PAST AND THE FUTURE

Most clients want to know what will happen to them in the future, while most existing dynamic therapies and therapists want to know what has happened to the client in the past (Szasz, 1965). This paradox is more acute with ethnic clients.

Many researchers have observed that therapists try to give insight and interpretations to ethnic clients that are irrelevant in the context of the ethnic client's life struggles (Rogler, Malgady, Constantino, & Blumenthal, 1987). Other researchers concur, and state "that certain socioeconomic groups and ethnic minorities do not particularly value 'insight'" (Sue, 1981, p. 6). A therapeutic model that emphasizes clarification and interpretation of (past) dynamics and attempts to provide insight appears inappropriate for the ethnic client. Therefore, these researchers maintain that therapy should emphasize concrete behaviors and future actions.

If a therapist espouses a theoretical model or the framework of traditional dynamic therapy, he or she is likely to emphasize insight into and interpretation of the client's past relationships and conflicts. According to this model, if one has insight into one's past conflicts and behaviors, future actions can be influenced. That is, it is the past that influences the future. If, however, the theoretical model of the therapist leans more toward the future, therapy is more likely to become action oriented for there is little to interpret in the future; there can only be anticipated actions. Thus the model of therapy with an ethnic client must emphasize actions and behavior, rather than insight and interpretation; it must take into account the culture and ethnicity, rather than ignore it; and it must be more flexible and unorthodox in its structural and interactional aspects. This in no way implies that the client's past must be shut out from discussion and exploration; however, the emphasis and focus in therapy must be changed.

USE OF CULTURAL THEMES AND PATTERNS IN THERAPY

A transcultural therapist should be able to utilize the ethnic patterns of interactions and relationships and the themes of the client's culture. It is even more important that the therapist be sensitive to and aware of the fact that in instituting approaches and modalities of therapy that are not in accord with the client's cultural themes, patterns of relationships and ideologies are likely to generate negative effects and reactions. Many examples of such negative effects have been given in the literature.

When Alergia was under French colonial rule, Franz Fanon, a black revolutionary psychiatrist in charge of Blida-Joinville Mental Hospital in Algeria, abolished the then-existing distinction between native African-Arab and European patients and tried to integrate the native Arab patients with the European-French patients. During this time the Algerian war of liberation was in progress. Algerian-Arab patients "became increasingly apathetic and hostile". The French patients welcomed the policy, and their discharge rate increased. To the Arab patients it meant that by "imposing such therapeutic arrangements, they [psychiatrists] were unwittingly implementing the colonial policy of assimilation and of non-reciprocity between cultures" (p. 269). Later, "Fanon hired indigenous story tellers for those (Algerian-Arabs) who could not read Notre Journal [journal of the hospital] and invited traditional healers to help in the treatment of patients" (Bulhan, 1980, p. 269). The latter approach was found to be quite successful with the African-Arab patients since it was commensurate with their cultural tradition.

Tsui (1985) discusses the dangers of using the same or similar sexual counseling techniques used for Anglo clients for the sexually dysfunctional Asian immigrants. She states:

> Asian immigrants do not talk about their personal issues directly. Rather such issues are usually disguised under special context. . . . Group therapy as recommended for orgasmic dysfunction . . . ejaculatory control . . . and erectile failure . . . are usually ineffective with Asian clients. To share one's problems with one individual (e.g., the therapist) is already shameful enough. To share it with a group of strangers . . . is extremely traumatic and aggravating. . . . The damage to one's self-esteem far outweighs the potential for support and group identification. (p. 360)

Various examples of and suggestions for successful utilization of ethnic patterns and themes have been mentioned in the literature. Church (1987) suggests the use of cultural patterns with Filipino clients.

Because Filipinos can be passive and modest with authority figures . . . the therapist may need to be more active and directive in the initial stages of therapy . . . clients expect a more authoritarian, directive role for the counselor. . . . Because Filipino clients tend to be family and small group oriented, it may be helpful to involve the significant members of the family or peer group in therapy. . . . Because Filipinos are sensitive and have strong needs for acceptance, emotional closeness, and security, the counselor needs to be warmer and paternalistic. (p. 283)

Espin (1985) suggests that in therapy with Hispanic women one could effectively utilize women's groups, because "Hispanic women rely on other women to discuss their personal problems, a fact that would suggest the development of women's groups as a viable form of therapy for Hispanic Women" (p. 170).

LeVine and Padilla (1980), discussing therapy with Hispanic clients, state:

The use of cultural themes, such as machismo, respecto, comadrazgo/ compadrazgo, the role of women, and personalismo, in therapy, especially family therapy, could prove extremely valuable in developing more adequate therapeutic models—the basic concept is that sex roles of Hispanic men and women are very rigidly defined: males value highly the virtues of courage and fearlessness (machismo); respect is given elders, and there is an adherence to traditional cultural norms and values (respecto); extended family relations, especially between godparents and godchildren, are ritualized and have a religious connotation (comadrazgo/compadrazgo); and interpersonal relations are based on trust for people mingled with a distaste for formal, impersonal institutions or organizations (personalismo). (p. 191)

Sue (1977), LeVine and Padilla (1980), Rogler et al. (1987) suggest various procedures and practices, more befitting the cultural patterns of ethnic clients, which should be taken into consideration in setting up mental health services for them. Mental health services should be located in the ethnic neighborhood it is supposed to serve. It should have bilingual and bicultural staff; paraprofessionals from the community should be used to help integrate the clinic in the community. Clinic should be open, not from 8:00 A.M. to 5:00 P.M., as most are, but during these hours that are most convenient for the community members.

Physical arrangement of the clinic, contrary to the existing ones, should be more akin to a family living room atmosphere where coffee is served and the receptionist can greet the troubled client in his native tongue. Walk-in service, where no prior appointment is needed, should be available. Fees should be flexible. Additionally, preventive services, consultation, and crisis intervention could be incorporated along with traditional services. The following case presents the application of some of the principles discussed here.

A 19-year-old married woman of East Indian origin was brought to therapy by her family members because she was suffering from "fits" (hysterical seizures) that required three or four family members to hold her down. She had been married for four months; her first "fit" developed two months prior to coming to therapy. She had been through three neurological examinations and a CAT scan in three different hospitals on the West coast. All findings were negative.

Hers was a semiarranged marriage. Her father and the husband's father were farmers in the same village in Punjab, India. Both had immigrated about 30 years ago. The girl's father moved to Coventry, England, where he worked as a laborer in a British Leyland motor factory; the husband's father moved to California, where, after many years of farm work, he bought his own farm. The parents had kept in touch with each other throughout the years, and when their children grew up (all born either in England or the United States), the parents thought it wise to arrange a marriage.

The husband (age 23) had a master's degree from the University of California. After his graduation, the parents suggested that he spend a month or so in Coventry to meet the girl and her family, which he did. He liked the girl. The girl agreed to marry him, partly to appease her parents and partly because she liked the future husband.

Neither the wife nor the husband had been to India, although the parents had made a few visits since their immigration. At home they spoke their native language. Themes and contents of parents' conversation and of their social group were farms back home, interaction of the joint family members, politics of their native land, and so on. Their food habits, tastes, and food preferences remained strictly east Indian. Their social circles and relationships were almost exclusively confined to the immigrant community. The client attended an English school, incorporated most of the English social values, and worked as a junior cashier at the factory. She did not believe the Indian people to be competent and sincere. Yet on the other hand she was charming, and affable, was liked and loved by the family members, had many friends, and was quite popular in the Indian social community. Thus her pattern of interaction and relationship and her values were both English and Hindu.

After her marriage she moved to her husband's home in California—a place she dreamt of immigrating to, away from English weather and society. She moved to a fruit-growing town, where everything she dreaded came true. She had to live in a joint family household, on a farm, in a farming community, surrounded by east Indian immigrants—accountants, lawyers, doctors, farm workers, many of whom were illiterate. She had very little contact with the American society. She was cut off from her English friends and relatives, did not have a home or apartment she could call her own, could not take a job outside the home because of the disapproval of her in-laws, and had no life of her own. Her husband went along with his parents in most matters. Two months after moving to California, as she began to realize her life situation, the emerging value conflicts, and her fear of rebelling against it, she began to have "fits." She came to therapy passively to appease her in-laws. During the first few sessions the entire family came with her.

In the first few sessions the therapist inquired of her life in England, both inside and outside her home, her relationship with the English community, and asked her to compare and contrast her perceptions and feelings of England and the United States. The therapist actively participated in discussion and conversation about the Indian community both in the United States and in Coventry, where the therapist had spent the summer a few years ago. The first session lasted for two hours. She gradually opened up and left in a better mood. The next few sessions covered much the same topics except that the therapist began to focus on her wishes, conflicts, hopes, trepidations, fears, likes, and dislikes.

Indirectly she began to express her distrust of the east Indian community. In the fourth session she mentioned that since the therapist was from India, she did not have much faith or confidence in improving. She began to talk of her disappointments in living arrangements, her being constricted and confined in her interactions and behaviors due to Hindu ethics and values, her difficulty in accepting social interactions within the framework of the joint family system, and her fear of breaking away, or rebelling against it.

The therapist spoke to the husband about the situation. The husband felt helpless, baffled, very upset about the situation, and suggested that the therapist speak to other family members. The therapist expressed his desire to speak to her in-laws. They insisted that the therapist should come to their home, which he did. They were confused and troubled about her condition and would do anything to help. The therapist raised the issue of her working outside the home. The in-laws said that they had no objection to her working outside, but the people of the east Indian community would accuse them of being cruel and greedy in putting the newly arrived daughter in-law to work, rather than allowing the newly wed to enjoy each other. A year or so after marriage, they would have no objection to her working. The therapist conveyed this to the client in the next session. She understood and was relieved. Therapy sessions with various members of the family were conducted either in the native language of the client's family, or English, or both.

In the next session with the in-laws, again at their home, the therapist asked them if they could talk to the client directly about their objections, for she was quite sensitive to these issues, and let her express her wishes. They did, and agreed that if after two weeks or so she still felt like taking a job, she should. The husband also supported this. She began to have hope, and her mood began to change. Two weeks later she got a job in a local bank.

After she started working, the therapist asked whether she had thought of the couple having their own apartment. She was hesitant to raise the issue with her husband for it was not her place in the hierarchy of the joint family system to do so. She asked the therapist to raise this issue with the husband in the next session. The therapist did. The husband was hesitant, but nevertheless he raised the issue with his parents. Four months later the couple moved into their own apartment. On a follow-up visit 18 months later, they reported they were happy.

THERAPISTS FEELINGS TOWARD THE CLIENT— THE COUNTERTRANSFERENCE

Perhaps one of the most critical problems in transcultural therapy is the therapist's feelings toward the client, which are likely to become a stumbling block in understanding the clients' struggles. In the literature such feelings have been called "countertransference." Some authors maintain that the "key elements in treatment of ethnic-minority clients are empathy and counter-transference" (Jones, 1985, p. 177).

Countertransference is quite common in therapy (Sharma, 1986). For many reasons the likelihood of countertransference becoming more intense and insidious with an ethnic client increases. The seven common sources of countertransference mentioned by Sharma (1986) are: (1) initial like or dislike of the client; (2) the therapist's countertransference to the client's negativity; (3) personality conflicts of the therapist; (4) the therapist's diffidence as a source of countertransference; (5) erotic countertransference of the therapist; (6) differences in values and ideology; and (7) money as a source of countertransference, we may mention a few more potential sources of countertransference with an ethnic client. In addition, there are three other sources of countertransference: (1) stereotyping, (2) distancing and anxiety, and (3) one's own culture.

Stereotyping

Many therapists have a stereotypical image of an ethnic client.

Stereotypes may be defined as rigid preconceptions we hold about all people who are members of a particular group, whether it be defined along racial, religious, sexual or other lines. The belief in a preconceived characteristic of the group is applied to all members without regard for individual variation. The danger of stereotypes is that they are impervious to logic or experience. All incoming information is distorted to fit our preconceived notions. (Sue, 1981, p. 44)

If a therapist holds a stereotypical view of a client, the therapist is likely to react to the client with somewhat predetermined feelings, emotions, and perceptions. He or she is likely to overlook or misinterpret the client's unique conflicts and emotions. This hinders the therapist's ability to be more empathic with the client, reduces understanding of the client's conflicts, and makes it difficult for the therapist to be effective.

Distancing and Anxiety

Differences in ethnic background and values may evoke anxiety in the therapist for many reasons. A therapist may feel that he or she does not fully understand the depth and complexity of the ethnic client's struggles; the client's struggles and/or problems may have an alien quality for the therapist; the client's struggles may evoke unfamiliar emotions in the therapist, which he or she cannot comfortably deal with; and so on. For these reasons a therapist may put a distance between himself or herself and the client's struggles. Therapy is then likely to become either "technique oriented" or sterile, devoid, and divested of feelings and emotion. Soon the client senses this and drops out.

One's Own Culture as a Source of Countertransference

Therapists may develop countertransference with clients of their own culture, just as strongly as they do with those of other cultures. There are many reasons for it. Some therapists want to disidentify with the beliefs and values, patterns of relationship and interaction, and the ideology of their own culture. An encounter with a client from his or her own culture, especially one who may not belong to the same socioeconomic class as the therapist, is likely to generate discomfort and anxiety in the therapist. To handle the anxiety, or countertransference, the therapist resorts to various devices. He or she may subtly push the client out of therapy; misdiagnose the client's psychopathology and/or put the client on drugs, pills, shocks, etc.; or minimize or exaggerate the client's problems. Littlewood and Lipsedge (1982) describe such a situation.

> We noticed that both our nursing colleagues from the Caribbean and the Asian junior psychiatrists were less than enthusiastic about cultural explanations of any type: for them witchcraft beliefs were always pathological and religious visions implied schizophrenia. To consider such experiences in any way normal was a negative reflection on their own culture. (pp. 7–8)

An opposite type of countertransference is also found when the therapist and the client have the same cultural background. Occasionally, a therapist is likely to overidentify with the client and/or his or her problems. The therapist, consciously or semiconsciously attempts to resolve, relive, rectify, or redeem his or her own past conflicts and/or dissatisfactions or even his or her own cultural values or heritage through the client. Thus the therapist loses the judging and the guiding distance from the client's problems and is not too successful in steering therapy in a direction that is helpful to the client.

ATTRIBUTES AND TRAINING OF A TRANSCULTURAL THERAPIST

So far the emphasis here has been on the factors, attitudes, and techniques that are likely to produce a negative atmosphere and poor outcome in transcultural therapy. We now discuss some of the factors that are likely to facilitate transcultural therapy, since frequently it requires a different combination of skills, processes, and goals.

Sue (1981) describes the attributes that are important for such a therapist. He states: "a culturally skilled counselor must posses specific knowledge and information about the group he/she is working with" (pp. 107–108). Second, such a therapist "has moved from being culturally unaware to being aware and sensitive to his/her cultural baggage" (p. 105). Third, he should be "aware of his values and biases and how they effect the minority clients" (p. 106). Finally, he should be "comfortable with the differences in beliefs and values that exist between the therapist and the client in terms of race and beliefs" (p. 106).

A second set of attributes required of transcultural therapists pertain to the theory and practice of psychotherapy. For various socio-historical reasons, few, if any, of the existing theories of therapy are comprehensive enough to encompass the dilemmas and conflicts of ethnic clients.

Hence a theoretical flexibility and eclecticism and an attempt at formulating innovative theories should become a part of the training process.

Further, a therapist should be aware of the limitations of therapy, while possessing a clear understanding and knowledge of the techniques and process of therapy. This seems to be of particular importance because many ethnic clients expect results from therapy that therapy cannot deliver, or they may not expect certain kinds of help that therapy can provide. Concomitantly, to suit the needs and requirements of an ethnic client, the therapist must learn to bend and modify the parameters of psychotherapy—that is, he or she must be able to be unorthodox without feeling uncomfortable about it.

Perhaps by far the most important struggle of a transcultural therapist is to transcend his or her own culture. This may require suspension of one's beliefs and value system, thereby giving the clients' beliefs and value systems an opportunity to emerge and attain the same significance as one's own value system.

To appreciate the client's cultural background and its role and significance in his or her conflicts and the possibility of utilizing his or her culture for therapeutic purposes, a naïve openness must be developed. It helps a therapist to better understand the clients' dilemmas. Lowenstein (1985) suggests that a transcultural therapist should be able to adopt

the same approach as many minorities who mix well with both the predominant and minority culture, by adopting certain attitudes and behaviors when in the company of different groups. Thus the West Indians in Great Britain will frequently seek to behave like British when in their company but upon returning to his or her own ethnic group reverts back to the same language and demeanor that is there. (p. 42)

TRAINING

It is difficult to prescribe guidelines for training of a transcultural therapist. Only a few suggestions can be made. An exposure to diverse cultures and cultural experiences helps in the development of a therapist. For training purposes, videotapes of therapy with different ethnic clients helps a trainee to become aware of whether he or she will be comfortable with the differences and similarities in values and ideology; it should help the trainee realize the potential difficulties. Other forms of exposures, such as case conferences on ethnic clients and tape recordings of therapy with ethnic clients, would be useful in training. In particular such techniques should help the trainee recognize his or her own values, biases, and attitudes toward other cultures. Such biases are generally submerged in the therapist's perceptions, formulations, and interpretations of clients' conflicts and problems.

Like other individuals, a therapist also has stereotypes of other ethnic groups. The therapist must be aware of this. Such awareness is best accomplished in the context of a case presentation and group supervision. The effect of stereotyping on the therapeutic process must be demonstrated; and the methods to correct the adverse effect of stereotyping must be suggested. Finally, a therapist should be trained to be unorthodox, so that he or she may be able to modify the rules and modalities of therapy structure when the situation warrants it, without compromising the integrity of therapy.

Questioning and suspension of one's value systems, attempts to transcend one's culture, and encountering one's ideology when it is not supported by external factors are difficult issues for most therapists, no matter what their cultural background may be. Unless a therapist is willing to engage in some of these activities, it is difficult to see how he can become a successful transcultural therapist.

CONCLUDING REMARKS

Transcultural therapy is a new and emerging aspect of the field of psychotherapy. Only in the last two decades has it been studied seriously, clinical observations reported, and a certain number of empirical investigations conducted. Because of the insufficient number of studies, many of its therapeutic principles have not been clearly worked out; only a few general guidelines can be proposed for a student.

What seems to be emerging from the reports and studies is that transcultural therapy is a difficult process for any therapist. First, the education and training a therapist receives may have a limited applicability in transcultural therapy. Reasons for this seem to be that many of the embedded assumptions and values of traditional therapy, upon which methods and techniques of therapy are built, may not be applicable. Similarly, many of the accepted tools used in therapy (e.g., diagnostic procedures and diagnostic tests) must be used with a great deal of caution. Therefore, sometimes new and innovative methods and procedures have to be devised.

The meaning and significance of the client's presenting complaints or the symptoms may be different in the client's life than what may be expected in the therapist's own culture, because meanings are derived from or given by the cultural context. Hence any interpretation of symptoms must be made after a considerable amount of data collection and with a great deal of caution.

To gain proper perspective on a client's struggles, the client's cultural way of viewing problems must be accepted by the therapist. If the therapist cannot do this, the client and the therapist begin to work at cross-purposes.

An additional factor that taxes a transcultural therapist is that he or she must inculcate various attitudinal qualities that he or she may not have to do with clients of one's own culture. A therapist must inculcate a naïve openness to other cultures, so that he or she may be able to appreciate them. He or she must gain a certain knowledge of and familiarity with the culture of other ethnic groups so as not feel uncomfortable or ill at ease with what the client is presenting. The therapist must become aware of biases and limits of his or her own culture since these are potentially likely to have a deleterious effect on therapy.

The transcultural therapeutic relationship generates many unfamiliar feelings and emotions in the therapist. A therapist may either deny them, become anxious, or channel them in a therapeutically helpful way. In any event, the therapist must do something with them. If these feelings are improperly handled, they tend to become a hindrance in understanding the client's struggles.

The same issues that during the course of transcultural therapy become a struggle for a therapist are also challenges for his or her professionalism and an opportunity for growth, both as a professional and as a human being. To develop certain attributes, learn new techniques, and acquire the ability to understand and help a client of a different culture is a rewarding experience for a therapist of any culture.

References

Abel, T., Metraux, R., & Roll, S. (1987). *Psychotherapy and culture.* Albuquerque: University of New Mexico Press.

Bloombaum, M. Yamamoto, J., & Evan, R. (1968). Cultural stereotypes amongst psychotherapists. *Journal of Counseling Clinical Psychology, 32,* 99.

Bockoven, J. S. (1963). *Moral treatment in American psychiatry.* New York: Springer.

Bulhan, H. (1980). Franz Fanon: The revolutionary psychiatrist. *Race and Class,* 3(3), 251–271.

Bulhan, H. (1985). The black American and psychopathology: An overview of research and theory. *Psychotherapy, 22,* 370–379.

Church, A. T. (1987). Personality research in a non-western culture: The Philippines. *Psychological Bulletin, 102,* 272, 292.

Cole, J., & Pilisuk, M. (1976). Differences in the provision of mental health services by race. *American Journal of Orthopsychiatry, 46,* 510–525.

Crosby, F., Bromley, S., & Saxe, L. (1980). Recent unobtrusive studies of black and white discrimination and prejudices: A literature review. *Psychological Bulletin, 88,* 546–553.

Draguns, J., & Phillips, L. (1971). *Psychiatric diagnosis and classification: An overview and critique.* Morriston, NJ: General Learning Press.

Egawa, J. E., & Tashima, N. (1981). *Alternative delivery model in Pacific/Asian American communities.* San Francisco: Pacific Asian Mental Health Research Project.

Espin, O. (1985). Psychotherapy with Hispanic women. Some considerations. In P. Pedersen (Ed.)., *Handbook of cross-cultural counseling and therapy* (pp. 165–173). Westport, CT: Greenwood.

Erikson, K. (1966). *Wayward puritans.* New York: Wiley.

Frank, G. (1975). *Psychiatric diagnosis: A review of research.* New York: Pergamon.

Gordon, S. (1965). Are we seeing the right patients? Child guidance intake. The sacred cow. *American Journal of Orthopsychiatry, 35,* 131–137.

Griffith, M. S. (1977). The influence of race on the psychotherapeutic relationship. *Psychiatry, 40,* 24–40.

Grob, G. (1975). Social origins of American psychiatry. In S. L. Sharma (Ed.), *The medical model of mental illness* (pp. 1–27). Woodland: Majestic Publishing Company.

Gross, H., Knatterud, G., & Donner, L. (1969). The effect of race and sex on the variation of diagnosis and disposition in the psychiatric emergency room. *Journal of Nervous and Mental Disease, 148,* 638–642.

Jones, E. (1985). Psychotherapy and counseling with black clients. In P. Pedersen (Ed.), *Handbook of cross-cultural counseling and therapy* (pp. 173–184). Westport, CT: Greenwood.

Jones, E., & Thorne, A. (1987). Rediscovery of the subject: Intercultural approaches to clinical assessment. *Journal of Consulting and Clinical Psychology, 55,* 448–497.

Karno, M., & Edgerton, R. (1969). Perception of mental illness in a Mexican American community. *Archives Of General Psychiatry, 20,* 233–238.

King, L. M. (1978). Social and cultural influences on psychopathology. *Annual Review of Psychology, 29,* 405–433.

Kline, L. Y. (1969). Some factors in the psychotherapeutic treatment of Spanish Americans. *American Journal of Psychiatry, 126,* 1664–1681.

Koh, S. D., & Upshaw, H. (1987). Assessment of affective disturbance in Asians and Americans. *Pacific Asian American Mental Health Center Research Review, 6,* No. 1/2, 1–4.

LeVine, E. S., & Padilla, A.M. (1980). *Crossing cultures in therapy.* Monterey, CA: Brooks/Cole Publishing.

Li-Repac, D. (1980). Cultural influences on clinical perceptions: A comparison between Caucasians and Chinese American therapists. *Journal of Cross-Cultural Psychology, 11,* 327–342.

Littlewood, R., & Lipsedge, M. (1982) *Aliens and alienists.* London: Penguin Books.

Lowenstein, L. F. (1985). Cross-cultural research in relation to counseling in Great Britain. In P. Pedersen (Ed.), *Handbook of cross-cultural counseling and therapy* (pp. 37–44). Westport, CT: Greenwood.

Malgady, R., Rogler, L., & Constantino, G. (1987). Ethno-cultural and linguistic biases in mental health evaluation of Hispanics. *American Psychologist, 42,* 228–234.

Marsella, A. F. (1985). The self, adaptation, and adjustment. In A. J. Marsella, G. DeVos, & F. L. K. Hsu (Eds.), *Culture and self* (pp. 279–307). New York: Tavistock Publication.

Mayo, J. A. (1974). The significance of sociocultural variables in psychiatric treatment of black outpatients. *Comprehensive psychiatry, 6,* 471–482.

Mokuau, N. (1985). Counseling Pacific Islander Americans. In P. Pedersen (Ed.), *Handbook of cross-cultural counseling and therapy,* (pp. 147–155). Westport, CT: Greenwood.

Nishio, K., & Bilmas, M. (1987). Psychotherapy with southeast Asian American clients. *Professional Psychology: Research and Practice, 18,* 342–386.

Olmedo, E. L. (1981). Testing linguistic minorities, *American Psychologist, 36,* 1017–1085.

Prizzia, R., & Villanueva-King, O. (1977). Central Oahu community mental health needs assessment survey. Part III. Survey of the general population. Honolulu: *Management Planning and Administration Consultant.*

Rogers, C. R. (1967). The condition of change from a client-centered viewpoint. In B. Berensen & R. Carkhuff (Eds.), *Sources of gain in counseling and psychotherapy* (pp. 71–85). New York: Holt, Rinehart and Winston.

Rogler, L., Malady, R., Constantino, G., & Blumenthal, R. (1987). What do culturally sensitive mental health services mean? *American Psychologist, 42,* 565–570.

Root, M. (1985). Guidelines for facilitating therapy with Asian Americans. *Psychotherapy, 22,* 349–356.

Sato, M. (1975). The shame factor: Counseling Asian Americans. *Journal of the Asian American Psychological Association, 5* (1), 20–24.

Sharma, S. L. (1986). *The therapeutic dialogue.* Albuquerque: University of New Mexico Press.

Sue, S. (1977). Community mental health services to the minority groups. *American Psychologist, 32,* 616–624.

Sue, D. (1981). *Counseling the culturally different.* New York: Wiley.

Sue, S., & McKinney, H. (1975). Asian Americans in the community mental health system. *American Journal of Orthopsychiatry, 45,* 111–118.

Sue, D., & Sue, S. (1987) Cultural factors in the clinical assessment of Asian Americans. *Journal of Consulting and Clinical Psychology, 55,* 479–487.

Sue, S., & Zane, N. (1987). The role of culture and cultural techniques in psychotherapy. *American Psychologist, 42,* 37–45.

Szasz, T. (1965). *Ethics of psychoanalysis.* New York: Basic Books.

Thomas, M., & Dansby, P. (1985). Black clients: Family Structure, therapeutic issues, and strengths. *Psychotherapy, 22,* 398–407.

Tsui, A. M. (1985). Psychotherapeutic considerations in sexual counseling for Asian immigrants. *Psychotherapy, 22,* 357–362.

Warren, R., Jackson, A., Nugarai, J., & Farley, G. (1973). Different attitudes of black and white patients towards treatment in a child guidance clinic. *American Journal of Orthopsychiatry, 3,* 384–393.

Yamamoto, J., & Acosta, F. (1982). Treatment of Asian Americans and Hispanic Americans: Similarities and differences. *American Academy of Psychoanalysis, 10,* 585–607.

18

Toward a Synthesis of Eastern and Western Psychologies

ROGER WALSH[1]

A great thorough-going man does not confine himself to one school, but combines many schools, as well as reads and listens to the arguments of many predecessors.

Kuo Hsi

WESTERN ETHNOCENTRICITY

That a book such as this has been written is a reflection of an increasing openmindedness within the culture in general, and among health professionals in particular, to non-Western world views, psychologies, and thought systems. This openmindedness is, unfortunately, a relatively new phenomenon and was preceded by a long history of ethnocentrism in which Western medicine and psychology alone were

[1]The author would like to thank Bonnie L'Allier for her excellent secretarial and administrative assistance and, as always, Frances Vaughan for her unswerving support.

deemed worthy of serious consideration. With rare exceptions, non-Western systems were viewed as unfortunate relics of primitive thinking, which would doubtless disappear when East met West and Easterners were able to recognize the clear superiority of Western thinking.

We are now beginning to appreciate that certain of the non-Western psychologies represent descriptions of human nature that in their own quite different ways may be as sophisticated as our own. Both East and West, it seems, may benefit from greater knowledge of each other. This is by no means to say that all things Eastern are valid or indeed that all things Western are either. It is simply to acknowledge that we appear to have underestimated the validity and profundity of aspects of certain non-Western psychologies and that we stand to gain a great deal from their careful study, as has been made clear in this book.

Why have Eastern psychologies been so misunderstood and underestimated? The major factor is probably simple ignorance. We appear to have dismissed the Eastern traditions in large part through ignorance and ethnocentricity, much like the 19th-century British envoy to India who made himself famous by remarking that he had never felt the need to learn the Indian language because he knew that the Indians had nothing worthwhile to say. Moreover, we have commonly assumed that only one psychology, almost invariably our own, described "the truth" and that competing models were false.

At first glance, these assumptions sometimes appeared to be confirmed when Western psychologists did undertake initial studies of Eastern systems, for Eastern descriptions of human nature and potentials sometimes run counter to basic Western assumptions and beliefs. Only recently with the emerging understanding of the problems of paradigm clash have we begun to appreciate the necessity of taking our own Western assumptions and world views into consideration when examining non-Western traditions (Tart, 1975b; Walsh, 1980). With this understanding we may be able to adopt a multiperspectivism from which we can appreciate that psychologies may address different aspects, perspectives, structures and levels of mind, consciousness, health, motivation, and the unconscious (Wilber, 1977, 1979, 1981).

IMPLICATIONS OF EASTERN PSYCHOLOGIES

This chapter is intended to provide a brief overview of the implications of certain Eastern psychologies, especially Buddhist and Hindu systems, and examine the possibilities for beginning to integrate them with Western psychology. Since the subject matter and its implications are so broad, only synoptic statements can be made here, which is an injustice to the topic. Many of the implications of Buddhist and Hindu psychologies are not only profound, but quite startling to our Western ways of thinking, and ideally they should be supported by considerable background data, logic, and discussion as is usually necessary when discussing paradigmatic assumptions different from the usually accepted ones (Kuhn, 1970). This support will be provided here simply by references. The reader should consult these if the validity of the claims appears dubious. Although many of the principles to be discussed are echoed in other Asian disciplines (e.g., Taoism, Neo-Confucianism, and Sufism), for the sake of simplicity this discussion will be confined to the psychological aspects of Buddhism and Hinduism's Yoga and Vedanta traditions.

The Nature of Mind

What are some of the central claims and implications of Buddhist and Hindu psychologies? First, let us examine their descriptions of the nature of mind. The central claim on which their existence and trainings are based is that in our usual states of consciousness our minds are far less under our control than we usually appreciate.

As the *Bhagavad Gita*, the "Hindu Bible" says

> Restless mans mind is,
> So strongly shaken
> In the grips of the senses
> Gross and grown hard
> With stubborn desire
> For what is worldly.
> How shall he tame it?
> Truly I think
> The wind is no wilder.
>
> (Prabhavananda &
> Isherwood, 1944, p. 68)

The result is said to be "that most of us, most of the time behave and act mechanically, like machines. . . . man merely imagines that he is in control of himself." (Schumacher, 1978, pp. 69, 29). These ancient claims have recently found support in the West from studies of cognitive processing, which suggest that "psuedothinking is more the rule than the exception" and that "there has been misdirected emphasis on people as rational information processors (Langer, Blank, & Benzion, 1978, pp. 638, 641). In fact, our minds are said to be so out of control that our usual perception, identity, and state of consciousness are so distorted that we do not even realize they are distorted. Therefore, the Eastern psychologies might be said to have extended Freud's (1917/1943, p. 252) observation that "man is not even master in his own house . . . his own mind."

Thus, whereas Freud shook the Western world by proclaiming that what we have taken to be "normality" is actually a culturewide form of neurosis, the Eastern psychologies shake it further by proclaiming that what we call "normality" is no less than a psychosis! Our usual Western definition of "psychosis" is a state of consciousness in which the mind is out of control and provides a distorted picture of reality in which the distortion is not recognized. Such, from the Asian perspective, is our usual state.

Thinkers of both East and West have acknowledged that our usual adult egoic mind state together with its limitations may be a developmentally necessary stage (Wilber, 1983). The problem is that at this time most of us do not recognize, correct, and develop beyond the limitations of this conventional stage even though such transconventional development is the very raison d'être of Eastern psychologies.

Identity

No less radical than the claim about our usual state of consciousness is the claim about our usual sense of identity. Most Western psychologies take for granted the idea that our usual egoic sense of identity is natural and appropriate. Yet these Asian psychologies point out that upon close examination, the ego is nowhere to be found. Rather, the sense of a continuous solid ego, when examined minutely as in Buddhist insight meditation, dissolves into (or in phenomenological terminology is deconstructed to) insubstantiality. Just as a movie presents an apparently continuous image, so too our lack of precise attention and careful introspection allows us to mistake a flux of individual thoughts, emotions, and fantasies for a solid continuous ego. This might be interpreted as an example of the "flicker fusion" phenomenon. For Buddhist and Hindu psychologies there is no "ghost in the machine," and those Western psychologies that are based on assumptions of ego identity are viewed as based on illusion.

Of course similar perspectives have occurred in the West. This dissection of experience and identity into a ceaseless flux is similar to the reports of Western introspectionists such as the philosophers David Hume, Henri Bergson, and William James. Hume, for example, concluded that the self is "nothing but a bundle of collections of different perceptions which succeed each other with an inconceivable rapidity and are in perpetual flux" (Needleman, 1984, p. 169). His description could easily be mistaken for a 2000-year-old Buddhist text.

Transpersonal Realization

The very raison d'être for these Asian systems, therefore, is to overcome the limits and distortions of "normality." The means for this is mind training, and the methods are quite precisely laid out as, for example, in the Buddhist eight-fold path or the eight limbs of yoga. These comprise regimes designed to cultivate ethics, concentration, emotional transformation, and wisdom; these four dimensions appear to be common to all effective contemplative disciplines. Only in the last few years have we begun to gain some understanding of the cognitive processes involved in these practices, and we now have some initial syntheses of Eastern meditative phenomenology and Western cognitive psychology (Brown, 1977; Brown & Engler, 1986; Goleman, 1988; Shapiro, 1980; Shapiro & Walsh, 1984).

The aim of these practices is claimed to be the realization of our true identity and potential, and that potential is said to be vast indeed. So radical are the states and experiences that result from deep mind training that, in their upper reaches, they are best described in terms that have traditionally been thought of as religious (e.g., "transcendent," "ineffable," "noetic," "blissful," "all-pervading"). Ultimately they go beyond words and are described as transverbal and transrational (Wilber, 1977, 1980a, 1980b).

All of us, claim Asian psychologies, have the potential for transcendent experiences. The great saints and sages of human history are said to differ from the rest of us by virtue of attainment and realization, not by some unsurpassable God-given ontological divide that forever sets them off from us as a different order of being. In the classical Buddhist texts the Buddha seems to have made no claims to have attained anything that was beyond our own realization, and an ancient Buddhist saying reminds us to "Look within, you are the Buddha."

The implications of Buddhist and Hindu psychologies are not merely theoretical, but eminently personal and practical. They claim that the trained mind is capable of levels of well-being, states of consciousness, depths of love, breadths of compassion, heights of joy, and clarity of perception far beyond those available to the untrained person (Walsh & Shapiro, 1983). Buddhist and Hindu psychologies point to these possibilities and claim to provide road maps for attaining them—maps whose validity can be experimentally tested in our own experience. Indeed, the proper testing ground for these psychologies lies within us and is us. To think that we can establish their validity or falseness by theory and scholarship alone is to confuse conceptual with contemplative knowledge and to commit what is known as a "category error" (Wilber, 1983).

A Contemporary View of Religion

These implications of Eastern psychologies point to a view and understanding of religion that is radically different from our traditional ones. At the heart of the great religions, particularly in their more mystical aspects, can be found a common core whose dimensions have been variously described as the perennial wisdom, the perennial philosophy (Huxley, 1944), the perennial religion (Smith, 1976) or transcendent unity of religions (Schuon, 1975), the consciousness disciplines (Walsh, 1980), and the perennial psychology (Wilber, 1977).

In light of our contemporary psychological understanding, the perennial wisdom of the great religions can be viewed as providing road maps or strategies for the induction of transcendent states of consciousness. Likewise, the various forms of the perennial philosophy and psychology can be viewed as philosophical and psychological analyses of the perspectives, insights, understandings, and world views afforded by these transcendent states. As Indian philosophers have remarked, one of the differences between Indian and Western philosophies is that the Western enterprise is conducted in, and descriptive of, only one state of consciousness, while several Indian systems claim to be products of, descriptive of, and only fully comprehended in multiple states of consciousness. The same general claim could be made of Indian and Western psychologies. The integration of Eastern and Western psychologies may provide us with new understandings of religion since studies of phenomena such as alternate states of consciousness, state dependent learning, meditation, and so on suggest that the perennial wisdom, philosophy, and psychology may be viewed as multistate disciplines designed to access and analyze transcendent states of consciousness and their corresponding world views.

THE RELATIONSHIP BETWEEN EASTERN AND WESTERN PSYCHOLOGIES

What, then, is the general nature of the relationship between Hindu and Buddhist psychologies and Western psychologies? Clearly there are areas of intersection and overlap between the two systems; these have been most fully investigated by the field of transpersonal psychology, which specifically aims at an integration of Eastern and Western perspectives (Vaughan, 1986; Walsh & Vaughan, 1980; Wilber, 1977). Several investigators have suggested that Western and Asian approaches may focus on different developmental levels (Vaughan, 1986; Wilber, 1980a). Likewise, others have noted that Western psychology has mapped psychopathologies in considerably greater detail than have Eastern systems, which have almost nothing to say about early development, the dynamic unconscious, or severe psychopathology (Russell, 1986; Wilber, Engler, & Brown, 1986). However, Asian psychologies appear to describe levels of development and well-being beyond those recognized in Western models other than the transpersonal (Goleman, 1988; Walsh, 1988; Walsh & Shapiro, 1983).

Thus it may be that Asian and Western psychologies may be partially complementary, with the Asian systems focusing on advanced stages of development and states of well-being and with the Western providing details of psychopathology and early development. Integrating the two perspectives, such as Ken Wilber (1980a) and his associates (Wilber et al., 1986) are doing, may thus provide us with the first "full spectrum" models of development, which trace development all the way from infancy through adulthood on into transpersonal, transconventional stages and then through the various stages of enlightenment.

Since they include a significantly wider range of states of consciousness, identity, and perceptual modes than do traditional Western psychologies, Buddhist and Hindu psychologies may offer broader models that encompass and extend the scope of traditional Western models. Indeed, the Western model may have a position in relationship to the Eastern comparable to the Newtonian model in relationship to the Einsteinian model in physics. For example, the Newtonian case applies to macroscopic objects moving at relatively low velocities compared to the speed of light. When applied to high-velocity objects, the Newtonian model no longer fits. The Einsteinian model, on the other hand, encompasses both low and high speeds; from this broader perspective, the Newtonian model and its limitations are all perfectly logical and understandable (employing Einsteinian and not Newtonian logic, of course). However, the reverse is definitely untrue, for Einsteinian logic is not comprehensible within a Newtonian framework. Furthermore, from a Newtonian perspective, reports of incongruous findings, such as the constancy of the speed of light and objects increasing in mass at high speed, are incomprehensible and suspect.

In terms of abstract set theory, the Newtonian model can be seen as a subset nested within the larger Einsteinian set. The properties of the subset are readily comprehensible from the perspective of the set, but the reverse is necessarily untrue. The general principle is that to try to examine a larger model or set from the perspective of a smaller is inappropriate and necessarily productive of false conclusions.

The implications of this for the comparison and assessment of Asian and Western psychologies should now be clear. From a multiple-states-of-consciousness model, the traditional Western approach is recognized as a relativistically useful model provided that, because of the limitations imposed by state-specific relevancy, learning, and understanding, it is not applied inappropriately to perspectives and states of consciousness and identity outside its scope. If it is so applied, then misinterpretations and misunderstandings may result.

Classic examples of such misunderstandings include the pathologizing interpretations of mystical experiences that were almost the norm, particularly among psychoanalysts, until recently. Thus, for example, mystical experiences have been variously interpreted as regressive psychopathologies due to artificially induced catatonia (Alexander, 1931), infantile helplessness (Freud, 1917/1943), regression to union with the breast (Lewin, 1950), or irrational thinking (Wilber, 1989). These interpretations are classic examples of the confusion of preegoic, prepersonal, prerational states with transegoic, transpersonal, transrational ones—a confusion that has become known as the "pre-trans fallacy" and that has been analyzed in considerable detail by Ken Wilber (1983). It results when traditional Western psychological models, which recognize only prepersonal and personal developmental stages and states, are applied to transpersonal phenomena. Since the transpersonal experiences are not personal, they are, logically enough, misclassified in the only other available category—the prepersonal. However, closer examination reveals clear differences. For example, Wilber (1980a, p. 78), when comparing the absence of self-other boundaries in infants and schizophrenics, on the one hand, and mystics, on the other, points out that schizophrenic or infantile fusion "is pre–subject/object differentiation, which means the infant cannot distinguish subject from object. But the mystic union (*sahaj samadhi*) is trans–subject/object, which means that it transcends subject and object, while remaining perfectly aware of that conventional duality." Both phenomenological (Kornfield, 1979) and conceptual analyses now make it clear that "pre and trans can be seriously equated only by those whose intellectual inquiry goes no further than superficial impressions" (Wilber, 1980a, p. 78).

A further implication of this Newtonian-Einsteinian analogy concerns the testing of Eastern claims about the information, insights, and perspectives that alternate states of consciousness afford (e.g., that the ego is illusory). It may be, just as the Eastern disciplines have long maintained, that full testing of the validity of these alternate-state claims may require entering them ourselves. Of course, this is not the *only* means of testing these Eastern claims, but we may not be able to evaluate them solely on the basis of our a priori assumptions based only on our usual-state experiences (Tart, 1975a, 1975b). For the Asian claim is that our usual-state experiences, perspectives, and world views may be radically reevaluated or recontextualized from the perspective of alternate states. This state-specific reinterpreting is known in Vedanta as "subrationing." A good discussion of subrationing and its philosophical implications is available in Deutsch (1969). To the extent these claims are accurate, Asian psychologies and philosophies may provide valuable metaperspectives on our Western perspectives and assumptions.

SOCIAL AND GLOBAL IMPLICATIONS

The Asian psychologies may also provide novel insights into a wide range of social phenomena. It is no secret that our species and planet are in grave danger. Each year, the problems and threats of ecological imbalance, nuclear warfare, starvation, resource depletion, and more appear to worsen (Brown, 1988). Twenty billion tons of TNT explosive power, a world population doubling every 40 years, 20 million dying of malnutrition every year, 600 million malnourished, ozone depletion, greenhouse warming, and more; the figures are truly staggering to anyone willing to appreciate their reality and implications. Even the more optimistic models and analyses of future trends such as *The Global 2000 Report to the President* (Council on Environmental Quality and the Department of State, 1980) predict problems of unprecedented scope and complexity within the next two or three decades unless major shifts in individual, cultural, national, and global priorities occur.

The unique feature of these threats to our collective well-being and survival is that they are all human caused. Indeed, what we think of as global problems are perhaps better thought of as global symptoms—symptoms of our individual and shared mind states (Walsh, 1984). "World is said to totter on brink of madness" cried the headline of an American Psychological Association (1983) publication reporting the conclusions of the World Congress on Mental Health. The Eastern psychologies would agree and would suggest that the recognition of this insanity is essential for its cure. Indeed, the horrendous condition of the world seems incomprehensible if we try to analyze it from the assumption that we are fully sane, but it becomes readily understandable in terms of the Asian claim that "normality" is no less than a psychosis fueled by the "three poisons" of greed, hatred, and delusion. Therefore, the insanity of the world reflects our individual and shared insanity, and from this perspective our culture can be seen as a form of collective psychosis.

This idea is hardly unique to Asia and has appeared in many forms. For Willis Harman (1962), culture is a shared hypnosis; for Ernest Becker (1973) and Otto Rank (1958), it is an immortality project supporting death denial; for Charles Tart (1986) it is a consensus trance; and for Ken Wilber (1980a, 1981), it is an expression of "the Atman project," the ego's self-defeating attempt to regain for itself the unitive transcendent consciousness or atonement (at-one-ment) from which it is separated by its very nature. One of the strongest statements is that of Ernest Becker (1973): "If we had to offer the briefest explanation of all the evil that men have wreaked upon themselves and upon their world since the beginning of time, it would be simply in *the toll that his pretense of sanity takes as he tries to deny his true condition*" (p. 24).

We are now at a new stage in human development. Whereas formerly our illusions and psychoses may well have caused vast suffering and premature death to untold numbers of individuals, now they threaten our entire species and planet. Our collective insanity appears to have produced a situation that threatens its own existence. The aim of the Buddhist and Hindu psychologies, philosophies, and religions has always been to awaken people from our collective trance, *maya* or *samsara*. Traditionally, this has occurred to only a very small minority, but it may be that we have established a condition in which large numbers of us will either begin to awaken together or die together, grow up together or blow up together. For we are perhaps at a stage where the palliative military and political responses that have been the norm until now are inadequate and where nothing less than radical reductions of the root causes of greed, hatred, and delusion may suffice to ensure our survival. We appear to have established an exquisite experiment in which we will mature and awaken at unprecedented rates or we will fall victims of our own disease. In either case, our psychological disorder appears to be self-limiting. Psychologists of both East and West may have much to offer here. They may be able to help us understand and correct the psychological roots of our contemporary crises and play an important role in ensuring human survival. Through integrating the insights of both East and West, they may be able to create a comprehensive and invaluable "psychology of human survival" (Walsh, 1984).

INTEGRATORS OF EAST AND WEST AS GNOSTIC INTERMEDIARIES

What are appropriate strategies for those of us seeking to understand and communicate the wisdom and relevance of Asian psychologies to Western psychology, culture, and individuals? The Asian psychologies are rich with suggestions, but to obtain them will demand that we familiarize ourselves with them deeply, both theoretically and experientially. There is a great need for good scholarship if the full depth, richness, and implications of these systems are to be appreciated and communicated to significant numbers of Westerners. Moreover, if they are to find widespread acceptance within the psychological community, then they must be translated, where possible, into Western language and concepts, and their claims must be subjected to experimental testing. For example, there is a crying need for more research to examine the effects of intensive meditation and the characteristics of advanced practitioners. Not that such laboratory evidence is necessarily important to Buddhist or Hindu practitioners, but it is important to Western psychologists.

Curiously enough, personal practice of Asian disciplines (e.g., meditation) may be just as important as scholarship and laboratory research for understanding Asian psychologies and philosophies. Whereas Western psychology aims primarily for objective knowledge (what we have), Asian psychologies aim for the cultivation of wisdom (what we are). For centuries, Asian practitioners have argued that their traditions—either religious, philosophical, or psychological—cannot be adequately understood, assessed, or communicated without personal experience; attempts to do so result in category error, misunderstanding, and pathologizing interpretations. In the words of Bhikku Vimalo, (1974), a contemporary Buddhist monk,

> Without practice, without contemplation, a merely intellectual, theoretical, and philosophical approach to Buddhism is quite inadequate. . . . Mystical insights . . . cannot be judged by unenlightened people from the worm's eye view of book-learning, and a little book knowledge does not really entitle anyone to pass judgment on mystical experiences.

Several Western psychologists have offered support for this claim from their own experience. They reported that their understanding of Asian psychologies deepened significantly as they undertook the corresponding contemplative practices such as meditation or yoga (Hendlin, 1979; Ram Dass, 1975; Shapiro, 1980; Walsh, 1977, 1978). Such claims are now comprehensible to Western psychology in light of the findings that state-specific learning places limits on our capacity to understand insights and information obtained in alternate states of consciousness (Tart 1975a, 1975b; Wolman & Ulman, 1986). Without personal practice and experience, we lack "adequatio" and are not fully adequate to the task of understanding, incorporating, or communicating the subtle insights that constitute the core of Asian wisdom.

To be optimal translators, scholars, and communicators of Eastern psychologies may require no less than that we become what Carl Jung termed "gnostic intermediaries." Gnostic intermediaries are people who imbibe a discipline or teaching so deeply that they can communicate and express it directly from their own experience into the language and conceptual network of the people to whom they are communicating. This role demands both contemplative practice and wisdom as well as a knowledge of Eastern and Western psychologies that is sophisticated enough for us to be able to understand both and build conceptual bridges between them. This is no small demand. Indeed, it requires a deeper commitment to wisdom and breadth of scholarship and understanding than almost any other tasks that a psychologist might face.

Never before in human history have those of us in the West had such access to Eastern psychologies nor possessed the psychological tools for understanding them. And never before has the need for practicing and understanding them been so great. The unique combination of these opportunities opens new frontiers to us, new possibilities of understanding and insight, new tools and techniques, new ways of viewing the world, our minds, and ourselves, and new methods of contributing. These opportunities are open to those willing to prepare themselves adequately for the task. There is exciting and important work to be done, and we are privileged to have the opportunity to do it.

References

Alexander, F. (1931). Buddhist training as an artificial catatonia (the biological meaning of psychic occurrences). *Psychoanalytic Review, 18,* 129–145.

American Psychological Association. (1983). *The Monitor, 14,* 8.

Becker, E. (1973). *The denial of death.* New York: Free Press.

Brown, D. (1977). A model for the levels of concentrative meditation. *International Journal of Clinical and Experiential Hypnosis, 25,* 236–273.

Brown, D., & Engler, J. (1986). The stages of mindfulness meditation: A validation study. Part II. Discussion. In K. Wilber, J. Engler, & D. Brown (Eds.), *Transformations of consciousness: Conventional and contemplative perspectives on development* (pp. 191–218). Boston: New Science Library/ Shambhala.

Brown, L. (1988). *State of the world.* New York: Norton.

Council on Environmental Quality and the Department of State. (1980). *The Global 2000 Report to the President.* Washington, DC: U.S. Government Printing Office.

Deutsch, E. (1969). *Advaita vedanta: A philosophical reconstruction.* Honolulu: East West Center Press.

Freud, S. (1943). *A general introduction to psychoanalysis.* Garden City, NY: Garden City Publisher. (Original work published 1917)

Goleman, D. (1988). *The meditative mind.* Los Angeles: Tarcher.

Harman, W. (1962). Old wine in new wineskins. In J. Bugental (Ed.). *Challenges of humanistic psychology* (p. 323). New York: McGraw-Hill.

Hendlin, S. J. (1979). Initial Zen intensive (sesshin): A subjective account. *Journal of Pastoral Counseling, 14,* 27–43.

Huxley, A. (1944). *The perennial philosophy.* New York: Harper & Row.

Kornfield, J. (1979). Intensive insight meditation: A phenomenological study. *Journal of Transpersonal Psychology, 11,* 41–58.

Kuhn, T. S. (1970). *The structure of scientific revolution* (2nd ed.). Chicago: University of Chicago Press.

Langer, E., Blank, A., & Benzion, C. (1978). The mindfulness of ostensibly thoughtful action: The role of "placebic" information on interpersonal interaction. *Journal of Personality and Social Psychology, 36,* 635–642.

Lewin, R. D. (1950). *The psychoanalysis of elation.* New York: Norton.

Needleman, J. (1984). *The heart of philosophy.* New York: Bantam.

Oppenheimer, J. R. (1954). *Science and the common understanding.* New York: Simon & Schuster.

Prabhavananda & Isherwood, (Trans.). (1944). *The song of God: Bhagavad Gita.* New York: New American Library.

Ram Dass, (1975). *The only dance there is.* New York: Doubleday.

Rank, O. (1958). *Beyond psychology.* New York: Dover.

Russel, E. (1986). Consciousness and the unconscious: Eastern meditative and Western psychotherapeutic approaches. *Journal of Transpersonal Psychology, 18,* 57–72.

Schumacher, E. (1978). *Small is beautiful.* New York: Harper & Row.

Schuon, F. (1975). *The transcendent unity of religions.* New York: Harper & Row.

Shapiro, D. (1980). *Meditation: Self regulation strategy and altered states of consciousness.* New York: Aldine.

Shapiro, D., & Walsh, R. (Eds.). (1984). *Meditation: Classic and contemporary perspectives.* New York: Aldine.

Smith, H. (1976). *Forgotten truth: The primordial tradition.* New York: Harper & Row.

Tart, C. (1975a). *States of consciousness.* New York: Dutton.

Tart, C. (Ed.). (1975b). *Transpersonal psychologies.* New York: Harper & Row.

Tart, C. (1986). *Waking Up.* Boston: New Science Library/Shambhala.

Vaughan, F. (1986). *The inward arc.* Boston: New Science Library/Shambhala.

Vimalo, B. (1974). Awakening to the truth. *Visaka Puja: Annual Publication of the Buddhist Association,* pp. 53–79.

Walsh, R. N. (1977). Initial meditative experience: I. *Journal of Transpersonal Psychology, 9,* 151–192.

Walsh, R. N. (1978). Initial meditative experiences: II. *Journal of Transpersonal Psychology, 10,* 1–28.

Walsh, R. (1980). The consciousness disciplines and the behavioral sciences: Questions of comparison and assessment. *American Journal of Psychiatry, 137,* 663–673.

Walsh, R. (1984). *Staying alive: The psychology of human survival.* Boston: New Science Library/Shambhala.

Walsh, R. (1988). Two Asian psychologies and their implications for Western psychotherapists. *American Journal of Psychotherapy, XLII,* 543–560.

Walsh, R., & Shapiro, D. H. (1983). *Beyond health and normality: Explorations of exceptional psychological wellbeing.* New York: Van Nostrand Reinhold.

Walsh, R., & Vaughan, F. (1980). *Beyond ego: Transpersonal dimensions in psychology.* Los Angeles: Tarcher.

Wilber, K. (1977). *The spectrum of consciousness.* Wheaton, IL: Theosophical Publishing House.

Wilber, K. (1979). *No boundary.* Boston: Shambhala.

Wilber, K. (1980a). *The Atman project.* Wheaton, IL: Theosophical Publishing House.

Wilber, K. (1980b). The pre/trans fallacy. *Revision, 3,* 51–72.

Wilber, K. (1981). *Up from Eden.* New York: Doubleday.

Wilber, K. (1983). *Eye to eye.* New York: Doubleday.

Wilber, K. (1989). Lets nuke the transpersonalists: A response to Albert Ellis. *Journal of Counseling and Development, 67,* 332–335.

Wilber, K., Engler, J., & Brown, D. (Eds.). (1986). *Transformations of consciousness: Conventional and contemplative perspectives on development.* Boston: New Science Library/Shambhala 1986.

Wolman, B., & Ulman, M. (Eds.). (1986). *Handbook of states of consciousness.* New York: Van Nostrand Reinhold.

Contributors

A. REZA ARASTEH, PH.D., formerly a faculty member of the Department of Psychiatry, School of Medicine, George Washington University, is the Director of the Institute for Psycho-Cultural Analysis in Bethesda, MD. Dr. Arasteh has also taught at Princeton University; Tehran University; the C. G. Jung Institute, Zurich, Switzerland; the University of Allahabad in India; and Toyo, Kogawa, and Komazawa Universities in Japan. He is an Affiliate Fellow of the Royal Society of Medicine, London, a Fulbright scholar, and one of the founding members of the Organization for Asian Psychology.

He is the author of several books in English, Persian, and Spanish, including *Toward Final Integration in the Adult Personality, Human Development and Creativity, Growth to Self-hood, Rumi the Persian,* and *Anxious Search: The Way to Universal Self.*

LORNE D. BERTRAND, PH.D., is Social Research Associate at the Canadian Research Institute for Law and the Family at the University of Calgary. He received his Ph.D. in Experimental Social Psychology at Carleton University in 1987. During his graduate training with Nicholas P. Spanos, he conducted research and published in the areas of memory alterations during hypnosis, the assessment of hypnotic susceptibility, and multiple personality. His current research interests include emerging redefinitions of the family, international and cross-cultural differences in criminality, and antecedent factors predicting youth involvement in criminal activity.

CROMWELL CRAWFORD, TH.D., is Chairman and Professor in the Department of Religion at the University of Hawaii. His specialties are religion and medicine, Indian studies, and comparative ethics. In 1972, he was named Fellow of the Royal Asiatic Society of Great Britain and Ireland.

Dr. Crawford lectures widely in international circles, and recently has organized two international conferences on religion and healing. He has contributed to several books and scholarly journals, and his books include *The Evolution of Hindu Ethical Ideals, In Search of Hinduism, Ram Mohan Ray, World Religions and Global Ethics, Dilemmas of Life and Death,* and *Hindu Ethics in a North American Context.*

557

LARRY DOSSEY, M.D., a highly distinguished physician and author, is the co-chairman of the Panel on Mind/Body Interventions, Office of Alternative Medicine at the National Institutes of Health and executive editor of the journal *Alternative Therapies in Medicine and Health*. He lectures widely in the United States and abroad; in 1988, he delivered the annual Mahatma Gandhi Memorial Lecture in New Delhi, India, the only physician ever invited to do so. Dr. Dossey has published numerous articles and is the author of five books, including *Space, Time & Medicine, Recovering the Soul, Mind and Medicine*, and *Healing Words*.

MARK EPSTEIN, M.D., is the author of *Thoughts Without a Thinker: Psychotherapy from a Buddhist Perspective*. He maintains a private practice in psychiatry in Manhattan. In 1981, Dr. Epstein in collaboration with Dr. Herbert Benson of the Harvard Medical School, traveled to Dharmsala, India to study the psychophysiology of advanced Tibetan meditation techniques. This research was supported by grants from the National Science Foundation and the American Institute of Indian Studies, and was conducted under the auspices of His Holiness, the Dalai Lama.

Dr. Epstein is the author of numerous articles on the relationship between the psychology of Buddhist meditation and psychodynamic thought.

DENISE L. HERZING, PH.D., President of the Wild Dolphin Society, is studying communication and behavior in dolphins at the World Dolphin Project in Florida. She received her graduate education in Behavioral Biology from San Francisco State University and worked as a Research Assistant in the Department of General Internal Medicine and Behavioral Medicine at the University of California School of Medicine, San Francisco.

ROBERT G. KUNZENDORF, PH.D., is Professor in the Psychology Department at the University of Lowell, Lowell, MA. Since the completion of his dissertation, *Imagery and Consciousness* in 1980, Dr. Kunzendorf has published over 50 articles dealing with the similarity of perceptual sensations and imaginal sensations, with the difference between conscious hallucinations and self-conscious images, and with the efficacy of health-related images and hypnotic hallucinations. Dr. Kunzendorf is co-editor of three books: *Psychophysiology of Mental Imagery: Theory, Research, and Application, Mental Imagery,* and *Hypnosis and Imagination*.

ROBERT G. LEY, PH.D., is Professor of Clinical Psychology at Simon Fraser University, Vancouver, Canada, and maintains a private practice. He has served as Fellow in Psychology at the Langley-Porter Psychiatric Institute at the University of California Medical School in San Francisco, and has had appointments in psychology at Baylor College of Medicine and at Texas Children's Hospital at the Texas Medical Center in Houston, Texas. Also, Dr. Ley is a recipient of the Dr. R. E. Harris Award for outstanding contributions to both clinical and experimental psychology.

Dr. Ley has done extensive work on cerebral laterality, emotions, and imagery, and has published many book chapters and journal articles on these topics.

ROBERT J. LUEGER, PH.D., is Associate Professor of Psychology and Chairman of the Department of Psychology at Marquette University. He received a Ph.D. in clinical psychology from Loyola University of Chicago in 1977. He has consulted for business, industry, and mental health organizations in addition to maintaining a private practice.

He is an active researcher and has published several chapters in edited books and numerous articles in professional journals. His current interest is in the area of psychotherapy outcome research and in making this research useful to practicing clinicians. His book, *Quality Assurance in Mental Health Treatment*, has received widespread attention.

CAROL E. McMAHON, PH.D., is in private practice in biofeedback and self-regulation. From 1974–1978, she did postdoctoral research in the history of psychosomatic medicine at the University of Buffalo. Support from the National Institutes of Mental Health enabled her to pursue her research at London's Wellcome Institute for the History of Medicine and at the libraries of Cambridge University; a grant from the American Philosophical Society supported further research.

Dr. McMahon has written numerous articles and book chapters, and, in 1986, she authored a self-help audiotape, *The Health State*. Her book, *Where Medicine Fails*, appeared in 1986, and another book, *Unconditional Happiness*, will be published soon.

PATRICIA NORRIS, PH.D., is the Clinical Director of the Biofeedback and Psychophysiology Center at the Menninger Clinic, and is on the faculty of the Karl Menninger School of Psychiatry. She was president of the Association for Applied Psychophysiology and Biofeedback from 1985–1986. From 1982 to 1985, she was an Associate Editor of the Association's Journal, *Biofeedback and Self-Regulation*. At this time, she serves on the Editorial Board. Dr. Norris is on the Board of Directors of the Institute for Adjunctive Career Therapy in Philadelphia, the Behavioral Medicine Institute of Santa Barbara, and the Drake Institute for Behavioral Medicine in Santa Monica.

DONALD M. PACHUTA, M.D., formerly Associate Professor of Medicine at the University of Maryland School of Medicine, practices in Kauai, Hawaii. He has studied Eastern philosophies, religion, and healing systems in depth and has combined this learning with Western medicine to create his own uniquely integrated system. Dr. Pachuta has served patients from around the world, many of whom had been previously considered hopeless. His work with imagery in the treatment of life-threatening illness has received widespread attention. He is the author of *The Life You Save May Be Your Own*.

KENNETH R. PELLETIER, M.D., PH.D., is Clinical Associate Professor at Stanford School of Medicine. He has published over 200 articles, and his books include *Consciousness: East and West; Mind as a Healer, Mind as Slayer; Toward a Science of Consciousness; Holistic Medicine: From Stress to Optimum Health; Longevity: Fulfilling Our Biological Potential; Healthy People in Unhealthy Places: Stress and Fitness at Work;* and *Sound Mind, Sound Body: A New Model for Lifelong Health*. His outstanding contributions have been the subject of reports on several television programs, such as the *Today* show, BBC's *The Long Search, Good Morning America,* and *MacNeil-Lehrer NewsHour*.

SUNDAR RAMASWAMI, PH.D., received his M.A. from the University of Newcastle, Australia, and his Ph.D. from Marquette University. He is working as a clinical psychologist at Fairfield Hills Hospital, Newtown, CT. Formerly, he was Acting Director of the Department of Psychology at St. Francis Medical Center, LaCrosse, WI, and Clinic Supervisor at the Nova University Clinic. Dr. Ramaswami is a native of Madras, India, where he studied with J. Krishnamurti.

LOBSANG RAPGAY, PH.D., is a Tibetan Buddhist monk physician and holds a Ph.D. in Tibetan medicine and Buddhist psychology from Visva Bharati University, India. He is the Director of the Tibetan Holistic Medical Center, New Delhi, and established the Institute for Tibetan Buddhist Wellness and Counseling in the Bay area, California. He has written several books and articles on Buddhist healing and psychology.

DAVID K. REYNOLDS, PH.D., formerly on the faculty of the University of Southern California School of Medicine and the University of California, Los Angeles, School of Public Health, is the Director of the Constructive Living Center in Coos Bay, Oregon. He is one of the leading authorities on Japanese systems of healing. His numerous books include *Morita Psychotherapy, Naikan Psychotherapy, The Quiet Therapies, Playing Ball on Running Water,* and *A Handbook for Constructive Living.*

SOHAN L. SHARMA, PH.D., Professor of Psychology, emeritus, obtained his doctorate from the University of Michigan, Ann Arbor. He has worked in several mental hospitals and outpatient clinics in Canada and the United States as staff psychologist and chief psychologist. He was Director of the Counseling Center, Department of Psychology for twenty years, and was also a Professor of Psychology at California State University for twenty-seven years. He is also in private practice, and is Director of The Sharma Center for Psychological Services in Sacramento. He is the editor of *The Medical Model of Mental Illness* and author of *The Therapeutic Dialogue.* Currently he is working on a new book, entitled *Depression and Being Depressed.*

ANEES A. SHEIKH, PH.D., Professor of Psychology at Marquette University, and Clinical Professor of Psychiatry and Mental Health Sciences and the Medical College of Wisconsin, is internationally recognized for his contributions to the field of mental imagery. A former editor of the *Journal of Mental Imagery,* he now edits the *International Review of Mental Imagery* and the *Imagery and Human Development Series.* His books include *The Potential of Fantasy and Imagination, Imagery: Current Theory, Research and Application, Imagination and Healing, Imagery in Education, Anthology of Imagery Techniques, Psychophysiology of Mental Imagery,* and *Death Imagery.* He is past president on the American Association for the Study of Mental Imagery.

KATHARINA S. SHEIKH, M.A., formerly on the faculty of Clara Schumann Schule, Bonn, Germany, Cardinal Stritch College, and St. Francis de Sales College in Milwaukee, is the President of the Institute for Human Enhancement.

For her undergraduate work, she attended the University of Western Ontario and the University of Strasbourg, France, and holds graduate degrees from the University of Toronto and Marquette University. Her publications include the book *Imagery in Education* which she coedited.

MAURA SMYLIE, PH.D., received her doctoral training in clinical psychology at Simon Fraser University, British Columbia, Canada. Currently, she is in private practice in Vancouver, Canada.

NICHOLAS P. SPANOS, PH.D., before his recent death, was Professor of Psychology at Carleton University. He received his Ph.D. at Boston University in 1974 and, after a period as Senior Research Scientist at the Medfield Foundation in Medfield, MA, he joined the faculty at Carleton in 1975. He published over 100 articles spanning most research topics in hypnosis and was co-author with Theodore X. Barber and John F.

Chaves of *Hypnosis, Imagination, and Human Potentialities,* and coeditor with Chaves of *Hypnosis: The Cognitive-Behavioral Approach.* His primary research interests included hypnotic analgesia, the modification of hypnotic susceptibility, psychological correlates of hypnotic susceptibility, and hypnotic amnesia.

ROGER WALSH, M.D., PH.D., is Professor in the Department of Psychiatry and Human Behavior at the University of California at Irvine. His areas of interest include the integration of different schools of psychology and psychotherapy, meditation, Asian psychologies and philosophies, the nature of psychological well-being, and the global problems currently threatening human welfare and survival. He is the coeditor of *Paths Beyond Ego: The Transpersonal Vision, Transpersonal Dimensions in Psychology, Meditation: Classic and Contemporary Perspectives,* and *The Spirit of Shamanism.*

Author Index

Subject Index